AN ADVANCED REVIEW OF SPEECH-LANGUAGE PATHOLOGY

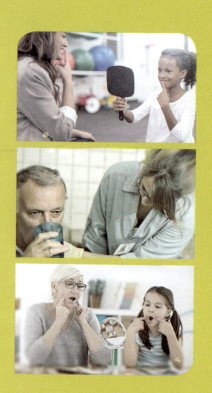

AN ADVANCED REVIEW OF SPEECH-LANGUAGE PATHOLOGY

PREPARATION FOR THE PRAXIS SLP AND COMPREHENSIVE EXAMINATION

Fifth Edition

CELESTE ROSEBERRY-MCKIBBIN

M. N. HEGDE

GLEN M. TELLIS

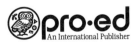

8700 Shoal Creek Boulevard
Austin, Texas 78757-6897
800/897-3202 Fax 800/397-7633
www.proedinc.com

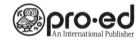

© 2019, 2016, 2011, 2006, 2000 by PRO-ED, Inc.
8700 Shoal Creek Boulevard
Austin, Texas 78757-6897
800/897-3202 Fax 800/397-7633
www.proedinc.com

All rights reserved. No part of the material protected by this copyright notice may be reproduced or used in any form or by any means, electronic or mechanical, including photocopying, recording, or by any information storage and retrieval system, without prior written permission of the copyright owner.

Library of Congress Cataloging-in-Publication Data

Names: Roseberry-McKibbin, Celeste, author. | Hegde, M. N., author. | Tellis, Glen M., author.
Title: An advanced review of speech-language pathology : preparation for the Praxis SLP and comprehensive examination / Celeste Roseberry-McKibbin, M.N. Hegde, Glen M. Tellis.
Description: Fifth edition. | Austin, Texas : PRO-ED, Inc., 2019 | Includes index.
Identifiers: LCCN 2018042705 (print) | LCCN 2018043183 (ebook) | ISBN 9781416411673 (ebook) | ISBN 9781416411666 (hc : alk. paper)
Subjects: LCSH: Speech disorders—Outlines, syllabi, etc. | Language disorders—Outlines, syllabi, etc. | Speech therapy—Outlines, syllabi, etc. | Audiology—Outlines, syllabi, etc.
Classification: LCC RC423 (ebook) | LCC RC423 .R66 2019 (print) | DDC 616.85/50076--dc23
LC record available at https://lccn.loc.gov/2018042705

Art Director: Jason Crosier
Designer: Bookbright Media
This book is designed in Bembo, Sofia Pro, Brandon Grotesque, Oswald, and Lato

Printed in the United States of America

3 4 5 6 7 8 9 10   27 26 25 24 23 22 21 20 19

In loving memory of
Beverly Wilson Roseberry
To whom this book is dedicated

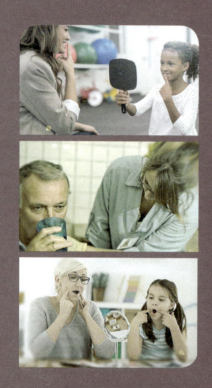

CONTENTS

Preface *xxi*

CHAPTER 1
Anatomy, Neuroanatomy, and Physiology of the Speech Mechanism   xxiv

Respiration: Structures and Processes   1
- Respiration Patterns During Speech Production   1
- Framework of Respiration   2
- Muscles of Respiration   6

Phonation: Structures and Processes   8
- The Larynx   8
- Laryngeal Structures and Cartilages   9
- Intrinsic Laryngeal Muscles   11
- Extrinsic Laryngeal Muscles   12
- Vocal Folds   13
- Physiology of Phonation   14
- Neuroanatomy of the Vocal Mechanism   16

Resonation and Articulation: Structures and Processes   17
- Fundamentals of Resonation   17
- Fundamentals of Articulation   18

Neuroanatomy and Neurophysiology: The Nervous System   30

Neurons and Neural Transmission   30
- Anatomy and Physiology of Nerve Cells   30
- Neural Transmission   31

The Peripheral and Autonomic Nervous Systems   33
- Peripheral Nervous System   33
- Autonomic Nervous System   43

The Central Nervous System   44
- Basic Principles   44
- The Brainstem   44
- Reticular Activating System   48
- Diencephalon   49
- Basal Ganglia   49
- The Cerebellum   50
- The Cerebrum   51
- Pyramidal System   56
- Corticobulbar Tract   57
- Extrapyramidal System   57
- Connecting Fibers in the Brain   60
- The Cerebral Ventricles   61

Protective Layers of the Brain   62
Cerebral Blood Supply   62

Chapter Highlights   67

Study and Review Questions   68

Study and Review Answers   70

CHAPTER 2

Physiological and Acoustic Phonetics: A Speech Science Foundation   72

Basic Principles and Definitions   73
Definitions   73

Phonetic Transcription   75
The International Phonetic Alphabet   75
Broad Phonetic Transcription   75
Narrow Phonetic Transcription   75

Production of Segmentals: Consonants and Vowels   77
Consonants and Vowels: The Syllable as a Unit   77
Classification Systems   78
Consonants   80
Vowels   84

The Effects of Context on Speech Sound Production   88
Dynamics of Speech Production   88
Suprasegmentals   88

Speech Science: Physiological Phonetics, Acoustic Phonetics, and Speech Perception   90
Acoustics: Basic Definitions   90

Introduction to the Study of Sound and Acoustic Analysis of Speech   92
Sound Wave Generation and Propagation   92
Frequency and Pitch   93
Amplitude and Loudness   94
Sound Pressure Level and Hearing Level   94
Introduction to the Acoustic Analysis of Speech   95

Chapter Highlights   96

Study and Review Questions   97

Study and Review Answers   100

CHAPTER 3

Language Development in Children   102

Terms and Definitions   103
- Morphology   103
- Syntax   105
- Semantics   106
- Pragmatics   108

Typical Language Development: Developmental Milestones   109
- Role of the Caregiver in Language Development   109
- Birth–1 Year   110
- 1–2 Years   112
- 2–3 Years   114
- 3–4 Years   117
- 4–5 Years   119
- 5–6 Years   120
- 6–7 Years   122
- 7–8 Years   123
- Language and Literacy Development in the School-Age Years   124

Theories of Language Development   125
- Behavioral Theory   125
- Nativist Theory   126
- Cognitive Theory   127
- Information-Processing Theory   128
- Social Interactionism Theory   131

Chapter Highlights   133

Study and Review Questions   134

Study and Review Answers   140

CHAPTER 4

Language Disorders in Children   142

Introduction to Children With Language Disorders   143
- Description of Language Disorders in Children   144
- Risk Factors for Language Disorders in Children   144

Children With Specific Language Impairment   145
- Characteristics of Children With Specific Language Impairment   145

**Children With Language Problems Associated
With Physical and Sensory Disabilities**   **149**

    Intellectual Disability   149

    Autism Spectrum Disorder   151

    Brain Injury   153

**Children With Language Problems Related
to Physical and Social–Environmental Factors**   **156**

    Language Problems Related to Poverty   156

    Language Problems Related to Neglect or Abuse   158

    Language Problems Related to Parental Drug and Alcohol Abuse   159

    Language Problems Related to Attention-Deficit/Hyperactivity Disorder   160

Assessment Principles and Procedures   **162**

    Language Assessment: General Principles and Procedures   162

    Assessment of Infants and Toddlers   166

    Assessment of Preschool and Elementary-Age Children   169

    Assessment of Adolescents   171

Treatment Principles and Procedures   **174**

    General Principles   174

    Specific Techniques and Programs   176

    Augmentative and Alternative Communication   181

Chapter Highlights   **184**

Study and Review Questions   **186**

Study and Review Answers   **192**

CHAPTER 5

Speech Sound Development and Disorders   194

Foundations of Articulation and Phonology   **195**

    Basic Definitions   196

Acquisition of Articulatory and Phonological Skills: Typical Development   **197**

    Theories of Development   197

    Infant Development: Perception and Production   199

    Typical Articulation Development in Children   201

    Overall Intelligibility   201

    Typical Phonological Development in Children   203

Speech Sound Disorders   **205**

    General Factors Related to Speech Sound Disorders   205

    Description of Articulatory Errors   207

    Organically Based Disorders   208

Assessment of Speech Sound Disorders   213
    Screening   213
    General Assessment Objectives   213
    Related Assessment Objectives   213
    Assessment Procedures   214
    Specific Components of an Assessment   215
    Scoring and Analysis of Assessment Data   217

Treatment of Speech Sound Disorders   220
    General Considerations in Treatment   220
    Motor-Based Approaches   222
    Linguistic Approaches   224
    Core Vocabulary (Consistency) Approach   226
    Phonological Awareness Treatment   227

Chapter Highlights   229

Study and Review Questions   230

Study and Review Answers   234

CHAPTER 6

Fluency and Its Disorders   236

Fluency and Stuttering: An Overview   237
    Definition and Description of Fluency   237
    Definition and Description of Stuttering   238
    Forms of Dysfluencies   239
    Theoretical and Clinical Significance of Dysfluencies   240
    Incidence and Prevalence of Stuttering   241
    Onset and Development of Stuttering   245
    Associated Motor Behaviors   246
    Associated Breathing Abnormalities   246
    Negative Emotions and Avoidance Behaviors   247
    The Loci of Stuttering   247
    Stimulus Control in Stuttering   248
    People Who Stutter and Their Families   249
    Theories of Stuttering   250

Assessment and Treatment of Stuttering   252
    Assessment of Stuttering   252
    Treatment of Stuttering   254

Neurogenic Stuttering   261
    Definition and Etiology of Neurogenic Stuttering   261

Description of Neurogenic Stuttering   262

Assessment and Treatment of Neurogenic Stuttering   262

Cluttering   263

Definition and Description of Cluttering   263

Assessment and Treatment of Cluttering   264

Other Types of Fluency Disorders   265

Chapter Highlights   265

Study and Review Questions   266

Study and Review Answers   270

CHAPTER 7

Voice and Its Disorders   272

Vocal Anatomy and Physiology   273

The Larynx   273

Voice Changes Through the Life Span   280

Vocal Pitch, Loudness, and Quality   282

Pitch   282

Loudness   283

Quality   283

Evaluation of Voice Disorders   285

Case History: Purposes and Goals   285

A Team-Oriented Approach   286

Instrumental Evaluation   286

Perceptual Evaluation   291

Quality of Life Evaluation   293

Disorders of Resonance and Their Treatment   294

Hypernasality   295

Hyponasality   296

Assimilative Nasality   296

Cul-de-Sac Resonance   296

Treatment Principles   297

Disorders of Phonation and Their Treatment   298

Carcinoma and Laryngectomy   299

Voice Disorders   303

Physically Based Disorders of Phonation   304

Idiopathic Voice Disorders   317

Neurologically Based Voice Disorders   317

Psychogenic Voice Disorders   321
　　　Behavioral Voice Therapy   322
　　　Gender Issues and the Voice   327
Chapter Highlights   329
Study and Review Questions   330
Study and Review Answers   335

CHAPTER 8

Neurologically Based Communicative Disorders   336

Aphasia   337
　　　Incidence and Prevalence of Aphasia   337
　　　Neuropathology of Aphasia   338
　　　Key Terms   339
　　　Definition and Classification of Aphasia   340
　　　Nonfluent Aphasias   340
　　　Fluent Aphasias   344
　　　Subcortical Aphasia   348
　　　Crossed Aphasia   348
　　　Aphasia in Bilingual Populations   348
　　　Assessment of Aphasia   349
　　　Treatment of Aphasia   354
　　　Alexia and Agraphia   359
　　　Agnosia   360

Dementia   360
　　　Definition and Classification of Dementia   361
　　　Dementia of the Alzheimer Type   361
　　　Frontotemporal Dementia   363
　　　Dementia Associated With Parkinson's Disease   366
　　　Dementia Associated With Huntington's Disease   367
　　　Infectious Dementia   368
　　　Other Forms of Dementia   371
　　　Assessment of Dementia   372
　　　Clinical Management of Dementia   373

Right Hemisphere Disorder   375
　　　The Right and the Left Hemispheres   375
　　　Symptoms of Right Hemisphere Disorder   375
　　　Assessment of Right Hemisphere Disorder   377
　　　Treatment of Right Hemisphere Disorder   378

Traumatic Brain Injury 379

Definition and Incidence of TBI 379

Common Causes of TBI 380

Types and Consequences of TBI 380

General Assessment of Persons With TBI 382

Assessment of Communicative Deficits Associated With TBI 383

Treatment of Persons With TBI 384

Chapter Highlights 386

Study and Review Questions 387

Study and Review Answers 390

CHAPTER 9

Motor Speech Disorders and Dysphagia 392

Apraxia of Speech 393

Definition and Distinctions 393

Neuropathology of AOS 394

General Symptoms of AOS 395

Communication Deficits in AOS 395

Assessment of AOS 396

Treatment of AOS 397

The Dysarthrias 398

Definition of the Dysarthrias 398

Neuropathology of the Dysarthrias 403

Communicative Disorders Associated With Dysarthria 403

Types of Dysarthria 404

Differentiating Apraxia of Speech From Dysarthria 412

Assessment of the Dysarthrias 412

Treatment of the Dysarthrias 414

Swallowing Disorders 416

The Nature and Etiology of Swallowing Disorders 416

Normal and Disordered Swallow 417

Assessment of Swallowing Disorders 419

Treatment of Swallowing Disorders 420

Chapter Highlights 424

Study and Review Questions 425

Study and Review Answers 428

CHAPTER 10

Cleft Palate, Craniofacial Anomalies, and Genetic Syndromes   430

Craniofacial Anomalies and Cleft Palate   431

Craniofacial Anomalies   431

Cleft Lip   431

Cleft Palate   432

Genetic Syndromes   444

Genetic Syndromes Associated With Communication Disorders   444

Chapter Highlights   453

Study and Review Questions   453

Study and Review Answers   458

CHAPTER 11

Communication Disorders in Multicultural Populations   460

Foundational Issues   461

General Cultural Considerations   462

ASHA Guidelines Regarding Multicultural Issues   463

Speech–Language Characteristics of CLD Clients   464

Dialects of American English   464

African American English   465

Characteristics of AAE Morphology, Syntax, and Articulation   466

Spanish-Influenced English   468

English Influenced by Asian Languages   471

Language Differences and Language Impairment   476

Differentiating Language Differences From Language Impairments   476

Acquiring a Second Language   477

Basic Interpersonal Communication Skills and Cognitive–Academic Language Proficiency   479

Assessment of EL Students   481

Legal Considerations   482

Considerations in the Use of Standardized Tests   482

Alternatives to Standardized Tests   485

Working With Interpreters in the Assessment Process   487

Treatment Considerations in Service Delivery to CLD Clients   488

Children With Language Impairments   489

Serving CLD Adults: Prevalence and Incidence Rates of Medical Conditions and Communication Disorders   490

Potential Sociocultural and Linguistic Barriers to Service Delivery   491

Adults With Neurologically Based Disorders of Communication   492

Chapter Highlights   495

Study and Review Questions   497

Study and Review Answers   503

CHAPTER 12

Audiology and Hearing Disorders   506

Anatomy and Physiology of Hearing   508

The Outer Ear   508

The Middle Ear   508

The Inner Ear   511

The Auditory Nervous System   513

Acoustics: Sound and Its Perception   515

The Source of Sound   515

Sound Waves   516

Frequency and Intensity   517

Sound Pressure Level and Hearing Level   518

The Nature and Etiology of Hearing Loss   519

Normal Hearing   519

The Nature of Hearing Impairment   520

Conductive Hearing Loss   520

Sensorineural Hearing Loss   525

Mixed Hearing Loss   528

Auditory Nervous System Impairments   528

Assessment of Hearing Impairment   531

Audiometry: Basic Principles   531

Pure-Tone Audiometry   532

Speech Audiometry   533

Acoustic Immittance   533

Other Methods   534

Hearing Screening   534

Assessment of Infants and Children   535

Interpretation of Hearing Test Results   535

Management of Hearing Impairment   539

Communication Disorders of People With Hearing Impairment   539

Aural Rehabilitation: Basic Principles   541

Amplification   542

    Communication Learning   547

Chapter Highlights   553

Study and Review Questions   554

Study and Review Answers   558

CHAPTER 13

Assessment and Treatment: Principles of Evidence-Based Practice   560

Evidence-Based Practice in Speech–Language Pathology   561

Standard Assessment Procedures   562

    Screening   562

    Case History   563

    Hearing Screening   565

    Orofacial Examination   565

    Interview   565

    Speech and Language Sample   566

    Obtaining Related Assessment Data   567

Principles of Standardized Assessment   568

    The Nature and Advantages of Standardized Assessment   568

    Limitations of Standardized Tests   569

    Prudent Use of Standardized Tests   570

    Types of Scores in Standardized Assessment   571

    Validity and Reliability of Standardized Tests   572

Rating Scales, Questionnaires, and Developmental Inventories   573

    Rating Scales   573

    Questionnaires and Interviews   573

    Developmental Inventories   573

Alternative Assessment Approaches   574

    Functional Assessment   574

    Client-Specific Assessment   575

    Criterion-Referenced Assessment   576

    Authentic Assessment   576

    Dynamic Assessment   577

    Comprehensive and Integrated Assessment   577

Treatment of Communication Disorders: Basic Concepts   578

    Treatment: Definition   578

    A Treatment Paradigm for Communication Disorders   579

    Basic Treatment Terms   579

    Reinforcers and Reinforcement   583

An Overview of the Treatment Process   585
  Selection of Treatment Targets   585
  Treatment Sequence   586
  Maintenance Program   587
  Follow-Up   588
  Booster Treatment   588

A General Outline of a Treatment Program   588
  Seven Steps of All Treatment Programs   589

Cultural–Linguistic Considerations in Assessment and Treatment   589
  The Need for Individualized Assessment and Treatment   590

Chapter Highlights   591

Study and Review Questions   592

Study and Review Answers   595

CHAPTER 14

Research Design and Statistics: A Foundation for Clinical Science   596

Essentials of the Scientific Method   597
  The Philosophy of Science: Basic Concepts   597
  Validity of Measurements   599
  Reliability of Measurements   600

Experimental Research   601
  Definitions of Terms   601
  Group Designs of Research   602
  Single-Subject Designs of Research   604

Varieties of Descriptive Research   608
  Basic Concepts   608
  Ex Post Facto (Retrospective) Research   609
  Survey Research   610
  Comparative Research   610
  Developmental (Normative) Research   610
  Correlational Research   611
  Ethnographic Research   612

Evaluation of Research   612
  Internal Validity   613
  External Validity   615
  Levels of Evidence for Evidence-Based Practice   616

Data Organization and Analysis: Principles of Statistics   618

Basic Concepts　618
　　Statistical Techniques for Organizing Data　619
　　Types of Measurement Scales　620
Chapter Highlights　621
Study and Review Questions　623
Study and Review Answers　628

CHAPTER 15

Professional Issues　630

ASHA and the Professions　631
　　The American Speech-Language-Hearing Association　632
　　The Professions of Speech–Language Pathology and Audiology　635
　　The Scope of Practice: Speech–Language Pathology　635
　　ASHA Accreditation　636

Issues in Certification and Licensure　637
　　Clinical Certification　637
　　Speech–Language Pathology Assistants　640
　　State Regulation of the Profession　641

Legislative Regulation of the Profession　643
　　Federal Legislation Affecting School Settings　643
　　Federal Legislation Affecting Employment Settings　645
　　Federal Legislation Affecting Health Care Settings　646
　　Future Trends　648

Chapter Highlights　649
Study and Review Questions　650
Study and Review Answers　653

Appendix　654

Study and Test-Taking Tips for the Praxis　655
　　The Nature and Purpose of the Praxis　655
　　Study Tips for Preparing for the Praxis　658
　　General Tips for Taking the Praxis　659
　　Understanding Computer-Generated Questions　662
　　Conclusion　663

Index　664
About the Authors　694

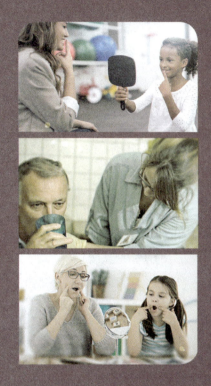

PREFACE

The idea for the first edition of this book was born some years ago when I (Celeste Roseberry-McKibbin) was part of a team that was conducting workshops for speech–language pathologists who needed to pass the Praxis so they could become licensed and certified in order to accommodate increasingly stringent professional state and federal requirements. These experienced clinicians, who had graduated from school 10–35 years ago, suddenly found themselves faced with the need to quickly learn (or retrieve from memory) a great deal of current information to pass a challenging examination. The task seemed formidable to many of them.

At the same time, my colleague at California State University–Fresno, Giri Hegde, and I were dealing with many graduate students who were experiencing great stress over the prospect of taking upcoming master's comprehensive examinations, as well as the Praxis (usually taken within the same time period). All of these people needed current information covering the entire field of speech–language pathology. Many of them did not have time to go to libraries, check out books, read through each book, and extract the most relevant and up-to-date information that was likely to be asked on the Praxis and on comprehensive examinations in graduate programs. As we reflected upon this situation, an idea was born. Why not write a book that would meet those needs? Why not gather current, relevant material into one book that would help students and practitioners review for examinations that would open career doors to them?

Several years later, the first edition of this book came together in one comprehensive package geared toward helping students and practitioners study for and pass the Praxis and comprehensive examinations in graduate programs. But there was, and still is, a third purpose for the book. We intend it to be not only a study guide but also a review for practitioners who want an update of the field for their professional growth. We have spoken with many practitioners in various professional settings, some of whom are aware that much of their knowledge has become dated but do not have the time or resources to obtain current knowledge in so many areas of an ever-expanding field. Thus, we have also written this book for experienced speech–language pathologists who would like to read current and comprehensive information for their own professional development.

It has been a joy to update a book that is unique in the field of speech–language pathology and has been a national and international bestseller for over 20 years. The book is written specifically to meet the needs of students taking comprehensive examinations and the Praxis, experienced practitioners taking the Praxis, and experienced practitioners who are seeking professional growth. When we have discussed the book with students and practitioners, the resounding response has been, "How soon will the book be out? I want to buy it! Please hurry and finish it!" (The last comment has also been heard from our spouses, but that is another story.) It is a great privilege for us to contribute the fifth edition of this book to our field, and we hope that it will open doors for those who are seeking further knowledge and opportunities.

The book includes unique pedagogical devices to facilitate the learning process. Each chapter has special features to help readers learn and retain the information presented. Chapters begin with a detailed "preview paragraph" to orient readers to chapter contents. Each chapter section contains both a brief introduction and an ending summary to help readers (a) become aware of what they will read, (b) read it, and (c) review what they have just read. We believe that repetition is one of the keys to learning and retaining information. At the end of each chapter, a "Chapter Highlights" section reviews and summarizes the most pertinent information. Readers who are studying for examinations can, soon before the examination, refresh their memories by rereading section introductions, summaries, and chapter highlights.

Test questions in multiple-choice format can be found at the end of each chapter. The multiple-choice questions are written in a manner similar to that of the questions on the Praxis, to help prepare readers for those questions. The newest version of the Praxis contains multiple-choice questions with answers in an A–D format, and we have updated our questions to reflect this. We have included many more "case study" type questions to reflect the current Praxis. Answers to multiple-choice test questions are located on the last page of each chapter. For readers who want more information about certain topics within a chapter, we have included a comprehensive list of current references and recommended readings by chapter at www.advancedreviewpractice.com. These lists have been substantially updated; the fifth edition of this book contains over 300 new, current references.

In the fifth edition of this book, we have also made content updates. All chapters have been revised to include current information and references. There is new information about the national Common Core State Standards; we tie child language information to the standards and discuss how speech–language pathologists can provide services that are current, relevant, and related to helping children with language impairments achieve the standards. In various chapters, we discuss iPad apps and how they can be used with persons with communication disorders. There is also new information about pediatric dysphagia and telepractice.

The information in the appendix has been almost entirely replaced with new information based on the new edition of the Praxis examination that was revised and updated in 2017.

We also have an updated online companion product, *An Advanced Review of Speech–Language Pathology–Fifth Edition: Practice Examinations*, which simulates the Praxis and tracks a student's results over multiple test sessions. This product has been continuously updated over several editions. My colleague Glen Tellis, Professor and Chair of the Speech-Language Pathology Department at Misericordia University, simultaneously suggested providing students with a digital product that simulates the actual Praxis SLP test and that covers all the major areas of the actual test. We have since combined the book with the online tests and have received wonderful feedback from students about the quality of the product.

The online tests are compatible with all browsers and most devices, the 1-year subscription allows a person to take multiple, varied practice tests. The tests simulate the actual Praxis SLP test and will break down results and provide information about a test taker's areas of strengths and weaknesses. Just like the new edition of the Praxis examination, this practice format includes questions from three content categories: (a) foundations and professional practice; (b) screening, assessment, evaluation, and diagnosis; and (c) planning, implementation, and evaluation of treatment. On completion of a test, students will be able to compare their current performance with previous performances. Test takers will see a screen that shows the: total time taken for the test, average time per question, total score, number of incorrect answers, and percentage of correct answers. Students will be able to review all results and print the incorrect answers. Students will not only be able to compare their scores with previous attempts at the test, but will also be able to compare their scores with others who took the exam nationally. Glen, thank you for your outstanding contribution! We are so grateful for the privilege of working with you and welcome you as the third author of the fifth edition!

We have been flattered by and most pleased with the success and acclaim that have greeted the first four editions of this book. Students and professionals from across the United States and even other countries have thanked us for writing this book, and we feel blessed to know that our work is providing help and support for so many readers. We have worked very hard to make this fifth edition even more useful.

A book such as this never happens without the help of many people. We would like to especially thank Beth Rowan, our editor at PRO-ED, for her patience, dedication, encouragement, and enthusiasm as we completed this fifth edition. Our student research assistants, Samantha Buldo, Abbey John, Quinn Kelley, Annette Ritzko, and Teri Vieira have spent countless hours in the lab to create many of the images in this text book. We would like to thank them for their invaluable efforts. We also thank our families, especially Mike and Mark McKibbin, Prema Hegde, and Cari Tellis, for their unconditional love and support.

Again, it is a privilege for us to contribute this work to our field. Thanks to the help and support of the aforementioned individuals, we are able to offer the fifth edition of this book to students and practitioners from all over the United States and abroad. It is our hope that it will open doors to those very deserving individuals who have dedicated their lives to serving persons with communication disorders.

CHAPTER 1

ANATOMY, NEUROANATOMY, AND PHYSIOLOGY OF THE SPEECH MECHANISM

Speech depends on an intricate and complex system of structures and functions working together to allow human beings to communicate with one another. **Respiration**, or breathing, supplies the energy for speech. **Phonation** is voicing with the structures and processes that help produce voice. **Resonation** is the modification of the voice produced at the laryngeal level, due to the dynamics of the various supralaryngeal cavities and structures. **Articulation** is production of speech sounds in isolation as well as in connected speech.

RESPIRATION: STRUCTURES AND PROCESSES

Respiration provides the necessary air supply to produce speech. It is made possible by a structural framework that includes the lungs, bronchi, trachea, spinal column, sternum, and rib cage. Respiration involves the cycle of inhalation (inspiration) and exhalation (expiration).

Respiration Patterns During Speech Production

Inhalation brings oxygen to the blood. Exhalation helps get rid of mixed air and gases that result from respiratory metabolism. When an excessive amount of carbon dioxide in the blood cells creates a need for oxygen, the **medulla oblongata** in the brainstem fires impulses to the respiratory muscles (Hixon, Weismer, & Hoit, 2013; Seikel, Drumright, & King, 2016).

- **Respiration** is the exchange of gas between an organism and its environment. **Inhalation** and **exhalation** create the rhythmic cycle of respiration.
- Inhalation draws air into the lungs, where an exchange of oxygen and carbon dioxide takes place. Through the contraction of the diaphragm and actions of other inspiratory muscles, we expand the chest cavity, and thus the lungs, to inhale air.
- As the lungs expand, the pressure within the lungs (alveolar pressure), compared to that outside the lungs (atmospheric pressure), is reduced. The air moves through the open laryngeal valve into the lungs, equalizing the pressure inside and outside the lungs.
- At that point, muscles contract to reduce the volume of the chest cavity and return the diaphragm to its resting position, creating a positive pressure within the lungs and causing exhalation. In this manner, the cycle of inhalation and exhalation automatically continues. In adults, this cycle occurs about 12–18 times per minute.

- Respiration provides the air supply needed to set the vocal folds into vibration for speech. Because speech is typically produced on exhalation, the duration of exhalations during speech tends to be longer than its duration during silent periods. Expiration is about 60% of the normal tidal breathing cycle, and inspiration is the remaining 40%; however, this ratio changes to 90% and 10%, respectively, when breathing for speech (Seikel et al., 2016). Longer and louder utterances may require deeper inhalations than usual. Singers often inhale deeply.
- Compared to quiet breathing, breathing for speech is more consciously monitored and adjusted to meet the demands of speech in various daily situations. Speech is created by dynamic and interconnected systems; a change in one system can influence another. During speech, movement of the articulators and vocal tract creates airflow resistance, causing the pressure within the lungs to fluctuate to expand and relax the lungs (Zemlin, 1998). To make these continuous and rapid adjustments, the respiratory structures must be intact.

Framework of Respiration

Respiration (inhalation and exhalation) is the basic energy source for speech. Humans generally inhale and then speak on exhaled air. The basic process of inhalation can be summarized as follows:

> **inhalation ➔ chest and lungs expand ➔ diaphragm lowers ➔ air flows in through the nose and mouth ➔ air goes down the pharynx and between the open vocal folds ➔ air continues downward through the trachea and bronchial tubes ➔ air reaches final destination of the lungs**

- The processes of inhalation, exhalation, and speaking are complex and require the support of many structures, including the lungs, bronchi, trachea, spinal column, sternum, and rib cage.

Lungs

The exchange of gas in respiration is accomplished in the lungs. Healthy lungs are soft, spongy, porous, elastic, and pink. They have a rich vascular supply and numerous air sacs.

- At rest, the lungs are partially inflated to approximately 40% of their total capacity (Hixon et al., 2013).
- The lungs are located in the thoracic cavity and take up most of the cavity's space. The right lung is shorter, broader, and bigger than the left lung, because the liver underneath it forces it into a slightly upward direction. The left lung is smaller because the heart takes up some of this space. The right lung has three lobes, whereas the left lung has two. The lungs are illustrated in Figure 1.1.

Bronchi

The **bronchi** are tubes that extend from the lungs upward to the trachea. They are composed of cartilaginous rings bound together by fibroelastic tissue.

- In the lungs, the bronchi subdivide into **bronchioles**, forming what is known as the bronchial tree. As the bronchi and bronchioles divide, they become less cartilaginous and more muscular in composition. The bronchioles repeatedly divide until they become very thin. They ultimately communicate with **alveolar ducts** that open into tiny air sacs in the lungs.

Trachea

As a person inhales, the air goes in through the larynx to the trachea to the lungs, which expand. When a person exhales, the air goes upward again through the **trachea**, a tube about 11 centimeters long formed by approximately 20 rings of cartilage (illustrated in Figure 1.1).

- These rings of cartilage are incomplete in the back, where the trachea comes into direct contact with the esophagus. The first tracheal cartilage is larger than the rest and connects to the inferior, or bottom, border of the cricoid cartilage.
- The trachea extends from the larynx, at the level of the sixth cervical vertebra, and the last tracheal ring splits in two, or **bifurcates**, into the left and right primary bronchi at the level of the fifth thoracic vertebra.

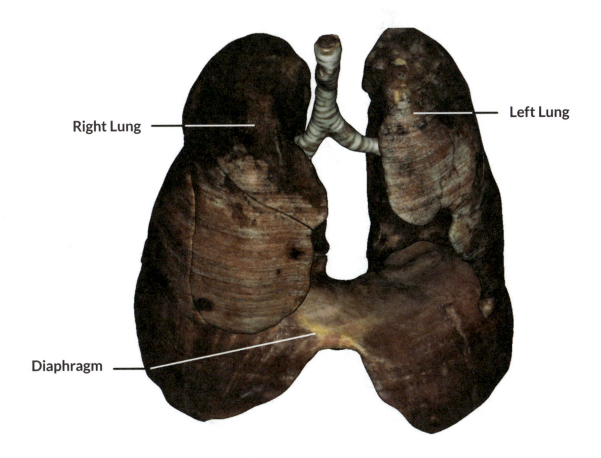

Figure 1.1 Lungs and diaphragm. Used with permission from Anatomage.

Spinal Column

The **spinal column** consists of 32–33 individual vertebrae. These vertebrae are divided into five segments (see Figure 1.2):

7 cervical vertebrae (C1–C7)
12 thoracic vertebrae (T1–T12)
5 lumbar vertebrae (L1–L5)
5 sacral vertebrae (S1–S5), fused in adults
3–4 coccygeal vertebrae (fused and called the coccyx)

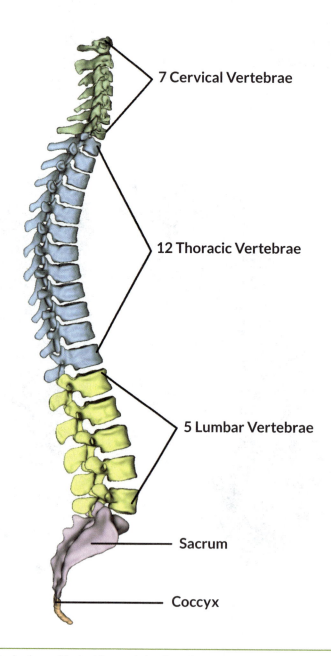

Figure 1.2   Vertebral column. Used with permission from Anatomage.

- **Cervical** vertebrae are small and are in the neck. The thoracic vertebrae provide points of attachment for the ribs. The lumbar vertebrae are the largest of the spinal column, which makes them suitable for weight-bearing functions. The five sacral vertebrae are fused together, forming the sacrum. Like the sacrum, the coccyx is formed by fused coccygeal vertebrae; it is often called the tailbone.

Sternum

The **sternum**, also called the **breastbone**, is located on the superior, anterior thoracic wall. The sternum consists of three parts: the manubrium, body, and xiphoid process.

- The **manubrium** is the uppermost segment of the sternum. The manubrium provides the attachment for the clavicle and the first rib.
- The body, or **corpus**, of the sternum is long and narrow. The cartilages of ribs 2 through 7 attach to the body of the sternum.
- The **xiphoid** (or ensiform) **process** is a small cartilaginous structure found at the bottom of the body of the sternum.

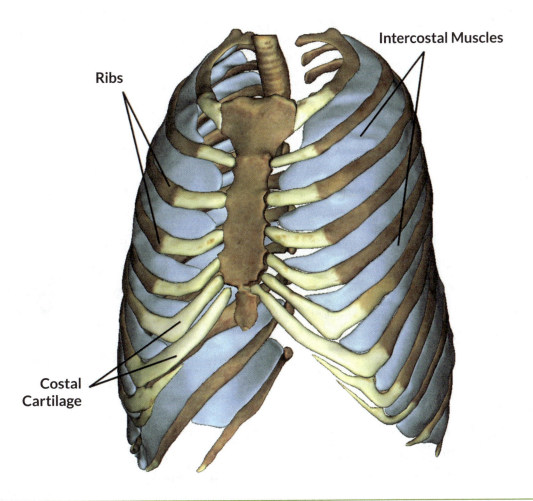

Figure 1.3 Rib cage. Used with permission from Anatomage.

Rib Cage

The **rib cage**, or **thoracic cage**, is usually called the chest. It consists of 12 pairs of ribs that articulate posteriorly with the vertebral column and anteriorly with the sternum to form a cylindrical structure. The ribs have a degree of mobility, which allows the rib cage to elevate during inspiration. The rib cage houses and protects such organs as the heart and lungs. Figure 1.3 shows a schematic of the rib cage.

- The rib cage is composed of several structures:

  The sternum in the anterior surface

  12 thoracic vertebrae in the posterior surface

  12 pairs of ribs that connect laterally from the vertebrae to their individual **costal cartilages**

Muscles of Respiration

Thoracic Muscles of Inspiration

The **diaphragm,** illustrated in Figure 1.1, is the floor of the chest cavity. It is a thick, dome-shaped muscle that separates the abdomen from the thorax. Because the lungs rest upon it, the diaphragm plays a major role in breathing and is considered the primary muscle of inspiration. Muscle fibers insert into the **central tendon** of the diaphragm and contract to pull the central tendon down and forward to expand the thoracic cavity.

- The **abdomen** houses structures such as the intestines, liver, and kidneys. Various abdominal muscles are critical in providing support for breathing.
- The **intercostal muscles**, the muscles between the ribs, illustrated in Figure 1.3, are also critical for respiration. The 11 paired **internal intercostals** pull the ribs downward to decrease the diameter of the thoracic cavity for exhalation, and the 11 paired **external intercostals** raise the ribs up and out to increase the diameter of the thoracic cavity for inhalation. Because they expand the thoracic cavity, the external intercostals provide a large amount of the total respiratory capacity, and therefore are crucial for speech breathing. The external intercostals and other inspiratory muscles also perform a *checking action* to control the flow of air leaving the lungs during speech (Wilson, Legrand, Gevenois, & De Troyer, 2001).
- Several other muscles also help elevate the rib cage. The **serratus posterior superior**, **levator costarum brevis**, **levator costarum longis**, and **external intercostal** muscles are all involved in rib cage elevation.
- A summary of these muscles, their innervations, and their functions follows (for more detailed information, see Seikel, Drumright, & King, 2016). (*Note*: The innervations basically arise from the vertebrae and their nerves and branches. For purposes of efficiency, only the vertebrae involved are listed—not the specific vertebral branches and nerves.)

Muscles and innervation	Function
Diaphragm (C3–C5)	Distends abdomen, enlarges vertical dimension of thorax, depresses central tendon of diaphragm
Serratus posterior superior (C7, T1–T4)	Elevates rib cage
Levator costarum brevis (T2–T12)	Elevates rib cage
Levator costarum longis (T2–T12)	Elevates rib cage
External intercostal (T2–T11)	Elevates rib cage

- Accessory muscles of the neck are also involved in the process of respiration. Three of the key neck muscles are the sternocleidomastoid, the trapezius, and the scalenes.
- The **sternocleidomastoid** elevates the sternum and thus, indirectly, the rib cage. The **trapezius** controls the head and elongates the neck, and thus indirectly influences respiration. The **scalenes** (anterior, middle, and posterior) stabilize and rotate the head. These muscles are attached to the first two ribs, and therefore indirectly enlarge the vertical dimension of the thorax (Davies & Davies, 2013).
- Muscles of the shoulder and upper arm act to move the rib cage and increase or decrease its dimensions. These muscles include the **pectoralis major**, **pectoralis minor**, **serratus anterior**, and **levator scapulae**.
- A summary of these muscles, their innervations, and their functions follows (for more detailed information, see Seikel et al., 2016). (*Note*: The innervations basically arise from the vertebrae and their nerves and branches. For purposes of efficiency, only the vertebrae involved are listed—not the specific vertebral branches and nerves.)

Muscles and innervation	Function
Pectoralis major (C4–T1)	Increases transverse dimension of rib cage through elevation of sternum
Pectoralis minor (C4–T1)	Increases transverse dimension of rib cage
Serratus anterior (C5–C7)	Elevates ribs 1–9
Levator scapulae (C3–C5)	Elevates scapula, supports neck
Rhomboideus major (C5)	Stabilizes shoulder girdle
Rhomboideus minor (C5)	Stabilizes shoulder girdle
Internal intercostal (T2–T11)	Depresses ribs 1–11
Innermost intercostal (T2–T11)	Depresses ribs 1–11
Transversus thoracis (T2–T6)	Depresses ribs 2–6

- Two posterior thoracic muscles are involved in respiration; they both support exhalation. The **subcostal muscle** depresses the thorax. The **serratus posterior inferior muscles**, when contracted, pull the rib cage down and thus aid in exhalation.

Abdominal Muscles of Expiration

Most muscles involved with breathing assist with inhalation. However, muscle action is also needed for exhalation of air. Muscles of expiration include the **latissimus dorsi**, **rectus abdominis**, **transversus abdominis**, **internal oblique abdominis**, and **quadratus lumborum**.

- A summary of these muscles, their innervations, and their functions follows (for more detailed information, see Seikel et al., 2016). (*Note*: The innervations basically arise from the vertebrae and their nerves and branches. For purposes of efficiency, only the vertebrae involved are listed—not the specific vertebral branches and nerves.)

Muscles and innervation	Function
Latissimus dorsi (C6–C8)	Stabilizes posterior abdominal wall for expiration
Rectus abdominis (T7–T12)	Flexes vertebral column
Transversus abdominis (T7–T12)	Compresses abdomen
Internal oblique abdominis (T7–T12)	Compresses abdomen, flexes and rotates trunk
Quadratus lumborum (T12, L1–L4)	Supports abdominal compression through bilateral contraction, which fixes abdominal walls

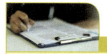

SUMMARY

- Respiration, the process of breathing involving an exchange of gas between an organism and its environment, is necessary for life and essential for speech.
- The framework of respiration supports the muscles necessary for respiration to take place. These muscles include two primary categories: the thoracic muscles of inspiration and the abdominal muscles of expiration.
- Respiration provides the energy for phonation (voice production).

PHONATION: STRUCTURES AND PROCESSES

Commonly known as the voice box, the larynx lies at the top of the trachea and houses the vocal folds, which vibrate to produce voice. Optimal laryngeal function and voicing depend upon the integrity of key laryngeal cartilages, as well as intrinsic and extrinsic laryngeal muscles. Certain neuroanatomical structures are also critical. These include cortical areas, the cerebellum, and cranial nerves VII and X (see the "Cranial Nerves" section of this chapter for more information).

The Larynx

During speech, the lungs supply the necessary air for phonation. The air flows upward through the trachea and comes toward the larynx. The **larynx** lies at the top of the trachea in the anterior portion of the neck.

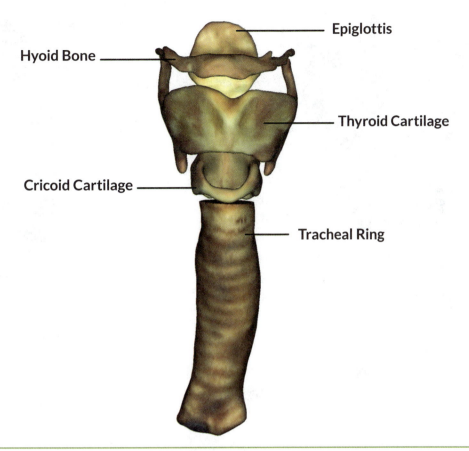

Figure 1.4 Structures of the larynx (thyroid and cricoid cartilages). Used with permission from Anatomage.

It is a valving mechanism that opens and closes. A few structures of the larynx (thyroid and cricoid cartilages) are shown in Figure 1.4.

- The larynx houses the **vocal folds**, which vibrate to produce sound. The vocal folds **adduct** (move toward the midline) and **abduct** (move away from the midline) as they vibrate. When a person is breathing quietly, the vocal folds are abducted.
- In addition to producing the sound needed for speech, the larynx has biological functions. These include (a) closure of the trachea so that food and other substances do not enter the lungs, (b) production of the cough reflex to expel foreign substances that accidentally enter the trachea, and (c) closure of the vocal folds to build subglottic pressure necessary for physical tasks such as excretion and lifting of heavy items.

Laryngeal Structures and Cartilages

The larynx is suspended from the U-shaped **hyoid bone**, which floats under the mandible, or lower jaw. The muscles of the tongue and various muscles of the mandible, skull, and larynx are attached to the hyoid bone.

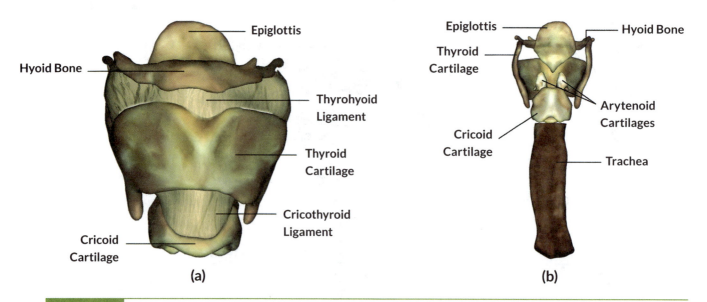

Figure 1.5 Front and back view of key laryngeal structures. Used with permission from Anatomage.

- The **epiglottis**, a protective structure, is a leaf-shaped piece of cartilage medial to the thyroid cartilage and hyoid bone. During swallowing, the epiglottis drops to cover the orifice of the larynx (Hixon et al., 2013). Figures 1.5a and b illustrate the epiglottis and other key laryngeal structures.

Key cartilages of the larynx include the thyroid, cricoid, and arytenoid cartilages.

- The **thyroid cartilage** is the largest laryngeal cartilage and forms the anterior and lateral walls of the larynx. It protects the larynx. The anterior surface of the thyroid cartilage is composed of two **laminae**, or plates, that meet at the midline to form the **thyroid angle**. Commonly called the "Adam's apple," the **thyroid notch** is the superior point of the thyroid angle. The thyroid cartilage is open posteriorly and has two pairs of horns, known as **cornu** (singular; plural *cornua*). The **superior cornua** extend upward to meet with the hyoid bone, and the **inferior cornua** extend downward to meet with the cricoid cartilage.
- The **cricoid cartilage**, which some view as the uppermost tracheal ring, is linked with the thyroid cartilage and the paired arytenoid cartilages. The cricoid cartilage completely surrounds the trachea and is larger in the back than in the front.
- The **arytenoid cartilages** are small, pyramid-shaped cartilages connected to the superior posterior cricoid through the cricoarytenoid joint, which permits sliding and circular movements. Many intrinsic laryngeal muscles connect to the arytenoid cartilages at two processes: the **vocal process** and the **muscular process**. The vocal folds are attached to the arytenoids at the **vocal process**. Muscles that both abduct and adduct the vocal folds attach to the arytenoids at the **muscular process**. Thus, the proper movement of the arytenoid cartilages is essential to voice production.
- The small, cone-shaped **corniculate cartilages** sit on the apex of the arytenoids. They assist in reducing the laryngeal opening when a person is swallowing. The tiny cone-shaped **cuneiform cartilages** are located under the mucous membrane that covers the aryepiglottic folds (defined in the "Vocal Folds" section of this chapter). The cuneiform cartilages serve to stiffen or tense the aryepiglottic folds.

Intrinsic Laryngeal Muscles

The **intrinsic laryngeal muscles** are primarily responsible for controlling sound production (Hixon et al., 2013). The intrinsic muscles of the larynx are the thyroarytenoid, lateral cricoarytenoid, transverse arytenoid, oblique arytenoid, cricothyroid, and posterior cricoarytenoid.

- The **thyroarytenoid** muscles are paired. Each thyroarytenoid is attached to the thyroid and arytenoid cartilages and is divided into two muscle masses: the internal thyroarytenoid and the external thyroarytenoid.
- The **internal thyroarytenoid** is the primary portion of the thyroarytenoid muscle, which vibrates and produces sound. It is generally referred to as the **vocalis muscle**, or more commonly, **vocal folds**. The vocal folds are illustrated in Figure 1.6. The external thyroarytenoid, also known as the **thyromuscularis muscle**, is lateral to the vocalis and, when contracted, aids in vocal fold adduction.
- Adductor muscles include the **lateral cricoarytenoid**, **transverse arytenoid**, and **oblique arytenoid**. These muscles act to bring the vocal folds together. The lateral cricoarytenoid increases medial compression of the vocal folds by rotating the arytenoids medially.
- The **cricothyroid muscle** is attached to the cricoid and thyroid cartilages. It lengthens and tenses the vocal folds, resulting in pitch change.

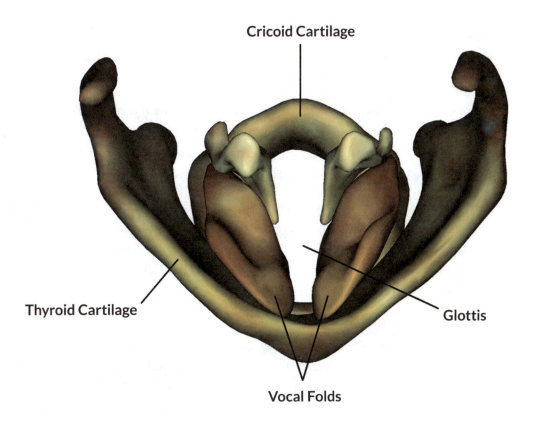

Figure 1.6 The vocal folds and surrounding structures. Used with permission from Anatomage.

- Figure 1.7a illustrates the **posterior cricoarytenoid muscle** and the **oblique** and **transverse arytenoid muscles**. Vocal fold adduction is supported when the oblique and transverse arytenoid muscles contract and pull the arytenoids closer together. Abduction of the vocal folds is accomplished when the posterior cricoarytenoid muscle contracts. The posterior cricoarytenoid muscle inserts into the muscular process of the arytenoid cartilage and is the only muscle responsible for vocal fold abduction.
- The intrinsic laryngeal muscles, the numeral of the cranial nerve that innervates them (e.g., "X" for the vagus nerve), and their functions are summarized below. Most intrinsic laryngeal muscles are innervated by the recurrent laryngeal nerve (RLN) branch of cranial nerve X, the vagus nerve. An exception is the cricothyroid, which is innervated by the external branch of the superior laryngeal nerve (SLN) branch of the vagus (Hixon et al., 2013).

Muscles and innervation	Function
Thyroarytenoid (X)	The internal thyroarytenoid is the primary portion of the thyroarytenoid muscle, which vibrates and produces sound.
Lateral cricoarytenoid (X)	Adducts vocal folds, increases medial compression
Transverse arytenoid (X)	Adducts vocal folds
Oblique arytenoid (X)	Pulls apex of arytenoids in a medial direction
Cricothyroid (X)	Lengthens and tenses vocal folds
Posterior cricoarytenoid (X)	Abducts vocal folds

A small opening that forms when the vocal folds are abducted is called the **glottis**. The glottis is not an anatomical structure; it is merely the name of that (opened) space between the vocal folds.

Extrinsic Laryngeal Muscles

The primary function of the **extrinsic laryngeal muscles** is to support the larynx and fix its position (Hixon et al., 2013). The extrinsic laryngeal muscles have one attachment to a structure within the larynx and one attachment to a structure outside the larynx. All extrinsic muscles are attached to the hyoid bone and lower or raise the position of the larynx within the neck.

- The **elevators**, or **suprahyoid muscles**, attach above the hyoid bone. Their primary function is elevation of the larynx. The suprahyoid muscles are the **digastric**, **geniohyoid**, **mylohyoid**, **stylohyoid**, **hyoglossus**, and **genioglossus**. The suprahyoid muscles are shown in Figure 1.7b.
- The **depressors**, or **infrahyoid muscles**, attach below the hyoid bone. Their primary function is depression of the larynx. The infrahyoid muscles are the **thyrohyoid**, **omohyoid**, **sternothyroid**, and **sternohyoid**.

  - The elevators and depressors and the numeral of the cranial nerves that innervate them are summarized in the following list. Innervations of these muscles are generally provided by branches of cranial nerve V (trigeminal), cranial nerve VII (facial), cranial nerve X (vagus), cranial nerve XII (hypoglossal), and portions of cervical spinal nerves C1–C3. (For more detailed information, see Seikel et al., 2016).

Anatomy, Neuroanatomy, and Physiology 13

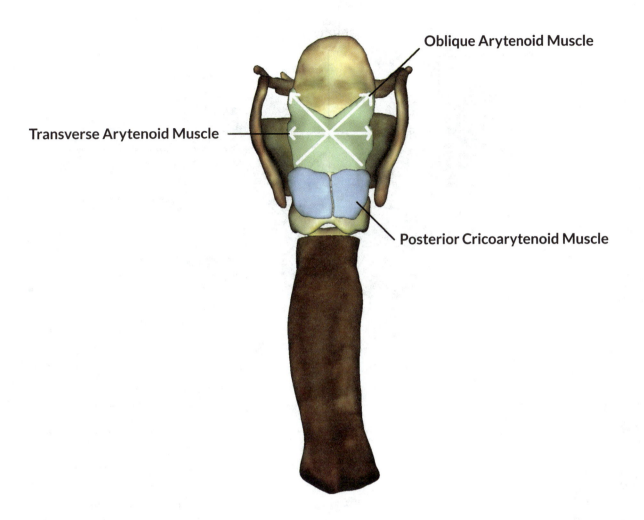

| Figure 1.7a | Posterior laryngeal muscles. Used with permission from Anatomage. |

Elevators and innervation (Suprahyoid)	Depressors and innervation (Infrahyoid)
Digastric (V, VII)	Thyrohyoid (XII, C1)
Geniohyoid (XII, C1)	Omohyoid (C1–C3)
Mylohyoid (V)	Sternothyroid (C1–C3)
Stylohyoid (VII)	Sternohyoid (C1–C3)
Hyoglossus (XII)	
Genioglossus (XII)	

Vocal Folds

The vocal folds have three layers: (a) the **epithelium**, or outer cover; (b) the **lamina propria**, or middle layer (which itself actually consists of three layers: superficial, intermediate, and deep); and (c) the **vocalis muscle**, or body, which provides stability and mass to the vocal fold.

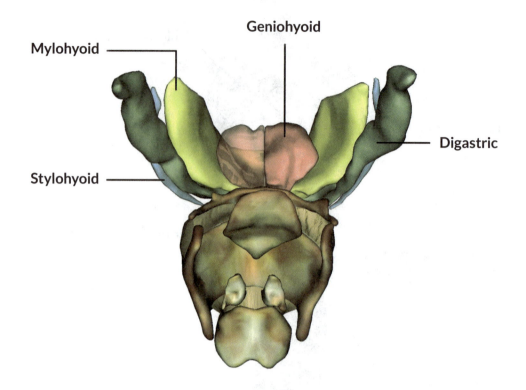

| Figure 1.7b | Suprahyoids muscles. Used with permission from Anatomage. |

- There are two other pairs of folds (see Figure 1.8):
  - **Aryepiglottic folds**. These are composed of a ring of connective tissue and muscle extending from the tips of the arytenoids to the epiglottis. They separate the laryngeal vestibule from the pharynx and help preserve the airway.
  - **Ventricular**, or **false**, vocal folds. The ventricular folds vibrate only at very low fundamental frequencies and usually not during normal or typical phonation. The ventricular folds compress during such activities as coughing and lifting heavy items.

Physiology of Phonation

Myoelastic–Aerodynamic Theory and Bernoulli Effect

The **myoelastic–aerodynamic theory** states that the vocal folds vibrate because of the forces and pressure of air and the elasticity of the vocal folds.

- The air flowing out of the lungs is temporarily stopped by the closed (or nearly closed) vocal folds. This builds up subglottal air pressure, which eventually blows the vocal folds apart. During this process, the folds are set into vibration, as well.
- The air then moves with increased velocity through the glottal opening. As the air moves swiftly through the open, but still somewhat constricted, vocal folds, the pressure between the edges of the vocal folds decreases, and, consequently, the folds are sucked together.
- The **Bernoulli effect** occurs when the velocity of a gas or fluid increases when it passes through a constriction, decreasing the pressure of the gas or fluid. In this case, the Bernoulli effect is caused by

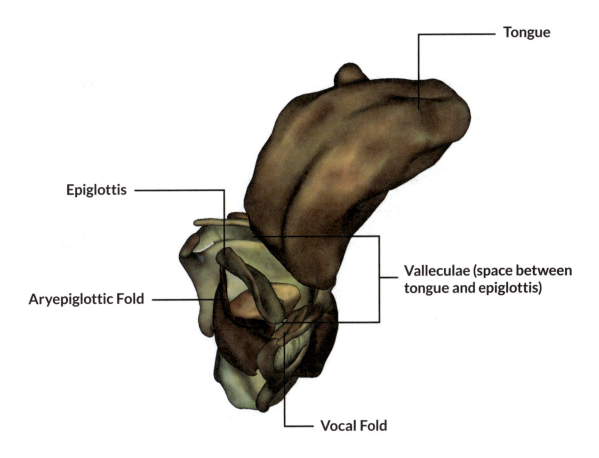

| Figure 1.8 | Valleculae and aryepiglottic fold. Used with permission from Anatomage. |

the increased speed of air passing between the vocal folds (the constriction). The resulting decrease in pressure between the vocal folds causes the "sucking" motion of the vocal folds toward one another.

- Once again, subglottal air pressure builds up and sets the folds in motion. Thus, there is a cycle of opening and closing of the vocal folds; this cycle is repeated more than 100 times per second during vocalization. The frequency at which the vocal folds vibrate depends on their length, tension, and mass and varies per individual (Zemlin, 1998).

Mucosal Wave Action

The mucosal wave is critical to vibration of the vocal folds. In **mucosal wave action**, the cover (epithelium and superficial lamina propria, also called Reinke's space) and the transition (intermediate and deep layers of the lamina propria) over the vocalis muscle slide and produce a wave.

- This wave travels across the superior surface of the vocal fold about two-thirds of the way to the lateral edge of the fold. Generally, the wave dissipates before reaching the inner surface of the thyroid cartilage. Without a mucosal wave, there is no vibration and thus no phonation.
- Vocal folds that have been stripped surgically to remove such abnormal vocal growths as nodules may be stiff and vibrate inefficiently due to alteration of the normal mucosal wave.

Neuroanatomy of the Vocal Mechanism

Cortical Areas

The primary cortical areas involved in speech–motor control, including phonation, are as follows:

- Area 4 (primary motor cortex)
- Area 44 (Broca's area)
- Areas 3, 1, 2 (somatosensory cortex)
- Area 6 (supplementary motor cortex)

Cerebellum

The function of the cerebellum is to regulate motor movement. It is critical in the control of speech movement.

- The cerebellum is key to the coordination of the laryngeal muscles for adequate phonation. It is also key to the effective functioning of other speech systems, such as respiration.

Cranial Nerves

Cranial nerve VII (the **facial nerve**) innervates the posterior belly of the digastric muscle.

- Cranial nerve X (the **vagus nerve**) includes the following primary branches, which innervate the larynx:
  - **Superior laryngeal nerve (SLN)**. The SLN has internal and external branches. The internal branch receives all sensory information from the larynx, and the external branch supplies motor innervation solely to the cricothyroid muscle.
  - **Recurrent laryngeal nerve (RLN)**. The RLN supplies all motor innervation to the interarytenoid, posterior cricoarytenoid, thyroarytenoid, and lateral cricoarytenoid muscles. It receives all sensory information below the vocal folds.

See a later section in this chapter, "Neuroanatomy and Neurophysiology: The Nervous System," for more information on speech–motor control and neural regulation of phonation.

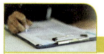

SUMMARY

Air for speech comes from the lungs, through the trachea, to the larynx and sets the vocal folds in motion for voicing. Adequate voicing depends upon the integrity of many laryngeal structures.

- Key laryngeal structures and cartilages provide protection to the larynx and aid in the process of vocalization.
- There are two sets of laryngeal muscles. The intrinsic laryngeal muscles have both their attachments within the larynx. The extrinsic laryngeal muscles have one attachment inside the larynx and one attachment outside the larynx.

- The myoelastic–aerodynamic theory and the Bernoulli effect explain the physiology of phonation. Mucosal wave action is critical to vocal fold vibration.
- Key neuroanatomical structures involved in vocalization include cortical areas, the cerebellum, and cranial nerves VII (facial nerve) and X (vagus nerve).

RESONATION AND ARTICULATION: STRUCTURES AND PROCESSES

As noted, respiration provides the energy for voicing. As the laryngeal tone travels upward past the larynx, it must be resonated by various structures, including the pharynx, the oral cavity, and the nasal cavity. The resonated tone is shaped and modified through articulation or production of speech sounds. Key structures involved in articulation include the pharynx, the soft palate, the hard palate, the mandible, the teeth, the tongue, the lips, and the cheeks. Functioning of these structures depends in part upon innervation by various cranial nerves.

Fundamentals of Resonation

The vocal folds vibrate to produce voice. **Resonation** is the modification of laryngeal tone by selective dampening or enhancement of specific frequencies. The resonant frequency is the frequency at which a cavity best vibrates and is dependent on the size and the shape of the cavity. The vocal tract is a cavity that changes size and shape based on movement of structures (or **resonators**), and therefore has a resonant frequency. Smaller cavities vibrate at a higher resonant frequency, whereas larger cavities vibrate at a lower resonant frequency. The resonators that thus modify laryngeal tone are the pharynx, the nasal cavity, and the oral cavity.

- The **pharynx** (throat) is part of the upper airway, extending from the nasal cavity to the vocal folds. It is located superiorly and posteriorly to the larynx. The size and shape of the pharynx are modified by the position of the tongue (forward or back) in the mouth and the vertical positioning of the larynx (high or low) in the neck (Peña-Brooks & Hegde, 2015).
- The **nasal cavity** has an important role in resonation. Only three sounds in English—/m/, /n/, and /ŋ/—are produced with nasal resonance. During the production of those sounds, the soft palate (velum), illustrated in Figure 1.9, is relaxed and lowered, **coupling** the nasal and oral cavities; they are not separated from one another.
- The **velum** is elevated and retracted for production of all other (oral) sounds in English. The raising and the retraction of the velum during the production of those sounds help make contact with the posterior pharyngeal wall, separating the oral cavity from the nasal cavity. The cavities are thus uncoupled, and the sounds are produced primarily with **oral resonance**.
- The **oral cavity** is the primary resonating structure for all English sounds, except /m/, /n/, and /ŋ/. The source-filter theory of vowel production—also known as the acoustic theory of vowel production—provides a widely accepted description of how the oral cavity is capable of producing speech sounds (Hixon et al., 2013).

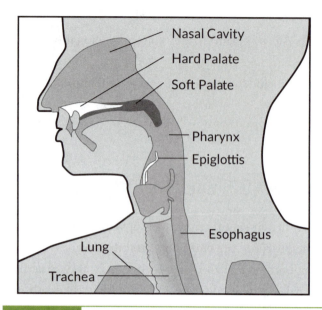 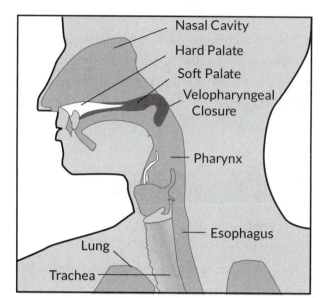

Figure 1.9 The velopharyngeal port, open and closed.

- The **source-filter theory** depicts the vocal tract as a series of linked tubes: the oral cavity, or mouth; the pharynx; and the nasal cavity (see Figure 1.10). These linked tubes provide the variable resonating cavity that helps produce speech.

  - The source-filter theory states that energy from the vibrating vocal folds (the **source**) is modified by the resonance characteristics of the vocal tract (the **filter**) (Behrman, 2012).
  - The vocal folds generate a voicing source. This voicing source is routed through the vocal tract, where it is shaped into speech sounds. Those speech sounds may be vowels when the source is phonation, and consonants when the sources include the turbulence of frication or combinations of turbulence and voicing.
  - Changes in the configuration and shape of the articulators (described in the next section of this chapter) govern the resonance characteristics of the vocal tract. The resonances of the vocal tract determine the sound of each specific vowel. Whether the produced sound is a consonant or a vowel, it passes through the filter of the oral cavity, which has been specifically configured for production of that sound (Hixon et al., 2013).
  - Structures within the oral cavity are shaped and moved to provide specific resonance for each sound. These structures are key in the process of articulation.

Fundamentals of Articulation

Articulation is the connection of movable parts or the joining of two elements. In speech, articulation refers to movements of speech structures to produce speech sounds. **Articulation** may also imply saying something clearly. In this section, the term *articulation* refers to the movement of joined anatomic parts, as well as the production of speech sounds that result from such movement.

- The larynx produces sound that is shaped into speech. The sound travels through the pharynx and the oral cavity (and the nasal cavity for nasal sounds). In the oral cavity, important structures

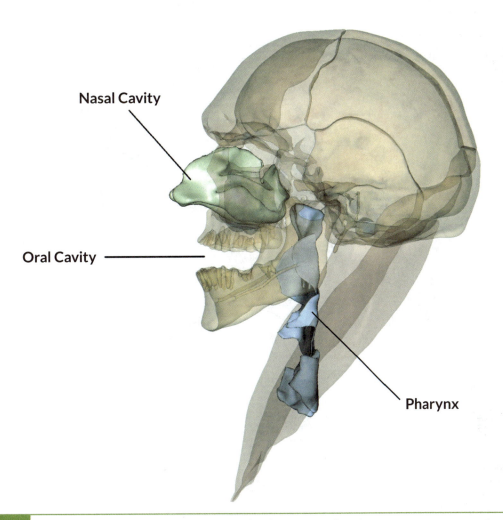

Figure 1.10 The pharyngeal, oral, and nasal cavities. Used with permission from Anatomage.

modify the sound into specific sounds for speech. These structures include the pharynx, the soft palate, the hard palate, the mandible, the teeth, the tongue, the lips, and the cheeks.

Pharynx

- The pharyngeal cavity is divided into three segments, which are illustrated in Figure 1.11:
  - The **laryngopharynx**, which begins immediately superior to the larynx and ends at the base of the tongue, is connected to
  - the **oropharynx**, which extends up to the soft palate and is connected to
  - the **nasopharynx**, which ends where the two nasal cavities begin.
- The laryngopharynx and the oropharynx add resonance to the sounds produced by the larynx. However, the nasopharynx adds noticeable resonance only to the nasals, /m/, /n/, and /ŋ/.
- The muscles of the pharynx are summarized in the following lists (Hixon et al., 2013). Most pharyngeal muscles are innervated by cranial nerve X (the vagus nerve) and cranial nerve XI (the spinal accessory nerve) via the **pharyngeal plexus**. The pharyngeal plexus is formed by the joining of cranial nerves X and XI; it supplies the upper pharyngeal musculature.

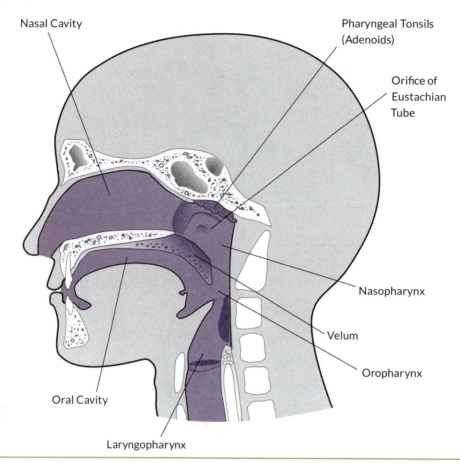

Figure 1.11 Diagram of the pharyngeal, oral, and nasal cavities.

Muscles and innervation	Function
Salpingopharyngeus (X, XI)	Elevates lateral pharyngeal wall and moves it medially
Stylopharyngeus (IX)	Elevates and opens pharynx
Superior pharyngeal constrictor (X, XI)	Constricts pharyngeal diameter, pulls pharyngeal wall forward
Middle pharyngeal constrictor (X, XI)	Narrows diameter of pharynx
Inferior pharyngeal constrictor, cricopharyngeus (X, XI)	Constricts superior orifice of esophagus
Inferior pharyngeal constrictor, thyropharyngeus (X, XI)	Reduces diameter of lower pharynx

Soft Palate

The soft palate, also called the **velum**, is a flexible muscular structure at the juncture of the oropharynx and the nasopharynx. It is located in the posterior area of the oral cavity and hangs from the hard palate (roof of the mouth). The **uvula** is the small, cone-shaped structure at the tip of the velum. The soft palate and other major structures of the oral cavity are shown in Figure 1.12.

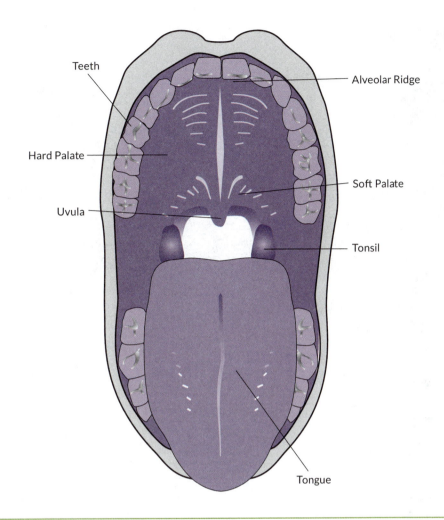

Figure 1.12 Major structures of the oral cavity.

- The soft palate is a dynamic structure of muscles that can be elevated or lowered. As previously stated, when the soft palate is lowered, there is coupling of the nasal and oral cavities for nasal sounds or quiet breathing through the nose.
- When the soft palate is raised and retracted, the muscles of the pharynx also move inward to meet the muscles of the soft palate. With this sphincter-like action, the nasal port is closed. This action is called **velopharyngeal closure**.
- If the muscular bulk of the soft palate is inadequate, the nasal cavity may remain open to some extent. Speakers with this condition sound excessively nasal because sound energy passes through the nasal cavities when it should not.
- The soft palate is composed of a number of muscles (see Figure 1.13). These include the **musculus uvulae**, **levator veli palatini**, the **tensor veli palatini**, the **palatoglossus**, and the **palatopharyngeus muscles**. These muscles, their innervations, and their functions are summarized in the following list (for more detailed information, see Hixon et al., 2013). The innervation "X, XI" refers specifically to the pharyngeal plexus, a structure arising from cranial nerve X, the vagus nerve, and cranial nerve XI, the spinal accessory nerve.

22 Chapter 1

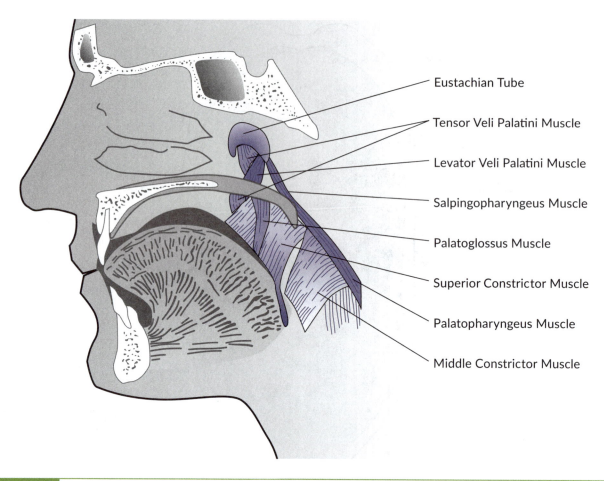

Figure 1.13 Muscles of the pharynx and soft palate.

Muscle and innervation	Function
Musculus uvulae (X, XI)	Embedded within the uvula, shortens velum
Levator veli palatini (X, XI)	Primary elevator of velum
Tensor veli palatini (V)	Tenses velum, dilates Eustachian tube
Palatoglossus (X, XI)	Also known as anterior faucial pillar, depresses velum, elevates tongue
Palatopharyngeus (X, XI)	Also known as posterior faucial pillar, narrows pharyngeal cavity, lowers velum, may help elevate the larynx

Hard Palate

The bony hard palate is the roof of the mouth and the floor of the nose. It is part of the maxillae (also called the paired maxillary bones). They are the largest bones in the face and form the entire upper jaw (Zemlin, 1998). The hard palate is illustrated in Figure 1.14.

- The front portion of the maxillary bone is called the **premaxilla**. The premaxilla houses the four upper front teeth known as the incisors.

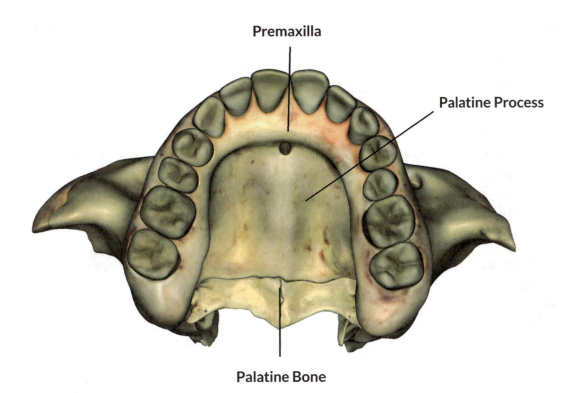

Figure 1.14   Hard palate. Used with permission from Anatomage.

- The portion of the maxillary bone that forms three-quarters of the hard palate is called the **palatine process**; it is the floor of the nasal cavity. The palatine process consists of two pieces of bone that grow and fuse at the midline during the fetal stage.
- The outer edges of the maxillary bone are called the **alveolar process**, which houses the molar, bicuspid, and cuspid teeth.
- For genetic and toxic environmental reasons, the premaxilla may fail to fuse with the maxillary bone. Also, the palatine process may fail to fuse at midline. These failures cause clefts of the palate in utero.
- Posteriorly, the maxillary bone joins with the **palatine bone** (different from the palatine process, which is part of the maxillary bone). The horizontal plate of the palatine bone comprises the remaining quarter of the hard palate. The soft palate attaches to the palatine bone.

Mandible

Also known as the lower jaw, the **mandible** is an important facial bone. It houses the lower teeth and forms the floor of the mouth. The mandible is formed by the fusion of two bones in the midpoint of the chin (also known as the **symphysis**) but is considered to be one bone in adults.

- The alveolar arch is the part of the mandible that houses the teeth. The two arches of the mandible are hinged to the skull with a set of muscles and tendons. The mandible is attached to the temporal bone of the skull by a joint called the **temporomandibular joint**.

- The muscles of the mandible serve two major functions: (a) opening and closing of the mouth, and (b) chewing food. Although its biological function is to chew food, the mandible is important for speech because it houses the lower teeth, serves as a framework for the tongue and lower lip, and is an integral part of the oral cavity. The tongue attaches to the mandible at several points. Though the jaw does not need to move more than a few millimeters for speech, precise movements of the mandible and tongue are integral to the production of varying speech sounds (Zemlin, 1998).
- The muscles of the mandible may be categorized as either elevators or depressors. They arise from branches of cranial nerves V (trigeminal nerve), VII (facial nerve), and XII (hypoglossal nerve). The geniohyoid also rises from the C1 spinal nerve. A summary of these muscles, their innervations, and their functions follows.

Elevators and innervation	Function
Masseter (V)	Elevates mandible, most powerful muscle of mastication
Temporalis (V)	Elevates mandible, draws mandible back if protruded (retraction)
Medial (internal) pterygoid (V)	Elevates mandible, protrudes mandible when contracted with lateral pterygoid

Depressors and innervation	Function
Anterior belly of digastric (V)	Depresses mandible in conjunction with posterior belly of digastric, pulls hyoid forward, aids in retraction of mandible
Posterior belly of digastric (VII))	Depresses mandible in conjunction with anterior belly of digastric, pulls hyoid back
Lateral (external) pterygoid (V	Depresses and protrudes mandible
Geniohyoid (XII, C1)	Depresses mandible, aids in retraction of mandible
Mylohyoid (V)	Depresses mandible, aids in retraction of mandible

Teeth

The lower dental arch is part of the mandible, and the upper dental arch is part of the maxillary bone. The major function of the teeth is **mastication** (chewing), but the teeth also help produce some speech sounds. For example, the labiodental sounds /f/ and /v/ require the lower lip to come in contact with the upper teeth. Therefore, the teeth are articulators.

- Teeth, illustrated in Figure 1.15, have specific names (e.g., molars, bicuspids) depending upon their location in the mouth. **Deciduous teeth** are temporary teeth that appear in a baby, usually around 6–9 months of age. Babies normally have 20 deciduous teeth, 10 in each arch. Of the 10, 4 are incisors, 2 are canine, and 4 are molar.
- Adults have 32 teeth, 16 in each arch. Of the 16 teeth, 4 are incisors, 2 are canine, 4 are premolar, and 6 are molar. The deciduous dental arch does not have premolars or the third molar.

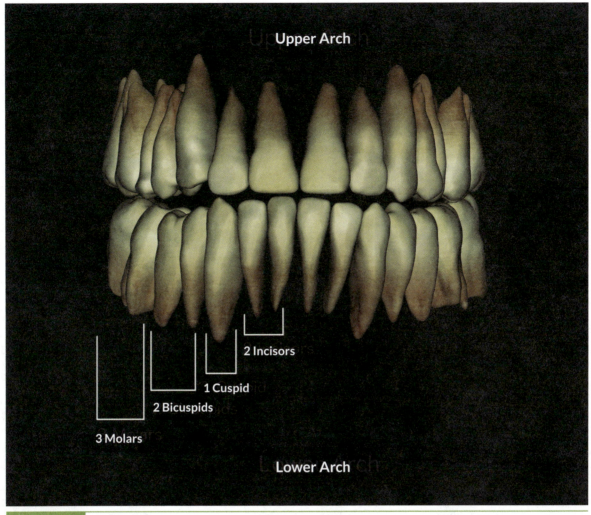

Figure 1.15 Types of teeth. Used with permission from Anatomage.

- **Occlusion** refers to the way the two dental arches come together when a person "bites down." Occlusion is normal if (a) the upper and lower dental arches meet each other in a symmetrical manner, and (b) if the individual teeth in the two arches are properly aligned.
- **Malocclusions** include deviations in the positioning of individual teeth and the shape and relationship of the upper and lower dental arches.

Tongue

The tongue plays an important role in eating and in speech production. The taste buds of the tongue help people taste their food, and the muscles of the tongue move food around in the oral cavity for efficient mastication and swallowing. Movements of the tongue are critical to articulation.

- For example, tongue movement is necessary to produce several classes of sounds, including the linguadentals (/θ/ and /ð/), lingua-alveolars (e.g., /t/, /d/, and /l/), and lingua-palatals (e.g., the fricative /ʃ/, the affricate /tʃ/). The tongue also constricts the air passage to create the friction needed to produce fricatives.

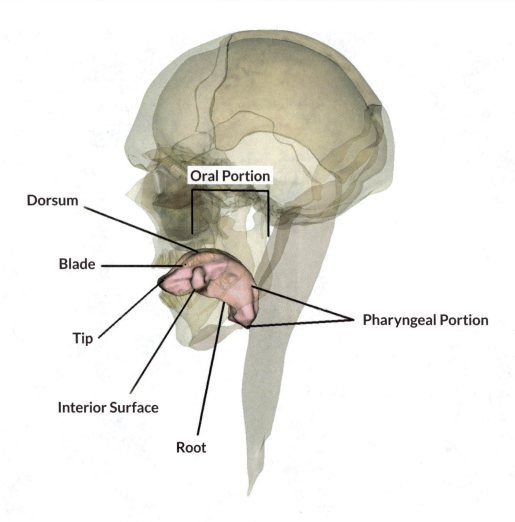

Figure 1.16 Major areas of the tongue. Used with permission from Anatomage.

- Anatomically, the tongue is divided into four major parts: tip, blade, dorsum, and root (see Figure 1.16).

  - The **tip** is the thinnest and most flexible part of the tongue and plays an important role in articulation.
  - The **blade** is a small region adjacent to the tip; in a resting position, it is the portion of the tongue that lies just inferior to the alveolar ridge.
  - The **dorsum** is the large area of the tongue that lies in contact with both the hard and soft palates. This is the area of the tongue that is visible upon protrusion.
  - The **root** is the very back and bottom portion of the tongue.
  - The **lingual frenulum** (or frenum) connects the mandible with the inferior portion of the tongue. This band of tissue may stabilize the tongue during movement.

There are two sets of important tongue muscles: **intrinsic** and **extrinsic**. As their name implies, intrinsic muscles are within the tongue itself, whereas extrinsic muscles connect the tongue to a structure outside the tongue. The extrinsic muscles are named based on the structures they attach to (e.g., hyoglossus connects the hyoid bone to the tongue). Upon contraction, the tongue muscles perform important functions in articulation. Extrinsic muscles are responsible for gross movement of the tongue, while the intrinsic muscles are responsible for fine movements. The tongue muscles are innervated by cranial nerve XII, the hypoglossal nerve. A summary of the muscles of the tongue, their innervations, and their functions follows.

Intrinsic or extrinsic	Tongue muscles and innervation	Function
Intrinsic	Superior longitudinal muscle (XII)	Shortens tongue, turns tip upward, assists in turning lateral margins upward
	Inferior longitudinal muscle (XII)	Shortens tongue, pulls tip downward, assists in retraction
	Transverse muscles (XII)	Narrow and elongate tongue
	Vertical muscles (XII)	Flatten tongue
Extrinsic	Genioglossus (XII)	Forms bulk of tongue; is able to retract tongue, draw tongue downward, draw entire tongue anteriorly to protrude tip or press tip against alveolar ridge and teeth
	Styloglossus (XII)	Draws tongue up and back, may draw sides of tongue upward to help make dorsum concave
	Hyoglossus (XII)	Retracts and depresses tongue; elevates hyoid bone
	Chondroglossus (XII)	Depresses tongue, elevates hyoid bone
	Palatoglossus	Sometimes considered a muscle of the velum, helps elevate posterior portion of tongue (but depresses velum)

- The **genioglossus muscle** forms the bulk of the tongue and allows it to move freely. It has both anterior and posterior fibers. Figure 1.17 illustrates the genioglossus and related muscles.

Face: Lips and Cheeks

Several major bones of the face have already been discussed. There are major facial muscles, involving the lips and cheeks, that are important for articulation (see Figures 1.18a, b, and c). These muscles assist in production of various sounds, especially the labial sounds /m/, /b/, and /p/.

- The primary muscle of the lips is the **orbicularis oris** muscle. The cheeks are primarily composed of the **buccinator muscle**, a large flat muscle whose inner surface is covered with mucous membrane.
- Most of the facial muscles are innervated by either the **buccal branches** or the **mandibular marginal branch** of cranial nerve VII, the facial nerve. These muscles, their innervations, and their functions are summarized in the following list (for more detailed information, see Seikel et al., 2016).

(text continues on page 30)

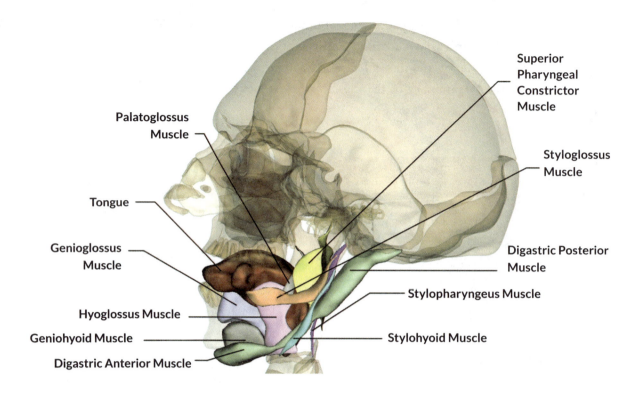

Figure 1.17 Muscles of the tongue and pharynx. Used with permission from Anatomage.

Muscles and innervation	Function
Mentalis (VII)	Pulls lower lip out, wrinkles and elevates chin
Platysma (VII)	Depresses mandible
Risorius (VII)	Retracts lips at corners
Buccinator (VII)	Constricts oropharynx; moves food onto grinding surfaces of molars
Depressor labii inferioris (VII)	Pulls lower lip down and out to dilate orifice
Depressor anguli oris (triangularis) (VII)	Helps to press lower and upper lips together, depresses corners of mouth
Zygomatic minor (VII)	Elevates upper lip, aids in lip protrusion
Zygomatic major (VII)	Retracts and elevates angle of mouth
Orbicularis oris inferioris and superioris (VII)	Pulls lips together, seals lips, serves as point of insertion for other muscles, interacts with other muscles to produce facial expressions, rounds lips
Levator anguli oris (VII)	Draws corner of mouth upward and medially
Levator labii superioris (VII)	Elevates upper lip
Levator labii superioris alaeque nasi (VII)	Elevates upper lip and ala of the nose, dilates the nose

Anatomy, Neuroanatomy, and Physiology * 29

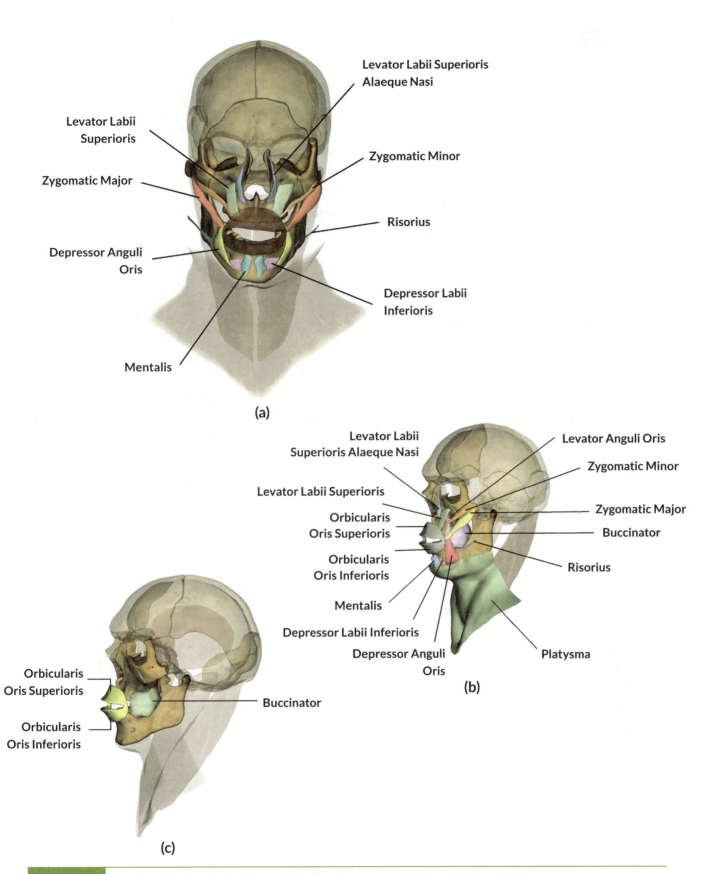

Figure 1.18 Muscles of the face. Used with permission from Anatomage.

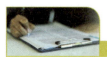

SUMMARY

Tones generated by the larynx travel upward and are resonated in the pharyngeal, oral, and nasal cavities. This process of resonation is explained by the source-filter theory.

- **Articulation** refers to the movement of speech structures to produce sounds. It depends upon the integrity of the following structures: the pharynx, soft palate, hard palate, mandible, teeth, tongue, lips, and cheeks.
- The cranial nerves innervating the muscles of articulation include cranial nerve V (trigeminal), VII (facial), X (vagus), XI (spinal accessory), and XII (hypoglossal).

NEUROANATOMY AND NEUROPHYSIOLOGY: THE NERVOUS SYSTEM

Neurology is the study of neurological disorders and diseases and their diagnosis and treatment. **Neuroanatomy** is a branch of neurology concerned with the study of structures of the nervous system. **Neurophysiology**, another branch of neurology, is concerned with the study of the function of the nervous system. In this section, basic neuroanatomy and neurophysiology of speech, language, and hearing are discussed. It is assumed that the reader has taken coursework in these areas; thus, this section provides only a basic review of some foundational ideas.

This section first covers **neurons** and **neural transmission**. It next discusses basic facts about the workings of the **peripheral** and **autonomic nervous systems**, including information about the cranial nerves. The main structures of the **central nervous system** (CNS) are then described: the brainstem, reticular activating system (RAS), diencephalon, basal ganglia, cerebellum, cerebrum, pyramidal system, extrapyramidal system, connecting fibers in the brain, cerebral ventricles, protective layers of the brain, and cerebral blood supply. (*Note*: The extrapyramidal system is not technically a part of the CNS; however, it is closely related to the CNS and is thus discussed under that heading.)

NEURONS AND NEURAL TRANSMISSION

The nervous system is composed of billions of specialized cells that function interconnectedly. Neurons are the most important of these cells. Sensory or afferent neurons carry sensory impulses toward the brain, whereas motor or efferent nerves transmit impulses away from the brain. Nerves may be organized into systems.

Anatomy and Physiology of Nerve Cells

The CNS is made up of different types of cells. **Glial cells** or **neuroglia** include astrocytes, **oligodendroglia**, ependymal cells, and microglia. The glia cells of the peripheral nervous system (PNS) are called **Schwann cells** and **satellite cells**. The neuroglia, or simply glia, cells do not transmit nerve impulses; they mainly support and protect the nerve cells (Bhatnagar, 2012).

- **Neurons** are the most important type of nerve cells. There are billions of neurons that receive information from other neurons, process that information, and then transmit the information to still other neurons.
- The neuron, or nerve cell, has two parts: (a) nerve fibers and (b) the soma, or cell body, which contains the nucleus. Figure 1.19a shows a basic (typical) neuron and 1.19b shows some common varieties of neurons.
- The core of the cell body is called the nucleus. The cell body is covered with a membrane. The axons and dendrites are projections of the cell body and specialize in receiving and conducting stimuli.
- **Dendrites** are short fibers that extend from the cell body. They receive neural impulses generated from the axons of other cells, and they transmit those impulses to the cell body. A single neuron can have a multitude of dendrites, which branch out to form a dendritic tree.
- Each cell has a single axon, which is wrapped in a myelin sheath (defined at the end of this section). Axons are longer fibers than dendrites and have **terminal**, or **end**, **buttons** at the tip. End buttons contain neurotransmitters. The end button of one neuron either makes close contact with or actually touches the dendrite of another neuron. Axons send out impulses generated within the neuron; these impulses are sent away from the cell body to other neurons.
  - Many axons, especially the larger axons of the CNS and those in the PNS, have a white insulating sheath called **myelin** around them. Schwann cells (in the PNS) and oligodendroglia (in the CNS) provide the myelin sheath around the axon. The myelin has breaks at the junction between the cells to facilitate the impulse transfer.
- Neurons are arranged in the form of fibers. A **nervous system**, on the other hand, is an organization of nerves according to specific spatial, structural, and functional principles. The peripheral, autonomic, and central nervous systems are often collectively referred to as the nervous system. In the next sections, each of these systems is explained.
- Neurons communicate with each other through junctions called **synapses**. An axon branches out into several smaller fibers, which form terminals. These terminals connect to a synapse, although this neural junction includes a small gap or space. Thus, a synapse consists of the terminal button of one neuron, the receptive site of another neuron, and the synaptic cleft or space between the two (Peña-Brooks & Hegde, 2015).

Neural Transmission

Neural transmission is a chemical process of information exchange at the level of the synapse. A **neurotransmitter**, a chemical contained within the terminal buttons, helps make contact between two cells by diffusing itself across the synaptic space.

- Such diffused neurotransmitters become bound to receptors in the postsynaptic membrane. The diffused neurotransmitter may cause the inhibition or excitation of the next neuron. **Dopamine** and **acetylcholine** are two important neurotransmitters in the motor system.
- Neurons have certain specialized functions. There are three basic types of neurons: **motor neurons**, **sensory neurons**, and **interneurons**.

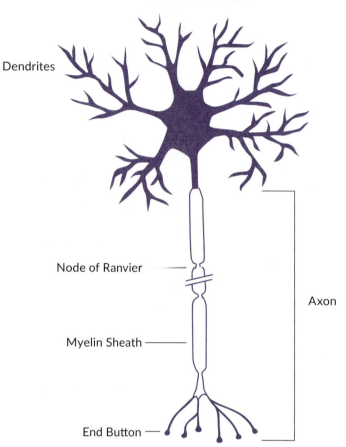
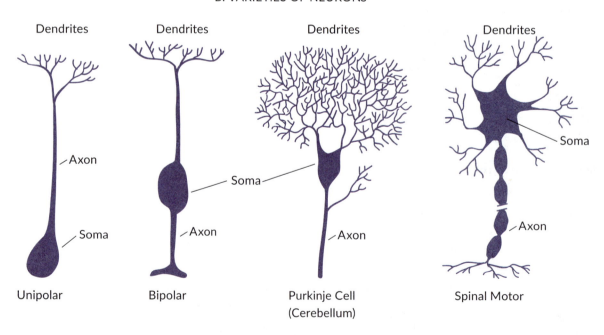

Figure 1.19 A typical neuron (a), and some of its varieties (b).

- **Sensory neurons**, also called afferent neurons, carry sensory impulses from the peripheral sense organs toward the brain.
- **Motor neurons**, also called efferent neurons, transmit impulses away from the CNS. Motor neurons cause glandular secretions or muscle contractions (movement).
- **Interneurons**, the most common type of neuron in the nervous system, link neurons with other neurons and, therefore, play an important role in controlling movement (Bhatnagar, 2012).

SUMMARY

Neurons, the central building blocks of the nervous system, are composed of a cell body, dendrites, and an axon.

Some of these nerves have myelin sheaths around them. Various types of nerves transmit impulses to and from the CNS.

THE PERIPHERAL AND AUTONOMIC NERVOUS SYSTEMS

The PNS, a collection of nerves outside the spinal column and skull, carries sensory and motor impulses back and forth from the brain to various parts of the body. The 12 pairs of cranial nerves are part of the PNS, and some of them are critical to language, speech, and hearing. The 31 pairs of spinal nerves are indirectly involved with speech because they control automatic functions, such as breathing. Part of the PNS is the autonomic nervous system (ANS), with its sympathetic and parasympathetic branches, which may have an indirect effect upon speech in certain situations. The CNS will be discussed in the next section.

The Nervous System

Peripheral nervous system	Central nervous system
Cranial nerves	Spinal cord
Spinal nerves	Brain
Autonomic nervous system • Sympathetic branch • Parasympathetic branch	

Peripheral Nervous System

Basic Principles

The **peripheral nervous system (PNS)** is a collection of nerves that are outside the skull and spinal column. These nerves carry **sensory** impulses, which originate in the peripheral sense organs, to the brain, and **motor impulses**, which originate in the brain, to the glands and muscles of the body.

- The PNS contains three types of nerves: the cranial, the spinal, and the autonomic. The nerves that make up the ANS are discussed later. There are 12 pairs of cranial nerves and 31 pairs of spinal

Table 1.1

Cranial Nerves

Nerve no.	Name	Function
I	Olfactory	Sense of smell (sensory)
II	Optic	Vision (sensory)
III	Oculomotor	Eye movement (motor)
IV	Trochlear	Eye movement (motor)
V	Trigeminal	Face (sensory); jaw (motor)
VI	Abducens	Eye movement (motor)
VII	Facial	Tongue (sensory); face (motor)
VIII	Acoustic	Hearing and balance (sensory)
IX	Glossopharyngeal	Tongue and pharynx (sensory); pharynx only (motor)
X	Vagus	Larynx, respiratory, cardiac, and gastrointestinal systems (sensory and motor)
XI	Spinal accessory	Shoulder, arm, and throat movements (motor)
XII	Hypoglossal	Mostly tongue movements (motor)

Note. From *Introduction to Communicative Disorders* (5th ed.), by M. N. Hegde, forthcoming, Austin, TX: PRO-ED. Copyright by PRO-ED, Inc. Reprinted with permission.

nerves. Of the three types of nerves, the cranial nerves are the most directly involved in speech, language, and hearing.

Cranial Nerves

The cranial nerves emerge from the brainstem and are attached to the base of the brain. They are part of the lower motor system, and they receive much of their innervations from the corticobulbar tract of the pyramidal system (discussed later in this chapter). The cranial nerves exit through **foramina**, or holes, in the base of the skull. They exit at different levels of the brainstem and the top portion of the spinal cord.

- The cranial nerves are numbered according to the vertical order in which they exit from the skull. They go out to connect to various sense organs and muscles of the neck and head. Table 1.1 lists the cranial nerves and their numbers and basic functions. Some students remember the cranial nerves by the following mnemonic: *On Old Olympus' Towering Top, A Finn And German Viewed Some Hops.*
- **Sensory nerves** are those cranial nerves that carry sensory information from a sense organ (e.g., the nose) to the brain. Sensory nerves also are called **afferent nerves**. **Motor** (movement-related) **nerves** carry impulses from the brain to the muscles that make those muscles move. Motor nerves also are called **efferent nerves**. Several cranial nerves are **mixed nerves** because they carry both sensory and motor impulses.
- There are 12 pairs of cranial nerves. The first two cranial nerves are related to the cerebral cortex. Cranial nerves III to XII originate from the brainstem and innervate the muscles of the pharynx, tongue, larynx, head, neck, and face. Figure 1.20 illustrates an inferior view of the brain showing cranial nerves, as well as other cerebral structures (described in the "Cerebrum" section of this chapter).

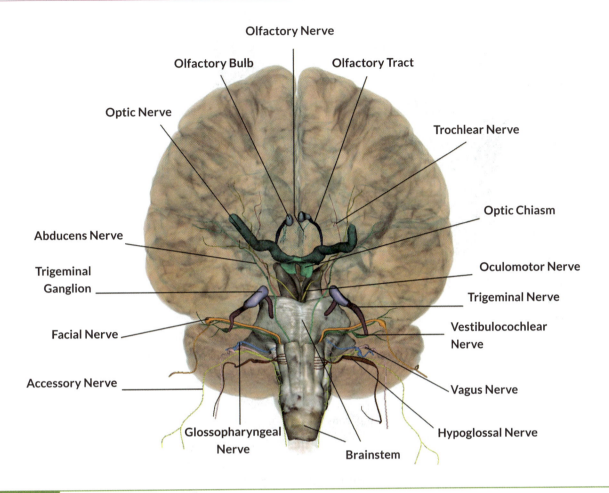

Figure 1.20 Cranial nerves. Used with permission from Anatomage.

Cranial nerves I, II, III, IV, and VI are not concerned with speech, language, or hearing.

- **Cranial nerve I (the olfactory nerve)** is a sensory nerve originating in the nasal cavity. It is involved with smell.
- **Cranial nerve II (the optic nerve)** is a sensory nerve originating in the retina. It is involved with vision.
- **Cranial nerve III (the oculomotor nerve)** and **cranial nerve IV (the trochlear nerve)** are motor nerves that originate in the midbrain area and innervate muscles corresponding to eye movement.
- **Cranial nerve VI (the abducens nerve)** is a motor nerve that controls eye movement.

Cranial nerves V and VII to XII *are* involved with speech, language, and hearing.

- **Cranial nerve V**, or the **trigeminal nerve**, is a mixed (both motor and sensory) nerve (see Figures 1.21a, b, and c).
- Its **sensory fibers** are composed of three branches: the ophthalmic, maxillary, and mandibular branches.
  - The **ophthalmic branch** has sensory branches from the nose, eyes, and forehead.

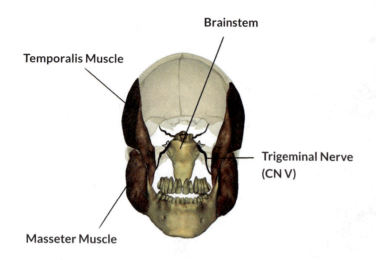

Figure 1.21a Anterior trigeminal innervation. Used with permission from Anatomage.

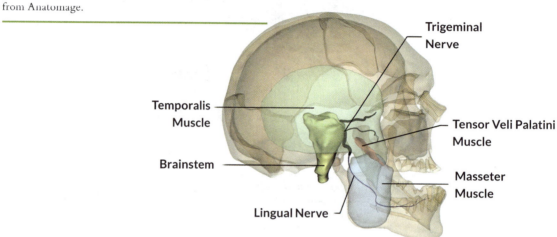

Figure 1.21b Lateral innervation of masseter and tensor veli palatini. Used with permission from Anatomage.

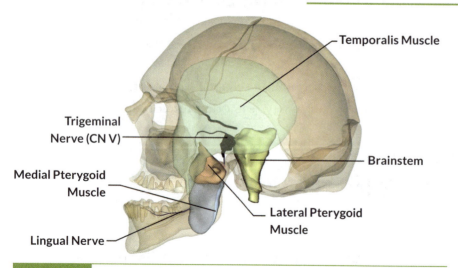

Figure 1.21c Lateral innervation of trigeminal pterygoids temporalis. Used with permission from Anatomage.

- The **maxillary branch** has sensory branches from the nose, upper lip, maxilla, upper cheek area, upper teeth, maxillary sinus, nasopharynx, and palate.
- The **mandibular branch** has sensory branches from the mandible, lower teeth, lower lip, tongue, part of the cheek, and part of the external ear. It transmits tactile, pain, and temperature (but not taste) stimuli from the anterior two-thirds of the tongue. The **mandibular branch** of cranial nerve V also has motor fibers, which innervate various jaw muscles, including the temporalis, lateral and medial pterygoids, masseter, tensor veli palatini, tensor tympani, mylohyoid, buccinator, and anterior belly of the digastric muscle.

■ The trigeminal nerve is bilaterally innervated, so unilateral upper motor neuron lesions minimally impact motor function. Unilateral damage to cranial nerve V will cause the jaw to deviate towards the affected side when the mouth is closed. Bilateral damage to cranial nerve V may result in an inability to close the mouth and difficulty in chewing. Damage to cranial nerve V may also cause **trigeminal neuralgia** (sharp pain in the facial area) (Hixon et al., 2013). **Cranial nerve VII**, the **facial nerve**, is also a mixed nerve (see Figures 1.22a, b, and c).

- The sensory fibers of the facial nerve are responsible for taste sensations on the anterior two-thirds of the tongue.
- The motor fibers of the facial nerve innervate muscles important to facial expression and speech. These muscles include the buccinator, zygomatic, orbicularis oris, orbicularis oculi, platysma, stapedius, stylohyoid, frontalis, procerus, nasalis, depressor labii inferioris, depressor anguli oris, auricular muscles, various labial muscles, and the posterior belly of the digastric muscle.
- The upper portion of the face is bilaterally innervated, so a unilateral upper motor neuron lesion will only paralyze the lower face. A person with bilateral damage to the facial nerve will be unable to move his or her upper and lower face, and will often have a mask-like appearance with minimal or no facial expression. When there is unilateral damage to the facial nerve, the smile is drawn to the undamaged side (Tate & Tollefson, 2006).

■ **Cranial nerve VIII**, the **acoustic** (or **vestibulocochlear**) **nerve**, is a sensory nerve for balance and hearing. It has two branches (vestibular and acoustic).

- The vestibular branch is primarily responsible for maintenance of equilibrium, or balance.
- The acoustic branch transmits sensory information from the cochlea of the inner ear to the primary auditory cortex of the brain, where it is interpreted.
- Damage to the vestibular branch of the acoustic nerve results in hearing loss, problems with balance, or both.

■ **Cranial nerve IX**, the **glossopharyngeal nerve**, is a mixed nerve. It has sensory, motor, and autonomic components.

- The **sensory** component of the glossopharyngeal nerve assists in processing taste sensations from the posterior third of the tongue. This component also provides general sensation for the tympanic cavity, ear canal, eustachian tube, faucial pillars, tonsils, soft palate, and pharynx.

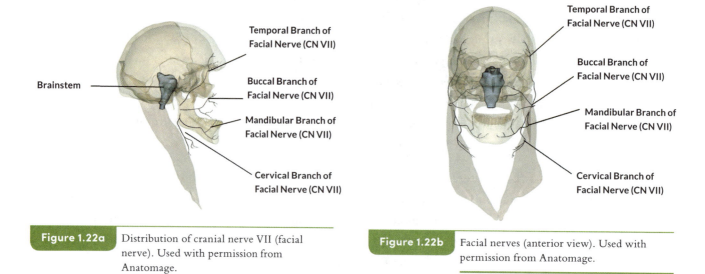

Figure 1.22a Distribution of cranial nerve VII (facial nerve). Used with permission from Anatomage.

Figure 1.22b Facial nerves (anterior view). Used with permission from Anatomage.

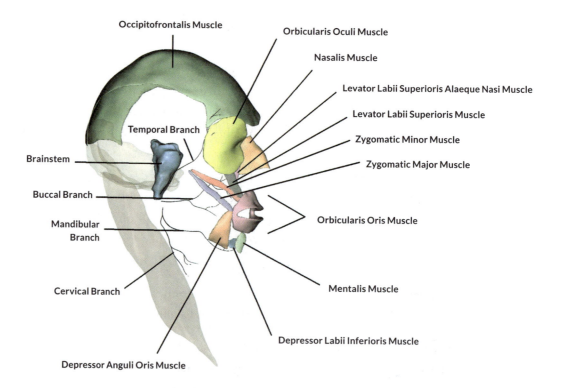

Figure 1.22c Facial nerves with muscles. Used with permission from Anatomage.

- The **motor** fibers of the glossopharyngeal nerve innervate the stylopharyngeus, a muscle that raises and dilates the pharynx.
- Experts differ on whether the motor fibers of the glossopharyngeal nerve also innervate the superior pharyngeal constrictor (Hixon et al., 2013). According to Zemlin (1998), the

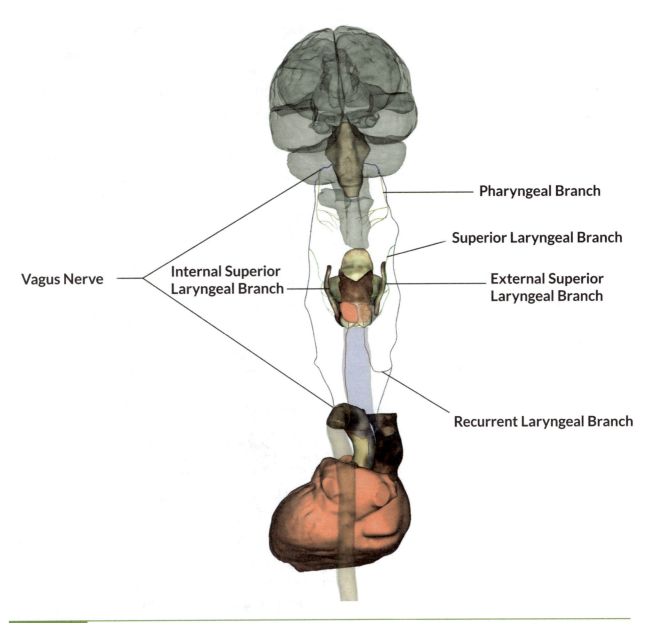

Figure 1.23 Distribution of cranial nerve X (vagus nerve). Used with permission from Anatomage.

glossopharyngeal nerve, along with fibers of the vagus nerve (X), supplies motor fibers to the **pharyngeal plexus**, which innervates the upper pharyngeal constrictor muscles.
- Lesions of the glossopharyngeal nerve may create difficulty in swallowing, unilateral loss of the gag reflex, and loss of taste and sensation from the posterior third of the tongue.

- **Cranial nerve X**, the **vagus nerve**, is a mixed nerve containing motor, sensory, and autonomic fibers (see Figure 1.23). It is called a wandering ("vagus") nerve because it extends from the neck into the chest and the stomach.

  - The **motor** fibers of the vagus nerve supply the digestive system, heart, lungs, pharynx, and larynx.

- The **sensory** fibers convey information from the digestive system, heart, trachea and bronchi, lower pharynx, larynx, and epiglottis. Sensory fibers also transmit pain, touch, and temperature sense from the skin covering the tympanic membrane and ear canal.
- The **recurrent laryngeal nerve (RLN)**, a branch of the vagus nerve, regulates the intrinsic muscles of the larynx, excluding the cricothyroid, which is supplied by the SLN branch. The RLN may be damaged during thyroid surgery, resulting in total or partial paralysis of the vocal folds. The left RLN courses under the heart and back up to the esophagus, trachea, and larynx. The left RLN may be damaged during cardiac surgery, resulting in paresis or paralysis of the left vocal fold.
- The **pharyngeal branch** of the vagus nerve supplies the pharyngeal constrictors. It also supplies all the muscles of the velum except the tensor veli palatini, which is innervated by the trigeminal nerve. It also transmits sensory information from the base of the tongue and pharynx.
- The **superior laryngeal nerve (SLN)**, another branch of the vagus nerve, is divided into internal (sensory) and external (motor) branches. The internal branch receives sensory information from the larynx above the vocal folds. The external branch innervates the cricothyroid muscle; damage to this branch results in the inability to change pitch.
- Due to its extensive course, damage to the vagus nerve includes a variety of sequelae, such as difficulty swallowing, paralysis of the velum (resulting in nasality issues), and voice problems (e.g., aphonia, breathiness, roughness, hoarseness, etc.) if the RLN is damaged.

- **Cranial nerve XI**, the **spinal accessory nerve**, is a motor nerve (see Figure 1.24). It is both a cranial and spinal nerve because of its cranial and spinal origin.

  - The spinal root supplies the trapezius and sternocleidomastoid muscles, which assist in head and shoulder movements.
  - In concert with the vagus nerve, the cranial fibers of the accessory nerve innervate the uvula and levator veli palatini muscles of the soft palate.
  - Lesions of the spinal accessory nerve may result in neck weakness, paralysis of the sternocleidomastoid, and consequent inability to turn the head, as well as an inability to shrug the shoulders or raise the arm above shoulder level (Zemlin, 1998).

- **Cranial nerve XII**, the **hypoglossal nerve**, is a motor nerve that runs under the tongue (see Figures 1.25a and b).

  - This nerve supplies all extrinsic tongue muscles except for the palatoglossus muscle.
  - The hypoglossal nerve also supplies all the intrinsic muscles of the tongue.
  - Lesions to the hypoglossal nerve can result in tongue paralysis, diminished intelligibility, and swallowing problems.

Spinal Nerves

The spinal nerves of the PNS are closely related to the ANS. Together, they control various bodily activities that are executed with little conscious effort or knowledge.

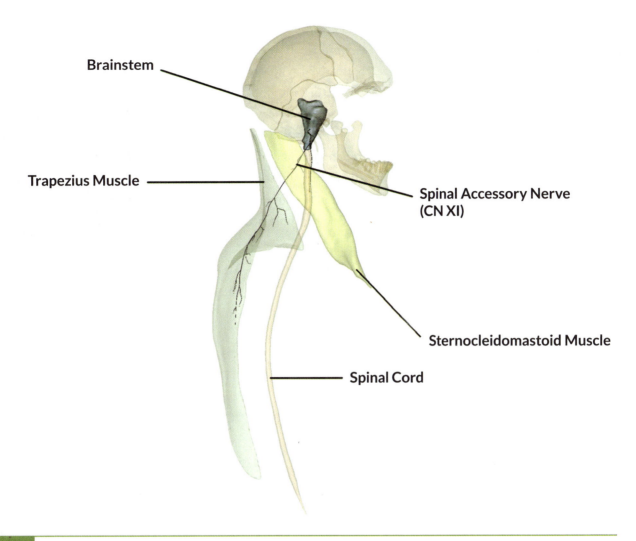

Figure 1.24 Distribution of cranial nerve XI (spinal accessory nerve). Used with permission from Anatomage.

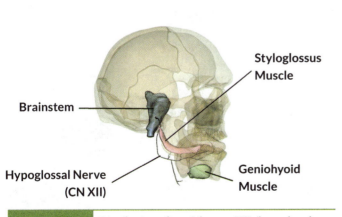

Figure 1.25a Distribution of cranial nerve XII (hypoglossal nerve), with innervation of geniohyoid and styloglossus muscles. Used with permission from Anatomage.

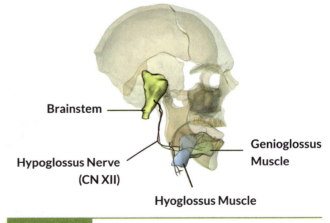

Figure 1.25b Hypoglossal innervation of hyoglossus and genioglossus muscles. Used with permission from Anatomage.

- The spinal nerves can be motor, sensory, or mixed. They transmit motor information from the CNS to the muscles and carry sensory information from peripheral receptors to the CNS.
- Not all the spinal nerves are directly involved with speech production; some nerves contribute to speech through innervation of the respiratory musculature. For example, the internal and external intercostals are innervated by the thoracic spinal nerves; the diaphragm is innervated by the motor branches of the C3–C5 spinal nerves (Peña-Brooks & Hegde, 2015).
- There are 31 pairs of spinal nerves. These nerves are attached to the spinal cord through two roots: one is efferent and ventral (toward the front), and the other is afferent and dorsal (toward the back).
- The 31 pairs of spinal nerves are divided into segments. They are named after the region of the spinal cord to which they are attached (cervical, thoracic, lumbar, sacral, and coccygeal; see Figure 1.26):

  - 8 pairs of cervical spinal nerves (C1–C8)
  - 12 pairs of thoracic spinal nerves (T1–T12)
  - 5 pairs of lumbar spinal nerves (L1–L5)
  - 5 pairs of sacral spinal nerves (S1–S5)
  - 1 pair of coccygeal spinal nerves (Co1)

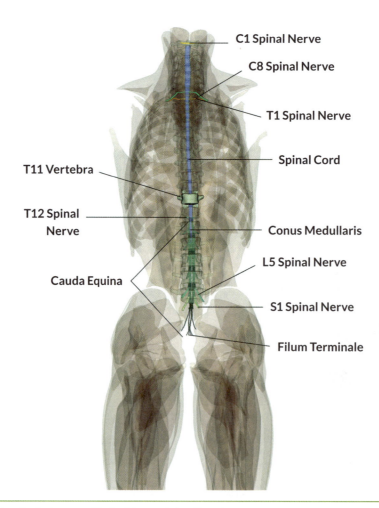

Figure 1.26 Spinal cord and spinal nerves. Used with permission from Anatomage.

- There are several other important spinal cord structures. One is the **conus medullaris**, where the spinal cord ends at the L1 vertebra level. The lowermost nerves are described as the **cauda equina** ("horse's tail"), which is above the **filum terminale** ("end filament"), where there are no spinal cord segments (Hixon et al., 2013).

Autonomic Nervous System

The **autonomic nervous system (ANS)** is generally viewed as part of the PNS. Here, it is presented separately for the sake of simplification.

- The ANS controls and regulates the internal environment of our bodies with its two branches: the sympathetic and the parasympathetic. For example, heartbeat and blood pressure are controlled by the ANS. The sympathetic and parasympathetic divisions of the ANS supply the body's smooth muscles and various glands that secrete hormones.

  - The **sympathetic branch** of the ANS mobilizes the body for "fight or flight" situations. Activation of the sympathetic branch accelerates the heart rate, dilates the pupils, raises the blood pressure, and increases blood flow to the peripheral body structures (e.g., the legs, which allow us to run from danger). Humans feel emotionally aroused when the sympathetic branch of the ANS is activated.
  - The **parasympathetic** branch of the ANS helps bring the body back to a state of relaxation. After the body has mobilized for highly charged situations, the parasympathetic branch lowers blood pressure, slows the heart rate, increases activity within the stomach, and generally relaxes the body. Humans feel relaxed and calm during activation of the parasympathetic branch of the ANS.

- The ANS does not have a direct effect upon speech, language, or hearing. However, the emotionally relaxed or aroused states created by ANS actions may have some effect on various parameters of communication.
- For example, people who stutter may become more dysfluent when the sympathetic branch is aroused. In another example, people who habitually speak too quickly and loudly, with consequent trauma to the vocal folds, might benefit from the feelings of relaxation provided from activation of the parasympathetic branch.

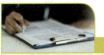

SUMMARY

The most important parts of the peripheral nervous system (PNS) in relation to communication are the cranial nerves. Cranial nerves V, VII, VIII, IX, X, XI, and XII are most directly connected with speech, language, and hearing.

- The spinal nerves of the PNS control automatic functions, such as breathing.
- The sympathetic and parasympathetic branches of the autonomic nervous system (ANS) have an indirect effect on speech when they cause speakers to feel emotionally relaxed or aroused.

THE CENTRAL NERVOUS SYSTEM

The central nervous system (CNS) is composed of the spinal cord and the brain. Key structures of the brain include the brainstem, the reticular activating system (RAS), the diencephalon, the basal ganglia, the cerebellum, and the cerebrum (Haines, 2012). Other key structures and systems include the pyramidal and extrapyramidal systems, connecting fibers within the brain, the cerebral ventricles, the protective layers of the brain, and structures that provide the cerebral blood supply. (As noted earlier, the extrapyramidal system is technically not part of the CNS but is included here because it is highly related and interconnected to CNS structures.)

Basic Principles

The brain gathers information about the environment from the PNS and then sends impulses that lead to actions. The peripheral systems and organs send and receive various kinds of information and possibly demand directions for action.

- The brain acts as a "central station" that coordinates this activity, integrates information, and issues commands.
- The CNS is composed of the brain and the spinal cord, as depicted in Figure 1.27a and b. The CNS acts as a motor command center for planning, originating, and carrying out the transmission of messages.
- The CNS is enclosed within the vertebral column and the cranial structure. The spinal cord is an elongated structure within the spinal canal of the vertebral columns.
- Pairs of spinal nerves branch out on either side of the vertebral column and reach most parts of the body. The upper portion of the spinal cord is continuous with the lower portion of the brain.
- The brain is the most important structure in the body for language, speech, and hearing. It is housed in and protected by the cranial cavity of the skull. The skull is made up of separate pieces of bone that eventually become a unified structure.
- Because the brain is so much more related to speech and language than the spinal cord, the rest of this section is devoted to a description of the structures and processes of the brain. Information about the spinal cord is integrated as necessary.

The Brainstem

The **brainstem** is said to be the oldest part of the brain. It connects the spinal cord with the brain via the diencephalon. It also serves as a bridge between the cerebellum and all other CNS structures, including the spinal cord, the thalamus, the basal ganglia, and the cerebrum. Many cranial nerves originate from the brain stem.

- Internally, the brainstem consists of **longitudinal fiber tracts**, **cranial nerve nuclei**, and the **reticular formation**. Outwardly, one sees the key structures of the brainstem—the midbrain, the pons, and the medulla—as illustrated in Figure 1.28.

Midbrain

The **midbrain**, also called the **mesencephalon**, is a narrow structure that lies superior to the pons and inferior to the diencephalon. The midbrain's **superior peduncles** help connect the brainstem and the

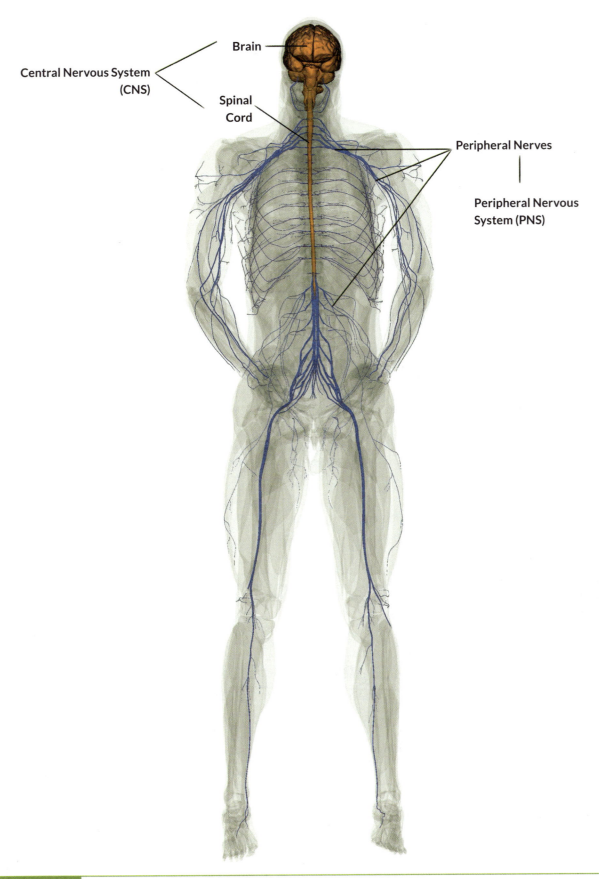

Figure 1.27a Central nervous system and peripheral nervous system. Used with permission from Anatomage.

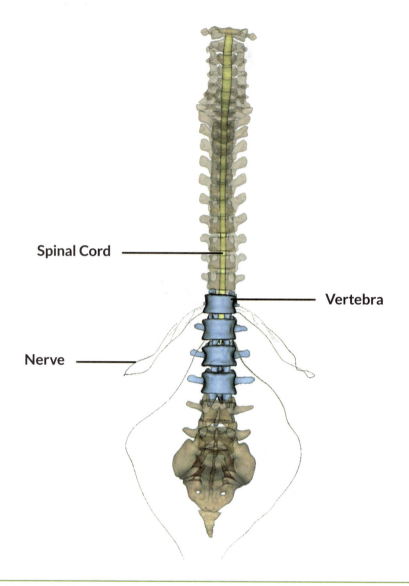

| Figure 1.27b | Spinal cord with vertebrae nerves. Used with permission from Anatomage. |

cerebellum. The **substantia nigra** (described in more detail in the "Basal Ganglia" section of this chapter) runs the vertical length of the midbrain at the level of the peduncles. Part of the brain's ventricular system, the cerebral aqueduct, runs through the midbrain.

- The midbrain's structures control many motor and sensory functions, including postural reflexes, visual reflexes, eye movements, and coordination of vestibular-generated eye and head movements.
- The midbrain contains the cranial nerve nuclei for the trochlear (IV) and oculomotor (III) nerves, neither of which is involved in speech production.

Pons

The **pons**, also called the **metencephalon**, is a roundish, bulging structure that bridges the two halves of the cerebellum. It is located directly inferior to the midbrain.

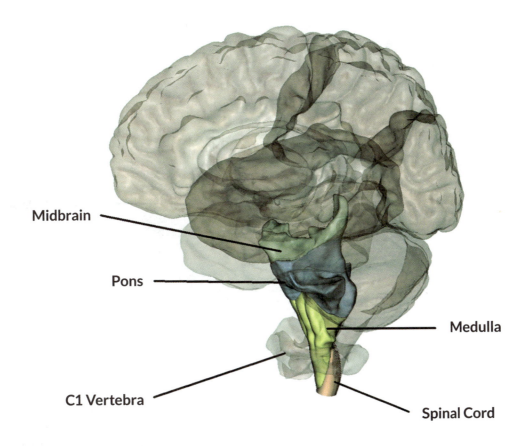

| Figure 1.28 | Brainstem. Used with permission from Anatomage. |

- The pons and the midbrain together serve as a connection point between the cerebellum and various cerebral structures through the **inferior** and **middle peduncles**. The pons transmits information relative to movement from the cerebral hemispheres to the cerebellum.
- The pons contains many descending motor fibers and is involved with hearing and balance. It also houses the nuclei for the trigeminal (V) and facial (VII) nerves, which are important for speech production.

Medulla

The **medulla**, also called the **myelencephalon**, is inferior to the midbrain and the pons. It is the uppermost portion of the spinal cord, which enters the cranial cavity through the **foramen magnum** at the base of the skull.

- The medulla contains all the fibers that originate in the cerebellum and cerebrum and move downward to form the spinal cord. It includes several centers that control vital, automatic bodily functions, such as breathing, digestion, heart rate, and blood pressure. The medulla also facilitates many reflexes, including sneezing, coughing, blinking, and vomiting (Zemlin, 1998).
- The medulla is very important for speech production because it contains descending fibers that transmit motor information to several cranial nerve nuclei.

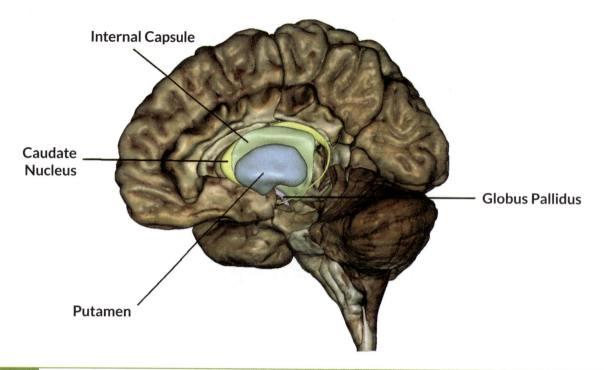

Figure 1.29 Basal ganglia and internal capsule. Used with permission from Anatomage.

- Cranial nerves whose nuclei are housed within the medulla include the vestibulocochlear (VIII), glossopharyngeal (IX), vagus (X), accessory (XI), and hypoglossal (XII) nerves.
- The medulla contains nerve fibers that carry commands from the motor center of the brain to various muscles. These fibers are called pyramidal tracts. The pyramidal tracts (described in more detail later, in the "Pyramidal System" section of this chapter) control many movements and supply some of the muscles that are involved in speech.
- At the level of the medulla, many of the pyramidal tracts from the left and right sides of the brain decussate, or cross over, to the other side. Thus, the right side of the body is primarily controlled by the left side of the brain and vice versa.

Reticular Activating System

The **reticular activating system** (RAS) is a structure within the midbrain, brainstem, and upper portion of the spinal cord. It integrates motor impulses flowing out of the brain with sensory impulses flowing into it.

- The RAS plays a role in the execution of motor activity. It sends diffuse impulses to various regions of the cortex and alerts the cortex to incoming impulses.
- The RAS is the primary mechanism of attention and consciousness; it arouses the cortex. It is important in controlling sleep–wake cycles. It plays a critical role in maintaining such states of consciousness as sleep, drowsiness, alertness, and excitement. Generally, the RAS may be viewed as the part of the CNS that responds to incoming information by affecting the state of a person's alertness and consciousness.

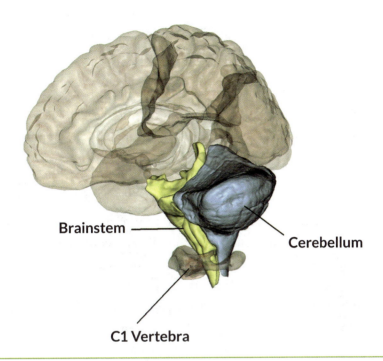

Figure 1.30 The cerebellum. Used with permission from Anatomage.

Diencephalon

The **diencephalon** lies above the midbrain and between the brainstem and the cerebral hemispheres.

- The thalamus and hypothalamus are the two main structures of the diencephalon.
- The **third ventricle**, a tall and narrow space filled with cerebrospinal fluid (CSF), is also found in the diencephalon.
- The **thalamus** is the largest structure in the diencephalon and is considered a primary sensory relay and integration center. It regulates the sensory information that flows into the brain and relays sensory impulses to various portions of the cerebral cortex.
  - The thalamus also receives information about motor impulses from the cerebellum and the basal ganglia and relays this information to motor areas of the cerebral cortex.
  - The thalamus is critical for maintenance of consciousness and alertness. The exact role of the thalamus in speech and language is unclear.
- The **hypothalamus**, which lies inferior to the thalamus, helps integrate the actions of the ANS. The hypothalamus also controls emotions.

Basal Ganglia

The **basal ganglia**, illustrated in Figure 1.29, are structures deep within the brain, near the thalamus and lateral ventricles. They are primarily composed of gray matter.

- The basal ganglia are a highly complex system of neural pathways that have connections with many subcortical and cortical areas. They receive input primarily from the frontal lobe and relay information back to the higher centers of the brain via the thalamus.

- Experts differ on the exact structure of the basal ganglia, but most agree that they consist of at least three nuclear masses: the globus pallidus, the putamen, and the caudate nucleus. **Corpus striatum** is the collective term for these structures.
- The basal ganglia are part of the **extrapyramidal system**. The extrapyramidal system helps regulate and modify cortically initiated motor movements, including speech. The **substantia nigra**, which is functionally related to (but not a part of) the basal ganglia, is an important part of the extrapyramidal system (Peña-Brooks & Hegde, 2015). Dopamine, a critical neurotransmitter, is produced in the substantia nigra and is projected to the corpus striatum. A lack of dopamine creates motor disorders, such as Parkinsonism (Zemlin, 1998).
- The extrapyramidal system, described in its own section later in this chapter, is considered an indirect activation system because motor movements are not directly controlled in the basal ganglia. The extrapyramidal system primarily affects motor movements by communicating with the cerebral cortex via other subcortical structures, such as the thalamus.
- Lesions in the basal ganglia can result in unusual body postures, dysarthria (described in Chapter 9), changes in body tone, and involuntary and uncontrolled movements (dyskinesias) that interfere with a person's voluntary attempts to walk, speak, or do many other activities (Hegde & Freed, 2017).

The Cerebellum

The cerebellum, illustrated in Figure 1.30, lies just below the cerebrum and behind the brainstem. Also called the "little brain," the cerebellum consists of two hemispheres (which are different from the cerebral hemispheres) separated by the **vermis.**

- Three primary fiber bundles serve as connections between the brainstem and the cerebellum. These are the **superior**, **middle**, and **inferior cerebellar peduncles**, which connect with the midbrain, the pons, and the medulla, respectively. All efferent and afferent fibers going to and from the cerebellum pass through these peduncles.

  - Afferent fibers travel through the inferior and middle cerebellar peduncles. These fibers mediate almost all sensorimotor information to the cerebellum.
  - Efferent fibers travel through the superior cerebellar peduncle. These fibers transmit information from the cerebellum to the brainstem; from there, the information is transmitted to the thalamus, motor cortex, and spinal cord.

- The cerebellum is not a primary motor integration or initiation center. It receives neural impulses from other brain centers and helps coordinate and regulate those impulses. Therefore, it acts as a "modulator" of neuronal activity through its efferent and afferent circuits. The cerebellum can be considered the error control device of the brain because it constantly fine-tunes movements by comparing the action to the intended movement and makes adjustments as necessary. **Purkinje cells**, large neurons found in the cerebellum, release gamma-aminobutyric acid (GABA), an inhibitory neurotransmitter, and therefore are crucial in the regulation and coordination of motor movements (Rogers, 2009). Purkinje cells are also the only output cells of the cerebellum (Purves et al., 2001).

- The cerebellum regulates equilibrium (balance), body posture, and coordinated fine motor movements. Because these movements are necessary for rapid speech, cerebellar intactness is very important to speech production.
- Damage to the cerebellum results in a neurological disorder called **ataxia**, found in some people with cerebral palsy and in people who have suffered cerebellar damage. These individuals are likely to show abnormal gait, disturbed balance, and a speech disorder called **ataxic dysarthria** (described in Chapter 9). Damage to the cerebellum also creates other communicative disorders, as described in Chapter 9.

The Cerebrum

Basic Facts

The **cerebrum**, or **cerebral cortex** (the terms are used interchangeably here), is the biggest and most important CNS structure for language, speech, and hearing. It is a complex structure of intricate neural connections that contains approximately 10–15 billion neurons and weighs about 3 pounds.

- The brain is often referred to as "gray matter" because the cerebrum has gray cells on top. This differs from the spinal cord and the brainstem, which have gray cells inside.
- The cortex includes the topmost portion of the brain but is actually arranged in six layers. Each layer consists of a different type of cell.
- The surface of the cerebrum appears wrinkled, because it is folded to accommodate as much tissue as possible in a small space. Billions of neural cells are packed into this structure and folded into ridges and valleys.
- A **gyrus** is a ridge on the cortex, and the cortex has many gyri (plural). A shallow valley is a **sulcus**, and there are many sulci on the surface of the brain. Deeper valleys are called **fissures**; there are fewer fissures than sulci. The fissures are the boundaries between the broad divisions of the cerebrum.
- The **longitudinal fissure** courses along the middle of the brain from front to back and divides the cerebrum into the left and right hemispheres; this fissure is deep and extends down to the corpus callosum. The **fissure of Rolando**, or **central sulcus**, is a major fissure that runs laterally, downward, and forward, and arbitrarily divides the anterior from the posterior half of the brain.
- The **Sylvian fissure**, or **lateral cerebral fissure** (sulcus), starts at the inferior portion of the frontal lobe at the base of the brain and moves laterally and upward. The areas of the brain surrounding the Sylvian fissure are especially critical in language, speech, and hearing.
- There are four lobes in the right hemisphere and four lobes in the left hemisphere of the cerebrum. The names of these lobes—the frontal, parietal, occipital, and temporal—are based on the cranial bones with which they are in contact. The four lobes each have their own function, but they are interconnected. The lobes are illustrated in Figure 1.31.

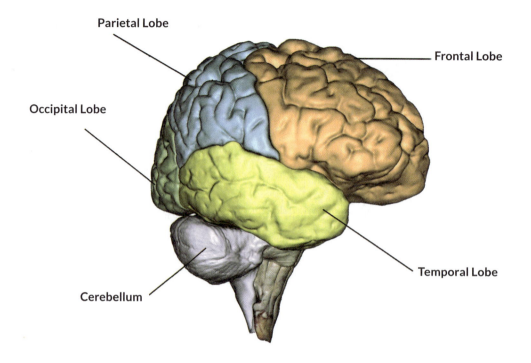

Figure 1.31 The lobes of the cerebral cortex. Used with permission from Anatomage.

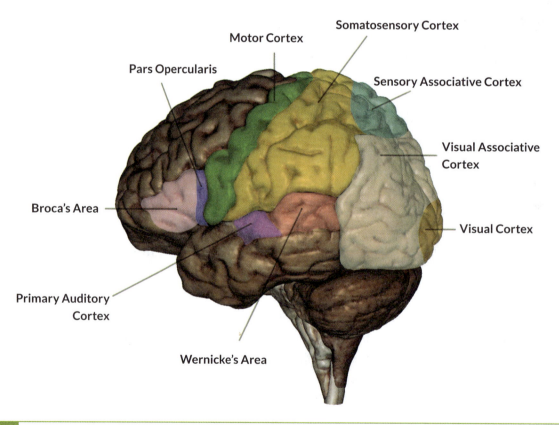

Figure 1.32 The major speech, language, and hearing areas of the brain. Used with permission from Anatomage.

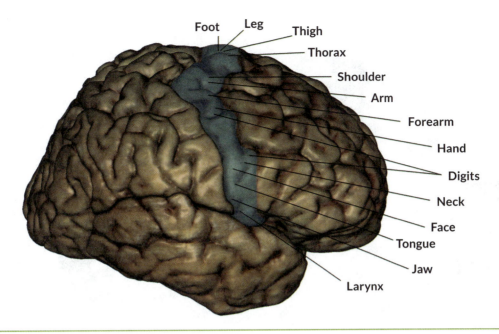

Figure 1.33 The right hemisphere showing regions of the motor cortex that govern motor activation of specific body regions. Used with permission from Anatomage.

Frontal Lobe

The frontal lobe is located on the anterior portion of the cerebrum in front of the central fissure and above the lateral fissure. It makes up approximately one-third of the surface area of the cerebrum.

- Intact frontal lobe functioning is critical to the deliberate formation of plans and intentions that dictate a person's conscious behavior. Therefore, people with damage to the frontal lobe have difficulty carrying out consciously organized activity (Bhatnagar, 2012).
- The frontal lobe contains areas that are especially critical to speech production. These include the primary motor cortex, a supplementary motor cortex, and Broca's area. The major areas pertinent to speech, language, and hearing are illustrated in Figure 1.32.
- The **primary motor cortex**, or **motor strip**, is located on the **precentral gyrus**, a large ridge that lies anterior to the central sulcus. This area controls voluntary movements of skeletal muscles on the opposite side of the body. This demonstrates the neurological principle of **contralateral motor control**, which means that each cerebral hemisphere controls the opposite side of the body.
- All muscles of the body, including those for speech production, are connected to the primary motor cortex through descending motor nerve cells. Figure 1.33 shows regions of the motor cortex that govern motor activation of specific body regions.
- When specific areas of the primary motor cortex are stimulated, corresponding motor responses (e.g., movement of the hand or lip) occur. A large area represents the larynx, jaw, tongue, and lips; this suggests the importance of cortical control of speech-related structures.
- The motor strip controls muscle movements through a neural pathway called the pyramidal system, mentioned earlier in this chapter. The motor impulses are modified by the extrapyramidal system, with its indirect and complex relay stations (Hegde, 2018).

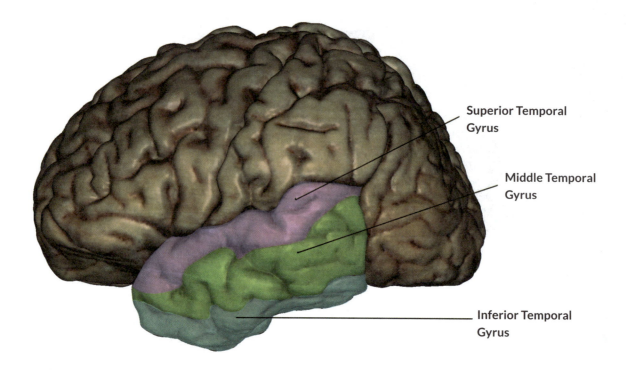

Figure 1.34 The temporal lobe. Used with permission from Anatomage.

- The **supplementary motor cortex** of the frontal lobe is believed to be involved in the motor planning of speech. It also plays a secondary role in regulating muscle movements.
- An important motor speech center is **Broca's area**, which is named after the 19th-century French anthropologist and neurosurgeon Paul Broca, who "discovered" it during a brain autopsy of a patient with aphasia.

  - Broca's area, known as the left inferior frontal gyrus, is located in the third convolution of the left cerebral hemisphere. It is anterior to the portion of the primary motor cortex that controls lip, tongue, jaw, and laryngeal movements.
  - Broca's area is also called the motor speech area because it controls motor movements involved in speech production. An intact Broca's area is important for production of well-articulated, fluent speech. Lesions in Broca's area cause motor speech problems, which are further described in Chapter 9.

Parietal Lobe

The parietal lobe is located on the upper sides of the cerebrum behind the frontal lobe and is the primary somatic sensory area. It integrates contralateral **somatic** sensations, such as pressure, pain, temperature, and touch. The parietal lobe also integrates information with other areas, predominantly with vision.

- The postcentral gyrus, also called the sensory cortex or sensory strip, lies just behind the central sulcus. It is the primary sensory area that integrates and controls somatic sensory impulses.

- Two specific areas of the parietal lobe are important for speech and language. These are the areas including and surrounding the supramarginal gyrus and the angular gyrus.

  - The **supramarginal gyrus** lies superior to the lateral fissure in the inferior portion of the parietal lobe. Its posterior portion curves around the lateral fissure. Damage to the supramarginal gyrus can cause conduction aphasia (described in Chapter 8) and agraphia, a writing disorder.
  - The **angular gyrus** lies posterior to the supramarginal gyrus. Damage to this area can cause writing, reading, and naming difficulties and, in some cases, transcortical sensory aphasia (described in Chapter 8).

Occipital Lobe

The occipital lobe lies behind the parietal lobe at the lower posterior portion of the head, just above the cerebellum. It is not very relevant to speech and hearing because it is primarily concerned with receiving and processing visual information.

- The major structure of the occipital lobe is the **primary visual cortex**. The remainder of the occipital lobe is composed of association visual cortices.

Temporal Lobe

The temporal lobe is the lowest one-third of the cerebrum (see Figure 1.34). It lies inferior to the frontal and parietal lobes and in front of the occipital lobe. There are three major gyri in the temporal lobe: the **superior (upper) temporal gyrus, the middle temporal gyrus,** and the **inferior (lower) temporal gyrus** (Bhatnagar, 2012).

- The temporal lobe contains two general areas that are critical to adequate hearing and speech. The first critical area, the primary auditory cortex, is located on the superior temporal gyrus.
- The second critical area, the auditory association area, lies posterior to the **primary auditory cortex. Heschl's gyri** is a term sometimes used in reference to the transverse convolutions that make up the **auditory association cortex** and the primary auditory cortex.
- The primary auditory cortex receives sound stimuli from the acoustic nerve (cranial nerve VIII) bilaterally. The auditory association area then synthesizes that information so that it can be recognized as whole units.
- In the dominant hemisphere (left hemisphere, for most people), the auditory association area generally analyzes speech sounds so that the person recognizes words and sentences. In the nondominant hemisphere (right hemisphere, for most people), the auditory association area generally analyzes nonverbal sound stimuli, such as environmental noises, music, and prosody (e.g., stress, rate, melody).

  - An important area within the left temporal lobe is **Wernicke's area**, named for Carl Wernicke, a famous German neuropsychiatrist of the late 19th and early 20th centuries. Wernicke's area is the posterior two-thirds of the superior temporal gyrus in the left hemisphere. It is close to the intersection of the parietal, occipital, and temporal lobes.

- Wernicke's area is critical to the comprehension of spoken and written language. It is connected to Broca's area through the arcuate fasciculus (described in the "Connecting Fibers in the Brain" section of this chapter).
- A lesion in the posterior portion of the left superior temporal gyrus causes **Wernicke's aphasia** (described in Chapter 8), in which the patient produces fluent but meaningless speech and experiences significant language comprehension problems.

■ The hippocampus is also located in the temporal lobe; this structure is responsible for recalling information and storing long-term memories. Lesions to the hippocampus can result in **anterograde** amnesia (the inability to create new memories) or **retrograde** amnesia (the inability to remember memories prior to the lesion).

Pyramidal System

Basic Facts

The **pyramidal system**, as previously stated, is the direct motor activation pathway that is primarily responsible for facilitating voluntary muscle movement (including speech).

■ The nerve fiber tract of the pyramidal system comes from the cerebral cortex to the spinal cord and brainstem to ultimately supply the muscles of the head, neck, and limbs. Voluntary movements needed to produce speech are initiated in the primary motor cortex.

■ The pyramidal system is composed of the corticobulbar and the corticospinal tracts. Because tracts are bundles of nerve fibers coursing through the CNS, one can imagine the pyramidal system and its two tracts as a group of myelinated nerve fibers carrying crucial neural impulses (Peña-Brooks & Hegde, 2015).

■ The corticospinal tracts terminate in the spinal cord, while the corticobulbar tracts terminate in the brainstem. The projection fibers of both the corticospinal and the corticobulbar tracts originate in the cerebral cortex, and the tracts are part of one unified system. However, these tracts are often discussed separately, if somewhat artificially, for purposes of simplification.

Corticospinal Tract

The **corticospinal tract** (see Figure 1.35) has nerve fibers that descend from the motor cortex of each hemisphere through the internal capsule. These fibers continue to course vertically through the midbrain and the pons. At the level of the medulla, approximately 80–85% of the fibers decussate.

■ The decussated fibers of the corticospinal tract synapse in the anterior horn (motor gray matter) of the spinal cord and communicate with the spinal nerves at different levels. Finally, the spinal nerves exit through the **vertebrae foramina** along the spinal column to innervate the muscles of the limbs and trunk.

■ Because of the decussation of fibers at the medullary level, the right side of the body is generally controlled by nerve fibers that originate in the left cerebral cortex, and vice versa. Left-hemisphere strokes, for example, result in weakness on the right side of the body.

Corticobulbar Tract

The **corticobulbar tract** is critical to speech production. The fibers of this tract control all the voluntary movements of the speech muscles (except the respiratory muscles).

- The corticobulbar tract originates primarily in the motor cortex. The fibers of this tract course downward vertically through the internal capsule and run along with the corticospinal tract fibers.
- The corticobulbar tract fibers terminate in the brainstem at the motor nuclei of cranial nerves III–XII (see Figure 1.36). These fibers then decussate at the level of the brainstem, where they terminate. For example, the fibers that terminate at the motor nuclei of the trigeminal nerve decussate in the pons. The fibers that terminate at the motor nuclei of the facial nerve decussate in the medulla (Peña-Brooks & Hegde, 2015).
- The cranial nerves involved in speech exit the skull via small foramina and innervate the muscles of the larynx, pharynx, soft palate, tongue, face, and lips. This innervation allows the muscles to function for production of speech.
- For practical clinical purposes, the corticospinal and corticobulbar tracts are further subdivided into lower and upper motor neurons. This division is clinically helpful in classifying the symptoms associated with lower versus upper motor neuron damage.
- **Lower motor neurons** are the motor neurons (efferent nerves) in the spinal and cranial nerves. They include nerve fibers that exit the neuraxis (spinal cord or brain) and communicate with the peripheral (cranial and spinal) nerves for innervation of muscles.

  - Lower motor neurons are part of the PNS and as such are the final route by which centrally mediated neural impulses are communicated to peripheral muscles. Lower motor neuron activity eventually results in muscular movement.

- **Upper motor neurons** are the motor fibers (efferent nerves) within the CNS. Upper motor neurons can be thought of as all the descending motor fibers that course through the CNS. As such, upper motor neurons include the pathways of both the pyramidal and the extrapyramidal systems.

Extrapyramidal System

A general distinction between the pyramidal and the extrapyramidal systems is that the pyramidal system is responsible for carrying the impulses that control voluntary fine motor movements. The extrapyramidal system transmits impulses that control the postural support needed by those fine motor movements (Hegde & Freed, 2017).

- The **extrapyramidal system** ("extra" referring to the motor tracts that are not part of the pyramidal system) is important in speech production. It is composed of different subcortical nuclei, including the red nucleus, the substantia nigra, the subthalamus, the basal ganglia, and the pathways that connect these structures to one another.
- Whereas the pyramidal system has a direct connection with lower motor neurons, the extrapyramidal system is considered a more indirect activation system that interacts with various motor systems in the nervous system.

(text continues on page 60)

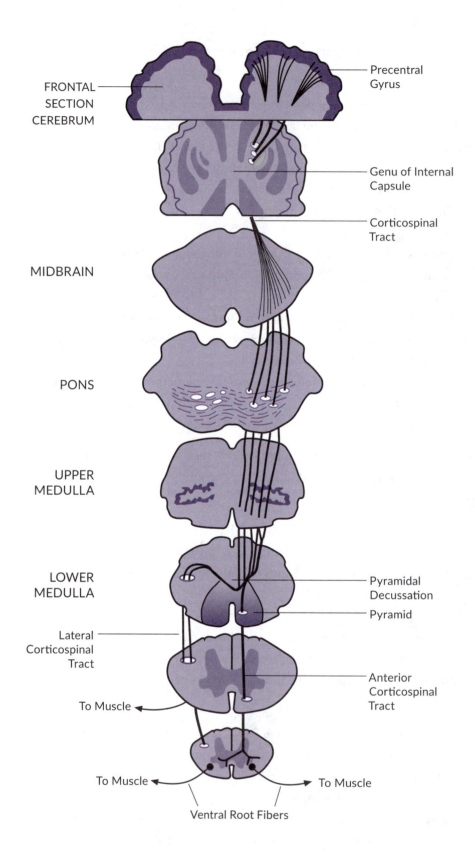

Figure 1.35 The corticospinal pathway as traced from the cerebral cortex to the spinal cord.

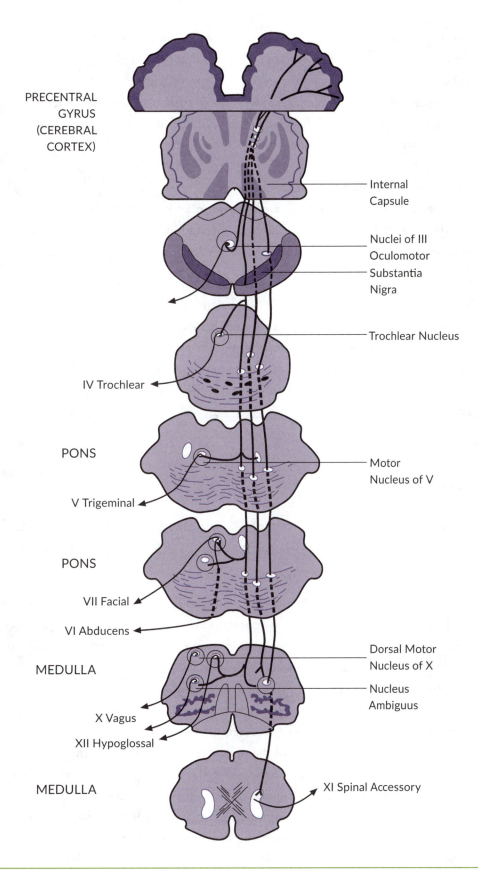

Figure 1.36 The corticobulbar tract as traced from the cerebral cortex to the cranial nerve nuclei.

- The neuronal activity of the extrapyramidal system begins in the cerebral cortex and ultimately influences lower motor neurons. The extrapyramidal system helps maintain posture and tone and helps regulate the movement that results from lower motor neuron activity.
- Damage to the extrapyramidal system creates motor disturbances that fall under the rubric of "involuntary movement disorders." Patients may show unusual movement patterns of various muscles (including facial muscles) and bizarre postures (Duffy, 2013).

Connecting Fibers in the Brain

The structures of the brain are connected with one another through specialized bundles of nerve fibers. These connecting fibers keep information flowing throughout the brain. This alerts various brain structures about sensory stimuli that have been received and actions that are planned and performed.

- Connecting fibers differ in length. Adjacent areas are connected by shorter fibers; distant areas are connected by longer fibers called **fasciculi** (singular **fasciculus**).
- **Intrahemispheric fibers** allow areas within each hemisphere to communicate with each other. **Interhemispheric fibers** permit communication between hemispheres and are composed mostly of myelinated axonal fibers, or white matter. Interhemispheric fibers form the medullary center of the brain. Depending upon the nature of their connections, the nerve fibers of the medullary center are divided into three types:

  - Projection fibers
  - Association fibers
  - Commissural fibers

Projection Fibers

Projection fibers create connections between the cortex and subcortical structures like the cerebellum, basal ganglia, brainstem, and spinal cord.

- Some fibers transmit motor information to the glands and muscles. Other fibers carry sensory information to the brain. The **internal capsule** contains the concentrated and compact projection fibers near the brainstem. The internal capsule transmits motor and sensory information to and from the cerebral cortex and between the basal ganglia and thalamus.
- The motor projection fibers originate primarily in the premotor and primary motor areas in the frontal lobe. They form the upper motor neuron system of the pyramidal tract, which is the direct activation pathway for voluntary motor movements.
- As projection fibers move upward toward the upper regions of the brain, they fan out in a structure called the corona radiata. Through the **corona radiata**, information is transmitted to other portions of the brain. The corona radiata consists of both afferent and efferent fibers.
- Afferent projection fibers relay sensory information (such as smell) from the peripheral sense organs (e.g., the nose) to the brain. Efferent projection fibers come together in the internal capsule and pass through the thalamus and basal ganglia. These efferent fibers relay motor commands to glands and muscles.

Association Fibers

Association fibers may be long or short; whatever their length, they connect areas within the same hemisphere. Association fibers assist in maintaining communication between the structures in a hemisphere.

- The most important of the association fibers is the bundle of **superior longitudinal fibers**, also called the **arcuate fasciculus**, that lies just below the surface of the cortex. The arcuate fasciculus arches backward from the lower part of the frontal lobe to the posterior superior part of the temporal lobe.
- The arcuate fasciculus connects Broca's area with Wernicke's area. It is important for verbal memory, language acquisition, meaningful language production, and repetition. Damage to this structure can cause conduction aphasia; in this form of aphasia, there are little to no receptive and expressive language deficits, but the individual is unable to repeat language presented auditorily (Seikel et al., 2016).

Commissural Fibers

The left and right hemispheres are divided by the medial longitudinal fissure. The **commissural fibers** are interhemispheric connectors; they run horizontally and connect the corresponding areas of the two hemispheres.

- The most important of the commissural fibers, the **corpus callosum**, is a thick, broad band of myelinated fibers that connects the two hemispheres at their base (see Figure 1.37):
- Damage to the corpus callosum disconnects the two hemispheres, resulting in **disconnection syndromes** characterized by problems in naming, reading, movement, and other functions.

The Cerebral Ventricles

The term **cerebral ventricles** refers to a system of cavities deep within the brain. These interconnected cavities are filled with CSF.

- This fluid is produced by the **choroid plexus**, which is composed of vascular membranous materials. The CSF circulates throughout the nervous system and nourishes the neural tissues, removes waste products, cushions the brain, and regulates intracranial pressure (Hegde, 2018).
- There are four cerebral ventricles:

  - The largest of the four ventricles are the two **lateral ventricles** (one in each hemisphere). Located immediately inferior to the corpus callosum, the lateral ventricles are C-shaped and course through the lobes of the cortex. The choroid plexuses of the two lateral ventricles produce the majority of the CSF.
  - The **third ventricle** is behind the lateral ventricles at the top of the brainstem. It looks like a broad disk and is connected with the lateral ventricles by the foramen of Munro.
  - The **fourth ventricle** is located between the cerebellum and the pons and is continuous with the central canal of the spinal cord below and the cerebral aqueduct above. The **cerebral aqueduct** connects the fourth and the third ventricles.

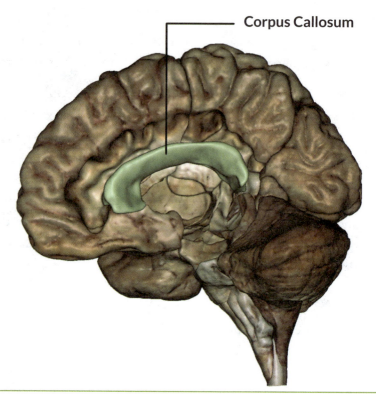

Figure 1.37 The corpus callosum. Used with permission from Anatomage.

Protective Layers of the Brain

The spinal cord of the CNS is protected by the vertebral column. The brain is protected by three structures: a layer of skin, the skull bones, and layers of tissue called the meninges.

- The **meninges** contain three layers of membranes (protective tissue) that cover the brain and spinal cord (see Figure 1.38):

  - The **dura mater** ("tough mother") is the thick, tough, outermost membrane, one side of which adheres to the skull and the other side of which adheres to the arachnoid.
  - The **arachnoid** ("spider web") is the semitransparent, thin, delicate, web-like, and vascular middle membrane; CSF fills the subarachnoid space between the arachnoid and the pia mater.
  - The **pia mater** ("tender mother") is the delicate, thin, transparent membrane that adheres to the brain surface and closely follows its gyri and sulci; many blood vessels penetrate the pia mater to enter the brain.

Cerebral Blood Supply

The brain makes up approximately 2% of the body's weight; however, it consumes 25% of the body's oxygen and requires 20% of the body's blood.

- The wonderfully complex and intricate brain is a highly vulnerable structure. If its blood supply is interrupted, consciousness may be lost within 10 seconds, electrical activity ceases after 20 seconds, and the brain is permanently damaged within 4–6 minutes.

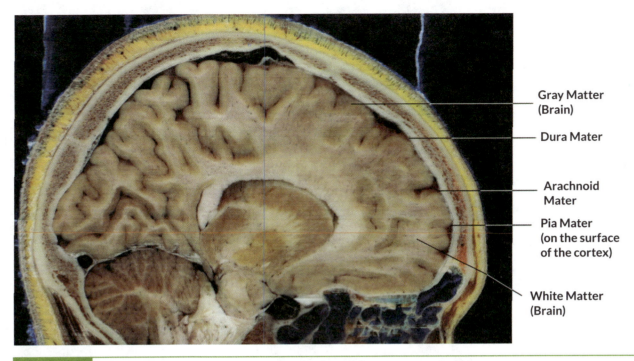

Figure 1.38 The relationship of the meninges to the brain and skull. Used with permission from Anatomage.

- The blood supplies oxygen and other nutrients to the brain. The major structures that supply blood to the brain are the aorta, the vertebral arteries, the carotid arteries, and the circle of Willis.

Aorta

The **aorta** is the main artery of the heart. It carries blood from the left ventricle to all parts of the body except the lungs.

- Just above the heart, the aortic arch divides into four branches. These branches are the two carotid arteries and the two subclavian arteries. Figures 1.39a, b, and c illustrate the major vascular supply of the cerebral cortex.

Vertebral Arteries

The right and left **vertebral arteries** branch out from the two subclavian arteries that emerge from the aortic arch. The subclavian arteries supply primarily the upper extremities.

- The vertebral arteries enter the skull and then branch out to supply the spinal cord and many organs of the body. As they move up to the lower level of the pons, the two vertebral arteries join to form the **basilar artery**.
- As the basilar artery moves toward the upper portion of the pons, it divides again into two **posterior cerebral arteries**. These arteries supply the lateral and lower portions of the temporal lobes and the lateral and middle portions of the occipital lobes.
- Several other branches of the basilar artery, such as the anterior, posterior, superior, and inferior cerebellar arteries, supply other structures, such as the inner ear, cerebellum, and pons.

Medial View

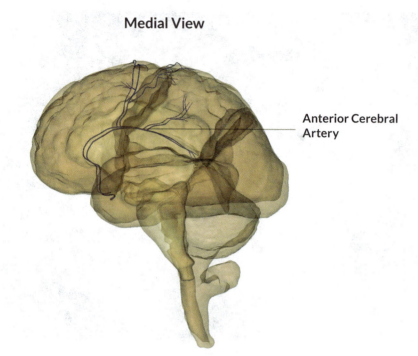

Figure 1.39a Anterior cerebral artery. Used with permission from Anatomage.

Lateral View

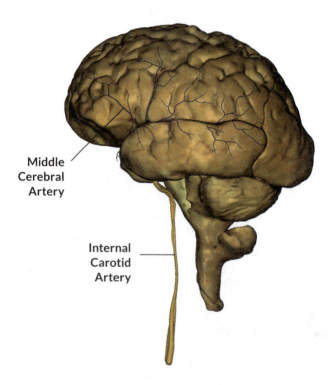

Figure 1.39b Middle cerebral artery and internal carotid artery. Used with permission from Anatomage.

Anatomy, Neuroanatomy, and Physiology 65

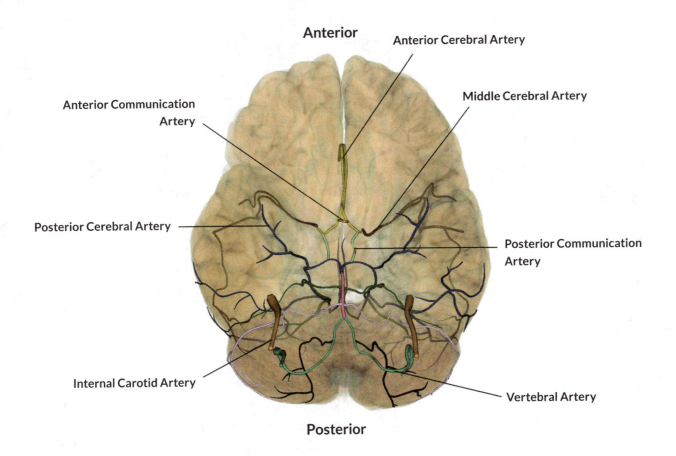

| Figure 1.39c | The major vascular supply of the cerebral cortex. Used with permission from Anatomage. |

Carotid Arteries

As the left and right **carotid arteries** (one on each side of the neck) enter the neck, each branches out into an internal carotid artery and an external carotid artery. The arteries enter the brain through the base of the skull and go through the dura mater and subarachnoid space.

- The **external carotid artery** moves toward the face and branches into smaller arteries. It supplies blood to the muscles of the mouth, nose, forehead, and face.
- The **internal carotid artery** is the major supplier of blood to the brain. This artery branches into several smaller blood vessels that supply different parts of the brain. Two key branches of the internal carotid artery are the middle cerebral artery and the anterior cerebral artery.
- The **middle cerebral artery** is the biggest branch of the internal carotid artery, and it supplies the entire lateral surface of the cortex, including the major regions of the frontal lobe.
  - The middle cerebral artery supplies blood to major areas involved with motor and sensory functions and language, speech, and hearing functions.

- The areas supplied by the middle cerebral artery include the motor cortex in the precentral gyrus, Broca's area, the primary auditory cortex, Wernicke's area, the supramarginal gyrus, the angular gyrus, and the somatosensory cortex.
  - Damage to the middle cerebral artery may result in strokes, causing aphasia, reading and writing deficits, contralateral hemiplegia, and an impaired sense of pain, temperature, touch, and position.

- The **anterior cerebral artery** supplies primarily the middle portion of the parietal and frontal lobes. It also supplies blood to the corpus callosum and basal ganglia. Branches of the anterior cerebral artery join with the posterior cerebral artery in the posterior medial areas of the brain.
  - Damage to the anterior cerebral artery can cause cognitive deficits, such as impaired judgment, concentration, and reasoning. Damage can also cause paralysis of the feet and legs.

Circle of Willis

The **circle of Willis** (**circulus arteriosus**), a sequence of anastomoses (connections between arteries), is formed at the base of the brain where the two carotid and the two vertebral arteries join. Shown in Figures 1.39a, b, and c, the circle is completed by the anterior and posterior communicating arteries. The posterior cerebral, anterior cerebral, and middle cerebral arteries branch out from the circle of Willis.

- The circle of Willis provides a common blood supply to various cerebral branches. If an artery is blocked above the circle, brain damage will occur because the brain has no alternate source of blood. If an artery is blocked below the circle of Willis, however, brain damage may be minimal because alternate channels of blood flow may be maintained to compensate for the lack of blood flow.

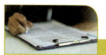

SUMMARY

The central nervous system, composed of the brain and the spinal cord, is a complex and intricate system that depends upon the intact functioning of and interconnections between many structures.

- These structures include the brainstem, the reticular activating system, the diencephalon, the basal ganglia, the cerebellum, and the cerebrum with its frontal, parietal, occipital, and temporal lobes.
- The pyramidal and extrapyramidal systems are concerned with movement. Projection, association, and commissural fibers connect key brain structures.
- Other critical components of the brain include the cerebral ventricles, meninges, and various arteries that supply blood to the brain and its structures.

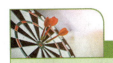

CHAPTER HIGHLIGHTS

- Respiration, or breathing, consists of a rhythmic cycle of inhalation and exhalation. Respiration provides the energy for voicing and ultimately for speech. The process of respiration relies upon the integrity of many structures. These include the lungs, bronchi, trachea, spinal column, sternum, rib cage, and muscles of inspiration and expiration.
- Voice is usually produced as exhaled air comes from the lungs through the trachea to the larynx. The larynx houses the vocal folds, which vibrate to produce voice. Optimal voicing relies upon key laryngeal cartilages and structures as well as the functioning of the intrinsic and extrinsic laryngeal muscles. The myoelastic–aerodynamic theory helps explain the physiology of phonation. Cranial nerves VII (facial nerve) and X (vagus nerve) are important in the phonation process.
- The vocal folds vibrate to produce voice, and the vocal sound travels upward to be modified or resonated by the pharynx and the oral and nasal cavities. English sounds have primarily oral or nasal resonance. The source-filter theory explains how speech sounds are ultimately produced through modification of the oral cavity and adjacent structures.
- Articulation for speech involves movements that produce particular sounds. Key structures for articulation in the oral cavity include the pharynx, soft palate, hard palate, mandible, teeth, tongue, lips, and cheeks. Cranial nerves primarily responsible for innervation of articulatory structures include V (trigeminal nerve), VII (facial nerve), IX (glossopharyngeal nerve), X (vagus nerve), XI (spinal accessory nerve), and XII (hypoglossal nerve).
- The nervous system, composed of neurons and other specialized cells, can be divided into two basic parts: the peripheral and central nervous systems. The peripheral nervous system (PNS) is composed of the spinal nerves and the cranial nerves. Cranial nerves most critical to speech, language, and hearing include the trigeminal nerve (V), facial nerve (VII), vestibulocochlear nerve (VIII), glossopharyngeal nerve (IX), vagus nerve (X), spinal accessory nerve (XI), and hypoglossal nerve (XII).
- The central nervous system (CNS) is composed of the brain and the spinal cord. The brain contains many structures, including the brainstem, reticular activating system (RAS), diencephalon, basal ganglia, cerebellum, and cerebrum. The brainstem, composed of the midbrain, pons, and medulla, connects the spinal cord with the brain via the diencephalon.
- The cerebellum helps coordinate and regulate neural impulses going to and from the brain. It regulates equilibrium, body posture, and coordinated fine motor movements. An intact cerebellum is critical to speech production, and people with cerebellar damage may show ataxia and dysarthria.
- The cerebrum, or cerebral cortex, has four lobes: the occipital, frontal, parietal, and temporal lobes. The occipital lobe is primarily concerned with vision. The frontal lobe contains motor

areas, such as Broca's area, that are critical to speech production. The parietal lobe, which integrates sensations such as pain, temperature, and touch, contains the angular gyrus and the supramarginal gyrus, which are critical to speech. The temporal lobe contains the key structures of the primary auditory cortex, the auditory association area, and Wernicke's area.

- The pyramidal and extrapyramidal systems are involved in motor movement. The pyramidal system, consisting of the corticospinal and corticobulbar tracts, is primarily responsible for facilitating voluntary movements of muscles, including speech muscles. The extrapyramidal system is a more indirect activation system, which helps maintain posture and tone as well as regulating movement.

- Important connecting fibers in the brain include projection fibers, association fibers, and commissural fibers. The corpus callosum, a critical commissural fiber, connects the two hemispheres. Other important brain structures include the cerebral ventricles, meninges, and structures that supply blood to the brain.

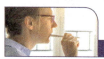

STUDY AND REVIEW QUESTIONS

1. Respiration relies on the muscles of inspiration and expiration. The thick, dome-shaped muscle that separates the abdomen from the thorax is called the

    A. sternocleidomastoid.
    B. levator costarum longis.
    C. pectoralis major.
    D. diaphragm.

2. Which branch of the vagus nerve (cranial nerve X) innervates the cricothyroid muscle?

    A. Superior laryngeal nerve
    B. Lateral laryngeal nerve
    C. Recurrent laryngeal nerve
    D. Pharyngeal branch

3. The primary muscle of the lips is the

    A. orbicularis oris.
    B. buccinator.
    C. risorius.
    D. levator labii superioris.

4. The neurons that transmit information away from the brain are called

    A. afferent neurons.
    B. efferent neurons.
    C. primary neurons.
    D. peripheral neurons.

5. An important structure adjacent to the brainstem that contains the hypothalamus (which controls emotions) and the thalamus (which relays sensory impulses to various portions of the cerebral cortex) is called the

    A. mesencephalon.
    B. diencephalon.
    C. superior cerebellar peduncle.
    D. postcentral gyrus.

6. The corpus striatum is composed of three nuclear masses, which are the

   A. globus pallidus, caudate nucleus, and putamen. ✓

   B. putamen, caudate nucleus, and basal ganglia.

   C. supramarginal gyrus, angular gyrus, and putamen.

   D. substantia nigra, angular gyrus, and globus pallidus.

7. The structure that regulates body posture, equilibrium, and coordinated fine motor movements is the

   A. angular gyrus.

   B. corticospinal tract.

   C. circle of Willis.

   D. cerebellum. ✓

8. The anterior cerebral artery supplies blood to the

   A. corpus callosum and basal ganglia. ✓

   B. corpus striatum.

   C. caudate nucleus and globus pallidus.

   D. lateral surface of the cortex.

9. The laryngopharynx and the oropharynx add resonance to sounds produced by the larynx. The nasopharynx adds noticeable resonance to which sounds?

   A. k, g, t, d

   B. r, l, y

   C. f, sh, s

   D. m, n, ng ✓

10. These are composed of a ring of connective tissue and muscle extending from the tips of the arytenoid cartilages to the epiglottis. They separate the laryngeal vestibule from the pharynx and help preserve the airway.

    A. Ventricular folds

    B. True vocal folds

    C. Lamina propria

    D. Aryepiglottic folds ✓

11. The cranial nerve that innervates the larynx and also innervates the levator veli palatini, palatoglossus, and palatopharyngeus muscles is

    A. cranial nerve X, the vagus nerve. ✓

    B. cranial nerve V, the trigeminal nerve.

    C. cranial nerve XI, the spinal accessory nerve.

    D. cranial nerve VII, the facial nerve.

12. Muscles that contribute to velopharyngeal closure through tensing or elevating the velum are the

    A. tensor veli palatini, levator veli palatini, and salpingopharyngeus.

    B. stylopharyngeus, salpingopharyngeus, and levator veli palatini.

    C. levator veli palatini, genioglossus, and salpingopharyngeus.

    D. palatoglossus, tensor veli palatini, and levator veli palatini. ✓

13. The structure at the inferior portion of the tongue that connects the tongue with the mandible is called the

    A. dorsum.

    B. root.

    C. blade.

    D. lingual frenum. ✓

14. When a person is producing voiced and voiceless /th/, the muscle that is most involved is the

A. palatopharyngeus.
B. sternocleidomastoid.
C. genioglossus. *(circled)*
D. styloglossus.

15. Which muscles from the list below are the most involved in adducting the vocal folds?

A. Lateral cricoarytenoids and transverse arytenoid *(circled)*
B. Digastrics
C. Cricothyroids
D. Posterior cricoarytenoids

References and Recommended Readings at www.advancedreviewpractice.com

STUDY AND REVIEW ANSWERS

1. D. The thick, dome-shaped muscle that separates the abdomen from the thorax is called the *diaphragm*.
2. A. The external branch of the superior laryngeal nerve innervates the cricothyroid muscle.
3. A. The primary muscle of the lips is the orbicularis oris.
4. B. The type of neurons that transmit information away from the brain are called *efferent neurons*.
5. B. An important structure adjacent to the brainstem that contains the hypothalamus (which controls emotions) and the thalamus (which relays sensory impulses to various portions of the cerebral cortex) is called the *diencephalon*.
6. A. The corpus striatum is composed of three nuclear masses, which are the globus pallidus, caudate nucleus, and putamen.
7. D. The structure that regulates body posture, equilibrium, and coordinated fine motor movements is the cerebellum.
8. A. The anterior cerebral artery supplies blood to the corpus callosum and the basal ganglia.
9. D. The laryngopharynx and the oropharynx add resonance to sounds produced by the larynx. The nasopharynx adds noticeable resonance to /m/, /n/, /ng/.
10. D. The aryepiglottic folds are a ring of connective tissue and muscle extending from the tips of the arytenoid cartilages to the larynx. They separate the laryngeal vestibule from the pharynx and help preserve the airway.
11. A. The cranial nerve that innervates the larynx and also innervates the levator veli palatini, palatoglossus, and palatopharyngeus muscles is cranial nerve X, the vagus nerve.

12. D. Muscles that contribute to velopharyngeal closure through tensing or elevating the velum are the palatoglossus, tensor veli palatini, and levator veli palatini.
13. D. The structure at the inferior portion of the tongue that connects the tongue with the mandible is called the *lingual frenum.*
14. C. The muscle that is most involved in producing the voiced and voiceless /th/ is the genioglossus.
15. A. The muscles most involved with adducting the vocal folds are the lateral cricoarytenoids and transverse arytenoid.

CHAPTER 2

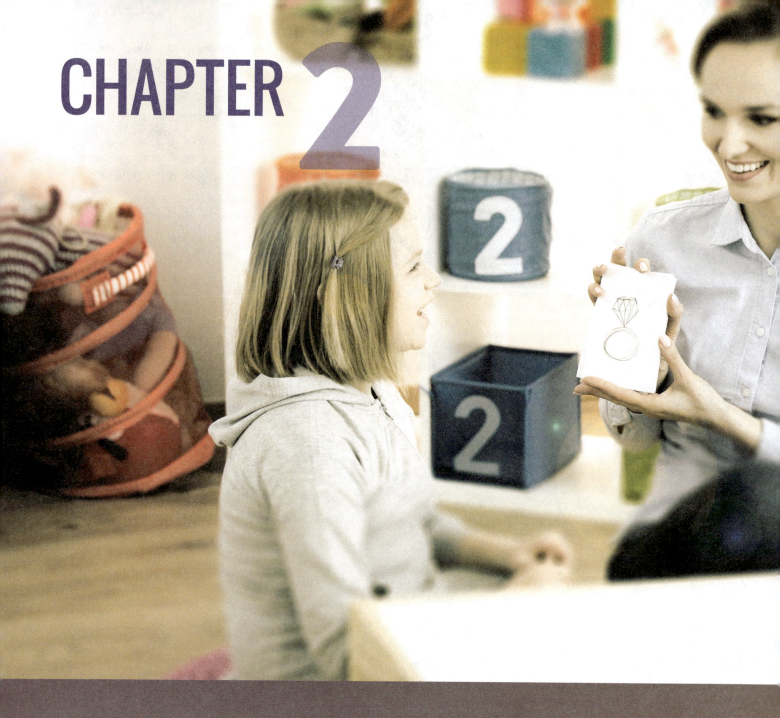

PHYSIOLOGICAL AND ACOUSTIC PHONETICS: A SPEECH SCIENCE FOUNDATION

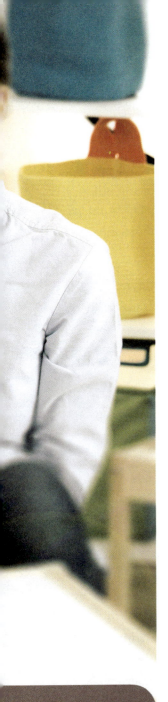

Speech science is the study of speech production at the acoustic and physiologic levels. Speech science helps make a comparative analysis of normal and disordered speech production. Speech sounds may be studied for their production as well as perception. The production of speech sounds is concerned with articulatory physiology—that is, how the physiological speech mechanism produces speech sounds. The perception of sounds is concerned with the relationship between the acoustic signal of speech and how it is understood by listeners. Phonetics, a branch of speech science, is the study of speech sounds and their production and perception in terms of their articulatory and physical characteristics (see Behrman, 2018; Garn-Gunn & Lynn, 2014; Raphael, Borden, & Harris, 2012; Speaks, 2018). Because much research effort in the speech sciences relates to issues in phonetics, phonetics is a central aspect of speech science. Thus, in this chapter, we integrate phonetic and related speech science information by describing physiological phonetics, which analyzes speech sound production, and acoustic phonetics, which studies the acoustic properties of sound waves that result when sounds are produced. Our discussion is relevant mostly to the production and perception of American English.

BASIC PRINCIPLES AND DEFINITIONS

Linguists describe language as a system with organized components. Phonetics, the study of speech sounds, organizes these sounds into systematic categories according to their perception and production. Speakers of any language need adequate respiration, phonation, resonation, and articulation to produce sounds for speech.

Definitions

- **Language**—a code or system of symbols used to express concepts formed through exposure and experience (linguistic definition). Speech is the production of language.
- **Language and speech**—verbal behaviors shaped and maintained by social communities (behavioral definition).
- **Phonology**—scientific study of the sound systems and patterns used to create the sounds and words of a language.
- **Phonemes**—the smallest units of sound that can affect meaning. For example, **man** and **fan** mean different things because of the different initial phonemes /m/ and /f/. Phonemes are families of sounds; the listener perceives members of a family as belonging to the same phoneme.

- **Allophones**—variations of phonemes that do not change word meanings, and, although one person's pronunciation can be measurably distinct from another person's, listeners still perceive the allophones as being the same. The phoneme /r/ sounds slightly different when speakers produce it in different linguistic contexts. For instance, the /r/ in *green* would be produced with more tongue retraction than the /r/ in *red*, which would be produced slightly more toward the front of the mouth. A speaker from New York would produce /r/ differently than a speaker from California. These different productions are allophonic variations of the /r/ phoneme, and such variations do not change the meaning of words in which they appear.

- **Phonemic**—as related to the abstract system of sounds; for example, the idealized and abstract description of /s/ is phonemic. Slash marks indicate phonemic representation of a sound or a general and abstract class of sounds.

- **Phonetic**—as related to concrete productions of specific sounds. Phonetic productions are enclosed in square brackets [ ], indicating specific sound productions of given speakers.

- **Phonetics**—the study of speech sounds in terms of their physical, physiological, and acoustic properties. It is derived from the word *phone*, which may or may not be a speech sound; the term refers generically to any sound that can be produced by the vocal tract. Usually, a phone is a single speech sound. Phonetics is divided into different categories (Behrman, 2018; Small, 2016), which may be summarized as follows:

  - **Acoustic phonetics**—the study of the relationship between articulation and the acoustic signal of speech and analyzes the acoustic properties of sound waves (e.g., periodicity and aperiodicity)
  - **Auditory phonetics**—the study of hearing, perception, and the brain's processing of speech
  - **Articulatory** or **physiological phonetics**—the study of speech sound production; emphasis is on how the physiological movements of the articulators produce individual sounds
  - **Applied (clinical) phonetics**—the study of the practical application of research in articulatory, perceptual, acoustic, and experimental phonetics to phonetic analyses of speech disorders
  - **Experimental phonetics**—analysis of speech sounds with objective laboratory and experimental techniques
  - **Descriptive phonetics**—the study and explanation of the unique sound properties of various dialects and languages

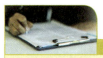

SUMMARY

- Every language has a system of sounds that is used to create words in that language. Phonetics is the study of speech sounds.
- To produce speech sounds, adequate respiration, phonation, resonation, and articulation are essential.
- Phonetics can be divided into six specific categories. This chapter concerns physiological and acoustic phonetics.

PHONETIC TRANSCRIPTION

Recording the sounds of the language as spoken by its people has been problematic because the letters of the alphabet often do not correspond strictly with the spoken sounds. Alphabets are written symbols of spoken sounds. A problem for many languages, including English, is that the same sound can be written, or spelled, in different ways. To deal with this challenge and to provide consistency across languages, the International Phonetic Alphabet (IPA) was developed. In this section, we describe the IPA and its broad and narrow symbols.

The International Phonetic Alphabet

- The IPA is a set of **orthographic symbols** that represent spoken sounds. Different orthographic symbols can be used to denote the same sound. Each IPA phonetic symbol represents a single speech sound accurately and consistently.
- Developed in 1888, the IPA is now used internationally. It was revised in 1993 and updated in 1996 and 2005 (www.internationalphoneticassociation.org).

Broad Phonetic Transcription

- When professionals use IPA symbols to transcribe words or sounds, they use **phonemic transcriptions**, which are indicated by enclosing phonemes between slash marks (e.g., /s/). These transcriptions are phonemic because variations in producing a phoneme are ignored. Sounds within slash marks are idealized phonemes.
- In **phonetic transcription**, allophones are indicated by placing them in brackets, as [s]. Sounds in brackets are actual productions of speakers.

Table 2.1 gives examples of IPA speech sound symbols for consonants, vowels, and diphthongs.

Narrow Phonetic Transcription

- Professionals use narrow phonetic transcription to record more detail about how a speaker produces a sound. Narrow phonetic transcription shows how speakers with such clinical conditions as a cleft palate, a severe phonological disorder, or hearing loss actually produce a phoneme.
- **Diacritical markers** are special symbols used in narrow phonetic transcription.

Table 2.2 shows the most widely used diacritical markers in the profession of speech pathology.

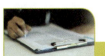

SUMMARY

- The International Phonetic Alphabet (IPA) is a system of representing speech sounds consistently and accurately.
- Speech–language pathologists can transcribe speech using broad as well as narrow phonetic symbols. Narrow phonetic symbols give increased detail about how individual speakers produce speech sounds.

Table 2.1

The International Phonetic Alphabet (IPA)

IPA symbol	Examples	IPA symbol	Examples
/p/	pot	/ʃ/	shine
/b/	bat	/ʒ/	vision
/m/	mat	/θ/	thin
/n/	net	/ð/	then
/ŋ/	sing	/tʃ/	chin
/d/	dime	/dʒ/	Jane
/t/	time	/v/	van
/g/	gum	/w/	wine
/k/	Kim	/l/	lean
/f/	fun	/j/	yawn
/s/	sun	/h/	hen
/z/	Zen	/r/	run
/ɑ/	fall	/ɛ/	bet
/æ/	fat	/e/	late
/ɔ/	fought	/o/	overcoat
/ə/	atop	/ʊ/	put
/ʌ/	fun	/u/	boot
/ɪ/	infect	/ɝ/	shirt
/i/	eat	/ɚ/	later
/eɪ/	main		
/aɪ/	lime		
/oʊ/	dome		
/aʊ/	how		
/ɔɪ/	boy		
/ɪʊ/	fuse		

Note. From *Introduction to Communicative Disorders* (4th ed., p. 139), by M. N. Hegde, 2010, Austin, TX: PRO-ED. Copyright 2010 by PRO-ED, Inc. Reprinted with permission.

Physiological and Acoustic Phonetics 77

Table 2.2

Diacritics

̥	Voiceless	n̥ d̥	̈	Breathy voiced	b̤ a̤	̪	Dental	t̪ d̪
̌	Voiced	s̬ t̬	̰	Creaky voiced	b̰ a̰	̺	Apical	t̺ d̺
ʰ	Aspirated	tʰ dʰ	̼	Linguolabial	t̼ d̼	̻	Laminal	t̻ d̻
̹	More rounded	ɔ̹	ʷ	Labialized	tʷ dʷ	̃	Nasalized	ẽ
̜	Less rounded	ɔ̜	ʲ	Palatalized	tʲ dʲ	ⁿ	Nasal release	dⁿ
̟	Advanced	u̟	ˠ	Velarized	tˠ dˠ	ˡ	Lateral release	dˡ
̠	Retracted	e̠	ˤ	Pharyngealized	tˤ dˤ	̚	No audible release	d̚
̈	Centralized	ë	̴	Velarized or pharyngealized	ɫ			
̽	Mid-centralized	ẽ	̝	Raised	e̝	(ɹ̝	= voiced alveolar fricative)	
̩	Syllabic	n̩	̞	Lowered	e̞	(β̞	= voiced bilabial approximant)	
̯	Non-syllabic	e̯	̘	Advanced tongue root	e̘			
˞	Rhoticity	ɚ ɑ˞	̙	Retracted tongue root	e̙			

Note. Diacritics may be placed above a symbol with a descender, e.g., ŋ̊ IPA Chart, http://www.internationalphoneticassociation.org/content/ipa-chart, available under a Creative Commons Attribution-Sharealike 3.0 Unported License. Copyright © 2015 International Phonetic Association.

PRODUCTION OF SEGMENTALS: CONSONANTS AND VOWELS

Speech sounds can be broadly classified into two categories: consonants and vowels. Variables related to production and perceptions of sounds relate to their description and classification. In speech–language pathology, consonants and vowels may be further classified in terms of (a) the distinctive features of sounds and (b) the place-voice-manner characteristics of sounds (Peña-Brooks & Hegde, 2015). (See also Chapter 5 for more information.)

Consonants and Vowels: The Syllable as a Unit
- Consonants and vowels may be defined by their role in the production of syllables. The **syllable** is defined as the smallest phonetic unit.
- Syllables may be considered **motor units** composed of three parts:
  1. **Onset.** This is the initial consonant or consonant cluster of the syllable, created by release of the syllable pulse through articulatory movements or action of the chest muscles.
  2. **Nucleus.** This is a vowel or diphthong in the middle of the syllable, created by vowel-shaping movements of the vocal tract.

Table 2.3

Comparisons of Vowels and Consonants

Vowels	Consonants
Always voiced	May be voiced or voiceless
May stand alone	Always combined with vowel
Velum always elevated	Velum elevated or lowered
Vocal tract open	Vocal tract modified or constricted
Airflow continuous	Airflow modified or stopped
May be described by: • distinctive features • tongue and lip position • tension vs. laxness	May be described by: • distinctive features • place-voice-manner

3. **Coda**. This is the consonant at the end of the syllable, created by arrest of the syllable pulse through articulatory movements, action of the chest muscles, or both.

- Nucleus and coda are collectively known as **rhyme**. In essence, vowels form the nucleus of syllables; consonants release and arrest syllables. Vowels may also stand alone to form syllables. For example, utterances such as *ah*, *oh*, and *I* are vowels and may stand alone. Consonants may not stand alone; they function only with vowels.

Table 2.3 illustrates basic comparisons between vowels and consonants. (See the "Consonants" and "Vowels" sections of this chapter for more on these comparisons.)

- Vowels may also be termed **syllabics** because they carry syllables. A few consonants have a syllabic nature in that they also can form the nucleus of a syllable (Small, 2016). These syllabic consonants are /l/, /n/, and /m/. The diacritical marker /ˌ/ is used to indicate the syllabic nature of these consonants. Examples follow:

/m̩/: love '*em*, leave '*em*
/n̩/: butto*n*, more '*n*' more
/l̩/: bott*le*, midd*le*

- Syllables may be open or closed. **Open syllables** end in vowels; *my*, *hey*, and *ski* are open syllables. **Closed syllables** end in consonants; *cook*, *lip*, and *hiss* are closed syllables.
- **Syllabification** is the skill of identifying the number of syllables in words. A knowledgeable speaker, for example, may count four syllables in *categorize* and a single syllable in *dog*.

Classification Systems

Distinctive feature analysis and place-voice-manner analysis are two systems for classifying speech sounds.

Table 2.4

The Chomsky-Halle Distinctive Features of English Consonants

	w	f	v	θ	ð	t	d	s	z	n	l	ʃ	ʒ	j	r	tʃ	dʒ	k	g	ŋ	h	p	b	m
Voiced	+	−	+	−	+	−	+	−	+	+	+	−	+	+	+	−	+	−	+	+	−	−	+	+
Consonantal	−	+	+	+	+	+	+	+	+	+	+	+	+	−	+	+	+	+	+	+	−	+	+	+
Anterior	+	+	+	+	+	+	+	+	+	+	+	−	−	−	−	−	−	−	−	−	−	+	+	+
Coronal	−	−	−	+	+	+	+	+	+	+	+	+	+	−	+	+	+	−	−	−	−	−	−	−
Continuant	+	+	+	+	+	−	−	+	+	−	+	+	+	+	+	−	−	−	−	−	+	−	−	−
High	−	−	−	−	−	−	−	−	−	−	−	+	+	+	−	+	+	+	+	+	−	−	−	−
Low	−	−	−	−	−	−	−	−	−	−	−	−	−	−	−	−	−	−	−	−	+	−	−	−
Back	−	−	−	−	−	−	−	−	−	−	−	−	−	−	−	−	−	+	+	+	−	−	−	−
Nasal	−	−	−	−	−	−	−	−	−	+	−	−	−	−	−	−	−	−	−	+	−	−	−	+
Strident	−	+	+	−	−	−	−	+	+	−	−	+	+	−	−	+	+	−	−	−	−	−	−	−
Vocalic	−	−	−	−	−	−	−	−	−	−	+	−	−	−	+	−	−	−	−	−	−	−	−	−

Note. From *Introduction to Communicative Disorders* (4th ed., p. 146), by M. N. Hegde, 2010, Austin, TX: PRO-ED. Copyright 2010 by PRO-ED, Inc. Reprinted with permission.

Distinctive Feature Analysis

- The **distinctive features** are a set of unique characteristics (features) of speech sounds of all languages. A phoneme is described in terms of a collection of independent features.
- Distinctive features help distinguish one phoneme from another (Chomsky & Halle, 1968; Jakobson, Fant, & Halle, 1952), although many phonemes share certain common features. Distinctive features also include considerations of place-voice-manner analysis.
- The main distinctive features that apply to English consonants are presented in Table 2.4.
- As shown in Table 2.4, each phoneme (consonant or vowel) is described as either having a feature (+) or not having it (−).

Place-Voice-Manner Analysis

- **Place-voice-manner analysis** categorizes consonants in terms of three parameters: place, voice, and manner of production.
- **Place of articulation** refers to the location of the sound's production within the speech production mechanism, indicating the primary articulators that shape the sounds. For example, /p/ is termed a bilabial because the place of its production is the two lips.
- **Voicing** refers to vocal fold vibration during production of sounds. Vocal folds vibration is present in voiced sounds, and absent in voiceless sounds. The /b/ is a voiced sound whereas the /p/ is a voiceless sound.
- **Manner of articulation** refers to the degree or type of constriction of the vocal tract during consonant production. For example, /p/ is termed a **stop** because it is produced by putting the lips together and completely stopping the airflow.

Table 2.5 illustrates the place-voice-manner classification of English sounds.

Table 2.5

Place-Voice-Manner Classification of English Consonants

Place of articulation	Manner of production						
	Nasals	Stops	Fricatives	Affricates	Liquids	Glides	Laterals
Bilabial	(m)	p (b)				(w)	
Labiodental			f (v)				
Linguadental			θ (ð)				
Lingua-alveolar	(n)	t (d)	s (z)		(l)		(l)
Linguapalatal			ʃ (ʒ)	tʃ (dʒ)	(r)	(j)	
Linguavelar	(ŋ)	k (g)					
Glottal			h				

Note. Voiced sounds are circled. From *Introduction to Communicative Disorders* (4th ed., p. 142), by M. N. Hegde, 2010, Austin, TX: PRO-ED. Copyright 2010 by PRO-ED, Inc. Reprinted with permission.

Consonants

- Consonants are those speech sounds that are produced by articulatory movements that modify the airstream in some manner—by interrupting it, stopping it, or creating a narrow opening through which it must pass.
- Consonants may be described according to either distinctive features or their place, voice, and manner of production (Tables 2.4 and 2.5).

Place-Voice-Manner Analysis

Consonants can be described according to the place, voice, and manner of production (Peña-Brooks & Hegde, 2015; Raphael et al., 2012; Shriberg & Kent, 2018).

Place of Articulation

- **Linguavelars** (also called velars) /g/, /k/, and /ŋ/ are produced when the dorsum of the tongue contacts the velum.
- **Linguapalatals** /j/, /r/, /dʒ/, /tʃ/, /ʒ/, and /ʃ/ are produced when the tongue blade is pressed against the hard palate to form the point of constriction just posterior to the alveolar ridge.
- **Lingua-alveolars** /s/, /z/, /n/, /l/, /t/, and /d/ are produced when the tip of tongue makes a contact with the alveolar ridge.
- **Linguadentals** /θ/ and /ð/ (also called interdentals) are produced by protruding the tongue tip slightly between the cutting edge of the lower and upper front teeth, forming a narrow

constriction, directing air through this constriction, and making light contact between the tongue and teeth.
- **Bilabials** /w/, /m/, /p/, and /b/ are produced by mutual contact of the upper and lower lips.
- **Labiodentals** /f/ and /v/ are produced by placing the lower edge of the upper central incisors on the upper portion of the lower lip, thus forming a narrow point of constriction.
- **The glottal**, only /h/ in English, is produced at the level of the glottis by open vocal folds through which the air passes through.

Voicing
- **Voicing** is a characteristic of vibrating vocal folds in producing certain consonants. Sounds such as /r/, /g/, and /z/ are voiced, whereas /k/, /t/, and /s/ are voiceless.
- **Cognate pairs** are sounds that are identical in every way except voicing. Place and manner of production are the same, but the feature of voicing is different. For example, /p-b/ and /k-g/ are cognate pairs in which one is voiced and the other is not.

Manner of Articulation
All sounds in each manner-of-articulation category are described not only according to manner, but also according to place and voice as well as distinctive features (Peña-Brooks & Hegde, 2015; Raphael et al., 2012; Shriberg & Kent, 2018).

Nasals: /m/, /n/, /ŋ/

- Nasals are produced by lowering the velum to keep the velopharyngeal port open. The open velopharyngeal port allows the sound produced by the vibrating vocal folds to pass through the nasal cavity.
- The vocal tract is lengthened, and there is an overall increase in the area for resonance. Thus, the resonance characteristic is changed by low-frequency components being added to the sounds.

/m/: place = bilabial
voice = voiced
manner = nasal
distinctive features = +voiced, +consonantal, +anterior, +nasal

/n/: place = lingua-alveolar
voice = voiced
manner = nasal
distinctive features = +voiced, +consonantal, +anterior, +coronal, +nasal

/ŋ/: place = linguavelar
voice = voiced
manner = nasal
distinctive features = +voiced, +consonantal, +high, +back, +nasal

Fricatives: /h/, /ʒ/, /ʃ/, /s/, /z/, /ð/, /θ/, /f/, /v/

- Fricatives derive their name from the friction—a hissing quality—that results from the continuous forcing of air through a narrow constriction.
- Two closely approximating articulators form a constriction through which a continuous airstream must pass. The constrictions in the vocal tract generate aperiodic noise as the airflow passes through them. The constrictions must be narrow enough and the airflow strong enough to create a turbulent airflow. This turbulent airflow creates noisy random vibrations, or frication. Firm velopharyngeal closure is necessary.

/h/: place = glottal
voice = voiceless
manner = fricative
distinctive features = +continuant, +low

/ʒ-ʃ/: place = linguapalatal
voice = /ʒ/ voiced, /ʃ/ voiceless
manner = fricative
distinctive features = +consonantal, +coronal, +continuant, +high, +strident

/s-z/: place = lingua-alveolar
voice = /s/ voiceless, /z/ voiced
manner = fricative
distinctive features = +consonantal, +anterior, +coronal, +continuant, +strident

/ð-θ/: place = linguadental
voice = /ð/ voiced, /θ/ voiceless
manner = fricative
distinctive features = +consonantal, +coronal, +anterior, +continuant

/f-v/: place = labiodental
voice = /f/ voiceless, /v/ voiced
manner = fricative
distinctive features = +consonantal, +anterior, +continuant, +strident

Affricates: /tʃ/, /dʒ/

- The affricates /tʃ/ and /dʒ/ have both a fricative and a stop component. These sounds begin as stops and are released as fricatives. The speaker makes alveolar closure for /d/ or /t/; when the closure is released, the tongue is retracted and shaped for the production of /tʃ/ or /dʒ/.
- Usually, the lips are slightly rounded as the fricative portion of the affricate sound is produced.

/tʃ-dʒ/: place = lingua-alveolar
voice = /tʃ/ voiceless, /dʒ/ voiced

manner = affricate
distinctive features = +consonantal, +coronal, +strident

Stops: /p/, /b/, /t/, /d/, /k/, /g/

- The stops are produced by complete constriction or closure of the vocal tract at some point, so the airflow is totally stopped. Stops are formed at three basic places: alveolar (closure between the tip of the tongue and the alveolar ridge), velar (closure between the tongue blade and roof of the mouth), and labial (closure of the lips).
- When the airflow is stopped, pressure builds up behind the point of contact; when the built-up air is released, there is a short audible burst of noise. Consequently, stops may also be called stop-plosives.

/p-b/: place = bilabial
voice = /p/ voiceless, /b/ voiced
manner = stop
distinctive features = +consonantal, +anterior

/t-d/: place = lingua-alveolar
voice = /t/ voiceless, /d/ voiced
manner = stop
distinctive features = +consonantal, +anterior, +coronal

/k-g/: place = linguavelar
voice = /k/, voiceless, /g/ voiced
manner = stop
distinctive features = +consonantal, +high, +back

Glides: /w/, /j/

- The glides, also called **semivowels** and **sonorants**, are produced by a quick transition of the articulators, as they move from a partially constricted state to a more open state for the vowels that follow them. The term **onglide** is used to describe this movement.
- In comparison to stops, fricatives, and affricates, glides are formed by a relatively transitory and unrestricted point of constriction.

/w/: place = bilabial
voice = voiced
manner = glide
distinctive features = +anterior, +continuant

/j/: place = linguapalatal
voice = voiced
manner = glide
distinctive features = +continuant, +high

Liquids: /r/, /l/

- The liquids are produced with the least oral cavity restriction of all the consonants. The vocal tract is obstructed only slightly more than for vowels.
- The /r/ is also called a **rhotic** and is commonly produced in two ways. One way is as a **retroflex**, made with the tongue tip retracted and approximating the hard palate; a second way is as a **bunched** /r/, in which the dorsum of the tongue is "bunched" or retracted and elevated toward the hard palate.

  /r/: place = linguapalatal
  voice = voiced
  manner = liquid
  distinctive features = +consonantal, +coronal, +continuant, +vocalic

- The /l/ is also called a **lateral** because when it is produced, the midsection portion of the tongue is relaxed and open, and thus air is directed through the sides of the tongue.

  /l/: place = lingua-alveolar
  voice = voiced
  manner = liquid
  distinctive features = +consonantal, +anterior, +coronal, +continuant, +vocalic

Consonant Clusters

- While many consonants are produced alone or adjacent to vowels, others are produced adjacent to some consonants. These **consonant clusters**, also known as **blends**, may occur in the initial, medial, or final position of words.
- Most consonant clusters in American English consist of two consonants. However, some three-consonant clusters also occur. Examples of two-consonant clusters are **mosquito**, **bless**, **silk**. Examples of three-consonant clusters are **burst**, **straw**, and **burnt**.

Vowels

- Vowels are produced with an open vocal tract. The vocal tract is open from the vocal folds to the lips, with no points of constriction.
- All vowels are voiced. Resonance patterns for the vowels are shaped by the vocal tract. Ongoing changes in the size and shape of the oral cavity result in unique resonance features of each vowel.

Distinctive Feature Analysis

Like consonants, vowels can be described according to their distinctive features (Peña-Brooks & Hegde, 2015; Raphael et al., 2012) and include the following features: (1) **vocalic**, (2) **sonorant**, (3) **voiced**, (4) **rounded**, (5) **tense**, (6) **front**, (7) **back**, (8) **high**, (9) **low**, and (10) **rhotic**.

Vowel Position Characteristics

- Vowel production may be described from a position of physiologic rest—that is, by the amount of mandibular, tongue, and lip movement away from physiologic rest that is necessary for production

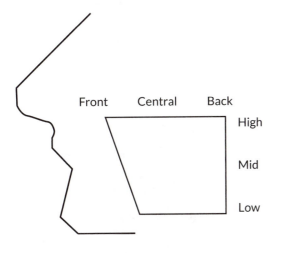
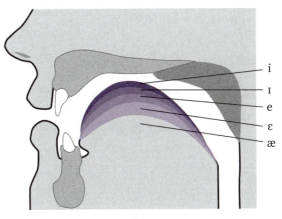
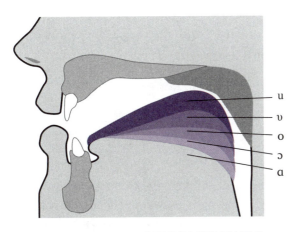
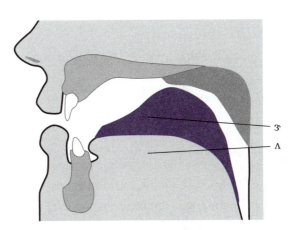

Figure 2.1 The vowel chart.

of each vowel. Figure 2.1 demonstrates the tongue positions with which vowels are typically produced.

- Using this concept, vowels can be characterized according to four dimensions:

  - **Lip position**. This causes vowels to be categorized as rounded or unrounded. For rounded vowels, the lips are protruded. For unrounded vowels, the lips are in a neutral or slightly retracted position.
  - **Tense/lax** qualities. Tense vowels have longer duration and are produced with increased tension, while lax vowels are of shorter duration and are produced with relatively less muscular tension.
  - **Tongue height**. This causes vowels to be categorized as high, mid, or low in terms of production within the oral cavity.
  - **Tongue forwardness** or **retraction**. This causes vowels to be categorized as front, central, or back in terms of production within the oral cavity.

In the following section, vowels are described according to these dimensions. Key words containing each vowel serve as examples.

Front Vowels: /ɪ/, /i/, /e/, /ɛ/, /æ/

- **High** front vowels /ɪ/ and /i/

  /ɪ/ : lax, unround; tongue is slightly lower and more posterior than for /i/. Key words: *bit, sick, tin.*
  /i/: tense, unround; tongue is in a high and forward position. Key words: *heat, meeting, see.*

- **Mid** front vowels /e/ and /ɛ/

  /e/: tense, unround; compared to production of /ɪ/, /e/ involves keeping the tongue lower and slightly more retracted. Key words: *make, later, fate.*
  /ɛ/: lax, unround; the /ɛ/ vowel is produced slightly lower than /e/. Key words: *let, ten, sent.*

- **Low** front vowel /æ/

  /æ/: lax, unround; one of the lowest vowels in English, produced with the tongue lower and more retracted than required for production of /ɛ/. Key words: *tan, matter, sat.*

Central Vowels: /ɜ/, /ɚ/, /ə/, /ʌ/

- The place of production varies for each of the central vowels, also called mid central vowels.
- /ɜ/ and /ɚ/

  /ɜ/: tense, half-round, retroflexed; the tongue blade is bunched and elevated toward the hard palate. The tongue is retracted toward /o/, and tongue height is approximately equivalent to that for /ɪ/ and /e/. The /ɜ/ is transcribed to represent /r/ production in syllables receiving primary stress (e.g., as in *certain*). Key words: *curtain, hurt, dirty.*
  /ɚ/: lax, half-round, and retroflexed. The /ɚ/, called schwar, is produced in the same manner as /ɜ/. However, schwar is transcribed to represent /r/ production in unstressed syllables, such as that in *butter*. Key words: *letter, color, ladder.*

- /ə/ and /ʌ/

  /ə/: lax, unround; the tongue blade is lowered in relation to /ɜ/. The unstressed /ə/ occurs in unstressed syllables such as that in *above*. Key words: *attempt, ahead, pizza.*
  /ʌ/: lax, unround; the /ʌ/ vowel is produced in a manner similar to that for /ə/, but the tongue is slightly more retracted toward /ɑ/. The /ʌ/ occurs in stressed syllables. Key words: *money, flood, up.*

Back Vowels: /u/, /ʊ/, /o/, /ɔ/, /ɑ/

- **High** back vowels /u/ and /ʊ/

  /u/: tense, round; the tongue is in the highest, most retracted position when a speaker is producing /ʊ/. Key words: *spoon, fruit, bruise.*

/ʊ/: lax, round; the /ʊ/ vowel is produced in a slightly lower and more forward manner than /u/. Key words: *took, put, foot.*

- **Mid** back vowels /ɔ/ and /o/

    /ɔ/: lax, round; the /ɔ/ vowel is produced a little lower than /u/. Key words: *fought, caught, shawl.*
    /o/: tense, round; in comparison to /u/, /o/ is produced slightly lower in the oral cavity. Key words: *coat, lower, soapy.*

- **Low** back vowel /ɑ/

    /ɑ/: lax, unround; the /ɑ/ vowel is produced with the lowest, most retracted tongue position of all the vowels. Key words: *calm, pocket, father.*

Diphthongs

- Diphthongs are produced as a slow gliding movement from one vowel (the **onglide**) to the adjacent vowel (the **offglide**). For example, in the diphthong /ɑI/, /ɑ/ is the onglide vowel, and /I/ is the offglide vowel. Diphthongs contain both an initial and a final segment.
- Diphthongs are represented phonetically by digraph symbols that highlight the initial and final segments. The diphthongs are:

/aI/ p**i**pe, m**y**, m**igh**t, r**i**te
/aʊ/ c**ow**, h**ou**se, t**ow**n, p**ou**t
/ɔI/ t**oi**l, b**oy**, m**oi**st, l**oi**ter
/eI/ v**a**cation, t**a**ke, f**a**ce
/oʊ/ l**oa**n, thr**o**ne, ph**o**ne

- **Phonemic** diphthongs /aI/, /ɔI/, and /aʊ/ cannot be reduced to pure vowels without changing word meaning. For example, /taIp/ and /tɑp/ represent two different meanings.
- Nonphonemic diphthongs /oʊ/ and /ɔi/ do not change word meanings. For example, the listener perceives /soʊp/ and /sop/ as the same words.

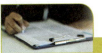

SUMMARY

- Consonants and vowels may be defined by their role in the production of syllables, the smallest phonetic unit.
- Two classification systems frequently used to describe consonants and vowels are distinctive features and place-voice-manner of articulation.
- Vowels may also be described according to lip position, tense–lax qualities, and tongue height and position within the oral cavity.

THE EFFECTS OF CONTEXT ON SPEECH SOUND PRODUCTION

Speech sound production is a dynamic process. The context of each sound and word influence the production of other sounds and words in the stream. In conversational speech, sounds are also influenced by suprasegmental parameters, which add variety and expression to speech.

Dynamics of Speech Production

- Sounds may be produced in two ways: in isolation or in the context of words, phrases, and sentences. Deliberate and isolated production of a sound is called the **citation form** of that sound. Sounds produced in a context, especially in connected speech, differ from their citation forms. **Phonetic context** or the effects sounds have on the neighboring sounds cause differences in phonetic sounds.
- Production of a sound is affected by the sound that immediately precedes and follows it. For example, the /m/ in *meek* is produced with more lip retraction than the /m/ in *moo*, which is produced with slight lip protrusion. The following vowel influences the production of /m/. To give another example, in the phrase "great zoo," the /z/ in **zoo** is devoiced because of the voiceless /t/ in the preceding word.
- The change a sound goes through in connected speech is described in terms of **coarticulation**. The sound /ð/ for example, may be produced distinctly in the word *them*. The same sound in the phrase *Them* in *Catch them* may be reduced to a mere "əm" as in [kætʃəm].
- Some phoneticians distinguish coarticulation from assimilation, while most use them synonymously. When distinguished, **assimilation** causes a sound to change to a different sound, as in *pomputer* for *computer*. As noted, coarticulation results in allophonic variations of the same sound.

Suprasegmentals

- **Suprasegmentals** are features of **prosody**, and add meaning, variety, and color to running speech. They involve larger units than such individual units (segments) as syllables, words, phrases, and sentences.
- Several variables, including a person's cultural and linguistic background, emotional state, gender, and age affect the suprasegmentals. The most commonly described suprasegmentals (prosodic features of speech) are length, stress, rate, pitch, volume, and juncture.
- **Length** of vowels and consonants is related to syllable perception and production. If syllables have long vowels, they tend to have short consonants. If syllables have short vowels, they tend to have long consonants.
- **Stress** is an important characteristic of syllables, for it can change the meanings of words. Stressed syllables are often called syllables containing **primary stress**, while unstressed syllables are referred to as those with **secondary** or **weak stress**.
- Stressed and unstressed syllables differ in four ways relative to each other:

Stressed syllable	Unstressed syllable
Loud	Soft
Longer	Shorter
Higher in pitch	Lower in pitch
Greater muscular effort	Less muscular effort

- Syllable stress helps differentiate noun and verb pairs that have identical sounds. For example, the words *object*, *permit*, *insult*, and *import* become nouns or verbs depending upon which syllables are stressed.
- **Rate** of speech refers to the speed of speech; it is a measure of the number of words or syllables produced per unit of time. Rapid speech tends to have reduced duration of vowels and consonants produced with less articulatory effort. Rate reflects the phonetic duration of both sound and silence and may be affected by the speaker's emotion.
- **Pitch** is the auditory sensation (typically called **perception**) of the frequency with which the vocal folds vibrate, whereas frequency is a physical property of the actual sound waves. Pitch is determined by mass, tension, and elasticity of the vocal folds. In English, pitch can be used to indicate different meanings of spoken units. For example, "We are having fun reading this book" can be a statement if the pitch falls at the end, a question if the pitch rises at the end.
- **Intensity** is sound pressure, and it is another physical property of sound. The sensory correlate of intensity is **loudness** (also generally described as **volume** of sound). This sensation or perception of loudness is related to amplitude, another physical property of the actual sound waves: the greater the amplitude of sound, the greater the sensation of loudness. A speaker's loudness may be influenced by many variables, including the amount of background noise, the speaker's feelings at the moment, and the speaker's or listener's hearing acuity.
- **Juncture**, also called **vocal punctuation**, is a combination of suprasegmentals, such as intonation and pausing, that mark special distinctions or grammatical divisions in speech. These distinctions affect the meaning of an utterance. For example, one would say, "What did you eat?" differently than one would say, "What, did you eat?" Or one might use juncture to make distinctions between such similar sounding words as *night rate* and *nitrate* or *I scream* and *ice cream*.

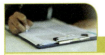

SUMMARY

- Speech sounds are generally produced within a context where they are influenced by one another.
- Suprasegmentals such as juncture, pitch, and stress add meaning and variety to speech as part of human interaction.

SPEECH SCIENCE: PHYSIOLOGICAL PHONETICS, ACOUSTIC PHONETICS, AND SPEECH PERCEPTION

Acoustics is the study of sound as a physical phenomenon. Mechanical vibrations of an object create waves of disturbance in the molecules of an elastic medium, which can be gas, liquid, or a solid object. These disturbances are called **sound waves**, and they may be periodic or aperiodic. Although sound waves are said to travel through the medium, there is no movement from point A to point B. Sound waves "travel" only in the sense that adjacent molecules are stimulated to move back and forth. To be scientifically studied, sound waves need not be audible to the human ear. **Acoustics**, a branch of physics, is the study of the physical properties of sound and how sound is generated and propagated.

Acoustics: Basic Definitions

- **Psychoacoustics** is the study of how humans respond to sound as a physical phenomenon; it is a branch of both psychology and acoustics.
- **Sound** may be defined both physically and sensorily (perceptually). Physically defined, it is the result of a vibration or disturbance in the molecules of a medium (air, gas, or liquid). Sensorily defined, it is a vibration or disturbance in the air that is potentially audible, although instruments can measure inaudible sound.
- **Sound waves** are movements of particles in a medium containing expansions and contractions of molecules.
- **Compression**, or **condensation**, is a phase of sound in which the vibratory movements of an object (e.g., the tines of a tuning fork) increase the density of air molecules because the molecules are compressed or condensed; it is the opposite of rarefaction.
- **Rarefaction** is the thinning of air molecules when the vibrating object returns to equilibrium; it is the opposite of condensation.
- **Simple harmonic motion**, also known as a **sine wave**, refers to the back-and-forth movement of particles when the movement is symmetrical and periodic.
- **Sinusoidal motion** or **wave** is a wave with horizontal and vertical symmetry because it contains one peak or crest and one valley or trough. A sinusoidal wave contains a single frequency and is a result of simple harmonic motion.
- **Periodic waves** are sound waves that repeat themselves at regular intervals and are predictable.
- **Aperiodic waves** are random vibratory patterns and therefore are difficult to predict from one time interval to the next.
- **Amplitude** is the magnitude and direction of displacement. The greater the amplitude, the louder the sound signal.
- **Intensity** is the quality of sound that creates the sensation of loudness. Physically, intensity is the amount of energy transmitted per second over an area of one square meter. It is measured in terms of watt per square meter and is also expressed in decibels (dB).
- **Bel** is a logarithmic unit of measure of sound intensity. It is a basic and relative reference measure that helps express the wide range of sound intensities to which the human ear is sensitive by means

of a compressed, logarithmic scale. **Decibel** (dB) is a measure of sound intensity that equals one tenth of a bel.

- **CSG system** is a metric system of measuring length in centimeters (cm), time in seconds (sec), and mass in grams (g); it can be contrasted with the MKS metric system of measuring length in meters (m), time in seconds, and mass in kilograms (kg).
- **Dyne** is a measure of force in the csg metric system; 1 dyne is the force required to accelerate a mass of 1 gram from a velocity of 0 cm per second to a velocity of 1 cm per second in 1 second.
- **Density** is the amount of mass per unit volume; density of matter serves as a medium for sound and affects sound transmission.
- **Displacement** is change in position; air molecules are said to be displaced because of the vibratory action of an object.
- **Oscillation** refers to the back-and-forth movement of the air molecules because of a vibrating object.
- **Force** is a vector quantity that tends to produce an acceleration of a body in the direction of its application; it is also defined as the product of mass and acceleration. Force is measured in terms of newton (Nt); 1 newton equals the force required to accelerate a mass of 1 kg from a velocity of 0 m per second to a velocity of 1 m per second in 1 second.
- **Elasticity** is a property that makes it possible for matter (which helps transmit sound) to recover its form and volume when subjected to distortion. All matter is subjected to distortion when force is applied to it.
- **Velocity** is a change in position of, for example, air molecules when an object is set to vibration. Velocity is measured in terms of the distance an object moves per the time and the direction it takes as it moves.
- **Frequency** is one of the two characteristics of vibratory motion. It is the rate of vibratory motion that is measured in terms of the number of cycles completed per second or, more recently, in terms of hertz (Hz). Hertz is the unit of measure for frequency and is the same as the cycle per second; 1 cycle per second is 1 Hz.
- **Natural frequency** is the frequency with which a source of sound normally vibrates. It is determined by the source's mass and stiffness. Mass is the quantity of matter and is not to be confused with weight, which is gravitational force exerted on mass. The mass of a medium of sound affects its transmission. Increased mass results in decreased frequency, and increased stiffness results in increased frequency.
- **Formant frequency** is a frequency region with concentrated acoustic energy. It is the center frequency of a formant, which is a resonance.
- **Fundamental frequency** is the lowest frequency of a periodic wave; it is the first harmonic.
- An **octave** is an indication of the interval between two frequencies. The intervals always maintain a ratio of 1:2; thus, each octave doubles a particular frequency (e.g., 200 Hz is 1 octave above 100 Hz, and 2000 Hz is 1 octave above 1000 Hz).
- **Impedance** is acoustic, mechanical, or electrical resistance to motion or sound transmission.
- **Newton's Laws of Motion** explain motion and its characteristics. Basically, sound involves motion. The law of inertia states that all bodies remain at rest or in a state of uniform motion unless

another force acts in opposition. In other words, a body in motion tends to remain in motion and a body at rest tends to stay at rest. The law of reaction forces says that every force is associated with a reaction force of opposite direction.
- **Pressure** is the amount of force per unit area. Force is measured either as dynes or as newtons and is important in understanding the amount of pressure sound waves exert on the eardrum.
- **Reflection** refers to the phenomenon of sound waves traveling back after hitting an obstacle, with no change in the speed of propagation.
- **Refraction** is the bending of the sound wave due to change in its speed of propagation; this happens, for example, when sound waves move from one medium (e.g., air) to another (e.g., water).
- **Resonance** is the modification of sound by other sources. In speech acoustics, resonance refers to modification of the laryngeal tone predominantly by the nasal and oral cavities.
- A **transmitting medium** is any matter that carries or transmits sound. Air, liquids, and solids can all transmit sound. The mass and elasticity of a transmitting medium affect sound (see the next section).

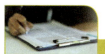

SUMMARY

- Acoustics, the study of sound, defines sound as a potentially audible vibration or disturbance in the air that creates sound waves. These waves may be periodic or aperiodic.
- Vibratory motion can be characterized according to intensity and frequency. Relative intensity is measured in decibels and frequency is measured in hertz.
- Sound may be resonated for speech by the nasal and oral cavities.

INTRODUCTION TO THE STUDY OF SOUND AND ACOUSTIC ANALYSIS OF SPEECH

Sound is the result of vibrations of an elastic object. Physically, sound is a compressional wave; sensorily, it is a compressional wave that produces a sensation. Sound exists both as a physical phenomenon and as a sensory experience (Behrman, 2018; Raphael et al., 2012; Speaks, 2018). Sound is perceived (or sensed) in terms of pitch and loudness. The acoustic analysis of speech is generally conducted through use of a sound spectrograph, which produces a spectrogram. The spectrogram displays various components, such as fundamental frequency and many other characteristics of vowels and consonants.

Sound Wave Generation and Propagation

- Sound or vibration propagation needs a medium, such as air, liquid, or gas. The two main properties of a medium that affect the transmission of sound are the mass (density) and the elasticity. More massive objects (sound media) require greater force to set them into vibratory motion because of their higher inertia.

- Vibratory motion is possible partly because of the elasticity of objects. For example, because of their elasticity, the tines of a tuning fork can be set into a back-and-forth motion by striking them. Elastic objects get distorted when a force is applied to them and, in due course, they recover their original form or position. As they change form or position, they create waves of molecular disturbances (vibratory motion).
- Vibratory motion has two important but independent characteristics that create distinctly different auditory sensation: frequency and amplitude.
- Vibrations repeat themselves in cycles or hertz. The number of times a cycle of vibration repeats itself within a second is the frequency of vibration. When a tone contains a single frequency, it is called a **pure tone**.
- **Simple harmonic motion** results in a tone of single frequency that repeats itself. Simple harmonic motion also is called sinusoidal motion. A graphical representation of a sinusoidal motion is called a sine wave.
- A **complex tone** is created when two or more single frequency tones of differing frequencies are combined. The vibrations that make up a complex tone are **periodic** or **aperiodic**. When waves repeat themselves at regular and predictable intervals, they are said to be periodic. When the vibratory patterns are random and the next pattern cannot be predicted from the previous pattern, the waves are said to be aperiodic. Although it is not always the case, aperiodic waves are equated with noise.
- Sound waves do not imply motion; there is no physical movement of matter. Instead, there is a transfer of energy. Sound is propagated because of the back-and-forth movements of molecules at which time the molecules are pressed either together (**compression**) or they move apart (**rarefaction**). Only the molecules swing back and forth to create a wave of disturbance that the human ear may detect as sound.
- The amount of molecular displacement per unit of time is measured in terms of **velocity**. A change in velocity is described as **acceleration** or **deceleration**. Acceleration also is related to direction of movement; when direction changes, velocity also changes.

Frequency and Pitch
- **Frequency** is a measure of the number of cycles per second, or **hertz**. A single cycle (or 1 Hz) consists of one instance of compression and one instance of rarefaction within a second.
- A related measure is called a **period**, which is the amount of time needed for a cycle to be completed. The frequency of vibration is a function of the properties of the vibrating object. For instance, the frequency of vibration of a tuning fork is determined by its metallic density and its length. The air molecules vibrate at the same rate as the vibrating object.
- The medium that transmits the sound does not affect the frequency of sound. However, it does affect the speed of sound. A more dense medium will retard the speed of sound transmission more than a less dense medium, which will propagate sound faster.
- A more elastic medium (even if it is more dense) will propagate sound faster than a less elastic (even if it is less dense) medium. Therefore, steel, which is more dense but also more elastic than air, will transmit sound faster than air, which is less dense but also much less elastic than steel.

- Variations in the frequency of vibration create variations in sensation we call **pitch**. Thus, pitch is a sensory (perceptual) experience related to changes in frequency, a physical event. A sound of higher frequency is perceived as a sound of higher pitch than a sound of lower frequency.
- The human ear is not sensitive to all frequencies of sound. The normal ear of a young adult can respond to 20 to 20000 Hz. The human ear is more sensitive to changes in lower frequencies (below 1000 Hz) than changes in higher frequencies.

Amplitude and Loudness

- **Amplitude**, the second important characteristic of vibratory motion, is a measure of the **magnitude** (intensity, strength) of the sound signal. In most cases, a measure of amplitude refers to sound pressure.
- Measured in **dynes** or **newtons**, sound pressure is the amount of force per unit area. Amplitude is the extent of molecular displacement; the greater the degree of molecular displacement, the higher the amplitude or intensity of sound.
- While amplitude, intensity, magnitude, and strength of a sound signal are physical concepts, loudness is a sensory concept. Loudness is a sensation related to physical amplitude or intensity of a sound. The higher the amplitude of a sound, the greater the perceived loudness of that sound.
- The human ear is sensitive to a wide range of sound intensity; perhaps 10 trillion units of intensity on a linear scale. Measuring this wide range presents a cumbersome problem; therefore, a logarithmic scale is used to express the intensity range to which the human ear is sensitive. On this scale, the ear is sensitive to 130 units called **decibels** (dB). As mentioned earlier, a decibel is one tenth of a **bel**, a unit of measure named after Alexander Graham Bell.

Sound Pressure Level and Hearing Level

- Instead of describing intensity, one can measure the pressure of sound. Therefore, intensity of a sound is expressed in terms of decibels at a certain **sound pressure level** (dB SPL). Sound pressure is the square root of power, which is measured in **watts**. The pressure itself is measured in terms of **pascals** (Pa).
- Sound should reach a certain minimum intensity to stimulate the human auditory system. This minimum level is called the **hearing level** (HL). Sounds of different frequencies need to reach different minimum levels before they stimulate the human ear.
- For example, sounds of 1000–4000 Hz can stimulate the auditory system at lower intensities than those at other frequencies. This differential sensitivity of the ear to different frequencies creates problems in the measurement of hearing and hearing loss. To solve this problem, the minimum SPL required to stimulate the auditory system is arbitrarily set at zero for all frequencies. This minimum level is known as the 0 dB HL.
- Loudness or intensity of speech also is measured in terms of dB SPL. Intensity of normal conversational speech varies between 50 and 70 dB SPL. Very intense sounds exceed 100 dB SPL and may induce pain.

Introduction to the Acoustic Analysis of Speech

- A variety of instruments are used in analyzing the acoustic properties of speech. Most instruments feed information to a computer that has specialized software to analyze the speech or other sound input (Behrman, 2018; Raphael et al., 2012).
- There are several basic techniques for acoustic recording and analysis of speech. Older methods include nondigital or analog methods. Newer methods include digital signal processing (DSP) techniques.
- The sound **spectrograph** is an electronic instrument that graphically records the changing intensity levels of the frequency components in a complex sound wave. The display of the running short-term spectrum is referred to as a **spectrogram**.
- In creating a sound spectrogram

  - a speaker speaks into a microphone which transduces the speech sample so that air pressure variations of the acoustic signal are put into the form of voltage variations.
  - the electrical signal is converted to an electromagnetic signal for storage on the magnetic drum of the spectrograph.
  - the stored magnetic pattern is converted back into an electrical signal for analysis as a spectrogram.
  - the signal is then filtered so that one can determine energy in various frequency regions.
  - the current of the electrical signal is amplified and fed to a marking stylus.
  - as the current flows from the stylus to the paper, there is localized burning of the paper. The burning produces a blackening of the paper in proportion to the current flowing through the stylus.

- The resulting spectrogram is a three-dimensional display of time, intensity, and frequency. Frequency is plotted on the vertical axis, increasing from bottom to top. Intensity is represented on the "gray scale," or the blackness of the pattern. Time appears on the horizontal axis and proceeds from left to right.
- One component of speech displayed on a spectrogram is fundamental frequency. **Fundamental frequency** (mentioned at the beginning of this chapter) can be defined as the lowest frequency of a periodic wave; it is the principal component of a sound wave and has the greatest wavelength. Fundamental frequency can further be defined as the tone produced by the vibration of the vocal folds before the air reaches any cavities. It is the first harmonic.
- In a periodic complex sound, all frequencies can be characterized as whole-number multiples of the fundamental frequency. These tones, called **harmonics** or **overtones**, occur over the fundamental frequency.
- In terms of acoustic analysis, vowels are generally easier to analyze acoustically than consonants. In a normal speaker who has no vocal pathology, vowels are associated with a steady-state acoustic pattern and a steady-state articulatory configuration. In addition, vowels are often described very simply according to the frequencies of the first three formants (F1, F2, and F3 frequencies).
- When extraneous factors such as suprasegmentals are controlled, the fundamental frequency of vowels varies with their height. On average, high vowels have a higher fundamental frequency than low vowels. For example, /i/ has a higher fundamental frequency than /ɑ/.

- A general rule in relating vowel articulation to vowel formant frequencies is that F1 varies mostly as a result of tongue height, and F2 varies mostly as a result of tongue advancement (variation in the anterior-to-posterior position of the tongue in the oral cavity).
- All vowels can be described with basically the same acoustic characteristics, such as formant pattern or duration. Consonants are more complex. They are analyzed according to parameters, such as voice onset time, formant transition (when a vowel follows the consonant), turbulent airflow (in the case of fricatives), and others.
- **Voice onset time** refers to the time between the release of the stop consonant (e.g., /k/) and the beginning of the vowel. It can be further described as the time required to initiate sound at the vocal fold level. **Voice termination time** refers to the time required to cease vocal activity.

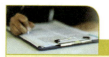

SUMMARY

- Sound, the result of vibrations of an elastic object, exists both as a physical phenomenon and as a sensory experience.
- Physically, sound is a compressional wave, which produces a sensation.
- The frequency of sound is measured by the number of cycles per second or hertz (Hz). The intensity of sound is expressed in units called decibels.
- The acoustic analysis of speech is generally conducted through use of a sound spectrograph, which produces a spectrogram. The spectrogram displays various components, such as fundamental frequency and many other characteristics of vowels and consonants.

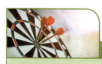

CHAPTER HIGHLIGHTS

- Phonetics is the study of speech sounds in terms of their physical, physiological, and acoustic properties. The main branches of phonetics include acoustic, articulatory/physiological, auditory, applied, experimental, and descriptive phonetics. This chapter is on acoustic and articulatory/physiological phonetics.
- The International Phonetic Alphabet, or IPA, is a set of internationally used phonetic symbols of vowels and consonants. Phonetic transcription of sounds can be broad, reflecting only vowels and consonants, or narrow, reflecting more detail about an individual speaker's sound production.
- Speech sounds can be broadly classified as consonants or vowels, which are described by their role in the production and perception of syllables. Syllables are motor units composed of an onset, a nucleus, and a coda.

- Speech sounds can be more narrowly classified according to two major approaches. The distinctive feature approach describes each phoneme according to a cluster of features that are either present (+) or absent (−) in that phoneme. The place-voice-manner approach describes consonants according to place, voicing, and manner of articulation.
- Sounds, or phonemes, produced within the context of conversational speech, get influenced by other sounds in the context, a phenomenon described as coarticulation.
- Such suprasegmentals as length of sounds, stress, rate of speech, pitch, volume, and juncture add variety and meaning to running speech.
- Acoustics, a branch of physics, is the study of sound as a physical phenomenon. Psychoacoustics is the study of how humans respond to sound as a physical phenomenon. Physically, sound is a compressional wave that causes a sensation. Sound exists both as a physical phenomenon and as a sensory (perceptual) experience.
- Sound, a result of vibrations of an elastic object, is propagated through waves of disturbances in molecules. A vibrating object is the source of sound, and media such as air, gas, water, and metal can transmit sound. Mass (density) and elasticity are two main properties of the medium that affect the transmission of sound.
- Vibrations repeat themselves (in frequencies, cycles, or hertz). Pure tones contain a single frequency and are the result of simple harmonic motion, also known as a sine wave or sinusoidal motion. Complex tones are a combination of two or more sounds of differing frequencies.
- Pitch is a sensory (perceptual) experience related to physical changes in frequency. The normal ear of a young adult can respond to frequencies within the range of 20 Hz to 20000 Hz. Loudness is a sensation related to physical amplitude or intensity of sound. Amplitude is measured in dynes or newtons. Intensity is often expressed in terms of decibels at a certain sound pressure level (SPL). A decibel (dB) is one tenth of a bel, a basic unit of measure.
- The minimum intensity of sound needed to stimulate the human auditory system, called the hearing level, differs for different frequencies. However, on all audiometers, the minimum required to stimulate the human ear is arbitrarily set at 0 dB for all frequencies. The intensity of normal conversational speech varies between 50 and 70 dB SPL.

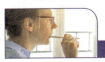

STUDY AND REVIEW QUESTIONS

1. The "typical" speaker of Standard American English would produce the word *emancipation* as

    A. /Imansʌpeʃʌn/.

    B. /imansʌpeIʃən/.

    C. /imænsəpeIʃən/.

    D. /Imʌnsʌpeʃn/.

2. The /r/ and /l/ sounds may both be categorized as

    A. rhotics.

    B. glides.

    C. laterals.

    D. liquids.

3. A semivowel that can be categorized as a voiced bilabial glide that is +anterior and +continuant is the

   A. /j/.
   B. /w/.
   C. /ʃ/.
   D. /r/.

4. The term coarticulation refers to

   A. speech sounds being modified due to the influence of adjacent sounds to the point that there are perceptible changes in sounds.
   B. the extent to which vocal tract configurations change shape during the production of consonants and vowels in running speech.
   C. the influence of one phoneme upon another in production and perception wherein two different articulators move simultaneously to produce two different speech sounds.
   D. the influence of various syllables upon one another when a client recites a phonetically balanced list of words.

5. Broad phonemic transcription involves

   A. the use of IPA symbols to transcribe phonemes by enclosing them within slash marks (e.g., /f/).
   B. the use of diacritical markers to transcribe phonemes by enclosing them within slash marks (e.g., /f/).
   C. the transcription of allophones by placing them within brackets (e.g., [f]).
   D. the transcription of allophones by the use of diacritical markers.

6. If a speaker said, "I just love 'em and leave 'em," the phrase "leave 'em" could be transcribed as

   A. [liv ʊm].
   B. [lev] [em].
   C. /liv ʊhm/.
   D. /liv m̩/.

7. The two properties of a medium that affect sound transmission are

   A. amplitude and intensity.
   B. mass and elasticity.
   C. compression and rarefaction.
   D. pressure and force.

8. A sinusoidal wave is a sound wave

   A. that is asymmetrical.
   B. with multiple peaks and valleys.
   C. with multiple frequencies.
   D. that is a result of simple harmonic motion.

9. A natural frequency is a frequency

   A. with which a source of sound vibrates naturally.
   B. that is unrelated to the mass and stiffness of the vibrating body.
   C. that is the center frequency of a formant.
   D. that refers to the simple harmonic motion.

10. An octave is

   A. the amount of molecular displacement per unit of time.
   B. the amount of time between cycles.
   C. an indication of interval between two frequencies.
   D. a measure of the magnitude (intensity, strength) of the sound signal.

11. The back-and-forth movement of air molecules because of a vibrating object is referred to as

   A. oscillation.
   B. amplitude.
   C. velocity.
   D. displacement.

12. The lowest frequency of a periodic wave is also known as

   A. the fundamental frequency or second harmonic.
   B. the fundamental frequency or first harmonic.
   C. the formant frequency or first harmonic.
   D. the first octave or the fundamental frequency.

13. When two or more sounds of differing frequencies are combined, the result is a

   A. complex tone whose vibrations may be periodic or aperiodic.
   B. complex tone; the vibrations are always periodic, where waves repeat themselves at regular intervals.
   C. pure tone, where the vibrations are usually periodic.
   D. pure tone, where the vibrations are always aperiodic.

14. When a speaker is producing a vowel and the vowel is being acoustically analyzed, one can state as a general rule that

   A. F2 varies mostly as a result of tongue height, and F1 varies mostly as a result of tongue position (variation in the anterior-to-posterior position of the tongue in the oral cavity).
   B. F2 varies mostly as a result of tongue height, and F3 varies mostly as a result of tongue advancement (variation in the anterior-to-posterior position of the tongue in the oral cavity).
   C. F1 varies mostly as a result of tongue height, and F3 varies mostly as a result of tongue advancement (variation in the anterior-to-posterior position of the tongue in the oral cavity).
   D. F1 varies mostly as a result of tongue height, and F2 varies mostly as a result of tongue advancement (variation in the anterior-to-posterior position of the tongue in the oral cavity).

15. In a periodic complex sound, tones that occur over the fundamental frequency and can be characterized as whole-number multiples of the fundamental frequency are called

   A. complex sinusoidal wave forms.
   B. autocorrelational periodic wave forms.
   C. harmonics.
   D. tonal configuration forms.

16. Diacritical marks are

  A. useful in making broad phonetic transcription.
  (B.) useful in making narrow phonetic transcription that gives more detailed information on a speaker's phonetic characteristics.
  C. Not useful in transcribing disordered speech.
  D. Used only in the analysis of speech with a foreign accent.

17. The term **coda** refers to

  A. the nucleus of the syllable.
  B. the initial sound in a syllable.
  (C.) the consonant at the end of the syllable.
  D. open syllables.

18. The **manner of articulation** refers to

  (A.) the degree of type of constriction of the vocal tract during consonant production.
  B. the actions of the primary articulators.
  C. the vocal fold vibrations during speech.
  D. a distinction between consonants and vowels.

19. During the typical speech production, vowels

  A. are often unvoiced.
  B. require interrupted airflow.
  C. require a lowered velum.
  (D.) may stand alone.

20. Compared to unstressed syllables, stressed syllables are typically

  A. softer in intensity.
  (B.) longer and higher in pitch.
  C. lower in pitch.
  D. shorter in duration.

References and Recommended Readings at www.advancedreviewpractice.com

STUDY AND REVIEW ANSWERS

1. C. The "typical" speaker of Standard American English would produce the word "emancipation" as: /imænsəpeɪʃən/.
2. D. The /r/ and /l/ sounds may both be categorized as liquids.
3. B. The /w/ sound is a semivowel that can be categorized as a voiced bilabial glide that is +anterior and +continuant.
4. C. Coarticulation is specifically defined as the influence of one phoneme upon another in production and perception wherein two different articulators move simultaneously to produce two different speech sounds.

5. A. Broad phonemic transcription involves use of IPA symbols to transcribe phonemes by enclosing them within slash marks.
6. D. If a speaker said, "I just love 'em and leave 'em," the phrase "leave 'em" could be transcribed as / liv m̩/.
7. B. The two properties of a medium that affect sound transmission are mass and elasticity.
8. D. A sinusoidal wave is a sound wave that is a result of simple harmonic motion.
9. A. A natural frequency is a frequency with which a source of sound vibrates naturally and that is affected by the mass and stiffness of the vibrating body.
10. C. An octave is an indication of the interval between two frequencies.
11. A. The back-and-forth movement of air molecules because of a vibrating object is referred to as oscillation.
12. B. The lowest frequency of a periodic wave is also known as the fundamental frequency or first harmonic.
13. A. When two or more sounds of differing frequencies are combined, the result is a complex tone; the vibrations that make up this complex tone may be said to be periodic or aperiodic.
14. D. F1 varies mostly as a result of tongue height, and F2 varies mostly as a result of tongue advancement (variation in the anterior-to-posterior position of the tongue in the oral cavity).
15. C. In a periodic complex sound, tones that occur over the fundamental frequency and can be characterized as whole-number multiples of the fundamental frequency are called *harmonics*.
16. B. Diacritical marks are useful in making narrow phonetic transcription that gives more detailed information on a speaker's phonetic characteristics.
17. C. The term *coda* refers to the consonant at the end of the syllable (arrest of the syllable pulse).
18. A. The *manner of articulation* refers to the degree or type of constriction of the vocal tract during consonant production.
19. D. During speech production, vowels may stand alone (not true of consonants)
20. B. Stressed syllables are longer and higher in pitch compared to unstressed syllables.

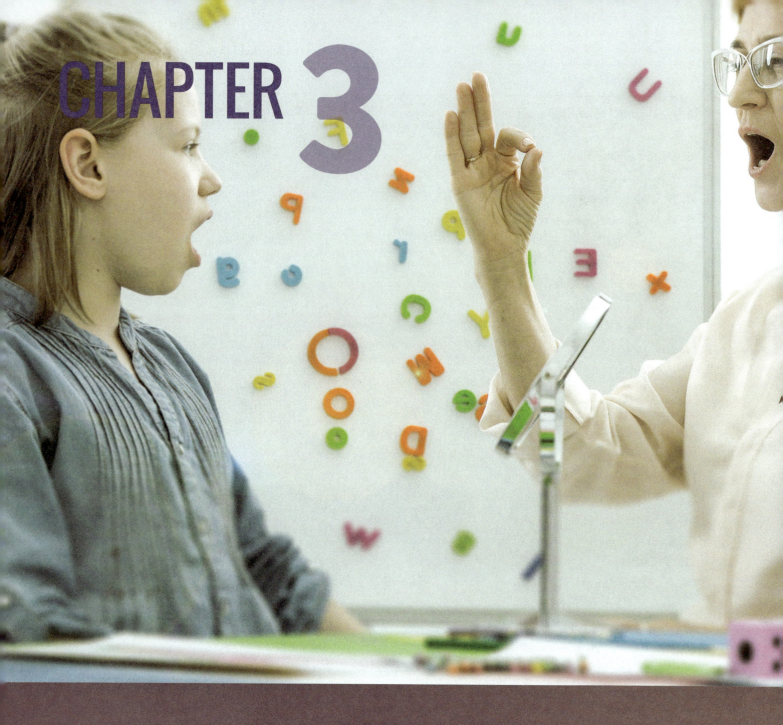

CHAPTER 3

LANGUAGE DEVELOPMENT IN CHILDREN

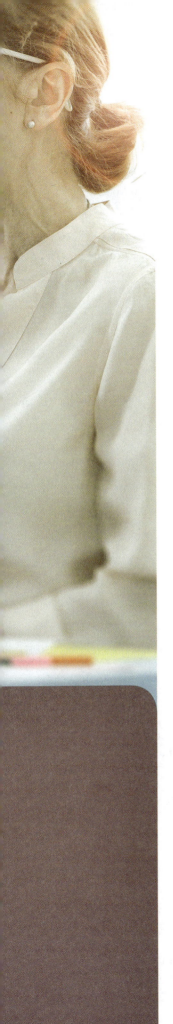

It is language that makes people so efficient at communication. It is language that provides people with a mechanism for social interaction and communication with one another. As societies have become more complex, organized, and interrelated, the ability to communicate effectively through language has become increasingly important. Good language skills are now crucial for even mundane occupational success and survival, as vocations have become more sophisticated and interrelated.

From a behavioral viewpoint, language can be defined as a form of social behavior that is shaped and maintained by a verbal community. The definition implies that language cannot be learned or maintained without the mediation of other people. From a linguistic viewpoint, language can be described as a code or system of symbols that represents concepts formed through exposure and experience. For example, the word *cookie* is a symbol for something sweet, small, and often round that children and adults like to eat for dessert. When children learn language, they learn words, or symbols, that represent concepts. For a child to learn the word *cookie*, it is helpful if he has actually had direct experience with cookies.

To understand what constitutes a language disorder in children, it is necessary to first understand typical language development. In this chapter, we discuss (a) basic definitions of aspects of language, (b) language development milestones in typically developing children, and (c) theories of language development.

TERMS AND DEFINITIONS

There are various approaches to the study of language. The behavioral approach, which will be described in a later section of this chapter, views language as verbal behavior. The linguistic approach describes different components of language. Linguistics is the study of language, its structure, and the rules that govern its structure. Linguists, specialists in linguistics, have traditionally analyzed language in terms of several subfields of study. These include morphology, syntax, semantics, pragmatics, and phonology. (Phonology is described in Chapter 5.)

Morphology

Morphology is the study of word structure. It describes how words are formed out of more basic elements of language called morphemes.

- A **morpheme** is the smallest meaningful unit of a language. Morphemes are considered minimal, because if they were subdivided any further, they would become meaningless. Each morpheme is different from the others because each signals a distinct meaning. Morphemes are used to form words.

- **Base**, **root**, or **free** morphemes are words that have meaning, cannot be broken down into smaller parts, and can have other morphemes added to them. Examples of free morphemes are *ocean*, *establish*, *book*, *color*, *connect*, and *hinge*. These words mean something, can stand by themselves, and cannot be broken down into smaller units.
- These words also can have other morphemes added to them. **Bound** or **grammatical morphemes**, which cannot convey meaning by themselves, must be joined with free morphemes in order to have meaning.
- In the following examples, the free morphemes are underlined; the bound morphemes are in capital letters:

    <u>ocean</u>S   <u>establish</u>MENT   <u>book</u>ED   <u>color</u>FUL   DIS<u>connect</u>   UN<u>hinge</u>

- Common bound or grammatical morphemes include the following:

    –ing, the present progressive (cook*ing*, writ*ing*)
    –s, the regular plural morpheme (cat*s*, basket*s*)
    –s, the possessive inflection (man*'s*, lady*'s*)
    –ed, the regular past tense (comb*ed*, wash*ed*)

- Bound morphemes can be divided into the subcategories of prefixes and suffixes. A **prefix** is added at the beginning of a base morpheme; a **suffix** is added at the end of a base morpheme. For example, see the table that follows:

Whole word	Prefix	Base word	Suffix
prearranged	pre	arrange	ed
disestablishment	dis	establish	ment
misunderstanding	mis	understand	ing

- **Allomorphs** are variations of morphemes; they do not alter the original meaning of the morpheme. For example, the plural morpheme can be denoted by the following allomorphs (with their sounds in parentheses): box*es* (ez), leav*es* (z), cat*s* (s).
- **Derivational morphemes** include prefixes and suffixes; they change whole classes of words. For example:

Happy	+	ily	=	Happily
(adjective)		(derivational morpheme)		(adverb)
Special	+	ness	=	Specialness
(adjective)		(derivational morpheme)		(noun)

- Inflectional morphemes are suffixes only, and they change the state of or increase the precision of the free morpheme. For example, plural –s and past tense –ed are inflectional morphemes. The noun *cat* + *–s* creates a new noun *cats*, meaning more than one. The verb *cook* + *–ed* creates a new verb *cooked*, meaning the action was done in the past.

- Morphemes are a means of modifying word structures to change meaning. The morphology of a given language describes the rules of such modifications. It describes what kinds of morphemic combinations are permissible in a given language.
- Speakers manipulate morphemes so that they can change the meaning of a sentence. For example, one can change "He cook*s* a meal" to "He cook*ed* a meal." By adding the past-tense *–ed* morpheme and omitting the third-person singular *–s*, the speaker changes sentence meaning.
- Sentence meaning is also conveyed by the order of the words in a sentence. This order is dictated by the rules of syntax.

Syntax

Syntax and morphology are concerned with two major categories of language structure. Morphology is the study of word structure; syntax is the study of sentence structure. The basic meaning of the word **syntax** is "to join," "to put together." In the study of language, syntax involves the following:

- The arrangement of words to form meaningful sentences
- The word order and overall structure of a sentence
- A collection of rules that specify the ways and order in which words may be combined to form sentences in a particular language

- Syntactic rules differ in different languages. For example, in English, one might use the phrase "the new car." In Spanish, one might say *"el carro nuevo"* ("the car new"). All languages are creative, and speakers can generate an infinite variety of structures.
- Structures, however, are governed by rules of syntax. Normally, speakers of a language do not produce structures with random and meaningless word order. For example, an English speaker could say, "He said he was going to come but didn't." Due to syntactic rules, a speaker could not say, "He going to was said he didn't but come."
- Sentences can be classified according to their functions, as follows:
  - **Passive** sentences, in which the subject receives the action of the verb ("The cat was petted by Mark.")
  - **Active** sentences, in which the subject performs the actions of the verb ("Mark petted the cat.")
  - **Interrogatives**, or questions ("Did you see that gorgeous sunset?")
  - **Declaratives**, which make statements ("The sunset was gorgeous.")
  - **Imperatives**, which state commands ("Shut the door.")
  - **Exclamatory** sentences, which express strong feeling ("I never said that!")
- As they mature in syntactic development, children begin to use compound and complex sentences, which can be defined as follows:
  - A **compound sentence** contains two or more **independent clauses** joined by a comma and a conjunction or by a semicolon. There are no subordinate clauses in a compound sentence. A **clause** contains a subject and a predicate.

- An **independent** or **main clause** has a subject and a predicate and can stand alone, as shown:

The policeman held up the sign,	and	the cars stopped.
(independent clause)	**(conjunction)**	**(independent clause)**
The dog ate her dog chow hungrily;		later she begged for more.
(independent clause + semicolon)		**(independent clause)**

- A **complex sentence** contains one independent clause and one or more **dependent** or **subordinate clauses**. A dependent or subordinate clause has a subject and predicate but cannot stand alone, as shown:

I will drive my car to Reno	if I have enough gas.
(independent clause)	**(dependent clause)**
You can comb your hair	after you have washed it.
(independent clause)	**(dependent clause)**

- Languages have different syntactic structures. In English, the basic syntactic structure is subject + verb + object. This structure, usually called the kernel sentence, can also be called the phrase structure or base structure.

Semantics

Semantics is the study of **meaning** in language. The semantic component is the meaning conveyed by words, phrases, and sentences.

- Semantics includes a person's **vocabulary** or lexicon. Vocabulary development depends heavily upon environmental exposure, as well as the individual capacity each child brings to the learning situation (Fogle, 2019).
- Important aspects of vocabulary development include knowledge of the following:
  - Antonyms, or opposites (e.g., *big–little*)
  - Synonyms, or words that mean similar things (e.g., *attractive–pretty*; *clear–transparent*)
  - Multiple meanings of words (e.g., *rock, pound*)
  - Humor (e.g., riddles, puns, jokes)
  - Figurative language, including

- Metaphors (He's drowning in money.)
- Idioms (It's raining cats and dogs. She kicked the bucket.)
- Proverbs (Don't put all your eggs in one basket.)

  - Deictic words, or words whose referents change depending on who is speaking (e.g., *this, here, that, come, go*)

- **Semantic categories** are used to sort words. Examples of a few of these categories are **recurrence** (concept of *more*), **rejection** (*no*), and **causality** (*cause and effect*). A child using recurrence might say, "More milk"; if that child didn't want any more, she might show rejection by saying, "No milk."

- Most words in a child's first 50 spoken words refer to things that the child can act upon (e.g., toys, objects). Young children may use **overextension** (e.g., all round items are balls; all tall men with glasses and brown hair are Daddy). They may also use **underextension** (e.g., only an Oreo is a cookie; only the family poodle is a dog, so a neighbor's German shepherd is not a dog).

- World knowledge and word knowledge are components of semantics. **World knowledge** involves a person's autobiographical and experiential memory and understanding of particular events. For example, a child might be able to discuss an aquarium because he has been to several and has been exposed to marine life. Such a child could use words, such as *octopus*, *jellyfish*, *seaweed*, and others, because he has seen them and experienced them personally. He has world knowledge of these words.

- **Word knowledge** is primarily verbal and contains word and symbol definitions. For example, a child might be able to name the planets in the solar system because she has learned them in kindergarten. She has not visited these planets, obviously, but has seen pictures of them and has memorized their names. She has word knowledge of the planets.

- A child's word knowledge depends heavily upon his or her world knowledge (Roseberry-McKibbin, 2013, 2018b). For example, a child who has never visited a zoo or been exposed to books about a zoo (world knowledge) might have difficulty understanding and using the word *zoo* (word knowledge).

- An important concept emphasized today in semantics is called **quick incidental learning**, or **fast mapping**. This refers to children's ability to learn a new word on the basis of just a few exposures to it. Typical children use fast mapping to rapidly expand their vocabularies.

- Another important semantic aspect of children's language development is developing the ability to categorize words. For example, children must learn that *tiger*, *lion*, *dog*, *cat*, *pig*, and *horse* fall under the category of *animals*.

- The use of categories helps bring order to the child's experiences. The child who successfully categorizes does not need to treat each experience as a totally new one. New experiences may be "filed" under preexisting categories or under mental constructs the child has that allow him or her to group similar items together.

- Vocabulary knowledge is an important indicator of language and literacy skills and, eventually, of overall academic success.

Pragmatics

Pragmatics is the study of rules that govern the use of language in social situations. In pragmatics, one focuses on use of language in social context. Pragmatics places greater emphasis on **functions**, or uses of language, than on structure.

- One can view pragmatics as the dimension of language that considers the **context** of the utterance (i.e., the situation, the listener–speaker relationship) and the **function** of the utterance (i.e., its purpose or goal).
- **Functions of language** (described in more detail later in this chapter) include the following:

  - **Labeling**—naming something; e.g., a child is playing with a puppy and says "tail"
  - **Protesting**—objecting to something; e.g., "Don't do that!"
  - **Commenting**—describing or identifying objects; e.g., "That's a cookie."

- Important functions of utterances include the following:

  - Providing listeners with adequate information without redundancy
  - Making a sequence of statements coherent and logical
  - Taking turns with other speakers
  - Maintaining a topic
  - Repairing communication breakdowns

- Language context involves the following:

  - Where the utterance takes place
  - To whom the utterance is directed
  - What and who is present at the time

- Children with effective pragmatic skills display adequate **cohesion**, or the ability to order and organize utterances in a message so that they build logically on one another.
- As they get older, children with effective pragmatic skills distinguish between and appropriately use **direct** and **indirect speech acts** or **requests**. For example, as a direct speech act or request, a child could say, "Bring me the ball." As a request, the child could say, "Will you bring me the ball?" Or as an indirect speech act, the child might say, "Wouldn't it be nice if I had the ball?"
- Indirect speech acts or requests are used to convey politeness. By the time a child is 6 years old, she can respond to many forms of indirect requests. She can also use indirect requests if she chooses to.
- Pragmatic skills also involve the appropriate knowledge and use of discourse. **Discourse** refers to how utterances are related to one another; it has to do with the connected flow of language. Discourse can involve a dialogue between two people, or even conversational exchange in a small group. When people talk with one another, they are engaging in discourse or conversation.
- **Narratives** are a form of discourse in which the speaker tells a story. The speaker talks about a logical sequence of events. This sequence can involve an actual episode from the speaker's life, such as a trip he or she took; it can involve a story about an event, such as a fairy tale or movie, that did not happen to the speaker directly.

- Pragmatic skills are heavily influenced by culture. For example, in Japanese culture, the use of indirect speech acts is believed to convey speaker sophistication and sensitivity. In American culture, people who use many indirect speech acts may be viewed as weak, unassertive, and unsure of themselves.
- Pragmatic skills are increasingly recognized as important for social, academic, and vocational success. Effective pragmatic skills enable speakers to relate successfully to others within their linguistic and cultural milieus.

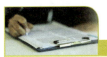

SUMMARY

- The linguistic approach analyzes language according to five components: morphology, syntax, semantics, pragmatics, and phonology. In this section, we have discussed the first four components.
- Morphology involves the study of word structure.
- Syntax includes rules for word order and rules for combining words into sentences.
- Semantics involves word meanings. A child's semantic skills are his vocabulary skills, which are influenced by word and world knowledge.
- Pragmatics are the social skills of language—how, where, when, and with whom language is used.

TYPICAL LANGUAGE DEVELOPMENT: DEVELOPMENTAL MILESTONES

The development of language rests upon several major variables that interact with one another. First, the individual child brings innate characteristics to the situation. Such characteristics may include, for example, a high IQ or a limited attention span. Second, the child's environment, including the caregivers in that environment, plays a major role (Owens, 2018; Moore & Montgomery, 2018; Roseberry-McKibbin, 2018a; Roseberry-McKibbin, 2018b). The more stimulating the environment, the better and faster children develop language skills. Language development also depends on cultural expectations. In some cultures, children are to be seen and not heard; those children may develop good visual skills, but their verbal skills may not develop at a rate expected by mainstream American professionals.

In this section, we describe language development milestones that represent a range of expectations for when children may develop certain language structures. These milestones depend heavily on the child's linguistic and cultural background, and cultures differ in their expectations for children's language development. This section focuses on the role of the caregiver and on semantic, syntactic, morphological, and pragmatic development as consistent with general mainstream American social expectations. (Chapter 5 contains detailed information about phonological development.) Developing literacy skills are briefly addressed.

Role of the Caregiver in Language Development

Caregivers play a crucial role in children's language development, particularly in the early years before school (Roseberry-McKibbin, 2018a). Caregivers can be the child's mother, father, grandparents, older siblings, day-care providers, and others. In the United States, in a child's very early months, often the primary caregiver is the mother.

- Ideally, a baby's mother or primary caregiver specifically gears communication to him by use of motherese. **Motherese**, or **child-directed speech** (CDS), refers to speech that includes several characteristics that help babies attend and respond to what they are hearing.
- First, in motherese, or CDS, utterances are produced with a higher pitch and greater pitch fluctuations. Babies tend to pay more attention to utterances that are higher pitched and that show variation. Utterances are also produced at a slower rate than normal speech and are usually clear and fluent.
- In addition, motherese is characterized by simpler utterances, longer pauses between utterances, and shorter utterances. Words used generally refer to events or objects in the here and now.
- Infants and young children also learn early turn-taking skills through interactions with their caregivers. Games such as peek-a-boo and pat-a-cake help infants learn rudimentary turn-taking skills that serve as the foundation of later conversational turn-taking.
- Eye contact is another important form of communication that begins in infancy. Parents frequently have more difficulty relating to children who are blind or have autism and thus avoid eye contact.
- If a baby cries and the caregiver responds immediately, this increases the baby's motivation to communicate.
- Motivated babies attempt more varied and frequent interactions. They often develop language at a more rapid pace than babies who are not motivated to communicate. Even babies who are only 3 months old begin to produce more speech-like sounds if an adult responds to their vocalizations.
- A child's language development is highly dependent on the quality of her interaction with her caregivers.
- High-quality interaction that begins in infancy helps children to develop language faster; frequently, such children's language shows early signs of sophistication. Conversely, children who are ignored or punished when they attempt to communicate may show delays or slowness in developing language skills.
- Research has consistently isolated two factors that are associated with more rapid, rich language development in infants and young children: (a) amount of talking and (b) caregiver responsiveness. Babies and young children who are exposed to greater amounts of talking and who have caregivers who respond immediately and positively to their initiations show more rapid development of language milestones and more extensive development of language skills, especially in the areas of syntax and semantics (Marklund, Marklund, Lacerda, & Schwarz, 2016).
- Caregivers who follow the infant's **line of regard** look at what the infant is looking at. For example, if the infant is looking at the family dog, the caregiver can follow her line of regard and look at the dog, also. It is helpful for the caregiver to comment about what the infant and caregiver are observing together.

Birth–1 Year

The following developmental milestones are observed in typically developing children from birth to 1 year of age (Newman, 2017; Owens, 2016; Paul, Norbury, & Gosse, 2018; Stoel-Gammon & Menn, 2017).

Birth–3 Months

Between birth and 3 months, the typical child shows the following developmental milestones:

- Displays startle response to loud sound
- Visually tracks, or moves eyes, to source of sound
- Attends to and turns head toward voice; turns toward sound source
- Smiles reflexively
- Cries for assistance
- Quiets when picked up
- Ceases activity or coos back when person talks (by two months)
- Vocalizes predominantly vowels

4–6 Months

At 4–6 months, the typical child reaches the following developmental milestones:

- Responds by raising arms when mother says, "Come here," and reaches toward child (by 6 months)
- Moves or looks toward family members when they are named (e.g., "Where's Daddy?")
- Explores the vocal mechanism through vocal play, such as growling, squealing, yelling, making "raspberries" (bilabial trills)
- Begins to produce adult-like vowels
- Begins marginal babbling; produces double syllables (e.g., "baba"); puts lips together for /m/
- Responds to name (5 months)
- Vocalizes pleasure and displeasure
- Varies volume, pitch, and rate of vocalizations

7–9 Months

At 7–9 months, the typical child reaches the following developmental milestones:

- Looks at some common objects when the objects' names are spoken
- Comprehends "no"
- Begins to use some gestural language; plays pat-a-cake, peek-a-boo; shakes head for "no"
- Uses a wide variety of sound combinations
- Uses inflected vocal play, intonation patterns
- Imitates intonation and speech sounds of others (by 9 months)
- Uses variegated babbling (e.g., "mabamaba") (at approximately 9 months)
- Uncovers hidden toy (beginning of object permanence)

10–12 Months

At 10–12 months, the typical child reaches the following developmental milestones:

- Understands up to 10 words, such as *no, bye-bye, pat-a-cake, hot*; understands one simple direction like "sit down," especially when command is accompanied by gesture

- Begins to relate symbol and object; uses first true word
- Gives block, toy, or object upon request
- Understands and follows simple directions regarding body action
- Looks in correct place for hidden toys (object permanence)
- Turns head instantly to own name
- Gestures or vocalizes to indicate wants and needs
- Jabbers loudly; uses wide variety of sounds and intonations; varies pitch when vocalizing

Pragmatics

As infants develop pragmatics skills, they typically go through the following stages:

- The child uses **perlocutionary behavior**, in which "signals" have an effect on the listener or observer but lack communicative intent. For example, if a child smiles reflexively, an observer may smile back or laugh, even though the child didn't intend to express pleasure or joy.
- At 9–10 months, the child uses **illocutionary behavior**, signaling to carry out some socially organized action, such as pointing and laughing; uses intentional communication.
- At approximately 12 months, the child enters the **locutionary stage**—begins to use words.
- The child establishes **joint reference**, or the ability to focus attention on an event or object as directed by another person. (Caregivers begin by establishing eye contact in the early months; later, they point to or name objects that both they and the child can focus on.)

1–2 Years

The following developmental milestones are observed in typically developing children between 1 and 2 years of age.

Syntax

Typically developing children between 12 and 18 months of age use one-word sentences and are in the **holophrastic** single-word phase, in which one word represents a complex idea. For example, "Up" might mean "Please pick me up because I don't want to sit here playing with the dog anymore." Average MLU (mean length of utterance) is 1.0–2.0 morphemes.

- The child also uses sentence-like words and communicates relationships by using one word plus vocal and body cues. The sentence-like word can serve several basic functions:
  - The emphatic or imperative statement ("Car!") (child telling you to look at a car)
  - The question ("Car?") (child asking if an object is a car)
  - The declarative statement ("Car.") (child saying an object is a car and not something else)
- Most children produce 50 words by 18 months of age. Between 18 and 24 months, they begin to put two words together.
- At 2 years, they may use three- or four-word responses, combining three- and four-word utterances about 50% of the time and using two-word utterances the other 50% of the time.

- At 24 months of age, a child uses 200–300 words expressively.
- Near 24 months of age, the child uses "and" to form a conjoined sentence.
- Approximately 51% of the child's utterances consist of nouns.

Semantics

- The 18–24-month-old child sometimes uses **holophrastic** speech, in which one word is used to communicate a variety of meanings. Around 18 months, the child produces 50 words. Two-word combinations become more common at this time.
- The child at 12–18 months shows understanding of some words and simple commands, including "no." Around 18 months, the child understands about 200 words.
- The child's most frequent lexical categories are nominals (e.g., *ball*, *Mommy*) and verbs (e.g., *drink*, *run*). These nominals are used in reference to things of greatest importance in the child's environment (e.g., objects, people, actions of immediate interest).
- The child also uses **semantic relations**, or utterances that reflect meaning based on relationships between different words (e.g., cause–effect relationships). The child begins with one-word utterances and gradually progresses to two-word utterances (see Tables 3.1 and 3.2).

The child also does the following during this period:

- Uses overextensions; for example, all brown-eyed, slender women are "Mommy"
- Answers the question "What's this?"; responds to yes–no questions by nodding or shaking head
- Says, "All gone" (emerging negation)
- Follows one-step commands or simple directions accompanied by gestures (e.g., "Give Mommy the spoon.")
- Follows directions using one or two spatial concepts, such as **in** or **on** (19–24 months)
- Points to one to five body parts on command; points to recognized objects (emerging nomination)
- Listens to simple stories; especially likes to hear stories repeated (19–24 months)
- Asks for "more"
- Refers to self with pronoun and name ("Me Johnny") (19–24 months)
- Verbalizes immediate experiences (e.g., "Bath hot!")
- Begins to use some verbs and adjectives

Pragmatics

The child uses verbal and nonverbal communication to control the behavior of others, satisfy needs and wants, interact with others, express emotions or interest, imagine, inform, and explore and categorize.

- **Presuppositions** emerge. Between 1 and 2 years of age, the child uses expressions that have shared meaning for the listener and speaker.
- The child begins to understand some rules of dialogue (e.g., "When someone talks, you need to listen"). The child is able to take the role of both speaker and listener.
- The child uses nonverbal as well as verbal communication to signal intent.

Table 3.1

Relations Expressed by Single-Word Utterances

Before children reach the two-word utterance stage, they typically use single words to express themselves. The relations expressed by single words are as follows:

Relation	Definition	Example
Attribution	Child uses an adjective; a property or characteristic of an event, person, or object	*Big* doggy *Clean* dolly Face *dirty*
Action	Child requests or labels an action; child indicates movement relationships between objects and people	*Open* box Kitty *run* *Close* door
Locative action	Child refers to a change in an object's location	*There* doggy Ball *up*
Existence	Child attends to an item or object present in the immediate environment, especially a novel one	What's *that*? *This* kitty
Nonexistence	Child expects an action or object to be present when it is not; something was present but disappeared	*All gone* juice *Bye-bye* Mom *No* doggy
Denial	Child denies a statement or previous utterance (e.g., in response to a parent saying, "Is this a kitty?")	*No* kitty
Rejection	Child does not want something to happen; child refuses an object or action	*No* bath *No* beans
Recurrence	An event happens again; an object reappears or replaces another	*More* cookie *Another* doggy
Possession	Child identifies something as belonging to him or her, or to another person	*His* block Doll *mine*

2–3 Years

The following developmental milestones are observed in typically developing children between 2 and 3 years of age.

Syntax

The typically developing child of 2–3 years

- uses word combinations; has beginning phrase and sentence structure.
- has an average MLU of 2.0–4.0; at 36 months, sentences often average 3–4 words.
- combines 3–4 words in subject-verb-object format (e.g., "Daddy throw ball").
- uses telegraphic speech; word order is often object–verb (e.g., "Doggy sit"), verb–object (e.g., "Push Barbie"), subject–verb. Most sentences are incomplete.
- asks *wh–* questions (e.g., "*Wh*at's that?" "*Wh*en go home?" "*Wh*y brush teeth?") and yes–no questions. Yes–no questions are asked by adding a rising intonation at the end of the sentence.
- expresses negation by adding "no" or "not" in front of verbs (e.g., "Me not do it." "He no bite").

Table 3.2

Semantic Relations Expressed by Two-Word Utterances

Semantic relation	Structure	Example
Notice	Hi + noun	Hi doggy
Nomination	Demonstrative + noun	That chair
Instrumental	Verb + noun	Write [with] pencil
Conjunction	Noun + noun	Knife spoon
Recurrence	More + noun	More juice
Action–object	Verb + noun	Pet kitty
Action–indirect object	Verb + noun	Give [to] Mommy
Agent–action	Noun (agent) + verb	Doggy bark
Agent–object	Noun (agent) + noun	Baby [drink] juice
Possessor–possession	Noun (possessor) + noun	Mommy sock
Attribute–entity	Adjective/attributive + noun	Red ball
Entity + locative	Noun + locative	Juice [in] glass
Action + locative	Verb + noun	Jump [on] bed

Semantics

Comprehension usually precedes production. At 30 months, the child comprehends up to 2,400 words.

- At 30 months, expressive vocabulary is 200–600 words; the average is 425 words.
- At 36 months, the child comprehends up to 3,600 words.
- Meanings seem to be learned in sequence: objects, events, actions, adjectives, adverbs, spatial concepts, temporal (time) concepts.
- First pronouns used are self-referents, such as *I* and *me*.
- The typically developing child of 2–3 years
  - answers simple *wh–* questions (e.g., "*Wh*at runs?"); generally understands questions; begins asking *wh–* questions of adults (30 months).
  - can identify simple body parts.
  - carries out one- and two-part commands, such as "Pick up the sock and give it to Mommy."
  - understands plurals.
  - can give simple account of experiences and tell understandable stories (36 months).

Morphology

The child's use of bound morphemes expands greatly between 2 and 3 years of age, when the child

- develops inflections, such as *–ing*, spatial prepositions *in* and *on*, plurals, possessives, articles, and pronouns (see Table 3.3).
- develops simple, irregular past tense (e.g., *went*).

Table 3.3

Average Order of Acquisition of 14 Grammatical Morphemes in Three Children

Order of acquisition	Morphemes	Examples	Average MLU	Stage	Age of mastery (in months)
1	Present progressive –*ing*	Mom com*ing*, Dog bark*ing*	2.25	II	19–28
2/3	Prepositions *in*, *on*	Toy *in* box, Book *on* table	2.25	II	27–30
4	Regular plural inflection –*s*	My crayon*s*, Dog bone*s*	2.25	II	24–33
5	Irregular past-tense verbs	*Came, ran, sat, broke*	2.75	III	25–46
6	Possessive –*s*	Daddy*'s* hat, Baby*'s* bottle	2.75	III	26–40
7	Uncontractible copula	Here *it is*, There *I am*	2.75	III	27–39
8	Articles	I want *a* cookie, Give me *the* ball	3.50	IV	28–46
9	Past-tense regular –*ed*	Mom pour*ed* juice, I color*ed* pictures	3.50	IV	26–48
10	Regular third-person –*s*	Daddy cook*s*, Kitty meow*s*	3.50	IV	26–46
11	Irregular third person	*Does, has*	4.00	V	28–50
12	Uncontractible auxiliary	She *was* working	4.00	V	29–48
13	Contractible copula	He *is* nice, or He*'s* nice	4.00	V	29–49
14	Contractible auxiliary	Mom *is* coming, or Mom*'s* coming	4.00	V	30–50

Note. Adapted from *A First Language: The Early Stages*, by R. Brown, 1973, Cambridge, MA: Harvard University Press.

- develops copular *were*.
- develops *is* plus adjective (e.g., "That is pretty").
- develops regular past-tense verbs (e.g., *walked*).
- overregularizes past-tense inflections (e.g., *goed, throwed, falled*).
- overgeneralizes plural morphemes (e.g., *feets, mouses*).
- uses some memorized contractions, such as *don't, can't, it's, that's*.

Pragmatics

The child's utterances, although occasionally egocentric, generally have a communicative intent.

- The child demonstrates rapid topic shifts; a 3-year-old can sustain the topic of conversation only about 20% of the time.

- Communication includes criticism, commands, requests, threats, questions, and answers.
- Interpersonal communication expands; the child learns to adopt a role to express his own opinions and personality.

3–4 Years

The following developmental milestones are observed in typically developing children between 3 and 4 years of age.

Syntax

The typically developing child of 3–4 years

- learns clause-connecting devices, including coordination (e.g., "and") and subordination (e.g., "because"), and uses them in sentences.
- begins using complex verb phrases (e.g., "I should have been able to do it").
- begins using modal verbs (e.g., *could, should, would*).
- begins using **tag questions** (e.g., "You want to go, *don't you?*").
- begins using **embedded** forms, which rearrange or add elements within sentences (e.g., "The man *who came to dinner* stayed a week").
- begins using passive voice (e.g., "She's been bitten by a dog").
- uses mostly complete sentences; at 48 months, sentences average 5–5.5 words per utterance. MLU is approximately 3.0–5.0.
- uses mostly nouns, verbs, and personal pronouns.
- acquires *do* insertions and ability to make transformations (e.g., "Does the kitty run around?").
- uses negation in speech (e.g., "Timmy can't swim").
- begins using complex and compound sentences (e.g., "I can sing and dance"); 7% of sentences are compound or complex.

Semantics

The typically developing child of 3–4 years

- comprehends up to 4,200 words by 42 months; up to 5,600 words at 48 months.
- uses 900–1,000 words expressively.
- asks how, why, and when questions.
- understands some common opposites (e.g., *day–night, little–big, fast–slow*).
- knows full name, name of street, several nursery rhymes.
- labels most things in the environment.
- relates experiences and tells about activities in sequential order.
- can recite a poem from memory or sing a song (by 48 months).
- answers appropriately questions such as "Which is the boy?" "Where is the dress?" "What toys do you have?" (by 42 months).
- can complete opposite analogies, such as "Daddy is a man; Mommy is a _____" (by 48 months).
- understands most preschool children's stories (by 48 months).

- uses pronouns *you*, *they*, *us*, and *them*, as well as others, such as *I*, *me*.
- understands concepts, such as heavy–light, empty–full, more–less, around, in front of–in back of, next to, big–little, hard–soft, rough–smooth (by 42 months).
- supplies last word of sentence (e.g., "The apple is on the _____") (closure).
- appropriately answers "What if" questions (e.g., "What would you do if you fell down?") (by 43–48 months).

Morphology

The typically developing child of 3–4 years

- uses irregular plural forms (e.g., *children*, *mice*, *feet*).
- uses third-person singular, present tense (e.g., "He runs").
- consistently uses simple (regular) past and present progressives (e.g., *is running*) and negatives (e.g., *not*).
- uses inflection to convert adjective to causative (e.g., *sharp*, *sharpen*).
- uses simple (regular) plural forms correctly (e.g., *boys*, *houses*, *lights*).
- begins to use *is* at beginning of questions.
- uses contracted forms of modals (e.g., *can't*, *won't*).
- uses *and* as a conjunction.
- uses *is*, *are*, and *am* in sentences.
- uses possessive markers consistently (e.g., *the boy's clothes*) (by 43–48 months).
- begins to use reflexive pronoun *myself* (by 43–48 months).
- begins to use conjunction *because* (by 43–48 months).

Pragmatics

The typically developing child of 3–4 years

- can maintain conversation without losing track of topic.
- begins to modify speech to age of listener (e.g., uses simplified language with a younger child).
- begins to produce indirectives (e.g., "Are the cookies done?" meaning "I want a cookie").
- uses requesting (e.g., yes–no questions, *wh-* questions).
- responds with structures, such as *yes*, *no*, *because*; expresses agreement or denial (e.g., "That's not really her dress"), compliance or refusal (e.g., "I won't take a bath!").
- uses conversational devices, such as
  - boundary markers, such as *hi*, *bye* (indicate beginning, end of communication).
  - calls, such as "Hey, Mommy!"
  - accompaniments, such as "Here you are."
  - politeness markers, such as *please*, *thanks*.
- uses communicative functions, such as
  - role-playing, fantasies.
  - protests and objections, such as "Don't touch that!"

- jokes, such as "I threw the juice in the ceiling!"
- game markers, such as "You have to catch me!"
- claims, such as "I'm first!"
- warnings, such as "Look out or you'll fall!"
- teasing, such as "You can't have this!"

4–5 Years

The following developmental milestones are observed in typically developing children between 4 and 5 years of age.

Syntax

The typically developing child of 4–5 years

- averages 6–6.5 words per sentence by 5 years; has an average MLU of 4.5–7.0 by 5 years.
- speaks in complete sentences.
- uses complex sentences; interprets complex sentences correctly. By 4.5 years, only about 8% of sentences are incomplete.
- uses future tense (e.g., "She will go to the store").
- uses *if, so* in sentences.
- uses passive voice (some children do; e.g., "The cat was fed by the man").

Semantics

The typically developing child of 4–5 years

- uses concrete meanings and words but responds to some abstract ideas appropriately.
- has an expressive range of approximately 1,500–2,000 words.
- comprehends about 5,600 words at 48 months, approximately 6,500 words by 54 months, up to 9,600 words by 60 months.
- can name items in a category (e.g., food, animals) and point to categorical items (e.g., fruit).
- uses most pronouns, including possessives (e.g., *mine, his, her*).
- uses *why* and *how*.
- understands time concepts, such as *early in the morning, tomorrow, after*.
- uses *what do, does, did* in questions.
- answers simple "when" questions like "When do you sleep?" (55–60 months).
- responds appropriately to "how often," "how long" questions (55–60 months).
- asks meaning of words.
- tells long stories accurately.
- can give whole name (first, middle, last).
- begins to understand right and left (5 years).
- can define 10 common words (4.5 years).
- shows objects by use and function, if directed (e.g., with "Show me what tells time." "Show me which one gives us milk").

- identifies past and future verbs, if asked (e.g., as in "Show me the man who kicked the ball." "Who will kick the ball?").
- demands explanations with frequent use of *why*.

Morphology
The typically developing child of 4–5 years

- uses comparatives (e.g., *bigger, nicer, taller*).
- uses *could, would* in sentences.
- uses irregular plurals (e.g., *mice, teeth*) fairly consistently.

Pragmatics
The typically developing child of 4–5 years

- modifies speech as a function of listener age (beginning at 4 years).
- begins to judge grammatical correctness and appropriateness of sentences.
- can maintain topic over successive utterances.
- uses egocentric monologue (that does not communicate information to the listener) about a third of the time.
- uses indirect speech acts, softens speech (e.g., "I think that goes in there," rather than "Put that in there.").
- begins to tell jokes and riddles (around 5 years).

5–6 Years
The following developmental milestones are observed in typically developing children between 5 and 6 years of age.

Syntax
The typically developing child of 5–6 years

- has an average MLU of 6.0–8.0.
- uses present, past, and future tenses consistently.
- uses conjunctions to string words together (e.g., "A bear and a wolf and a fox").
- asks "how" questions.
- uses auxiliary *have* correctly at times.
- uses "if" sentences (e.g., "If I had a cookie, I'd eat it").
- increases understanding and use of complex sentences; decreases grammatical errors as sentences and vocabulary become more sophisticated.
- comprehends verb tenses in the passive voice (e.g., "The bus was hit by the car." "The cat was fed by the man").
- uses a language form that approximates the adult model.

Semantics

The typically developing child of 5–6 years

- knows spatial relations and prepositions, such as *on top, behind, far, near.*
- can distinguish *alike, same, different.*
- distinguishes right and left in self, not in others.
- knows complete address.
- knows most common opposites (e.g., *hard–soft, fat–thin, high–low*); understands "opposite of" (e.g., "What's the opposite of *cold*?").
- defines objects by use, composition (e.g., "Napkins are made of paper; you wipe your mouth with them").
- tells long stories; retells tales of past and present events.
- comprehends 13,000–15,000 words (by age 6).
- can answer "What happens if?" questions.
- understands concepts such as yesterday–tomorrow, more–less, some–many, several–few, most–least, before–after, now–later.
- can state similarities and differences of objects.
- can name position of objects: first, second, third.
- can name days of week in order.
- comprehends *first, last.*
- knows functions of body parts.

Morphology

The typically developing child of 5–6 years

- knows indefinite pronouns—*any, anything, anybody, every, both, few, many, each,* and others.
- uses irregular plurals with general consistency.
- uses possessives and negatives consistently.
- uses all pronouns consistently.
- uses superlative *–est* (e.g., *smartest*).
- begins to use adverbial word endings (e.g., *–ly*).

Pragmatics

The typically developing child of 5–6 years

- understands humor, surprise.
- corrects potential errors by modifying the message.
- can recognize a socially offensive message and reword it in polite form.
- modifies speech according to listener's needs.
- begins to use and understand formal levels of address (e.g., *Mr., Mrs.*).
- gains greater facility with indirect requests (e.g., "I would like a sticker," instead of "Gimme a sticker").

- can differentiate 80% of the time between polite and impolite utterances.
- uses expressions, such as "Thank you" and "I'm sorry."
- often asks permission to use objects belonging to others.
- contributes to adult conversation.

6–7 Years

The following developmental milestones are observed in typically developing children between 6 and 7 years of age.

Syntax

The typically developing child of 6–7 years

- uses *if* and *so*.
- uses reflexive pronouns (e.g., *himself, myself*).
- begins to use perfect-tense forms (e.g., *have, had*).
- has full use of passive voice.
- has an average MLU of 7.3 words.
- uses embedding more frequently (e.g., "The girl *who bought the dress* went to the party").

Semantics

The typically developing child of 6–7 years

- comprehends 20,000–26,000 words.
- understands the seasons of the year and knows what you do in each.
- forms letters left to right (reversals and inversions are common).
- prints alphabet and numerals from previously printed model.
- recites the alphabet sequentially, names capital letters, matches lower- to uppercase letters.
- rote counts to 100.

Morphology

The typically developing child of 6–7 years

- uses most morphological markers fairly consistently.
- uses irregular comparatives (*good, better, best*) more correctly.
- continues to improve in correct use of irregular past tense and plurals.
- begins to produce **gerunds** (a noun form produced by adding *–ing* to a verb infinitive, e.g., *fish* becomes *fishing*).
- acquires use of **derivational morphemes**, in which verbs are changed into nouns (e.g., *catch* becomes *catcher*).

Pragmatics

The typically developing child of 6–7 years

- becomes aware of mistakes in other people's speech.
- is apt to use slang and mild profanity.

7–8 Years

The following developmental milestones are observed in typically developing children between 7 and 8 years of age.

Syntax

The typically developing child of 7–8 years

- has an MLU of approximately 7.0–9.0.
- uses predominantly complex and compound sentences.

Semantics

The typically developing child of 7–8 years

- interprets jokes and riddles literally.
- anticipates story endings.
- uses some figurative language.
- uses details in description.
- creates conversation suggested by a picture.
- enjoys telling stories and anecdotes.
- retells a story, keeping main ideas in correct sequence.

Morphology

The typically developing child of 7–8 years

- uses most irregular verb forms, though with some mistakes in irregular past tense.
- uses superlatives (e.g., *biggest*, *prettiest*).
- uses adverbs regularly.

Pragmatics

The typically developing child of 7–8 years

- initiates and maintains conversation in small groups.
- is able to role-play, to take the listener's point of view.
- determines and uses appropriate discourse codes and styles (e.g., informal with friends, formal with adults).

- uses nonlinguistic and nonverbal behaviors—posture, gestures—appropriately.
- takes more care in communicating with unfamiliar people; announces topic shifts.
- can sustain a topic through a number of conversational turns, but topics tend to be concrete.

Language and Literacy Development in the School-Age Years

It is expected that during the preschool years, children have had adequate exposure to prereading and prewriting skills and activities (e.g., coloring, being read to). Such exposure affects a child's development of **emergent literacy** or **preliteracy skills**, which are foundational to later reading and writing in school. Preschool language knowledge has been shown empirically to be a reliable predictor of later academic achievement (Einarsdottir, Bjornsdottir, & Simonardottir, 2016).

- After children enter kindergarten, they develop literacy skills in the areas of phonological awareness, print knowledge, reading, and writing. In recent years, experts have emphasized the importance of children developing adequate morphological awareness skills as well (Apel, Brimo, Diehm, & Apel, 2013; Owens, 2016).
- **Phonological awareness** refers to a child's specific ability to detect and manipulate sounds and syllables in words. Phonological awareness encompasses the ability to be aware of sounds and syllables apart from whole words.
- **Print knowledge** refers to children's emergent knowledge about functions and forms of written language. For example, a child needs to be able to distinguish uppercase from lowercase letters.
- **Morphological awareness** is the recognition, understanding, and use of word parts that carry significance. For example, students need to understand that prefixes, suffixes, inflections, and root words are all morphemes that can be taken away from or added to words to change their meaning.
- Phonological awareness, morphological awareness, and print knowledge are foundational to reading and writing skills. Children develop skills in all of these areas as they grow and mature.
- In recent years in the United States, there has been a much greater emphasis on literacy skills at the preschool level. Some preschools now actively teach the alphabet, for example.
- The Common Core State Standards (National Governors Association Center for Best Practices, 2010), adopted by 42 out of 50 states, emphasize development of oral and literate language skills in school-age students in kindergarten–12th grade. Major goals of the standards are as follows:
  - To create globally competitive citizens in the 21st century
  - To prepare students for college
  - To create critical readers who "read deeply"
  - To help students become responsible citizens who use evidence for deliberation

- Many school-based speech-language pathologists today use the English Language Arts Common Core State Standards as their rubric for creating curriculum-based expectations for language achievement in children (Schmitt, Logan, Tambyraja, Farquharson, & Justice, 2017).

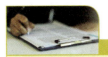

SUMMARY

- Children develop language based on their innate characteristics, the environment they are exposed to, and the expectations of their cultures.
- Children's caregivers play an important role in language development. Ideally, a baby's caregivers use motherese, or child-directed speech, speech geared specifically to help babies attend and respond to what they hear.
- The development of syntactic, semantic, morphological, and pragmatic skills depends in large part on children's innate characteristics, as well as interaction with their caregivers. Each child develops at his or her own rate, and variation among children is to be expected.
- Children develop literacy skills as they grow. Phonological awareness, print knowledge, and morphological awareness are foundational skills for competent reading and writing.
- Today, many school-based speech-language pathologists use the English Language Arts portion of the Common Core State Standards as a standard for expectations for children's performance.

THEORIES OF LANGUAGE DEVELOPMENT

Theories influence clinical practice to varying extents. The way clinicians conduct assessment and treatment depends greatly on their orientation to theoretical viewpoints. Some clinicians are eclectic in their approach; that is, they blend aspects of several theories to achieve what they see as a balanced approach to language assessment and treatment. Other clinicians depend primarily on, and operate from, one theory. Still other clinicians, thinking that most theories are at best only partially supported, may be totally atheoretical. In this section, we describe five major theories of language development: behavioral, nativist, cognitive, information-processing, and social interactionism. These theories differ in describing how language is developed and in their implications for (a) areas that clinicians should target in assessment and intervention and (b) what procedures should be used to facilitate language learning (Bohannon & Bonvillian, 2017).

Behavioral Theory

Behavioral theories focus on observable and measureable aspects of behavior. They emphasize language **performance**, or what we can see and hear, over language **competence**, which cannot be observed.

- Behavioral psychologist B. F. Skinner's (1957) system of behavioral analysis explained the acquisition of verbal behavior. **Verbal behavior** is a form of social behavior maintained by the actions of a verbal community. Verbal behaviors are acquired under appropriate conditions of stimulation, response, and reinforcement.
- Behavioral scientists suggest that learning, not innate mechanisms, plays a major role in the acquisition of verbal behaviors; they offer evidence that caregivers perform a variety of actions that promote language learning in children.

- Behavioral scientists find little or no evidence of innate language acquisition devices (LADs) that figure in linguistic theories.
- To behavioral scientists, the events in the child's **environment** and **social interactions** are important. Children learn only the language they are exposed to; severe social deprivation results in language deprivation, as well.
- Verbal behavior is characteristically produced under social stimulation. An audience is necessary; the audience, or persons interacting with the speaker, sets the stage for speech. This is why verbal behavior is defined as a form of social behavior shaped and maintained by the members of a verbal community.
- Practically all forms of verbal behaviors can be increased or decreased experimentally. Social reinforcement, for example, can increase babbling, word and phrase responses, and the production of grammatic features.
- For example, if a child says something like "Want bath," the caregiver might say, "You want a bath! Good girl! Let's have a bath right now." The caregiver reinforces the statement by responding verbally and then starting to run the bathwater. If the caregiver ignores or punishes the child, the child is much less likely to express this request again. Thus, behaviorists question the nativist assumption that the environment offers little assistance to the child in acquiring language.
- In treatment, most speech–language pathologists teach verbal behavior to children by modeling correct responses and reinforcing children's correct productions.
- Clinicians who conduct language treatment according to principles of the behavioral theory believe that one can teach language by targeting any observable behavior and manipulating the elements of a stimulus, a response, and some type of reinforcement.
- In treatment, the clinician selects specific target responses, creates appropriate antecedent events, and reinforces correct responses. There is a clearly established criterion for success (e.g., 8 out of 10 responses produced accurately).
- For example, a clinician teaching a child to use plural –s might create a game using toy cars. If the clinician points to the cars and asks, "What are these?" and the child says, "Cars," the clinician might respond with "Good job!" Much of the clinical work in speech–language pathology supports the role of appropriate stimulation and reinforcement in teaching language skills to children with language disorders.

Nativist Theory

The nativist theory is an influential theory of syntax proposed by Noam Chomsky in the late 1950s. This theory has influenced both linguistics and speech–language pathology.

- Chomsky (1957) stated that syntactic structures are the essence of language and that language is a product of the unique human mind. He said that there are universal rules of grammar that apply to all languages.
- The nativist theory states that children are born with a **language acquisition device** (LAD). The LAD is assumed to be a specialized language processor that is a physiological part of the brain. The LAD knows about languages in general, because it contains the universal rules of language.

- The child's environment provides information about the unique rules of the language to which the child is exposed. The LAD then integrates the universal rules and the unique rules of that language, and thus helps the child learn language in a relatively short time.
- Nativists believe that children are born with an innate capacity to learn language and that, because the basic knowledge necessary to acquire language is already present at birth, language is not learned through environmental stimulation, reinforcement, or teaching.
- Because Chomsky (1957) believed that such creative transformation of sentence forms is the essence of language, his theory was often called the **transformational generative theory of grammar**. According to Chomsky, with knowledge of the rules of grammar and the use of transformations, speakers can generate an endless variety of sentences.
- A revision of Chomsky's theory was proposed in the early 1980s. The **government binding theory** attempts to describe the way the mind represents the autonomous system of language. Chomsky wanted to present a theory that accounted for the variety in human languages and explained the development of grammars on the basis of limited input (Owens, 2014). According to Owens, too few child studies have been performed to make a definite statement about the contribution of government binding theory to our understanding of language development.
- Chomsky (2002) presented his theory as the Minimalist Program. In this view, he reduced the language faculty to its narrowest form, wherein the only components are a level of representation for meaning, a level of representation for sound, and a recursive element called "merge" that provides the mechanism for joining words or phrases. It is this element that accounts for the linguistic novelty of children's productions (Gerber & Wankoff, 2014).
- The nativist theory and its variants lead to few specific implications for assessment and treatment of children who have language disorders. However, Chomskyan theorists believe that in therapy, it is necessary to focus heavily on syntax in selecting treatment goals.
- In therapy to increase a child's language skills, reinforcement is unnecessary. Because language knowledge is innate, reinforcing a child for talking would be tantamount to reinforcing a child for walking. Manipulating the child's environment, as the behaviorist does, is unlikely to be successful, according to this theory.
- Clinicians, however, have found that reinforcement and environmental manipulations are necessary to teach language skills to children who have not acquired them in a typical fashion.

Cognitive Theory

Described as a variant of the nativist theory, the cognitive theory emphasizes **cognition**, or knowledge and mental processes, such as memory, attention, and visual and auditory perception. Cognitivists focus on the child's regulation of learning and on internal aspects of behavior.

- According to cognitive theory, language acquisition is made possible by cognition and general intellectual processes. Language is only one expression of a more general set of cognitive activities, and proper development of the cognitive system is a necessary precursor of linguistic expression.
- Thus, a child must first acquire concepts before producing words. For example, a child who has not been exposed to a *dog* or a *triangle* is not likely to say those words.

- Proponents of the **strong cognition hypothesis** believe in cognitive precursors to language. They state that there are cognitive abilities that are essential prerequisites to language skills. Without these prerequisite cognitive abilities, language skills will not be optimally developed. Language development is dependent on cognitive development.
- Piaget (1954), a supporter of the strong cognition hypothesis, described four stages of cognitive development that children must go through (see Table 3.4). He believed that children successively acquire the necessary cognitive operations that, in turn, lead to higher levels of language development. Children must master the features of one stage in order to progress to the next.
- Children pass through each cognitive stage in the order given but may show variation in the **rate** at which they progress through the stages.
- Although researchers have not produced convincing evidence that there is a causal relationship between cognitive and language skills, it has been observed that certain language skills develop at about the same time as certain cognitive skills. For example, children's use of "all gone" (a disappearance phrase) is associated with the emerging understanding of object permanence.
- The **weak cognition hypothesis** states that while cognition accounts for some of a child's language abilities, it cannot account for all of them; some aspects of language do not develop directly as a result of underlying cognitive skills.
- Cognitive theorists believe that while nonlinguistic, cognitive precursors are innate, language is not. Thus, because they believe that language is neither innate (nativist view) nor learned (behaviorist view), they view language as emerging as a result of cognitive growth.
- A clinical implication of the cognitive theory is that clinicians must assess cognitive precursors to language and facilitate the development of those precursors before working on language itself. Language will not improve until cognitive precursors are developed.
- For example, a young child may not have developed object permanence, or the ability to know that an item exists even when it goes out of sight. Therefore, before teaching that child to say any words, the clinician would establish object permanence. Once object permanence is firmly established, the clinician would teach the child to say words.

Information-Processing Theory

Proponents of the information-processing theory are mostly concerned with cognitive **functioning**, not cognitive structures or concepts. In other words, information-processing theorists are interested in **how** language is learned.

- Information-processing theorists view the human information-processing system as a mechanism that encodes stimuli from the environment, operates on interpretations of those stimuli, stores the results in memory, and permits retrieval of previously stored information.
- Of primary concern are the steps involved in handling or processing incoming and outgoing information. These steps include organization, memory, transfer, attention, and discrimination. Long- and short-term memory are especially important (Owens, 2014). Language learning relies on information-processing mechanisms; this view has also been called **cognitive connectionism**.

Table 3.4

Piaget's Stages of Cognitive Development

Sensorimotor (0–2 years)

Usually divided into six substages

Substage 1: Birth–2 months
- Child displays reflexive vocal behavior.
- Child displays reflexive sensorimotor behavior.

Substage 2: 2–4 months
- Child makes coordinated eye–hand movements.
- Child makes coordinated hand–mouth movements.

Substage 3: 4–8 months
- Child acts on objects and begins to search for objects.
- Child imitates some sounds and babbles.

Substage 4: 8–12 months
- Child starts walking.
- Child uses first word.
- Child searches for objects based on her memory of where she last saw them.
- Child begins to recognize that he has the ability to cause objects to move.

Substage 5: 12–18 months
- Object permanence becomes evident.
- Child walks with confidence.
- Child may imitate another person's behavior when that person is present (e.g., claps hands or plays peek-a-boo).
- Child experiments with the properties and functions of objects (e.g., uses a spoon to eat cereal, to bang on the table, to drop in front of the dog, etc.).

Substage 6: 18–24 months
- Child uses words when referents are not present (e.g., says "Mommy" even when Mommy is not in the room).
- Child uses thought to solve problems.
- Basic cause–effect relations are acquired.
- Child uses symbolic play, using one item to represent another (for example, using a tissue as a doll's blanket, using a stick as a gun).

Preoperational (2–7 years)

Frequently divided into two stages: preconceptual (2–4 years) and intuitive (4–7 years)

Preconceptual: 2–4 years
- Child is egocentric, has difficulty taking perspective of others.
- Child overextends word meanings (all men are "Daddy").
- Child underextends word meanings (only the family pet, Rover, is a "dog").

Intuitive: 4–7 years
- Egocentrism continues.
- Child displays concreteness of thought (e.g., in Monopoly, the child has a hard time recognizing that five $100 bills represent the same amount as one $500 bill).
- Perceptions guide thoughts.
- Child deals with only one variable at a time.
- Classification skills have improved but are still inadequate.
- Child displays lack of conservation (e.g., lack of ability to see that a ball of clay can be rolled into a snake shape and still be the same amount of clay).

(continues)

Table 3.4 (continued)
Concrete operations (7–11 years)
• Child is less egocentric, has increasing ability to see others' points of view. • Child acquires seriation and conservation skills. • Child employs logical causality. • Child uses effective classification skills.
Formal operations (more than 11 years)
• Child displays lack of egocentricity, is able to see others' point of view. • Child displays ability to think and speak in the abstract. • Child can use inductive and deductive thought processes. • Child can use verbal reasoning and make "if . . . then" statements. • Child is able to use hypothetical reasoning.

Note. Adapted from *An Introduction to Children with Language Disorders* (3rd ed., p. 33), by V. A. Reed, 2005, Boston, MA: Allyn & Bacon.

- Recent literature has included a great deal of discussion about the relationship between information processing and language disorders. Specifically, researchers have been interested in whether or not children with language disorders have concomitant information-processing problems. The role of working memory has been especially scrutinized (e.g., Adlof & Patten, 2017; Boudreau & Costanza-Smith, 2011; Ebert, 2014; Kohnert, 2013). Working-memory deficits in children with language impairments are described in more detail in Chapter 4.
- Ellis Weismer and Evans (2002) suggest that there are two broad categories of information processing related to children's language disorders: phonological processing and temporal auditory processing.
- **Phonological processing** deals with the processes involved in the ability to mentally manipulate phonological aspects of language, such as word rhyming, word segmentation, syllabication, and others. A child who has difficulty rhyming words or knowing that "c-a-t" means "cat" has phonological processing problems.
- **Temporal auditory processing** deals with the ability to perceive the brief acoustic events that comprise speech sounds and track changes in these events as they happen quickly in the speech of other people.
- In research on the temporal auditory processing skills of children, researchers have been interested in children's (a) overall processing capacity and (b) speed of processing. In a simple example, researchers might ask whether a child with a language disorder is able to listen to someone quickly say "5-9-3-6-2," remember this digit string, and repeat it immediately and accurately. The child may have difficulty with the length of the digit string, the speed with which the string was said, or both.
- Children with difficulties in temporal auditory processing often have difficulty with other tasks, as well. These include remembering and following long and complex directions; repeating sentences verbatim; repeating lists of real and nonsense words; and other tasks that tap the ability to hear, remember, and give back information that they have heard—especially if the information was given rapidly.

- Foundational to adequate auditory processing is normal auditory sensitivity. When normal auditory sensitivity is established, some clinicians use their treatment programs to address the components of auditory processing, which follow:

  - **Auditory discrimination.** These skills enable children to identify differences between sound stimuli. Popular available tests ask children, for example, "Listen: *cat–bat*. Are these words the same or different?" The validity of these tests has been questioned by many professionals. Although the role of auditory discrimination in language development is heavily debated, researchers have found that children with language impairments have poorer auditory discrimination skills than their typically developing peers.
  - **Auditory attention.** This is the ability to ignore irrelevant acoustic stimuli and focus on important information. Children with poor auditory attention have difficulty filtering relevant and irrelevant stimuli. Without appropriate auditory attention, they may focus equally on all incoming stimuli, thus experiencing sensory overload. Optimal language learning cannot take place under such conditions, as children cannot sort out and attend to the important aspects of speech.
  - **Auditory memory.** This refers to the ability to mentally store speech stimuli or remember what one has heard. Many clinicians and researchers have found that children with language impairments have difficulty with auditory memory, also referred to as working memory.
  - **Auditory rate.** This refers to the ability to process acoustic stimuli that are presented at different rates or speeds. Much research has suggested that children with language impairments have difficulty processing incoming stimuli presented at rapid rates and that if the rate of incoming information is slowed down, they can process it more easily.
  - **Auditory sequencing.** This is the ability to identify the temporal order in which auditory stimuli occur. Although the role of auditory sequencing in language development has been debated, it has been found that children with language disorders do more poorly on auditory-sequencing tasks than children who are developing in a typical fashion.

- Researchers today believe that in therapy for children with language impairments, directly targeting working memory and speed of processing skills is helpful (Boudreau & Costanza-Smith, 2011; Kohnert, 2013). It is also believed that intensive language treatment may facilitate cognitive processing skills (Ebert, 2014). More will be said about this in Chapter 4.

Social Interactionism Theory

The social interactionism theory does not focus on innate linguistic competence (nativism). Rather, this theory stipulates that the structure of human language has arisen from language's social–communicative function in human relations (Bohannon & Bonvillian, 2017). Although the theory does not explicitly use the behavioral concepts (e.g., reinforcement contingencies) in explaining language learning, it is similar to the behavioral view that language is possible only because of social interactions.

- Proponents of social interactionism emphasize language function, not structure. They give credence to the situations in which social interactions occur, believing that interactions vary depending on the situation.

- Social interactionists believe that language develops because people are motivated to interact socially with others around them. For example, infants seek out human faces and respond to them. Thus, the environment and its inherent social experiences are crucial to the emergence of language.
- Proponents of social interactionism believe that the child, as well as his or her caregivers and the environment, plays an active role in language acquisition.
- Lev Vygotsky (1962), a Russian psychologist, believed that language is a tool for social interaction. He saw language as being intrinsically linked with the social–interactive context.
- According to Vygotsky, language knowledge is acquired through social interaction with more competent and experienced members of the child's culture. Therefore, Vygotsky emphasized the importance of verbal guidance and adult modeling.
- Vygotsky (1962) stated that a child's conversational partners, including the parents, are significant contributors to the language-acquisition process. These partners contribute by scaffolding, or supplying the necessary communicative structure that allows the child to communicate despite limited communication skills.
- Parents play a critical role in supporting language development by adjusting their linguistic input to an appropriate level for the child and by responding contingently to the child's output.
- Unlike Piaget (1954), who believed that cognitive development preceded language development, Vygotsky (1962) thought that children first learned language in interpersonal interactions and then used that language to structure thought.
- Vygotsky further believed that as children's language develops, they increasingly use language internally to structure their actions and direct their thoughts. For example, small children playing house by themselves may be observed talking to themselves as they play. Eventually, as they mature, children use language silently internally to mediate thought.
- According to Vygotsky (1962), cultural tools play a critical role in children's language development. For example, in a culture that only uses Roman numerals, certain ways of thinking mathematically are not possible. But in a culture where people have ready access to calculators and computers, various high levels of mathematical thinking are possible. Children's learning is guided by the cultural tools available and by the social interactions around these tools.
- Social interactionism suggests that language, both oral and written, continues to develop across the span of a person's life. Adolescents, for example, continue to refine their skills in figurative language and pragmatics as they mature. Adults who change jobs or vocations must learn the vocabulary relevant to their new station in life.
- Clinicians whose practice is driven by social interactionism focus on children's motivation for communication. Treatment sessions are built around increasing children's motivation to communicate.
- To motivate a child to use language, clinicians supply external situations and contexts, both verbal and nonverbal, that encourage the child to use language to meet his or her needs. For example, a clinician might withhold an attractive bottle of bubbles until the child says, "I want bubbles."

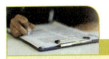

SUMMARY

- The nativist, cognitive, behavioral, information-processing, and social interactionism theories have been briefly described. Although other models of language development exist, these five theories have greatly influenced research and practice.
- Most speech–language pathologists, rather than allowing their practice to be driven by a single theory, incorporate aspects of all five theories to allow an eclectic blend to serve as a foundation for optimal assessment and treatment of children with language impairment.

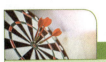

CHAPTER HIGHLIGHTS

- Language is a form of social behavior that is shaped and maintained by a verbal community. Language can also be defined as a system of symbols used to represent concepts that are formed through exposure and experience.
- Linguists have traditionally analyzed language in terms of morphology (the study of word structure), syntax (rules specifying how words may be combined to form meaningful sentences), semantics (the study of meaning), and pragmatics (the study of rules that govern language use in various social situations). (Phonology, frequently studied under the aegis of language, is defined and discussed in Chapter 5.)
- Language development in children depends on several factors: the innate characteristics the individual child brings to the situation (e.g., a high IQ, a limited attention span), the child's environment and social interactions, and cultural expectations. High-quality interaction with caregivers is critical to optimal language acquisition, and this type of interaction should begin in infancy.
- Clinicians use language developmental milestones to guide their expectations about the language characteristics of children at certain chronological ages. However, a great deal of individual variability exists among children, so developmental milestones can serve only as a *general* guide and frame of reference. Most schools have a set of expectations for students to demonstrate increasingly sophisticated language skills as they progress through the grades.
- Theories of language development provide the foundational underpinnings for assessment and treatment of children with language problems. Key theories that have affected clinical practice include the behavioral theory (Skinner), the nativist theory (Chomsky), the cognitive theory (Piaget), the information-processing theory, and the social interactionism theory (Vygotsky).
- The behavioral theory was proposed by Skinner (1957), who explained language acquisition as the development of verbal behavior. He suggested that learning, not an innate and unmeasurable mechanism such as a language acquisition device (LAD), plays a major role in language

development. He emphasized the importance of environmental contingencies (appropriate stimulus conditions, including motivation, verbal responses, and social consequences for those responses) in language learning.
- According to the nativist theory, proposed by Chomsky (1957), children are born with an LAD that contains the universal rules of language. Chomsky described the concepts of language competence and language performance. More recently, he narrowed his theory into what he termed the Minimalist Program.
- Proponents of the cognitive theory state that cognition and intellectual processes make language acquisition possible. Piaget (1954), a supporter of the strong cognition hypothesis, stated that children pass through four overlapping developmental cognitive stages: the sensorimotor, preoperational, concrete operations, and formal operations stages.
- The information-processing theory focuses on *how* language is learned—that is, on what types of cognitive functioning are necessary for language learning. A strong emphasis of this theory is auditory processing, composed of the components of auditory discrimination, attention, memory, rate, and sequencing. Research has also proposed the categories of phonological processing and temporal auditory processing. Recently, there has been a strong interest in the role of working memory skills in children's language development.
- Proponents of the social interactionism theory, influenced by Vygotsky (1962), emphasize language function over language structure. Social interactionists believe that language develops as a function of social interaction between a child and his environment (including significant others in that environment). Motivation is considered to be key in using language.

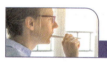

STUDY AND REVIEW QUESTIONS

1. A child says, "Red crayon." This is an example of which type of semantic relations?

A. Attribute + entity
B. Action + locative
C. Agent + action
D. Attribute + locative

2. You have been asked to give a workshop to a group of parents of infants who attend a developmental nursery. The parents are interested in what they can do to communicate more successfully with their infants. Most of the infants are between 1 and 10 months of age. Most of the parents do not have much money or access to toys and objects, but you are told that they do spend plenty of time with their babies. You are asked to speak about what specifically these parents can do to successfully interact with their infants in daily routines, such as bathing, dressing, and eating. You will tell these parents which of the following?

A. When your baby starts to cry, let him do so for 5–10 minutes before you respond; this will teach the baby independence and motivate him to express himself in words later on (instead of crying).

B. Ideally, speak to the baby in utterances (child-directed speech) that are higher pitched and have greater pitch fluctuations than ordinary speech.

C. Babies do not benefit from activities used to build turn-taking skills until they are 2 years old, so do not bother with games that focus on turn-taking.

D. Babies do not usually say their first word until 18 months of age, so do not worry if your child is 12 months old and not saying any words.

3. A child using **recurrence** would say which of the following?

A. "Face dirty."
B. "All gone juice."
C. "More cookie."
D. "Doll mine."

4. An example of a sentence using an **embedded form** would be which of the following?

A. The boy who got a haircut looks nice.
B. The girl ate a cookie, three crackers, and some fruit.
C. Mom and Dad are going to the store to buy some groceries.
D. Because he was on time, they were happy with him.

5. A mother comes to you, concerned because her son Jake was born prematurely and had to spend the first few months of his life in a neonatal intensive care unit. Now Jake is 9 months old, and his mother wants to make sure that his language development is "on target for his age." You go to Jake's home to observe him, and you also ask his mother to give you a detailed description of his communication patterns. As you evaluate Jake's language development, you need to remember that one of the following does NOT occur between 8 and 10 months of age in the typically developing child. Which one is it?

A. Comprehension of *no*
B. Using the phrase "all gone" to express emerging negation
C. Using variegated babbling (e.g., "madamada")
D. Uncovering a hidden toy (beginning of object permanence)

6. You are conducting an assessment with an incoming kindergartener, Jason E., who has difficulty with word endings. Specifically, he tends to omit endings like *–est* (saying "sad" instead of "saddest"), *–ily* (saying "angry" instead of "angrily"), etc. He is having difficulty with which specific aspect of language?

A. Syntax
B. Pragmatics
C. Semantics
D. Morphology

7. A 7-year-old girl, Ashton, is referred to you by her second-grade classroom teacher, Mr. Alvarez. Mr. Alvarez says that Ashton "doesn't always get along with her peers" and "doesn't know how to hold a decent conversation." You assess Ashton personally and also observe her on the playground during recess and in the cafeteria at lunchtime. You see that Mr. Alvarez is right. Ashton has difficulty in conversational exchanges with her peers, and they frequently ignore her. You notice that when talking to you, she seems uncomfortable and doesn't say much, even when you use a variety of interesting games and toys. In therapy, your first priority with Ashton will be to

   A. teach her the appropriate use of compound and complex sentences in appropriate contexts.
   B. teach her the appropriate use of allomorphs when presented with pictures of different people and activities.
   C. increase her skills in quick incidental learning so that she can expand her vocabulary.
   D. increase her skills in discourse.

8. You observe a clinician working with a child who has a language impairment. They are making cookies together, and the clinician is saying things like "Look, the dough goes *in* the bowl; the spoon is *beside* the bowl. We will set the bowl *on top* of the counter, and then make the cookies. We'll put them *in* the oven and take them *out* when they are done." The clinician is working on developing the child's skill in the area of understanding

   A. indirect requests.
   B. locatives.
   C. pragmatics.
   D. gerunds.

9. A 5-year-old child has been referred to you for a language assessment. There is a concern about his expressive language skills, and you decide to gather a language sample to assess expressive morphology and syntax. At one point, when looking at a book, the child points to a book character and says, "Him no eat cookies." This is an example of

   A. four words, five morphemes, personal pronoun + one negative + one verb + one plural noun.
   B. four words, six morphemes, modal + one negative + one verb + one auxiliary.
   C. four words, four morphemes, personal pronoun + one copula + one negative + one noun.
   D. four words, five morphemes, negative + one personal pronoun + one copula.

10. Which one of the following Piagetian stages, which include object permanence, corresponds with the emergence of a typically developing child's first word?

    A. Preoperational
    B. Formal operations
    C. Sensorimotor 10 - 14 months
    D. Concrete operations

11. Which one of the following is NOT a goal of the Common Core State Standards?

    A. To create globally competitive citizens in the 21st century
    B. To prepare students for college
    C. To ensure that all students speak at least two languages so they become more competent global citizens
    D. To help students become responsible citizens who use evidence for deliberation

12. A fourth-grade child, Alex, has been referred to you for language testing by his teacher. His parents are concerned and upset with the teacher because they feel that Alex needs more help in reading and writing skills than he is receiving. They tell you that the math and science homework assignments are too difficult for him, and they feel that the fourth-grade teacher is making unreasonable demands. You find out that Alex did not attend preschool, and even in kindergarten, the teacher wrote on his first-trimester progress report that he "began school not knowing basic concepts; he didn't talk as much as the other children either." You will tell Alex's parents that

   A. the teacher really is being unreasonable and demanding too much.
   B. Alex definitely has a language delay and needs therapy.
   (C.) you would like to conduct an assessment of Alex's language skills in a variety of domains to see whether he needs support services in oral and written language.
   D. Alex definitely needs a psychological evaluation to see if he has an intellectual disability.

13. You are asked to assess Tina, who has Down syndrome. She is 4 years 10 months old, and her parents tell you that they wish for her to begin kindergarten in the fall (it is July, and school begins in September). You assess Tina's receptive and expressive language skills and find that she has an average MLU of 3.0 and an expressive vocabulary of 350 words. She sustains a topic of conversation about 20% of the time and overregularizes past-tense inflections. You will tell Tina's parents that

   A. Tina's overall language skills are very generally within normal limits for her age.
   B. though Tina's language skills are approximately 6 months delayed for her age, she will be able to participate in a regular kindergarten classroom.
   (C.) Tina's language skills are generally commensurate with those of a 2- to 3-year-old child and starting kindergarten in the fall would probably be difficult for her.
   D. Tina's language skills are generally commensurate with those of a 1-year-old, and, thus, she needs to be in a preschool setting with very young children.

14. You are observing a clinician in a private practice setting. He specializes in child language disorders and serves elementary-age children from a variety of local public schools. When you observe this clinician doing therapy, you see that he has a well-structured reward system for each child. Some children receive a fruit loop for each correct response they make; others work to earn stickers and even small toys. This clinician has written down each specific behavior that he wishes to elicit from each child, with a percentage of accuracy attached. For example, an objective for one child reads, "When presented with a picture of two or more objects, Jimmy will label the picture using plural –s 80% of the time." This clinician probably subscribes to which theory of child language development?

   A. Information processing   C. Social interactionist
   (B.) Behaviorist   D. Government binding

15. You are asked to work with a 3-and-a-half-year-old child whose language has been somewhat slow to develop. Matthew is the youngest of four children, and his parents tell you that his older siblings often talk for him. After assessing Matthew's language, you find that he consistently uses the following morphemes: present progressive *–ing*, prepositions *in* and *on*, and regular plural *–s*. His parents would like to enroll him for therapy because they want him to go to a local preschool, and they want him to "sound like the other kids and have good grammar." Which of the following morphemes would you begin with when Matthew starts therapy?

    A. Possessive *–s*
    B. Irregular past-tense verbs
    C. Articles *the, a, an*
    D. Contractible auxiliary

16. A first-grade teacher refers 6-year-old Mandy to you for an assessment. The teacher is concerned, because reportedly Mandy has problems with remembering what she hears. The teacher tells you, "Sometimes I have to give the children three or four directions, and I have to do it quickly because we have to go somewhere, like an assembly. Mandy is the only one in my class who doesn't remember what I tell the kids to do." Based on this brief description, you suspect that Mandy might have difficulties in which of the following areas?

    A. Temporal auditory processing
    B. Divergent semantic production
    C. Phonological processing
    D. Convergent semantic production

17. A young child who says "down" when a cup of juice spills off of the dinner table is using the relation of

    A. action.
    B. possession.
    C. locative action.
    D. attribution.

18. A child has been referred to you for an assessment of his pragmatic skills. The chief complaint of adults and children with whom he interacts is that he frequently gives commands and sounds rude and bossy. His classroom teacher says she is "fed up with his bossiness," and peers do not include him in their games. His father tells you that the boy frequently says things like "Take me to Pizza Palace" and "Get me the *Spiderman* DVD." The father would like intervention to help his son say things like "I wonder if we could get a *Spiderman* DVD at the store," instead of giving orders. In therapy, you know you will need to work on the boy's facility with

    A. passive sentence transformations.
    B. cohesion.
    C. narrative skills.
    D. indirect requests.

19. A young child who often says things like "my doggy" or "her ball" is using the relation of

    A. recurrence.
    B. possession.
    C. location.
    D. denial.

20. You have been asked to assess the language skills of 6-year-old Jennifer, who has been referred by her classroom teacher. The teacher says that Jennifer "talks in these really short sentences. I don't know if she is just shy or if there is more going on." The teacher has worked on oral language skills daily with her class. The end of the year is coming soon, and the teacher is concerned about how Jennifer will perform in second grade. You decide to conduct an informal language screening to decide whether you need to formally evaluate Jennifer's expressive language skills. You find that she uses many sentences, such as "He has a ball" and "I like Pokémon." She uses few compound or complex sentences. You talk with her parents and find that this performance is also typical at home. Your next step would be to

- A. tell the teacher and parents that Jennifer is within normal limits for her age, and that a formal language evaluation is unnecessary.
- B. inform the teacher and parents that Jennifer may have autistic-like tendencies and that she needs to be formally evaluated by a team of special educators.
- C. tell the teacher and parents that you will take a "wait and see" approach. If the second-grade teacher has concerns similar to those of the first-grade teacher, you will follow up with a formal evaluation of Jennifer's language skills.
- **D.** tell the teacher and parents that you would like to formally evaluate Jennifer's language skills because at 6 years of age, she should have an average MLU of 6.0–8.0, and her language should approximate the adult model.

21. In order to begin producing two-word combinations, how many words does a toddler need to have in his expressive vocabulary?

- **A. 50**
- B. 20
- C. 100
- D. 10

22. A baby, Jason, is looking at the family cat. His grandma sees him looking at the cat and directs her gaze toward the cat, also. She prepares to comment about the cat. Jason's grandma is

- A. using presupposition.
- **B. following Jason's line of regard.**
- C. intuiting Jason's thoughts about felines.
- D. preparing to use a holophrase.

References and Recommended Readings at www.advancedreviewpractice.com

STUDY AND REVIEW ANSWERS

1. A. When a child says, "Red crayon," this is an example of attribute + entity.
2. B. Ideally, speak to the baby in utterances (child-directed speech) that are higher pitched and have greater pitch fluctuations than ordinary speech.
3. C. A child using recurrence would say, "More cookie."
4. A. Embedding refers to adding or rearranging elements within sentences; in this example, the phrase "who got a haircut" makes the sentence one that uses an embedded form.
5. B. Most children use "all gone" to express emerging negation between 1 and 2 years of age.
6. D. Jason is having difficulty with morphology, because he is deleting bound morphemes from the ends of words.
7. D. Based upon your observations and the teacher's report, your first priority in therapy will be to work on Ashton's discourse skills, or skills in the give-and-take of conversation.
8. B. The clinician is working on increasing the child's skill in using locatives; she is saying and physically demonstrating locatives, such as *on top*, *in*, *beside*.
9. A. If you are conducting a language sample with a 5-year-old and the child says, "Him no eat cookies," this is an example of four words, five morphemes, personal pronoun + one negative + one verb + one plural noun.
10. C. Children usually use their first word between 10 and 14 months of age, which corresponds to the sensorimotor cognitive development stage.
11. C. Though bilingualism is a highly desirable goal, it is not written in the Common Core State Standards that schools must ensure that all students speak at least two languages so they become more competent global citizens
12. C. You tell the parents that you would like to conduct an assessment of Alex's language skills in a variety of domains to see whether he needs support services in oral and written language. It is important for you to evaluate Alex's language skills to see if he needs intervention, because there are several red flags, such as his difficulties that began in kindergarten and his struggles with the fourth-grade curriculum.
13. C. According to language development milestones, Tina's language skills are commensurate with those of a 2–3-year-old; in kindergarten, she would be learning along with typically developing children who are 5–6 years of age.
14. B. This clinician bases his therapy on the behaviorist theory, which promotes the concept of stimulus, response, and reinforcement of behaviors that are observable and measurable.
15. B. According to Brown's list of morphemes, irregular past-tense verbs would be next to develop; thus, this would be a good starting point for therapy.
16. A. Mandy's difficulties with remembering directions probably indicate problems with temporal auditory processing.
17. C. When the cup of juice spills off the dinner table and the child says "down," she is using the relation of locative action.

18. D. The ability to say something like "I wonder if we could get a *Spiderman* DVD at the store" indicates facility with indirect requests.
19. B. Utterances such as "my doggy" and "her ball" represent the relation of possession.
20. D. Based on your screening results, it will be important to conduct a formal, in-depth assessment of Jennifer's language skills. She definitely should be using longer, more complex utterances that approximate the adult model.
21. A. In order to begin putting two words together, a toddler must have at least 50 words in his expressive vocabulary.
22. B. By seeing the baby look at the cat and then looking at the cat as well, Jason's grandma is following his line of regard.

CHAPTER 4

LANGUAGE DISORDERS IN CHILDREN

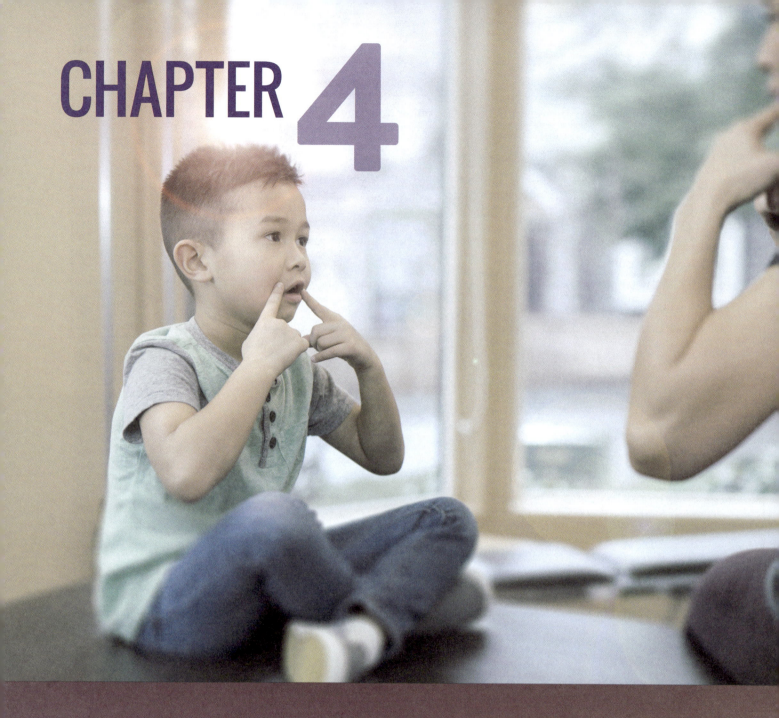

As stated in the previous chapter, behavioral theory defines language as a form of social behavior that is shaped and maintained by a verbal community. Linguistics defines language as a system of symbols used to represent concepts that are formed through exposure and experience. Children with impairments or disorders of language have limited language skills. (Note: In this chapter, the terms *language disorders* and *language impairments* are used interchangeably. Many experts today prefer the term *language impairment*, as the term *disorder* is not consistently recognized across educational and medical settings.)

Both the comprehension and production of language may be impaired in these children. Children with these impairments cannot interact with their families, communities, or cultures in a manner consistent with that of their peers or with societal expectations. Throughout their lives, children with language disorders find themselves at a disadvantage in personal, academic, and occupational settings. Roughly 12–14% of school-age children exhibit language disorders. More boys than girls exhibit language disorders.

Language disorders are caused by or associated with several factors. There are many theoretical models from which to view these problems, their causes, and associated factors. In this chapter, we discuss three broad categories of children with language problems: (a) children with specific language impairment (SLI; also known as primary language impairment); (b) children with language problems associated with other clinical conditions, including intellectual disability (ID), autism spectrum disorder (ASD), and acquired brain injury; and (c) children who have language difficulties related to a combination of factors, including poverty, neglect or abuse, alcohol or drug exposure in utero, and attention-deficit/hyperactivity disorder. We then discuss assessment and treatment principles and procedures that can be used when serving children with language problems and describe the use of augmentative alternative devices for children with complex language needs.

INTRODUCTION TO CHILDREN WITH LANGUAGE DISORDERS

Language problems in children are described by many terms: language delay, language disorder, language impairment, primary language impairment, and SLI. The *Diagnostic and Statistical Manual of Mental Disorders–Fifth Edition* (DSM-V) of the American Psychiatric Association (2013) uses the term **language disorder**. Various early risk factors are known to be associated with later language disorders in children. Children with language problems have certain distinguishing characteristics that clinicians need to be aware of as they provide services to these children.

Description of Language Disorders in Children

Children with language disorders exhibit the following kinds of deficiencies (Fogle, 2019; Moore & Montgomery, 2018; Roseberry-McKibbin, 2018b; Rudolph, 2017):

- **Limited amount of language**. A significant deficiency in the quantity of language learned and understood (e.g., vocabulary) is a major, general characteristic of children with language disorders.
- **Deficient grammar**. Another major characteristic of children with language disorders is deficient grammar. Both syntactic structures and morphologic features may be difficult for these children to learn and produce under normal conditions.
- **Inadequate or inappropriate social communication**. Deficiencies in social communication, often described as pragmatic aspects of language, also constitute a significant component of language disorders. The social communicative behaviors of children with language disorders may be inadequate or even inappropriate. For example, they may not appropriately take turns in conversations.
- **Deficient nonverbal communication skills**. Children with language disorders may be deficient in nonverbal communication, as well. Their use of gestures, facial expressions, and proper body language may be limited.
- **Deficient literacy skills**. Children with language disorders are known to experience academic problems in school, including difficulties in reading, writing, and spelling.
- **Cognitive deficits**. Children with language disorders may have deficits in the areas of working memory, attention, and speed of processing.

Risk Factors for Language Disorders in Children

Various early risk factors are known to be associated with later language disorders in children; some important risk factors include the following:

- Prenatal conditions such as maternal drug abuse (including alcohol and nicotine) and maternal infections (e.g., rubella, herpes simplex, and HIV)
- Perinatal conditions such as abnormally long labor, precipitated or uncontrolled labor, abnormal presentation of the infant; any condition that causes brain injury during delivery
- Neonatal conditions such as premature birth, low or very high birthweight, poor feeding, infections of the newborn, and the presence of physical and sensory abnormalities
- Presence of any one of many genetic syndromes (e.g., Down syndrome, fragile X syndrome); family history of language disorders
- Environmental factors, including poverty in the home and neglect and/or abuse
- Prelinguistic communication deficits, which include avoidance of eye contact, limited or no babbling, frequent crying, little interest in such gestures as "bye-bye," and showing little or no emotion
- Failure to point by 12 months of age
- Failure to follow such simple instructions as "Go get your shoes"

- Delayed production of the first words, including "Mama" and "Dada"
- Lack of social smile and lack of, or little interest in, social play
- Reduced use of gestures or, conversely, communicating only through gestures
- Impaired learning of speech sounds

CHILDREN WITH SPECIFIC LANGUAGE IMPAIRMENT

A language disorder in a child who is otherwise typically developing is described as a specific language impairment (SLI), also known as a primary language impairment. The majority of children with language disorders exhibit SLI. About 7–8% of kindergarten children exhibit SLI. Children with SLI have certain characteristics that distinguish them from other populations.

Characteristics of Children With Specific Language Impairment

General Characteristics of Children With Specific Language Impairment

Past and current research has delineated characteristics of children with SLI. Most researchers agree upon the following:

- Children with SLI manifest an impairment specific to language. This impairment is not secondary to other developmental disabilities.
- Children with SLI have no known etiology or associated condition, such as sensorimotor problems, ID, or significant neurological impairments. Some children with SLI have cognitive deficiencies, although their general intelligence may be within the normal range.
- The sequence of language development in children with SLI is the same as that of typically developing children. However, problems may be seen with various components of language, such as morphology.
- Children with SLI display varied profiles. Some have great difficulty in syntax but relatively normal pragmatic performance and moderate difficulty with semantic skills, for example. Children with SLI represent a widely varied and heterogeneous group.
- There are two major explanations of SLI. The first explanation is that SLI reflects the **normal variation** in linguistic skills and that children with SLI are at the lower end of the normal continuum of language skills. Just as some people have poor math or musical skills, some people have poor linguistic skills (Leonard, 1991, 1998).
- The second explanation is that of **underlying deficits**. In this view, SLI is due to deficits in cognitive, auditory, perceptual, and intellectual functions that underlie language. Currently, it is believed that there are biological and genetic components to SLI.
- Today, most experts believe that the neurological underpinnings of language impairment have been identified in language-specific areas of the brain: Heschl's gyrus and the asymmetrical planum temporale.
- Frontal lobe abnormalities, especially in the inferior frontal regions, are also common in children with SLI. These abnormalities are linked with deficits in cognitive processing, including executive functioning.

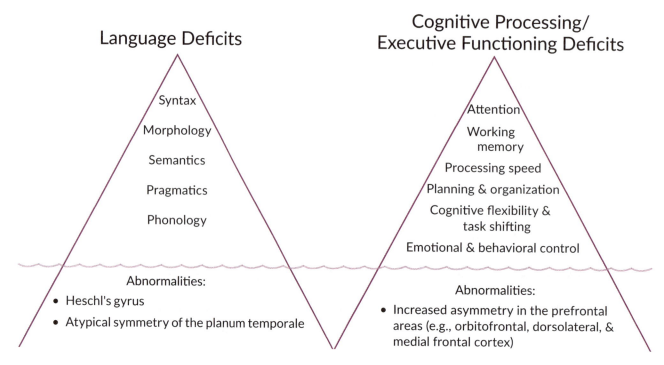

Figure 4.1 The "dual iceberg" model of specific language impairment.

- Thus, children with SLI have abnormalities in two specific areas of the brain: (a) language-specific areas and (b) frontal brain areas that influence development of executive functioning skills (see Figure 4.1). Today, many researchers believe that common cognitive processes may underlie both verbal and nonverbal performance in children with SLI.

Specific Characteristics of Children With Specific Language Impairment

Speech and Language Deficits
- Children with SLI often have **articulatory and phonological problems**, currently also called **speech sound disorders**. They may have poor speech intelligibility and may exhibit the use of **phonological patterns** (e.g., final consonant deletion) longer than typically developing children.
- Children with SLI may use less-complex syllable structures; for example, they may use more consonant–vowel (CV) combinations than same-age peers who are using CVCV combinations. Children with SLI may also have fewer consonants in their phonetic repertoires.
- Children with SLI are often late starting to talk. They have a slow rate of word acquisition, especially between 18 and 24 months of age, when children typically show a great vocabulary spurt. For example, most typically developing children have 50 words in their expressive vocabularies by

18 months of age and 200–300 words by 24 months of age. Children with SLI may reach their second birthday saying as little as 30–40 words.

- Children with SLI may either **overextend** words (e.g., calling all adult males "Daddy") or **underextend** words (e.g., calling only the family pet "dog" and failing to use the term for other dogs). In another example of underextension, only an Oreo may be a "cookie"; a chocolate chip cookie, frosted wafer, or animal cookie may not be labeled "cookie" because they are not Oreos.
- Children with SLI often demonstrate **word finding** or **word retrieval problems**. These word finding problems may result in dysfluencies, such as pauses and interjections or fillers, such as "um" and "you know." Word finding problems may also result in the use of vague or general words (e.g., "this," "that," "thing") instead of specific referents.
- Learning abstract or figurative words is often hard for children with SLI. They frequently use concrete, not abstract, words to express themselves. For example, a child with SLI might say, "I'm mad," instead of "I feel frustrated with this situation."
- The majority of children with SLI have marked morphological problems, as follows:

  - **Perceptual problems**. Children do not perceive morphological features as well as they do other features, because those features are produced with less stress and lower intensity.
  - **Syntactic problems**. The syntactic complexity involved in sentence comprehension and production may have a negative effect on morphology.

- Morphological problems include omissions of the following:

  - Regular and irregular plural morphemes (e.g., *cats*, *trees*; *mice*, *geese*)
  - Possessive morphemes (e.g., Dadd*y's* hat, big brothe*r's* bike)
  - Present progressive *–ing* (e.g., swing*ing*, play*ing*, eat*ing*)
  - Third-person present tense singular (e.g., "He play*s* ball" or "She dance*s* ballet.")
  - Articles (*a*, *an*, *the*)
  - Auxiliary and copula verbs (e.g., the auxiliary *is* in "She is running"; the copula *is* in "She is smart")
  - *Regular past-tense inflections and irregular past-tense words (cooked, typed; rode, ate)*
  - Comparatives and superlatives (e.g., *–er* in *smaller* and *–est* in *smallest*)

- Children with SLI frequently use shorter utterances than typically developing children. That is, their mean length of utterance, or MLU, is shorter than that of typically developing peers.
- Children with SLI use transformations and complex and compound sentences less frequently or not at all; simple, declarative sentences may predominate.
- The speech of some young children with SLI is **telegraphic**. Instead of saying, "The cat is eating her food," the child might say, "Cat eat food." The child preserves the meaning of the utterance while omitting the smaller grammatical elements.
- Understanding or comprehending complex sentences is difficult for many children with SLI. This especially presents problems in the classroom setting, where SLI students spend much of their time in large groups of typically developing children who understand complex teacher talk.

- The pragmatic skills of children with SLI vary greatly. While some have fairly normal pragmatic language skills, others have difficulty initiating and sustaining topics of conversation.
- Many children with SLI are passive—that is, unassertive and unresponsive—in communicative interactions. Other children with SLI are assertive yet unresponsive; they initiate conversations but are unaware of and unresponsive to their partners' needs.
- Children with SLI may have difficulty with the following aspects of pragmatic skills:
  - Topic initiation
  - Topic maintenance
  - Turn taking
  - Appropriate conversational repair strategies (e.g., asking, "What do you mean?" when a speaker's utterances are not understood or changing one's own productions when a listener fails to understand)
  - Discourse (conversation) and narrative skills
  - Staying relevant during conversation
- Narratives of children with SLI are less complete, contain fewer utterances, and show more communication breakdowns than those of typically developing children.
- Young children with SLI are at risk for later problems with spelling, reading, and writing.
- Children with SLI may have difficulty with utterances requiring attention to **order of mention**. In some cases, they may literally follow commands as they are given in sequence, rather than following the commands as they are intended. For example, if a caregiver says, "Before you eat lunch, wash your hands," the child may eat lunch first and wash his hands afterward because he is following the exact sequence of the utterance.

Cognitive Processing/Executive Functioning Deficits

- Recent research has focused upon subtle cognitive deficits of children with SLI (Boudreau & Costanza-Smith, 2011; Ebert, 2014; Owens, 2014; Rispens & Baker, 2012; Wittke, Spaulding, & Schectman, 2013).
- These deficits fall under the umbrella term **executive functioning**. **Executive functioning** is a broad term that encompasses the domain of cognitive abilities responsible for initiating, planning, sustaining, and inhibiting behavior and thoughts.
- Specific executive functioning challenges for children with SLI include the following:
  - **Speed of processing**. Children with SLI process information more slowly than typically developing children.
  - **Attention to task**. Research consistently shows that children with SLI have difficulty focusing for appropriate periods of time on necessary tasks.
  - **Working memory**. This is a domain-general system that controls attention and processing of information; it involves information that is in an active and/or accessible state and is used to complete some form of mental activity. Real-life activities that draw on working memory include following multistep directions; repeating or writing verbatim sentences just heard;

repeating back strings of digits, syllables, or nonwords; and following the actions of multiple characters over the course of a story. These tasks are hard for children with SLI.

- **Emotional control**. A child's inability to modulate his emotions to successfully and appropriately engage in social interaction often leads to problems relating to peers. Difficulty regulating emotions, which is related to behavior problems, can negatively affect such things as vocabulary learning (Schmitt, Justice, & O'Connell, 2014).
- **Task shifting**. Children with SLI have more difficulty switching tasks with ease than typically developing peers; they also become more easily taxed.
- **Planning and organization**. This executive functioning skill requires using problem-solving ability to organize, formulate, evaluate, select, and implement a sequence of thoughts and actions to achieve a desired outcome (Wittke et al., 2013). Children with SLI often manifest disorganization and lack of ability to plan effectively.

■ Again, as previously stated, experts today believe that common cognitive processes may underlie both verbal and nonverbal performance in children with SLI. Thus, it is important to assess and treat children with SLI in the areas of language and executive functioning (Ebert, 2014).

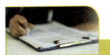

SUMMARY

- Children with SLI manifest an impairment specific to language. This impairment is not due to known etiological factors or associated conditions, such as sensorimotor problems or intellectual deficiencies. However, certain early risk factors are associated with later language impairment.
- Children with SLI generally show specific difficulties in all aspects of language skills: syntax, morphology, phonology, semantics, and pragmatics. They also manifest executive functioning, or cognitive processing, deficits.
- However, there is great heterogeneity in the SLI population, with children manifesting different profiles of problems with various language and cognitive components.

CHILDREN WITH LANGUAGE PROBLEMS ASSOCIATED WITH PHYSICAL AND SENSORY DISABILITIES

Language disorders in some children are associated with other kinds of disabilities. For instance, ID, ASDs, hearing loss, traumatic brain injury (TBI), and cerebral palsy (CP) are associated with language disorders. Language problems coexist with these disabilities.

Intellectual Disability

Intellectual disability (ID), the term now preferred to **mental retardation**, is defined by the American Psychiatric Association (2013) as a "disorder with onset during the developmental period that includes both intellectual and adaptive functioning deficits in conceptual, social, and practical domains" (p. 17).

- Children with ID are a diverse group. Some are affected by inherited genetic syndromes, such as Down syndrome, which is due to a chromosomal abnormality; others are affected by environmentally induced genetic abnormalities (e.g., fetal alcohol syndrome).
- A variety of prenatal factors can cause ID: rubella, maternal lead poisoning, maternal anoxia, and prenatal trauma. Fetal anoxia, or oxygen deprivation during the birth process, can also cause ID.
- Postnatal factors that can cause ID include lead poisoning, TBI, low birthweight, endocrine and metabolic disorders (e.g., hypothyroidism and phenylketonuria), and cranial abnormalities (e.g., micro- and macrocephaly).
- The severity of communication problems in children varies with the extent of the ID. Most experts agree that language is the area that is the most impaired in these children. The language of children with ID is deficient in phonologic, morphologic, semantic, syntactic, and pragmatic components.
- It is generally believed that the language of children with ID is **delayed** rather than deviant. That is, children with ID follow the same **sequence** of language development as typically developing children. However, they reach language milestones more slowly.
- Profoundly intellectually disabled children may show **echolalia** (parrotlike repetition of what others say), which is uncommon in children who are learning language normally. **Immediate echolalia** (immediate repetition of another person's utterance) may be present. For example, if a mother says "Chelsea, see the kitty?" the child might immediately say "Chelsea, see the kitty?"
- Some children with ID have concomitant problems, such as the following:
  - Distractibility and a short attention span
  - Congenital microcephaly ("small head")
  - Difficulties with gross and fine motor skills
  - Physical structural deficits, such as a cleft palate
- Cognitively, children with ID tend to have depressed skills. These children are very concrete and have difficulty with abstract concepts. This is thought to affect language skills, particularly semantic skills.
- Children with ID have semantic difficulties, in that they frequently have smaller, more concrete vocabularies than typically developing children. There may also be a gap between comprehension and expression skills, with comprehension being superior to expression.
- Morphologic skills are especially poor in most children with ID. Due to difficulty with the abstract nature of bound morphemes, the speech of many children with ID is telegraphic. Such children tend to omit bound morphemes and **function words**, or the small words that help make up sentences (e.g., instead of saying "The man is going to the store," a child with ID might say, "Man go store").
- The syntax of children with ID is reduced both expressively and receptively. They master syntactic constructions like typically developing children do, but at a slower pace. They frequently use short and simple syntactic structures and have difficulty understanding long and complex sentences.
- Pragmatically, children with ID may be passive in interacting with others. Or, because of their reduced communication skills, they may be physically aggressive and communicate physically rather than verbally.

- Because many children with ID have other problems (e.g., medical, gross motor), it is usually necessary to use a multidisciplinary approach to assessment and treatment.

Autism Spectrum Disorder

Leo Kanner (1943), an Austrian child psychiatrist, originally described **autism** as a profound emotional disorder of childhood. It was believed for many years that autism was a form of child psychosis. Currently, most experts support genetic or neurophysiological theories of autism, including hypotheses that cortical or subcortical dysfunction, or both, may be involved.

- In 1944, another Austrian psychiatrist, Hans Asperger, also described a group of children with unusual behaviors and called their condition **autistic psychopathy**.
- It is now believed that Kanner and Asperger described the same clinical condition, except that Kanner's children generally had IQs below 70 and Asperger's children had IQs above 70. (Note: The term **Asperger's syndrome** is still informally used in some but not all circles; it represents children who are high functioning and on the autism spectrum. It is not used as much today because of the new definition in the DSM-V described below.)
- Because of the wide variations in the symptom complex of autism, the phenomenon is described under the single title of **autism spectrum disorder** (ASD). According to the DSM-V (American Psychiatric Association, 2013), **ASD** is defined as "persistent deficits in social communication and social interaction across multiple contexts, as manifested by the following" (p. 27):
  - Deficits in social–emotional reciprocity
  - Deficits in nonverbal communicative behaviors used for social interaction
  - Deficits in developing, maintaining, and understanding relationships
- The DSM-V specifies, "Individuals with a well-established DSM-IV diagnosis of autistic disorder, Asperger's disorder, or pervasive developmental disorder not otherwise specific should be given the diagnosis of autism spectrum disorder" (p. 29). Because of inconsistencies in diagnosis, the DSM-V collapses the previous categories under the umbrella of ASD.
- However, because the categories of Asperger's syndrome and others have proven to be helpful for assessment and intervention, many professionals continue to use those labels as previously indicated.
- The estimated prevalence of children with ASD is 1 in 59 children—1 in 37 for boys and 1 in 151 for girls. The prevalence of autism is rising, and experts are unsure about the cause(s) of that. Numerous studies have shown that childhood vaccines, for example, do not cause autism (Autism Science Foundation, 2017). Today, it has been shown that autism has a genetic component.
- Characteristics of children with ASD generally include the following:
  - Generally below-average intelligence (IQ 70 or below)
  - Lack of responsiveness to and awareness of other people
  - Preference for solitude and objects rather than people
  - Lack of interest in nonverbal and verbal communication
  - Stereotypic body movements, such as constant rocking
  - Insistence on routines, strong dislike of change

- Dislike of being touched or held
- Self-injurious behaviors, such as head banging (in some children)
- Unusual talent in some area, such as arithmetic (in some children)
- Seizures (in about 25% of children)
- Hyper- or hyposensitivity to sensory stimulation

■ Language problems associated with autism include the following:

- Inadequate or lack of response to speech
- Lack of interest in human voices and better response to environmental noises; fascination with mechanical noises
- Slow acquisition of speech sound production and language, reflecting general disinterest in interaction with others
- Use of language in a meaningless, stereotypic manner, including echolalia
- Echolalia may be immediate or delayed (in **delayed echolalia**, the child imitates a previous utterance after a few minutes, days, weeks, or even years)
- Perseveration on certain words or phrases
- Faster learning of concrete than abstract words, including more ready learning of words that refer to objects as opposed to emotions
- Deficits in comprehension and use of figurative language
- Lack of generalization of word meanings
- Lack of understanding of the relationships between words
- Pronoun reversal (use of *you* for *I* and *I* for *you*; referring to self as *he*, *she*, *him*, or *her*)
- Use of short, simple sentences; occasional use of incorrect word order
- Omission of grammatical features, such as plural inflections, conjunctions
- Social communication problems, including lack of eye contact, difficulty maintaining conversational topics, reduced initiation of conversation, and lack of assertiveness
- Difficulty establishing joint reference

■ Children with autism may have associated problems, such as motor deficits, ID, abnormal electrical activity of the brain, and hearing loss. Because of these associated problems, it is frequently necessary to use a multidisciplinary team approach to assessment and intervention.

■ Treatment for autism has emphasized social skills training (Moore & Montgomery, 2018). Systematic and prolonged language training has resulted in meaningful communication patterns in many children. Behavioral management techniques, when combined with behavioral language training, have been shown to be effective.

■ Today, it is estimated that 20–50% of individuals with ASD do not develop functional natural speech, so the use of alternative, augmentative communication devices may be warranted (Finke et al., 2017).

■ Asperger's syndrome is characterized by the following:

- Characteristics similar to those of autism except for communication skills and intellectual levels, which are higher (IQ 70 or above)

- Impaired social interactions similar to those of autism
- Repetitive and stereotyped behaviors similar to those of autism

■ As previously stated, the DSM-V does not officially recognize the term **Asperger's syndrome** today. However, because some professionals continue to use the term informally, communication deficits of children with Asperger's syndrome are described as follows:

- Generally, children with Asperger's syndrome acquire language skills better than those with autism; they may have excellent vocabularies and seemingly typical syntactic skills. However, their social communication is quite atypical.
- Children with Asperger's show idiosyncratic and restricted behavioral patterns and interests. They may talk obsessively about their preoccupations; their speech is often more a monologue than a dialogue; they may not allow others to take conversational turns; they may not grasp that their listeners are bored or in a hurry.

■ Communication treatment of children with Asperger's syndrome is usually concerned mostly with their pragmatic deficits. These deficits often present significant challenges to children with Asperger's syndrome as they attempt to interact with family, peers, and teachers. Social skills training is currently popular for children with Asperger's.

■ One popular treatment paradigm is called the SCERTS model (Prizant, 2004). The SCERTS acronym emphasizes the importance of targeting goals in social communication (SC) and emotional regulation (ER) by implementing transactional supports (TS). These transactional supports include visual supports, environmental arrangements, and communication style adjustments.

■ More recently, naturalistic interventions have been emphasized. In these approaches, social skills are taught in informal settings not primarily designed for instruction (e.g., the child's home). In the developmental–social pragmatic perspective, there is a focus on increasing the adult's responsiveness to a child and establishing balanced turns between the child and the adult.

■ Studies indicate that there is strong evidence that helping parents increase their responsiveness to their children's behavior can increase joint engagement and support development of social communication skills (Ingersoll, Meyer, Bonter, & Jolinek, 2012).

Brain Injury

Children can have brain injury due to various causes. Children with brain injury can be classified into various subgroups depending on the injury's cause and sequelae. Two major subgroups of brain-injured children include those who sustain injury due to head trauma (with resulting TBI) and those who have CP. Traumatic brain injury is treated in greater detail in Chapter 8; here, we summarize information relevant to children's language disorders.

Traumatic Brain Injury

■ TBI in children refers to cerebral damage caused by external physical force. The injury is not congenital, nor is it a result of a neurological disease. A **focal injury** is restricted to one area of the brain; **diffuse injury** involves multiple areas because damage is widespread.

- TBI in children is most frequently caused by vehicular and sports-related accidents, falls, physical abuse, assaults, domestic violence, and gunshot wounds. The highest rates of injury occur among low-income children, possibly because of increased exposure to violence, gunshot wounds, decreased supervision, and lack of knowledge of preventative care.
- In 2012, an estimated 329,290 children (age 19 or younger) were treated in U.S. emergency departments for sports and recreation-related injuries that included a diagnosis of concussion or TBI. From 2001 to 2012, the rate of emergency department visits for sports and recreation-related injuries with a diagnosis of concussion or TBI, alone or in combination with other injuries, more than doubled among children (age 19 or younger). In 2013, assaults were the leading cause of TBI-related death for children ages 0–4 years (Centers for Disease Control and Prevention, 2017).
- A multidisciplinary team approach to assessment and treatment is always necessary. Medical personnel may be especially involved.
- Immediate effects of TBI include coma or loss of consciousness and confusion and posttraumatic amnesia (memory loss). Abnormal behaviors, including aggression, anxiety, irritability, hyperactivity, lethargy, and withdrawal, may be present. There may also be motor dysfunctions such as tremors, rigidity, spasticity, ataxia, and apraxia.
- Cognitive and language difficulties may be associated with TBI. Some of these are observed only initially and may resolve; others may be long term. Problems associated with TBI include the following:
    - Comprehension problems, especially of sentences
    - Word retrieval problems leading to reduced fluency
    - Syntactic problems, including limited MLU, fewer utterances, and difficulty expressing and understanding long, complex sentences
    - Reading and writing problems, poor academic performance
    - Pragmatic problems, such as difficulty with turn taking and topic maintenance (often related to poor inhibition and lack of self-monitoring)
    - Inability to recognize one's own difficulties
    - Reduced speed of information processing
    - Difficulties with reasoning, organization, and memory
    - Distractibility and difficulty focusing
    - Low tolerance for frustration
- Children with TBI have unique needs. Frequently, the effects of TBI persist over time. One challenge for children with TBI is that traditional, standardized language tests used in schools are often not sensitive to the special problems these children manifest.
- In recent years, an increasing trend is for speech–language pathologists (SLPs) to become more actively involved with students with mild TBI due to sports-related injuries (Moore & Montgomery, 2018).
- Children with TBI need to be assessed regularly in natural settings to determine how they are functioning in those settings. Such children should be served through a comprehensive team approach that helps them integrate into school and society.

Cerebral Palsy

Cerebral palsy (CP) is a disorder of early childhood in which the immature nervous system is affected. This results in muscular incoordination and associated problems. Cerebral palsy is not a disease; it refers to a group of symptoms associated with brain injury in children.

- CP occurs in 2.3–3.6 out of every 1,000 children. Spastic CP is most common, making up 61–76.9% of all CP cases (cerebralpalsy.org, 2017).
- Associated problems may include orthopedic abnormalities, seizures, feeding difficulties, hearing loss, perceptual disturbances, and intellectual deficits. However, not all children with CP have all these problems.
- CP is not a progressive disease. It generally occurs for the following reasons:
  - **Prenatal brain injury** due to maternal rubella, mumps, accidents, or other factors
  - **Perinatal brain injury** due to difficulties in the birth process, such as prolonged labor, prematurity, and breech delivery
  - **Postnatal brain injury** due to anoxia, accidents, infections, and diseases, such as scarlet fever and meningitis
- Children with CP can manifest paralysis of various body parts. These may be categorized as follows:
  - **Hemiplegia**—one side of the body, the right or left, is paralyzed
  - **Paraplegia**—only the legs and lower trunk are paralyzed
  - **Monoplegia**—only one limb or a part thereof is paralyzed
  - **Diplegia**—either the two legs or the two arms are paralyzed
  - **Quadriplegia**—all four limbs are paralyzed
- Although many types of CP have been described, most professionals categorize CP into three major types:
  - **Ataxic CP**, which involves disturbed balance, awkward gait, and uncoordinated movements (due to cerebellar damage)
  - **Athetoid CP**, which is characterized by slow, writhing, involuntary movements (due to damage to the indirect motor pathways, especially the basal ganglia)
  - **Spastic CP**, which involves increased spasticity (increased tone, rigidity of the muscles), as well as stiff, abrupt, jerky, slow movements (due to damage to the motor cortex or direct motor pathways)
- Speech and language problems associated with CP depend heavily on the type of CP and the presence of associated problems, such as ID or hearing loss. Some children with CP have typical language skills, while others have severe language problems. Dysarthria, described in greater detail in Chapter 8, is common among children with CP.
- Treatment for children with CP should involve a multidisciplinary team approach and the use of alternative, augmentative methods of communication if necessary.

- Today, iPad applications, or "apps," are quite popular for use with children with CP. These apps often have excellent pictures, icons, and other features that enable children with CP to communicate more quickly and easily. Anecdotally, some clinicians and parents have found that an iPad is much "cooler" than a bulky, old-fashioned augmentative alternative communication device.

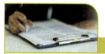

SUMMARY

- Children who have physical and sensory disabilities, such as intellectual disability (ID), autism spectrum disorder (ASD), and TBI, manifest unique language characteristics that tend to coexist with the disabilities.
- Children whose disabilities are severe may require the use of augmentative, alternative communication devices.
- A comprehensive team approach to assessment and treatment is necessary for children whose language problems co-occur with physical and sensory disabilities.

CHILDREN WITH LANGUAGE PROBLEMS RELATED TO PHYSICAL AND SOCIAL–ENVIRONMENTAL FACTORS

Some children manifest language difficulties that are related to a combination of physical and social–environmental factors, such as poverty, neglect or abuse, alcohol or drug exposure in utero, and attention-deficit/hyperactivity disorder. Researchers and clinicians are seeing increasing numbers of children who have a wide variety of language problems that coexist with these factors (Roseberry-McKibbin, 2013, 2014, 2015).

Language Problems Related to Poverty

There is no demonstrated causal relationship between poverty and language-learning difficulties. Professionals should be careful never to equate poverty with dysfunction. Many children from low-income backgrounds have excellent language skills because their home environment stimulates and supports language learning.

- Other children, however, show problems in language learning. Research shows that while not directly causing language problems, limited access to health care, low socioeconomic status, and low educational levels of caretakers are associated with limited early language experience for children. Language that children from lower socioeconomic and educational levels hear at home may be limited both in quantity and quality (Hart & Risley, 1995; Palafox, 2017; Roseberry-McKibbin, 2014, 2018b).
- Socioeconomic status is more critical to language development than ethnic background. The factor most highly related to socioeconomic status is the mother's educational level.

- According to the Pew Research Center (2017), today 21.8% of poor Americans are children under the age of 18. Poverty is heaviest in the southern United States. Current statistics indicate that in the United States, Hispanic and African American children experience poverty at higher rates than White children (Pew Research Center, 2017). Many of these children have limited access to health care.
- Limited access to health care can affect language skills because of the following:
  - Children who are often sick and do not get adequate medical treatment miss much school, thus limiting academic and language exposure.
  - Children who come to school sick have difficulty concentrating and learning.
  - Children who do not have access to medical care frequently have untreated ear infections.
  - Mothers of low-income children often get inadequate prenatal care, which affects the neural development of the fetus.
  - Mothers who receive inadequate prenatal care tend to have premature or low-birthweight babies; prematurity and low birthweight are associated with language and cognition problems.
- Research has documented a strong correlation between education and income level. For example, long-term welfare dependency is strongly associated with lack of a high school diploma and low literacy levels. Three out of four people on welfare can't read (Literacy Project Foundation, 2017). This may affect the language development of children from low-income homes, because some caregivers may not provide the following:
  - Adequate oral language stimulation for the children
  - Opportunities for literacy
  - A variety of enriching experiences (e.g., trips to zoos, museums)
  - Toys and books that stimulate language development
- Children from backgrounds of poverty show wide variation in their language skills. Some have excellent language skills. Others show such deficits as the following (Roseberry-McKibbin, 2013, 2014, 2018b):
  - Difficulty in reading and writing
  - Difficulty referencing time and temporal concepts due to a lack of routine and structure in the home
  - Lack of familiarity with "school-type" tasks, such as reciting the alphabet, singing rhyming songs, reading books
  - Delayed vocabulary skills due to lack of language stimulation and lack of exposure to a variety of experiences; difficulty with abstract vocabulary is very common
  - Delayed morphosyntactic skills
  - Less verbal elaboration and overall verbalization

Intervention for children in poverty with potential and actual language impairments often involves enriching and building oral and literate language skills. Providing access to literacy materials is particularly needed, since so many low-socioeconomic-status children have no books at all in the home. Teaching parents strategies to increase children's oral and literate language skills should be particularly emphasized.

Language Problems Related to Neglect or Abuse

Statistics indicate that increasing numbers of children come from backgrounds in which they experience neglect, abuse, or both (NA). NA can be found across all socioeconomic levels and ethnic groups but may be somewhat more prevalent in low-income communities because of the stressors associated with poverty.

- According to Safe Horizon (2017), 75% of the child victims who come to the attention of Child Protective Services are victims of neglect, 17% are victims of physical abuse, and 8% are victims of sexual abuse. Seventy-eight percent of child fatalities in the United States involve at least one parent as the perpetrator. Children with disabilities are especially vulnerable to abuse.
- Research has shown a relationship between communicative disorders (particularly those associated with physical anomalies and disabilities) and NA. Parents of children with special needs tend to become frustrated more easily than parents of typically developing children. Frustration creates stress, which can lead to NA.
- The effects of NA on language depends greatly upon the **extent** and **severity** of the NA. A child who regularly undergoes severe physical, emotional, or verbal abuse, or all of these, will have more severe language problems than a child who experiences neglect without abuse.
- While it is difficult to make generalizations about this heterogeneous group of children, certain trends have emerged characterizing the effect of NA on language development and skills.
- Among mother–child pairs in which abuse has been identified, mothers have been observed to be less likely to engage in reciprocal interactions with their infants. In addition, some of these mothers have been found to punish the exploration and risk taking that accompany normal development (Nelson, 2010).
- Children who experience NA are frequently deprived of adequate language stimulation related to **isolation**. Physical or social isolation, or both, reduce the human contact needed to acquire language optimally. Children's opportunities for hearing and practicing a variety of language structures are reduced. Thus, their expressive and receptive language skills are underdeveloped.
- Children who undergo abuse tend to have **expressive language delays**. Some of these children are hit or yelled at when they speak; thus, they speak less and therefore do not develop oral language optimally.
- These children often have poor conversational skills; an inability to discuss feelings; fewer descriptive utterances; and shorter, less complex utterances. They are likely to use terse, practical language to "get the job done," with little elaboration. Little social affect may be observed.
- To best serve children who experience NA, SLPs may serve on multidisciplinary teams that address the emotional and physical, as well as the language, needs presented by these children.
- In addition, today many SLPs serve on teams that work with parents to teach them basic discipline and behavior management skills that they can implement with their children. For example, parents

can be taught that instead of hitting their children for disobedience, they may effectively use time-outs and verbal problem-solving to shape behavior.

Language Problems Related to Parental Drug and Alcohol Abuse

Speech–language pathologists participate in multidisciplinary teams to serve increasing numbers of children who have language problems related to maternal alcohol consumption or drug use during pregnancy. Children who have been prenatally exposed to drugs, alcohol, or both present a wide variety of problems, depending on the extent, pattern, and type of exposure to such substances.

- Recent research has shown that **paternal** alcohol consumption, drug use, smoking, or exposure to environmental toxins can also negatively affect fetal development. Sperm can be damaged by cigarette smoke, marijuana, and alcohol. Men exposed to those teratogens have a greater chance of fathering babies with abnormalities like hydrocephalus, Bell's palsy (paralysis of cranial nerve VII), and mouth cysts.
- Today, it is estimated that 1 out of every 500–600 babies has fetal alcohol spectrum disorder (FASD). FASD is a pattern of mental, physical, and behavioral defects that develop in infants born to some women who drank alcohol during the pregnancy. FASD is a leading cause of intellectual disabilities in the Western world.
- FASD causes direct language problems and creates difficulties in areas associated with language development. Problems associated with FASD include the following:
  - Pre- and postnatal growth problems; abnormally low birthweight and length; small head size (microcephaly)
  - Central nervous system dysfunction; delayed motor development, mild–profound ID or learning disabilities
  - Abnormal craniofacial (skull and face) features
  - Malformations of major organ systems, especially of the heart; possibly a small trachea and kidney problems
  - Behavior problems, including hyperactivity and attention-deficit disorder
  - Poor play and social skills, including poor organizational responses to environmental stimuli
  - Learning and academic problems; poor reading, writing
  - Speech problems such as articulation delay; may have cleft palate or oral–motor coordination problems
  - Swallowing problems, including impaired sucking reflex at birth
  - Language delay
  - Cognitive problems—difficulties with reasoning, memory, learning
  - Auditory processing problems
  - Hearing problems—conductive and sensorineural losses
- **Fetal alcohol effects** (FAE) are signs (e.g., mild physical and cognitive deficits) that have been linked to the mother's drinking during pregnancy. Babies with FAE do not meet the diagnostic criteria for FASD.

- Children who are prenatally exposed to drugs also have difficulties in language and related skills (Kjellmer & Olswang, 2013; Lewis et al., 2013), including the following:

  - **Motor and neurological problems** such as poor visual tracking, gross and fine motor delays, tremors, and seizures
  - **Affective and behavioral problems** such as mood swings, great difficulty with transitions and changes, refusal to comply with simple commands, and testing of limits
  - **Social attachment and related problems** such as limited eye contact, separation anxiety, indiscriminate attachment to new people, aggressiveness with peers, and decreased responsiveness to praise and rewards
  - **Cognitive skill impairments** such as poor on-task attention, distractibility, and difficulty with immediate, short-term, and long-term memory
  - **Language learning problems** such as delayed language acquisition, decreased use of words and increased use of gestures to communicate wants and needs, word finding problems, and difficulty following directions

- Children prenatally exposed to drugs and alcohol may have language problems that are not readily detected by standardized language measures. Thus, such children may be denied services in the public schools because they do not fit a recognized category, such as **learning disability** or **intellectual disability**.
- Early intervention is critical for children who are prenatally exposed to drugs and alcohol. These children appear to especially benefit from structure and routine. Caregivers must be involved as much as possible in treatment efforts.
- An enriched environment may help to ameliorate some effects of early exposure to cocaine; for example, some studies have shown that the caregivers of cocaine-exposed children in foster or adoptive care had higher vocabulary scores than biological caregivers. Cocaine-exposed children in foster or adoptive care attained IQ scores similar to those of children with no cocaine exposure (Lewis et al., 2013).

Language Problems Related to Attention-Deficit/Hyperactivity Disorder

Speech–language pathologists are seeing increasing numbers of students with language problems related to **attention-deficit/hyperactivity disorder** (ADHD). Children with ADHD are at elevated risk for language impairment in pragmatic, syntactic, and semantic skills. Thus, SLPs are increasingly collaborating with multidisciplinary teams that identify and serve students with ADHD.

- According to the DSM-V (American Psychiatric Association, 2013), ADHD is characterized by difficulties in two major areas: (a) inattention and (b) hyperactivity and impulsivity. The behaviors in these two areas must be long lasting and evident for at least 6 months, with onset before age 7. It is estimated that 13.2% of boys and 5.6% of girls have ADHD.
- Increasingly, ADHD is being studied in the context of executive functions. Students with ADHD are described as having chronic difficulties in the areas of impulsivity, attention, and overactivity to a

degree inappropriate to their age and developmental level. They are more likely to receive lower grades in academic subjects, and over half of children with ADHD will fail at least one grade by adolescence.

- Students with ADHD are at risk because they frequently experience academic and behavior problems. In some cases, language and auditory-processing difficulties contribute to or coexist with those problems. It is important for clinicians to provide intervention in cases where these factors are present.
- Behavioral characteristics of ADHD students include fidgeting, distractibility, difficulty waiting for one's turn, and difficulty sustaining attention in tasks or activities.
- Research and clinical experience indicate that students with ADHD tend to manifest the greatest amount of difficulty in social interaction skills. Specifically, these students exhibit the following behaviors:

  - Often blurt out answers to questions before the questions have been completed
  - Have difficulty following through on instructions
  - Often do not seem to be listening
  - Often talk excessively, interrupting others and manifesting poor turn-taking skills
  - Frequently manifest false starts because they change their minds while structuring a response
  - Use an excessive number of fillers and pauses because verbal expression occurs with minimal planning
  - Have difficulty describing things and telling stories in an organized, coherent manner; have general difficulty with expressive language organization
  - Have difficulty with social entry (limited knowledge of how to successfully initiate or join ongoing interactions)
  - Use inappropriate register; for example, use the same interactive style with adults and peers
  - Perceive or act inappropriately upon interlocutors' nonverbal cues

- If students with ADHD are evaluated with traditional language tests that ignore the area of pragmatics, they probably will not qualify for language intervention in the schools. Speech–language pathologists must become actively involved in interdisciplinary, collaborative teams that create effective assessment and service delivery models for students with ADHD.
- Goals of treatment may include work on auditory processing skills, pragmatics, and expressive language organization. A combination of behavioral and pharmacological approaches to treatment often yields the best results.

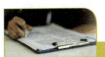

SUMMARY

- Increasing numbers of children have language problems related to physical and social–environmental factors, such as poverty, neglect or abuse, alcohol or drug exposure in utero, and attention-deficit/hyperactivity disorder.
- Speech–language pathologists are increasingly serving on multidisciplinary teams that address the comprehensive profile of needs presented by these children.

ASSESSMENT PRINCIPLES AND PROCEDURES

Language assessment is a process of observation and measurement of a child's language behaviors to determine (a) the existence of a clinically significant problem, (b) the nature and extent of the problem, and (c) the course of action that must be taken to help the child and the family. In this section, we discuss common procedures and principles that can be applied to children of any age; use of standardized and alternative forms of assessment; and specific recommendations for infants and toddlers, preschool and elementary-age children, and adolescents.

Language Assessment: General Principles and Procedures

Whatever the age of the child being assessed, clinicians typically follow a set of common procedures that serve as the foundation for the assessment. Procedures common to assessing any disorder in clients of any age are described in Chapter 13. Here we will summarize what is especially relevant to assessing language disorders in children.

- Typically, clinicians need to do the following as part of general procedures for assessment of children of all ages:

  - Obtain results of visual or audiological evaluations
  - Obtain any available relevant medical data that might be important
  - Obtain psychological data, including the results of cognitive functioning and intelligence testing
  - Interview family members (especially the parents or other primary caregivers) to better understand the problem as they see it, obtain information about the child's language development, assess family communication patterns, and ascertain caregiver preferences about treatment targets

- For elementary-age and adolescent students clinicians need to do the following:

  - Obtain assessment data on educational achievement that might suggest learning disabilities
  - Talk to the teacher about the academic demands the child faces in the classroom relative to the Common Core State Standards and select potential treatment targets based on the teacher's recommendations

- Language assessment generally falls into three broad categories: screening, standardized assessment, and alternative assessment approaches.

Screening

Screening is a process of quickly obtaining a general overview of a child's language skills.

- Most clinicians use screening initially to decide whether further assessment is necessary.
- Screening usually indicates one of two things: (a) The child's language skills fall within the normal range, and, therefore, no further assessment needs to be completed, or (b) there is a possible language impairment, and further assessment is needed.

- Many clinicians use informal measures to screen language. These are often constructed by individual clinicians and consist of simple activities, such as conversational samples, that quickly test children's expressive and receptive language skills. Published screening tests are also available.

Standardized Assessment

Standardized tests provide clinicians with a quantitative means of comparing the child's performance to the performance of large groups of children in a similar age category.

- Standardized tests are preferred by many clinicians because they yield quantitative scores that may be converted into such other measures as language age, percentile rank, standard score, and standard deviation. Many school district guidelines require the use of these normatively based quantitative measures for placement of a child into special education services within the public school system.
- When selecting standardized tests, clinicians must consider their inherent limitations. Some of the serious limitations include an inadequate national sampling in the normative process, inadequate response sampling (e.g., only one or two opportunities to produce a grammatical feature), contrived test situations that do not represent naturalistic communication, limited participation of families in assessment when tests are the main source of information, and general inappropriateness for culturally and linguistically diverse children (Moore & Montgomery, 2018; Roseberry-McKibbin, 2018b) (Other limitations of standardized tests are described in Chapter 13.)
- Clinicians must avoid using standardized tests as the sole measure for making clinical judgments about children's language skills and the presence of a language impairment. In fact, clinicians should consider standardized tests as supplements to language samples and other alternative assessment approaches.

Alternative Assessment Approaches

Although the use of standardized language tests is widespread in the United States, many researchers and clinicians are increasingly turning to various alternative assessment approaches.

- Limitations of standardized tests are the main reason for considering alternative approaches, which are especially relevant to assess clients who are culturally and linguistically diverse. Alternative approaches also tend to sample more naturalistic communication skills and expand the scope of assessment to include more information about the child's daily functioning.
- Several useful alternative approaches are described in Chapters 11 and 13. These approaches include **criterion-referenced assessment**, **dynamic assessment**, **assessment of information processing skills**, and **portfolio assessment**. Because no alternative is complete by itself, it is essential to combine the most desirable and necessary elements of each approach and individualize the assessment instruments used to the needs of the individual child.
- Clinicians must be familiar with these approaches so their assessment is relevant to all clients, avoids a false positive or false negative diagnosis, and generates reliable and valid data on which treatment

Table 4.1

Rules for Counting Morphemes

Count as two morphemes

Structure	Examples
Regular past-tense –*ed*	wash*ed*, wav*ed*, look*ed*
Present progressive –*ing*	writ*ing*, decorat*ing*, runn*ing*
Possessive marker –*'s*	Mommy*'s*, teacher*'s*, friend*'s*
Plural marker –*s*	cookie*s*, present*s*, glass*es*
Third-person singular present tense marker	swim*s*, flie*s*, drink*s*

Count as one morpheme

Structure	Examples
Compound words (2 or more free morphemes)	birthday, hotdog, railroad
Proper names	Dr. Cho, Mr. Cook, Uncle Ed, Wile E. Coyote
Each recurrence of a word for emphasis	no, no, no; awesome, awesome, awesome!
Ritualized reduplications	night-night, choo-choo
Contracted negatives	won't, can't, don't
Diminutives	dolly, horsie, kitty
Irregular past-tense verbs	swam, ate, wrote
Auxiliary verbs	is, will
Catenatives	gotta, hafta, wanna

Do not count

Structure	Examples
Fillers	um, ah, er, uh
Dysfluencies, except the one complete form	l-l-l-lollipop

Note. Adapted from *A First Language: Early Stages,* by R. Brown, 1973, Cambridge, MA: Harvard University Press, and *Language Disorders: A Functional Approach to Assessment and Intervention* (4th ed.), by R. E. Owens, 2004, Boston, MA: Allyn & Bacon.

plans may be based. Such assessment data also help document the progress clients make during treatment.

- Language sampling is a popular, widely used alternative assessment approach that avoids the drawbacks of standardized tests.

Language Sampling

Language sampling is a measure of communication skills vital to a diagnosis of language impairment in children. This is a procedure of recording a student's language under conditions that are relatively typical, and appropriate for the client, which usually involve conversation.

- Put differently, language sampling ideally obtains language as the child directly uses it in specific situations. Ideally, the language sample is representative of the child's everyday usage.
- The clinician's main task in obtaining a language sample is to stimulate the child to speak as freely and naturally as possible. This can be accomplished through the use of a variety of toys, books, stories, pictures, and games. Other conversation partners, such as peers and family members, may interact with the child. Ultimately, the language sample should be representative of the child's daily language use.
- Clinicians must remember that a single language sample is not sufficient; additional samples must be obtained. Brief language samples should be recorded subsequent to the first sample.
- Clinicians may informally analyze a language sample or use a number of published protocols that are available. These include the *Language Assessment, Remediation, and Screening Procedure* (LARSP; introduced in Crystal, Fletcher, & Garman, 1976); *Developmental Sentence Scoring* (DSS; introduced in Lee, 1974); and the *Language Sampling, Analysis, and Training* procedure (LSAT; introduced in Tyack & Gottsleben, 1974).
- Some language sampling programs are available as computer software; these include *Computerized Profiling* (Long, Fey, & Channell, 2004), *Lingquest 1* (Mordecai & Palin, 1982), and *Systematic Analysis of Language Transcripts* (SALT; Miller & Chapman, 1983).
- Many clinicians use a language sample to obtain a measure of a child's **mean length of utterance** (MLU), which is usually calculated in morphemes through the following method:

$$\text{MLU} = \frac{\text{number of morphemes}}{\text{number of utterances}}$$

- Clinicians can analyze not only the child's MLU but also the presence or absence of Brown's 14 grammatical morphemes (see Chapter 3, Table 3.3). There is a set of generally accepted rules for counting morphemes, which are summarized in Table 4.1.
- As an example of how to calculate MLU based on morphemes, suppose an SLP collects a 50-utterance language sample that contains 225 morphemes. The child's average MLU would be 4.5. In another example, suppose the SLP records 50 utterances and obtains a language sample that consists of 300 morphemes. This child's average MLU would be 6.0.
- Language samples can also be analyzed through a **type-token ratio** (TTR), which is calculated as follows:

$$\text{TTR} = \frac{\text{number of different words in a sample}}{\text{number of words in sample}}$$

- TTR represents the variety of different words the child uses expressively, thus assessing the child's semantic or lexical skills. To calculate TTR as shown above, the clinician first counts all the words in the sample (even if they are repeated). These words become the denominator. The clinician then counts each different word in the sample—for example, if *dog* occurs 10 times, it is only counted once. The number of different words the child uses becomes the numerator.

- For children 3–8 years of age, the TTR is typically 1:2, or 0.5. In other words, the total number of words spoken by the child during the language sample is usually about twice the number of different words in the sample.

Assessment of Infants and Toddlers

The assessment and treatment of infants and toddlers has taken on increasing visibility in past years. There are several reasons for this.

- First, laws, such as P.L. 99-457, Preschool Amendments to the Education of the Handicapped Act, 1986, have provided incentives at the state and federal levels for SLPs to identify and treat infants and toddlers with established risk of language disorders or who experience conditions that put them at risk for developing language disorders.
- Specifically, Part C of the Individuals with Disabilities Education Act (IDEA, 2004) is called The Program for Infants and Toddlers with Disabilities. It is a federal grant program that assists states in operating a comprehensive statewide program of early intervention services for infants and toddlers with disabilities, ages birth through age 2 years, and their families. In order for a state to participate in the program, it must assure that early intervention will be available to every eligible child and its family.
- Due to advances in medical science, many more medically fragile pre-term infants are surviving; these infants often have multiple disabilities, including speech, language, and motor skill problems. The assessment of infants and toddlers holds special challenges for clinicians, who must account for risk factors as well as overt language problems.

Risk Factors for Language Disorders in Infants and Toddlers

Factors involving an **established risk** of developing language disorders are mostly biological or disease related. These factors include the following:

- Congenital malformations (e.g., cleft palate, spina bifida)
- Genetic syndromes (e.g., Down syndrome)
- Atypical developmental disorders (e.g., autism)
- Sensory disorders (e.g., hearing loss, visual impairment)
- Neurological disorders (e.g., cerebral palsy, muscular dystrophy)
- Metabolic disorders (e.g., Tay-Sachs disease, pituitary diseases)
- Chronic illnesses (e.g., diabetes, cystic fibrosis)
- Severe infectious diseases (e.g., HIV, encephalitis)
- Severe toxic exposure (e.g., lead poisoning, fetal alcohol syndrome)

Prelinguistic Behavioral Deficiencies in Infants and Toddlers

There are early warning signs that a child may have a language impairment. Infants who may later be diagnosed with language impairment frequently show one or more of the following:

- Difficulty establishing eye contact, mutual gaze, and joint reference; lack of pointing by 12 months

- Communication of needs through greater use of gestures and vocalizations than words and phrases; frequent delays in onset of first word and onset of two-word combinations
- Reduced amount of babbling, fewer consonants in babbling, and less complex babbling

Late Talkers

In recent years, there has been increasing interest in a group of children labeled "late talkers." These children are characterized by a significant expressive language delay at 24–30 months of age.

- These children are generally less vocal and verbal than their peers, exhibiting smaller consonant and vowel inventories, delays in morphosyntactic development, smaller vocabularies, and problems with narratives.
- An ongoing point of discussion about late talkers is whether they will spontaneously outgrow their language delays and catch up with their typically developing peers.
- Although many late talkers appear to eventually catch up to their typically developing peers, recent research reveals that even children who appear to have recovered by age 4 from early delay are at modest risk for continuing difficulties. It is recommended that they receive continued monitoring, even if they are in the low-normal range for language development.
- For example, Hammer et al. (2017) analyzed data from a longitudinal study involving 9,600 children. They found that being a late talker (at 24 months of age) increased children's risk of low vocabulary at 48 months and low school readiness at 60 months. Late talkers had more difficulty in kindergarten.

General Assessment Guidelines and Procedures for Infants and Toddlers

- Make a family-centered communication assessment of infants and toddlers in both home and clinical settings.
- Begin assessment as early as possible and repeat assessments throughout the childhood period. Assess the family constellation, family resources, family strengths and limitations, and family communication patterns, including bilingual–bicultural status (Karanth, Roseberry-McKibbin, & James, 2017b).
- Work on a team with other professionals. Make interdisciplinary decisions regarding which assessment materials and methods to use and how assessment results will be used.
- Conduct interviews and gather an extensive case history, including maternal health during pregnancy, circumstances of the birth, and early development patterns of the infant (e.g., fine and gross motor skills, speech and language).
- Take into consideration the cultural practices in family communication patterns, child rearing, caretaker–child interactions, and accepted roles for children in adult–child interaction.

Specific Assessment Guidelines and Procedures for Infants and Toddlers

With infants and toddlers (depending upon the age), clinicians generally need to assess comprehension and production of language, hearing, readiness for communication, infant–caregiver interaction, and play activities. This is often accomplished through the use of parent questionnaires designed to use parent report to establish the presence or absence of certain language behaviors.

Language-Related Skills

- Assess the infant's attentional and physiological state (including alertness, drowsiness, light or deep sleep states, eye opening, crying, toleration of handling, etc.).
- Assess the infant's readiness for communication (e.g., whether the baby shows reciprocal interaction with the environment).
- If necessary, refer the infant to an audiologist.

Language Comprehension and Verbal Communication

Use language development milestones (see Chapter 3) to assess the presence or absence of verbal communication behaviors, as well as language comprehension skills. This can be done through direct observation, parent report, or both.

Infant–Caregiver Interaction

Materials exist for evaluating caregiver–infant interactions (e.g., Brookes Publishing publishes observation tools). These instruments help assess caregiver behaviors such as how they visually focus on the baby, how quickly they respond when the baby vocalizes or otherwise indicates need, and how the caregivers express affection for the baby.

Play Activities

- Observe the child engaged in play with one or several other children (Karanth et al., 2017a; Owens, 2018). Observe the child's pattern of interaction during play and evaluate whether the child does any of the following:

  - Exhibits aggressive or uncooperative behaviors
  - Refuses to share toys
  - Talks little during play
  - Passively watches others play
  - Plays cooperatively with other children
  - Engages in isolated or parallel play
  - Engages in constructive activities with or alongside other children
  - Engages in pretend play and role-playing

- There are several types of play that may be evaluated:

  - **Solitary play.** The child is completely engrossed in playing and does not seem to notice other children. This is often seen in children between 2 and 3 years old.
  - **Parallel play.** The child mimics other children's play but doesn't actively engage with them. For example, she may use the same toys but not interact with the other children who are playing with those toys.
  - **Associative play.** Children are more interested in each other than in the toys they are using. This is the first category that involves strong social interaction between the children while they play.

- **Collaborative (cooperative) play.** Some organization enters children's play—for example, the playing has some goal, and children often adopt roles and act as a group (around 4 years old). For example, children might say things like "Let's have a store. I'll be the cash register person and you be the customer. You can be the mommy who is buying groceries."

Assessment of Preschool and Elementary-Age Children

Language problems often become apparent during the elementary school years. They are frequently brought to the surface by reading and writing deficiencies that cause academic problems and even failure. Children who experience academic difficulties are usually referred for speech–language assessment. In ideal circumstances, language problems would be noted and treated when children are in preschool.

Description of Language Disorders in Preschool and Elementary-Age Children

Language problems of preschool and elementary-age children can be associated with a variety of factors, such as SLI, ID, environmental factors, and others. Characteristics of such children with language problems may include the following:

- **Difficulty in comprehending spoken language.** This includes problems with comprehending syntactically longer and more complex productions, as well as difficulty comprehending the meaning of complex words, phrases, sentences, and abstract terms.
- **Slow or delayed language onset.** This can include delayed babbling, slower vocabulary growth rate, delayed acquisition of vocabulary, slowness in combining words into phrases and sentences, and overall slower acquisition of language milestones.
- **Limited language output or expressive language.** This includes generally limited verbal repertoire, lack of complex or longer word productions, limited amount of vocabulary produced and comprehended, and lack of abstract words in the child's repertoire.
- **Problematic syntactic skills.** This includes use of shorter instead of longer sentences, simpler instead of more complex sentences, single words or phrases in place of sentences, and a limited variety of syntactic structures.
- **Problematic pragmatic skills.** This includes difficulty with initiating and maintaining conversations, turn taking, using conversational repair strategies, maintaining eye contact, and using narrative skills.
- **Problematic learning of grammatical morphemes.** This includes difficulty with comparatives and superlatives (e.g., *smaller, smallest*), omission of bound morphemes (e.g., past-tense *–ed*, plural *–s*), and incorrect use of learned grammatical morphemes, including overgeneralizations (e.g., *womans/women, goed/went*) past the appropriate developmental point.

General Assessment Guidelines and Procedures for Elementary-Age Children

- Begin by screening language to determine whether a more detailed assessment is needed; do this through brief language sampling or through formal screening measures.

- Use social assessment methodologies; conduct interviews as appropriate and necessary. Obtain information from parents, teachers, and peers about the child's communication patterns.
- Evaluate semantic, syntactic, morphologic, and pragmatic aspects of both expressive and receptive oral language.
- Evaluate reading and writing skills if relevant and relate communication skills to academic demands and performance if relevant. Relate communication skills especially to Common Core State Standards, and ask if the child's oral and written communication skills are adequate to meet the standards.
- Assess the family constellation and communication patterns. Consider factors related to bilingualism, second-language acquisition, and use of a social dialect if relevant (Roseberry-McKibbin, 2018b).
- Suggest treatment targets based on findings generated by use of these assessment procedures.

Specific Assessment Guidelines and Procedures for Elementary-Age Children

- Obtain an extended speech and language sample for a typical analysis of language functions. Language samples can be collected on different days with different interlocutors (e.g., peers, teachers, family members) over a period of time to obtain the most representative sample of the child's language.
- Language samples can be analyzed and a description given of the child's semantic, morphologic, syntactic, and pragmatic skills (Pavelko & Owens, 2017). Language comprehension can also be analyzed.
- To assess **syntactic skills**, calculate the child's MLU, as well as the complexity of utterances. Evaluate the child's use of noun, verb, and prepositional phrases. In addition, evaluate the child's use of various types of sentences, such as simple, declarative, compound, complex, active, questions, negatives, and requests.
- To assess morphologic skills, use pictures, toys, and questions to assess production of plurals, comparatives and superlatives, possessives, and use of present progressive –*ing*.

  - Evoke past-tense constructions by telling a story through pictures and then asking the child to use the pictures to retell the story.

- To assess semantic skills, ask parents to list the words the child uses at home (if the child only uses a few words). Ask the child to name and describe pictures, toys, and objects as you show them.

  - Note phenomena, such as unusual word usage, over- and underextensions of words, signs of misunderstanding words, and the use of general terms (e.g., *this, that, thing*) for more specific ones.

- To assess **pragmatic skills**, observe the child's eye contact and other nonverbal behaviors, topic initiation and maintenance, turn-taking (including not interrupting), and ability to remain on topic.
- To assess language comprehension, do the following:

  - Note inappropriate or irrelevant responses that indicate lack of comprehension.

- Note the complexity level at which comprehension breaks down (e.g., comprehension of words and phrases, but not sentences).
- Give specific commands that gradually increase in length and complexity (e.g., "Point to the blue square," "Point to the small, blue square," "Point to the blue square and the green triangle," "Point to the big, blue square and the small, green triangle").
- Ask the child to point to correct pictures that help assess comprehension of grammatical morphemes (e.g., "Show me *the dog is barking*," "Show me *the ball is in the bag*," "Show me *three shoes*").
- Assess comprehension of abstract statements by asking the child to explain the meaning of common proverbs (e.g., "Tell me what 'A penny saved is a penny earned' means"). It is important to remember that proverbs and other figurative language expressions are extremely culture bound.

Standardized Tests for Elementary-Age Children

Various school district guidelines may require the use of formal scores, gathered from formal tests, for the diagnosis of a language impairment in a preschool or elementary-age child. Frequently, these tests evaluate a child's language knowledge. Thus, the tests may or may not be valid for children who are English language learners or who come from low-income backgrounds where they did not obtain the core background knowledge—especially vocabulary—assumed by the tests (Roseberry-McKibbin, 2018b).

Response to Intervention

Today, many school districts are incorporating a response to intervention (RtI) model of assessment for students suspected of language impairment. In this model, at-risk students who are struggling in classrooms are given increasing amounts of targeted individual and small-group support within the classroom setting before a special education referral is made. Students' progress is monitored, and there is increasingly intense and differentiated instruction (Moore & Montgomery, 2018).

- If the students do not respond to this instruction through increased success in academic performance, they are then referred for special education evaluation, including evaluation for potential language impairment.
- RtI is a form of dynamic assessment in which personnel evaluate a student's ability to learn when provided with instruction; this is much more effective and nonbiased than traditional standardized testing.
- A major advantage of RtI is that it is much more effective than traditional standardized testing for students, such as those in poverty and those of English learner status.

Assessment of Adolescents

Language disorders often persist from the early childhood years into adolescence. Research increasingly shows that unless treated, these language disorders usually carry over into adulthood and have an impact upon the person's life in multiple areas: academic, vocational, social, and personal. Language learning and language disorders in adolescents are receiving increased attention in speech–language pathology because of their far-reaching effects. (*Note*: In referring to adolescents, the terms **student** and **client** are used interchangeably.)

General Assessment Guidelines and Procedures for Adolescents

- Begin by screening language to determine if a more detailed assessment is needed; do this through brief language sampling or through formal screening measures.
- Obtain a case history.
- Use social assessment methodologies. For example, conduct interviews with parents, teachers, and peers about the adolescent's everyday communication patterns.
- Evaluate syntactic, semantic, morphologic, and pragmatic receptive and expressive language skills.
- Evaluate reading and writing skills and assess how those skills relate to the demands of the classroom.
- Relate written and oral communication skills to potential vocational needs and demands.
- Consider factors related to second-language acquisition, bilingualism, and use of a social dialect.
- Create treatment targets based upon test results; ensure that targets will result in improved functional written and oral communication.
- Remember that adolescent language assessment may take more time than assessment of language in a younger child because of the need to obtain extended narratives, writing samples, and interviews with people in the adolescent's environment.

Specific Assessment Guidelines and Procedures for Adolescents

- Clinicians should use a combination of formal and naturalistic measures to assess syntactic, semantic, pragmatic, and reading and writing problems, which are common in adolescents with language disorders.
- Clinicians should obtain an extended speech and language sample to analyze the client's language as it occurs naturally in the environment.
- Clinicians should also obtain a sample of a conversation between the client and such interlocutors as a teacher, one or more peers, and a family member or members.
- To assess **syntactic skills**, use the following methods:

  - Assess the use of vague, wordy, and roundabout expressions instead of more precise (thus shorter) expressions.
  - Assess the use of connectives or cohesion devices; note the contexts in which the student should have used such devices but did not.
  - Assess agreement (e.g., noun–verb agreement) in oral and written language.
  - Conduct an analysis of syntactic skills through the use of speech and language samples, narratives, and writing samples.
  - Assess sentence length in **C-units** (communication units) or **T-units** (terminable units). (Both C-units and T-units contain an independent clause and subordinate clauses, but the C-units also may be incomplete sentences produced in response to questions. Count the number of words per unit and calculate both the mode—the most frequently observed length—and the mean.)

- Assess **semantic skills** as follows:
  - **Word definition skills.** Obtain a list of words from the student's teachers and textbooks; ask the student to define them.
  - **Word retrieval problems.** Take note of such dysfluencies in conversational speech as pauses, revisions, false starts, repetitions, and so forth; take note of words that are retrieved with more or less difficulty.
  - **Word-relation problems.** Ask the student to define and contrast synonyms (e.g., *pretty–beautiful*) and antonyms (*pretty–ugly*).
  - **Difficulty in using precise terms.** During conversation, narrative tasks, and writing, take note of the frequency with which the student uses such vague expressions as *stuff, thing, this, that, you know*.
  - **Difficulty in understanding and correctly using figurative language.** Make a list of common idioms, proverbs, and metaphors (e.g., "Don't count your chickens before they hatch"; "fit as a fiddle"; "kicked the bucket") and then ask the student what they mean.

- To assess **pragmatic skills**, employ the following:
  - Assess the frequency with which the client asks you to repeat information; frequent requests suggest poor listening skills.
  - Assess the use of correct register depending on the situation (e.g., use of slang register with peers and more formal register with authority figures).
  - Note any inappropriate body language during conversation (e.g., standing too close, using inappropriate gestures).
  - Introduce various topics and evaluate the student's ability to maintain those topics over successive utterances.
  - Ask the student to read a story and then retell it; ask the student to orally narrate a story; evaluate the student's ability to correctly sequence events in a manner understandable to the listener.
  - Count the frequency of maze behaviors, such as false starts and repeated attempts to express the same idea.
  - Note interruptions, irrelevant comments, and non sequiturs.
  - Make some vague and nonspecific statements to the student, and evaluate whether the student makes requests for clarification.

- To analyze **reading and writing skills**:
  - Ask the student to read grade-level material; analyze the type and frequency of reading errors made.
  - Ask questions about the material the student read to evaluate reading comprehension.
  - Analyze multiple writing samples and look for difficulty forming letters and other handwriting problems, spelling and punctuation errors, syntactic errors, cohesion and overall organization, and appropriateness of content, including the adequacy of information offered and details given.

Standardized Tests for Adolescents

- A problem with many formal, published adolescent language tests is that they contain sections that evaluate aspects of language that develop at much younger ages in typically developing children. For example, some adolescent language tests evaluate students' production of Brown's grammatical morphemes.
- Thus, many clinicians prefer to use nonstandardized procedures to assess language problems in adolescents. However, specific school district guidelines may require the use of formal scores, gathered from formal tests, for the diagnosis of a language disorder in an adolescent.

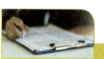

SUMMARY

- Language assessment is used to observe and measure children's language behaviors. The purpose of assessment is to ascertain whether a clinically significant problem exists and what direction to take in treatment if a problem does exist.
- Assessment can involve the use of standardized instruments as well as nonstandardized alternative measures of language.
- Children of different age levels require (a) common foundational assessment procedures, such as hearing screening and a case history, and (b) specialized procedures reflecting the special needs of children in certain age groups.

TREATMENT PRINCIPLES AND PROCEDURES

A wide variety of programs and procedures are available for serving children with language problems. Clinicians may select from different service delivery models to provide the most cost-effective and comprehensive services possible. These models include individual therapy, therapy in small groups, therapy carried out in the classroom setting one-on-one or with a small group, and therapy carried out by nonprofessional people (e.g., parents, interpreters) who have been trained by the clinician. In this section, we describe (a) general language treatment principles, (b) specific language intervention techniques and programs that may be modified according to the age and individual needs of the child being served, and (c) augmentative and alternative communication principles for children with severe disorders of language.

General Principles

- It is important to involve the family in therapy as much as possible. Family members should take part in selecting treatment targets for the child and should be educated in the treatment procedures to be used. Family involvement is especially important for the generalized production of language skills in natural settings and maintenance of skills over time in such natural settings as the home and classroom.

- Clinicians should focus on **academic** and **social** language—the language needed for success in school and the language needed to be socially competent, respectively. The ultimate goal of therapy is social and vocational success (Roseberry-McKibbin, 2018b).
- Clinicians should select literacy—reading and writing—skills when appropriate. Literacy skills may often be incorporated into the traditional speech and language treatment. Because literacy skills are language based, SLPs have much to contribute to the improvement of reading and writing skills in children.
- Various kinds of literacy skills may be taught in the context of speech and language therapy, as described later in this chapter in the "Teaching Literacy Skills" section. Children who are regularly introduced to books and reading will not only develop better language skills but also perform better in the classroom.
- Clinicians should select language treatment targets that are culturally and linguistically appropriate for the child and the family. The child's cultural and linguistic background affects many variables, including the language skills to be taught, the appropriateness of stimulus materials, and possibly certain treatment procedures (Roseberry-McKibbin, 2018b).
- Clinicians must specifically target language behaviors that create social penalties for children. For example, an adolescent who constantly interrupts others will probably be excluded from important peer groups, and reducing such inappropriate language behaviors will facilitate more effective peer interactions.
- Clinicians should use a multimodal approach to treatment. Most children benefit from hearing, seeing, and touching. Instead of focusing exclusively on the auditory modality, clinicians need to use visual and tactile stimulation to reinforce language targets being taught.
- For children who are reluctant to speak, **communicative temptations** can be used (Paul, Norbury, & Gosse, 2018). These are elicitation tasks that increase the likelihood that a child will verbalize to meet her needs. For example, a clinician can set a very attractive toy just beyond a child's reach and not give the toy to the child until she verbally requests it.
- To learn and retain language treatment targets, most children need **multiple exposures to multiple exemplars** of those targets; they also need to be **actively engaged**. For instance, instead of the clinician showing a picture of a Labrador and teaching the child the word *dog*, the clinician needs to have many pictures of different dogs and perhaps even some toy dogs for the child to play with. Rather than just being a passive observer, the child needs to be actively engaged in activities that promote learning (e.g., games, books, worksheets, etc.).
- Clinicians must remember that a child's chronological age does not necessarily dictate specific treatment procedures. The child's current skill level (developmental level) is a much more reliable indicator of what treatment procedures and goals will be appropriate.
- Computer-assisted language therapy is an option for many clinicians. Several companies publish software that addresses a variety of language needs. The iPad is a popular tool, and many apps are available for SLPs to use to build students' oral and literate language skills (Kraemer & Bryla, 2017).
- Collaboration with the classroom teacher is extremely important in bridging classroom language requirements with treatment targets. Children will experience much better carryover of language

targets if those targets are reinforced in the classroom. Clinicians can use classroom materials in therapy, go into the classroom to conduct therapy, and collaborate in many other ways.

- Today, clinicians must help all students with language impairments achieve the Common Core State Standards to the extent possible. The overarching goal of the standards is to create college-ready, globally competitive citizens in the 21st century. The standards address English language arts and math. English language arts consists of four areas: reading, writing, speaking and listening, and language (Common Core State Standards Initiative, 2014). Some clinicians choose to focus their Individualized Education Program (IEP) goals on speaking and listening standards.

- SLPs also need to help elementary-aged and adolescent students succeed with the "hidden curriculum" of the classroom setting, where instructional discourse is used. Instructional discourse, used by teachers, is decontextualized and involves connected utterances used in a sustained exchange (Roseberry-McKibbin, 2015).

- Being flexible and considering the child's current skill level, clinicians can use one or a combination of the following delivery models:

  - Indirect intervention, in which the clinician sets the goals and a peer, parent, teacher's aide, interpreter, or other person carries out the treatment
  - One-on-one intervention in a pull-out model in the therapy room
  - Small-group intervention in a pull-out model in the therapy room
  - One-on-one or small-group intervention in the child's classroom (classroom-based intervention)

- Today, many SLPs conduct classroom-based intervention instead of or in addition to pull-out therapy. In the classroom-based intervention model, SLPs go into the classroom and work with students with language impairments individually or in small groups, helping these students achieve curriculum goals. For example, the SLP might conduct therapy using the classroom language arts book, focusing on the story that the class is currently reading.

- Some experts today believe that classroom-based intervention is superior to pull-out intervention in terms of helping students with language disorders to generalize treatment targets to real-world settings (Moore & Montgomery, 2018). The clinician's goal is to help students become more independent, competent learners across the curriculum (Ukrainetz, 2017).

Specific Techniques and Programs

The following specific techniques and programs can be modified for both group and individual therapy. They can also be modified based upon the child's developmental level, individual needs, and associated clinical conditions.

Discrete Trial Procedure

- Discrete trials are useful in the initial stages of treatment, when skills have to be shaped or established. However, they are not efficient for ensuring that a skill generalizes to the child's natural environment. Therefore, in the later stages of treatment, the clinician should use a more naturalistic method.

- In discrete trial training, the clinician does the following:
  - Places a stimulus picture in front of the child (e.g., a picture of two cups)
  - Asks the child a relevant question (e.g., "Antonio, what do you see?")
  - Immediately models the correct response for the child (e.g., "Say 'two cups'") and waits for a few seconds for the child to imitate the modeled response
  - Reinforces the child for correct imitation (verbal praise, token, smile, etc.)
  - Gives corrective feedback if the child missed the target response (e.g., *two cup*) by saying "No, that is not correct."
  - Records the response on a recording sheet
  - Waits for a few seconds and initiates the next trial

Expansion
- In expansion, the clinician expands a child's telegraphic or incomplete utterance into a more grammatically complete utterance. For example, the child says, "Doggy bark," and the clinician says, "Yes, the doggy is barking."
- It is often more effective to have the child imitate the longer production and reinforce it than to simply display a longer production for the child.

Extension
- In extension, the clinician comments on the child's utterances and adds new and relevant information. For example, a child says, "Play ball." The clinician says, "Yes, you are playing with a big, red, plastic ball that bounces."
- Research extensively supports the efficacy of the use of extensions to build children's expressive language skills (Roberts & Kaiser, 2011). Extensions are easy to fit into caregivers' daily routines and can be used by speakers of any language.

Focused Stimulation
- In focused stimulation, the clinician repeatedly models a target structure to stimulate the child to use it. This is usually done during a play activity that the clinician designs to focus on a particular language structure (e.g., the plural morpheme *–s*).
- The clinician uses various stimulus materials, talks about them, and repeatedly models the plural constructions (e.g., "Look, here are two *pigs*. I see two *pigs* here. Over here are some *boys* playing. The *boys* are drinking from *cups*. The *cups* have *flowers* on them.").
- The clinician does not correct the child's incorrect responses but instead models the correct target (e.g., the child says, "I see two duck swimming," and the clinician says, "Yes, *two ducks* are swimming in the pond").

Milieu Teaching
- Milieu teaching refers to a group of techniques that have been experimentally evaluated and shown to be effective in teaching a variety of language skills to children.

- Milieu teaching teaches functional communication skills through the use of typical, everyday verbal interactions that arise naturally and uses effective behavioral procedures in naturalistic settings. A popular specific technique is incidental teaching in the child's natural environment.
- In the incidental teaching method, the adult waits for the child to initiate a verbal response and
  - pays full attention to the stimulus that prompts a response from the child (e.g., looks at the child pointing to a ball);
  - prompts an elaboration of the response (e.g., "What do you want?") or models an elaboration ("You want that ball! What do you want?"); if the child fails to elaborate, a traditional model ("Say . . .) may be used;
  - praises the child and hands over the desired object when the child elaborates (spontaneously or imitatively).
- Incidental teaching can be used by parents or others who work with the child (e.g., day-care providers).

Joint Book Reading (Dialogic Reading)

- In joint book reading, the clinician stimulates language in children through the use of systematic storybook reading. Joint, or dialogic, book reading allows for repetitive use and practice of the same concepts and phrases.
- It is also helpful for establishing joint attention (in which the clinician and the child are focused on the same thing). It can be used to teach morphologic structures as well (Maul & Ambler, 2014).
- Children listening to a story are encouraged to participate actively in the experience. The adult encourages participation through the use of specific questions, such as those involving recall, completion, and others.
- The clinician selects appropriate storybooks with attractive, colorful, culturally appropriate pictures. He or she reads the same story several times during several sessions, so that the children memorize it.
- The clinician uses prosodic features frequently to draw attention to specific language structures. For example, the clinician might emphasize the past-tense –*ed* morpheme through increased emphasis on words containing that morpheme (e.g., "The man *looked* out the window and *opened* his eyes wide when he *viewed* the snowman.").
- When the children are quite familiar with the story, the clinician stops at points containing target language structures and prompts the children to supply the appropriate words, phrases, or sentences (e.g., "The woman was driving her _____"). Clinicians can manipulate the activity by pausing at different junctures, so children supply different language structures or produce progressively longer utterances.
- Children can be asked eventually to "read" (recite from memory but looking at the text and pictures) and pause while other children supply words, phrases, or sentences. Joint book reading helps develop vocabulary acquisition, as well as a sense of story grammar in children.

- Joint, or dialogic, book reading promotes language and literacy skills in children. It is also helpful if the adult who is reading to the child engages in print referencing, encouraging the child's attention to and interactions with the print on the page. For example, the adult can focus the child's attention on how various letters are formed, how print moves from left to right, and so on.
- The foundational print referencing skill that children develop first is distinguishing pictures from print on a page. This is a good starting point for developing children's print awareness skills.

Narrative Skills Training

- **Narratives** are speakers' descriptions of events (episodes, stories) and experiences. They have specific story grammar characteristics, which include aspects of macrostructure and microstructure.
- Children with language disorders frequently have difficulty with the structure of narratives and need specific instruction in appropriate aspects of macrostructure and microstructure.

Macrostructure

- This can be thought of as the picture frame of the story. It involves:
  - *Characters*—those who perform the actions in the stories
  - *Setting*—time and place where the story occurred
  - *Initiating events*—episodes that begin the story
  - *Internal response*—the characters' thoughts, emotions, reactions
  - *Plan or goals of the characters*—what the characters are trying to accomplish
  - *Attempts*—actions the characters take to achieve their objectives
  - *Direct consequences*—results of characters' actions
  - *Conclusion*—how everything turns out, the lessons or morals learned from the story

Microstructure

- This is the inside of the story "picture." Microstructure involves the details of the story.
- Microstructure involves cohesion, or how each proposition or statement relates to the text as a whole.
- The microstructural level of a narrative concerns the linguistic structures (e.g. embedded clauses, conjunctions, noun phrases) the child uses in the construction of the narrative.
- Microstructure also involves complexity measures, such as the total number of words the child used and the number of different words that the child used. Sentence complexity is also important.
- Clinicians can use various materials (e.g., picture cards, books, and even videos) to help children develop appropriate macrostructure and microstructure narrative skills.

Parallel Talk

- In parallel talk, the clinician plays with the child and describes and comments upon what the child is doing and the objects the child is interested in. For example, the clinician says, "You are putting the lady in the truck," or "That cow you have is brown and white."

Recasting

- Recasting children's limited productions into longer or syntactically different forms can be useful in teaching complex grammatical forms. The child's own sentence is repeated in modified form, but the clinician changes the modality or voice of the sentence rather than simply adding grammatical or semantic markers.
- For example, the child says, "The baby is hungry." The clinician asks, "Is she hungry?" (Changed to question form.) Child: "The dog chases the cat." Clinician: "The cat is chased by the dog." (Changed to passive voice.)

Self-Talk

- In self-talk, the clinician describes her own activity as she plays with the child. Using language structures that are appropriate for that child, the clinician might say something like, "Look, I'm putting the dress on the doll. See, I'm putting the dress on her."

Teaching Literacy Skills

- The clinician should work with family members to educate them about the importance of a literacy-rich home environment and to provide the child with books, pens, paper, and other literacy-related materials to promote reading and writing at home.
- The parents should be asked to be role models by engaging in literacy activities themselves and to include their children in such activities (Roseberry-McKibbin, 2018a).
- The parents should be trained to read more to the child and encourage printing of the alphabet and writing simple words at an early age.
- The clinician should offer effective intervention for oral language disorders to provide a foundation for literacy skills and to prevent reading and writing problems. Written language goals (e.g., specific goals for increasing students' skills in reading, writing, and spelling) can be specifically targeted or can be informally incorporated into therapy for building oral language skills.
- The clinician should select language targets in consultation with the teacher to better integrate language teaching with classroom curriculum content. As stated, it is ideal to help students with language impairment achieve mastery of Common Core State Standards.
- To incorporate literacy training into language intervention, the clinician should use printed words that accompany pictorial and other stimuli used in teaching words, phrases, and sentences; while modeling oral productions, the clinician should point to the corresponding printed words, phrases, or sentences.
- The clinician may use storybooks to promote complex language skills, as well as print recognition, by pointing to words as she reads the stories.
- Targeting vocabulary skills will help increase reading comprehension and fluency and build oral language, as well.
- Research evidence shows that literacy skills can be increased through directly targeting morphological awareness skills (Apel, Brimo, Diehm, & Apel, 2013; Maul & Ambler, 2014). Morphological awareness is the recognition, understanding, and use of word parts that carry significance (Apel &

Lawrence, 2011). For example, students need to understand that prefixes, suffixes, and root words are all morphemes that can be removed from or added to words to change their meaning.

- Targeting phonological awareness skills is also important, as these are foundational for literacy. Phonological awareness, discussed in Chapter 5, refers to the explicit awareness that words are created from sounds, syllables, and their combinations; it is the child's knowledge of underlying sound representations in the mind.
- Research consistently supports the efficacy of targeting phonological awareness skills. Specific phonological awareness skills to be targeted in therapy include the following:

  - **Rhyming**—e.g., correct identification of words that sound alike (*cat–hat*)
  - **Syllable awareness**—knowledge of how many syllables are in a word
  - **Phoneme isolation**—identifying whether the sound is at the beginning, middle, or end of a word
  - **Sound blending**—blending two or more sounds that are temporally separated by a few seconds into a word (e.g., "d-o-g—what animal is that?")

Targeting Executive Functioning/Cognitive Processing Skills

- It was stated earlier in this chapter that children with language impairment (LI) have specific deficits in two basic areas: language and executive functioning (EF), or cognitive processing, skills. The question is whether attempting to improve the EF/cognitive weaknesses in children with language impairment produces improvement in language skills.
- Research has shown that targeting EF as well as language skills can create improvement in both areas; cross-domain interactions exist, as shown by treatment studies (Ebert, 2014; Ebert, Kohnert, Pham, Rentmeester Disher, & Payesteh, 2014; Gillam et al., 2008; Stevens, Fanning, Coch, Sanders, & Neville, 2008).
- Specifically, SLPs can help students with LI improve their working memory, attention, and processing speed through targeted tasks designed to directly address these areas. For example, it has been shown that training children with LI to repeat increasingly long strings of nonsense syllables can help improve their working memory (Boudreau & Constanza-Smith, 2011; Ebert et al., 2014).
- In another example, a research study showed that when students with LI were supported in increasing attention to task and overall behavior regulation, their vocabulary skills improved. There was a positive association between behavior regulation and vocabulary gain (Schmitt et al., 2014).

Augmentative and Alternative Communication

Basic Principles

Augmentative and alternative communication (AAC) is a multimodal intervention approach that uses forms of communication, such as picture communication boards, manual sign language, and computerized or electronic devices that produce speech; these are called speech-generating devices.

- AAC methods supplement deficient oral communication or provide alternative means of communication for children with extremely limited oral communication skills. Children with severe physical impairments, autism, and severe ID are often candidates for AAC.
- AAC methods and materials may also benefit adults and children with apraxia, aphasia, CP, laryngectomy, glossectomy, tracheostomy, spinal cord injury, and other conditions.
- AAC is not necessarily a last-resort approach; it may be the primary and preferred method of communication for certain individuals.
- The major purposes of AAC are helping the child (a) express wants and needs, (b) transfer information, (c) promote social closeness, (d) participate in social etiquette routines (e.g., greetings and leave-takings), and (e) communicate with oneself (e.g., writing down a reminder about an appointment the next day).
- Today, SLPs are being encouraged to provide AAC devices and strategies to children as early as infancy and toddlerhood in order to maximize their communication potential (Davidoff, 2017).
- Increasingly, AAC options are used not only to replace spoken language, but also to supplement an individual's speech and facilitate language development (Lund, Quach, Weissling, McKelvey, & Dietz, 2017).
- AAC devices can be **low-technology devices**, such as notepads or message boards, which do not use electronic instruments. **High-technology devices**, or methods that use electronic instruments, such as computers, may also be used.
- When AAC users want to communicate messages, they use **displays**, systems or devices that show the messages to their communication partners. Displays range from communication boards to computer screens.
- Symbols used by AAC users may be iconic or non-iconic. **Iconic symbols** look like the object or picture they represent. For example, a hieroglyphic picture of a house is an iconic symbol indicating the word *house*.
- **Non-iconic symbols** are arbitrary, abstract, and geometric. They do not resemble the objects they represent and must be specifically taught. Flexible plastic shapes and chips are examples of non-iconic symbols.
- Regardless of the type of AAC device used, users of the device send messages through two means: direct selection and scanning.
- In **direct selection** the user selects a message by touching a keypad, touching an item or object, depressing an electronic key, pointing, or some other direct means.
- In **scanning**, the user is offered available messages by a mechanical device or communication partner. The messages are offered sequentially until the AAC user indicates the messages he or she wants to communicate.
- Speech–language pathologists may, as part of treatment, help children learn to use AAC devices in a variety of settings outside the treatment room. These settings include the home, classroom, and various places in the community.
- Today, iPad technology is increasingly being used by children with multiple communication needs. iPad apps are often ideal because they can provide meaningful, fun contexts for interaction, expand

output options to include animation or voice, and provide options for personalization. All of these qualities are important in motivating children to use AAC technology (Kraemer & Bryla, 2017).
- A child's willingness to use AAC technology is also affected by response efficiency. Response efficiency involves response effort, as well as quality, rate, and immediacy of reinforcement.
- In both assessment and treatment of children who use AAC devices, a team approach is extremely important. Team members may include a speech–language pathologist, physical therapist, occupational therapist, psychologist, social worker, engineer, vocational counselor, teacher, and nurse. The team may work with the child to use one of several forms of AAC: gestural (unaided), gestural-assisted (aided), or neuro-assisted (aided) methods.

Gestural (Unaided) AAC

- In **gestural** (**unaided**) AAC, no instruments or external aids are used. Rather, the child uses gestures and other patterned movements, which may be accompanied by some speech. Gestures play a major role in communication of messages. Examples of widely used current gestural (unaided) forms of AAC are:

  - **Pantomime**—mostly uses gestures and dynamic movements that involve the entire body or parts of the body. The child uses transparent messages, facial expressions, and dramatizations of meanings. **Transparent messages** are those likely to be understood with no additional cues by an observer without special training. Balandin (2005) describes transparency as "ease of deciphering what the symbol means" (p. 387). Conversely, a message or symbol that is **opaque** is one that is not easily decipherable.
  - **American Sign Language (ASL)**—consists of manual signs for the 26 letters of the alphabet, as well as signs for words and phrases. Recognized as a separate language, ASL may be used alone or with oral speech. Sign language can be effective and useful as a method of AAC for babies and toddlers with disabilities (Davidoff, 2017).

Gestural-Assisted (Aided) AAC

- In **gestural-assisted** (**aided**) AAC, gestures or movements are combined with an instrument or message-display device. Gestures are used (a) to display messages on a mechanical device, such as a computer monitor, or (b) to scan or select messages displayed on a nonmechanical device, such as a communication board.
- Mechanical devices tend to involve high technology and sophisticated electronics. These devices are often run by software, and they generate printed messages or speech.
- Speech-generating devices typically display pictures that represent what the child wants to say. When a specific picture is pressed on a speech-generating device, it generates speech with a synthesized (computerized) or digitized (recorded) form that the communication partner can hear.
- Nonmechanical devices use no electronic technology, and there is no message storage, speech output, or printed output.

- Messages on both mechanical and nonmechanical devices take various forms. Examples of common types of symbols are:

  - **Rebuses**—pictures that represent events or objects along with words, grammatical morphemes, or both.
  - **Picture Exchange Communication System (PECS)**—a low-technology method of communication that is known to be effective. The clinician initially teaches the child to exchange specific pictures to communicate with a partner (e.g., hands the picture of a glass of water to the partner to request water); it is known that PECS eventually promotes spontaneous verbal expressions, as well.

Neuro-Assisted (Aided) AAC

- **Neuro-assisted** (**aided**) AAC is useful for children who have such profound motoric impairments and limited hand mobility that they cannot use a manual switching device. This type of AAC uses bioelectrical signals, such as muscle-action potentials, to activate and display messages on a computer monitor.
- The electrical activity of the muscles associated with their contraction is used to activate switching mechanisms. Electrodes attached to the child's skin pick up electrical discharges that are then amplified, so they can activate special kinds of switches (called **myoswitches**) or specific displays.
- The user receives feedback (e.g., onset of sound or light) when a switch or display is activated. The user then learns, through biofeedback, to use muscle-action potentials for activating messages.
- Equipment for users of neuro-assisted (aided) AAC is expensive and can be challenging to maintain.

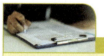

SUMMARY

- Clinicians can use several service delivery models and treatment programs to serve children with language problems.
- Treatment must always be individualized to meet the needs of each child, with family and classroom involvement being an intrinsic part of therapy.
- Some children have extremely limited oral communication skills because of conditions such as autism and cerebral palsy. For these children, augmentative and alternative communication methods can supplement oral communication or provide alternative means of communication.

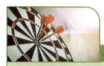

CHAPTER HIGHLIGHTS

- In some children, language deficits are the only major problem. Children with specific language impairment (SLI) may appear typically developing except for their language deficits, which are not associated with a known etiology or clinical condition. Children with SLI have deficits in two major areas: language and executive functioning/cognitive processing.

- In other children, language deficits may be associated with specific physical and sensory disabilities, such as intellectual disability (ID), autism, hearing impairment, and brain injury. It is important to provide individualized assessment and treatment based on those children's particular needs. A comprehensive team approach is especially critical, because those children often have multiple disabilities and multiple needs.
- Some children have language problems related to physical and social–environmental factors. These factors include poverty, neglect and abuse, maternal or paternal drug or alcohol use, and attention-deficit hyperactivity disorder. Speech–language pathologists are seeing increasing numbers of children with language problems related to these factors. Early intervention and prevention are critical components of treatment.
- Assessment of language skills involves observation and measurement of a child's language behaviors to determine whether a clinically significant problem exists. Assessment can involve screening; the use of formal, standardized measures; the use of alternative, nonstandardized measures; or a combination of these.
- Formal, standardized measures provide clinicians with a means to quantitatively compare a child's performance to the performances of large groups of children in a similar age category. Many clinicians rely on these measures because they yield quantitative data (e.g., percentile ranks), which many school districts require before a child can receive treatment in the public school system.
- Because of the problems inherent in using formal, standardized measures, clinicians have increasingly turned to alternative, nonstandardized measures. Language sampling is an excellent way to evaluate children's language skills in natural settings.
- Clinicians are increasingly serving infants and toddlers who have an established risk of language disorders or who experience conditions that put them at risk for developing language disorders. Working with families and with interdisciplinary teams is critical in providing comprehensive, appropriate services.
- Many children with language problems are identified in preschool or elementary school. These children usually have difficulties with multiple aspects of language, including morphologic, syntactic, phonologic, semantic, and pragmatic aspects. In elementary schools, language disorders are associated with literacy problems (reading, writing, and spelling problems).
- Language problems from childhood frequently carry over into adolescence. Assessment of adolescent language can be challenging because language problems affect all aspects of the adolescent's life: social–personal, academic, and, potentially, vocational.
- Treatment of language disorders must be individualized to meet children's needs. Varied service delivery models, programs, and procedures exist for meeting those needs. Clinicians are increasingly collaborating with classroom teachers to promote generalization of language treatment targets into classroom settings. Clinicians are increasingly incorporating literacy skills into speech–language therapy. Children with severe language disorders may use augmentative and alternative communication devices to assist them with communication.

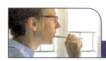

STUDY AND REVIEW QUESTIONS

1. A clinician is working with parents on home language-stimulation activities for their 3-year-old daughter, Hannah, whose language is delayed. Among other things, Hannah needs to increase her expressive language skills to a level more commensurate with her chronological age. Her mean length of utterance is restricted, and her utterances are more typical of a young 2-year-old child. The clinician has recommended that at home, the parents use a technique in which they play with Hannah and describe and comment upon what she is doing and the objects she is interested in. For example, the parents might say, "You are making the car go fast," or "That pig is pink." The parents are using the technique of

    A. self-talk.
    B. expansion.
    C. expatiation.
    D. parallel talk.

2. You are seeing a 6-year-old child, Tyler, with specific language impairment. When you assess Tyler, you find that he has adequate language comprehension. He is able to follow directions, understand vocabulary, and comprehend sentences of appropriate length and complexity for his age. However, his teacher and parents report that he has "no friends" and that they are concerned about his social skills. When you observe Tyler several times on the school playground, in the classroom, and in the school cafeteria, you see that, while he is well behaved and nondisruptive, he does not initiate interactions with others. Treatment should focus on

    A. increasing mean length of utterance.
    B. working on bound morphemes.
    C. increasing assertiveness in conversation.
    D. increasing sentence complexity.

3. You are seeing a 9-year-old boy, Emile, whose *Peabody Picture Vocabulary Test–Fourth Edition* score is one year above age level. Emile appears to be performing adequately in the classroom. His teacher reports that he is at grade level in most subjects. However, he often interrupts others and irritates his listeners; as a result, he is avoided by many peers. His mother reports that he is not invited to other children's birthday parties and that she has heard that other mothers view him as rude and disrespectful. Treatment should focus on increasing

    A. pragmatic skills.
    B. syntactic skills.
    C. morphologic skills.
    D. semantic skills.

4. You are working with an adolescent, Alyssa, who has receptive and expressive language problems. She is getting Ds in most of her classes at the junior high school and has few friends. In therapy, it would be best to target

    A. increasing auditory memory skills.
    B. increasing the use of complex sentences containing subordinate clauses.
    C. increasing social use of language and collaborating with the classroom teachers.
    D. increasing the understanding and use of figurative language.

5. A child who shows slow, writhing, involuntary movements has which type of cerebral palsy?

    A. Spastic

    B. Mixed

    C. Ataxic

    (D.) Athetoid

6. Which one of the following is *not true*?

    A. Standardized language tests provide a means of quantifiable comparison of a child's performance to that of large groups of children in a similar age category.

    (B.) Standardized language tests help sample behaviors adequately, providing multiple contexts for sampling target-language behaviors.

    C. With young children, we want to examine play skills (among other things).

    D. In language sampling, some clinicians calculate a type-token ratio (TTR), which represents the variety of different words a child uses expressively.

7. You are assessing the expressive language skills of a 4-year-old with delayed language. One of the things he says is "My birthday party was fun—we ate cake and cookies!" This would count as

    A. 10 words, 10 morphemes.

    B. 10 words, 12 morphemes.

    (C.) 10 words, 11 morphemes.

    D. 10 words, 9 morphemes.

8. You move to a new elementary school and begin seeing the children on the caseload at this school. One child, who is being treated to "increase semantic skills," has four goals listed on her IEP. Which one of these goals is inappropriate?

    A. Increase types and numbers of words the child uses in the classroom

    B. Increase specific word usage and decrease usage of nonspecific words, such as *this, that, thing*

    C. Decrease overextensions of words

    (D.) Increase use of appropriate discourse skills, turn taking, and conversational repair strategies → pragmatics

9. A child with traumatic brain injury would most likely manifest which of the following?

    A. A higher familial incidence

    B. Echolalia and obsessive talking

    C. Hypersensitivity to touch, insistence on routines, lack of interest in human voices

    (D.) Impaired word retrieval and comprehension, lack of attention, and memory problems

10. Which of the following is *not true* with regard to treatment of children with language disorders?

    (A.) Because many children with language disorders have difficulties with working memory, clinicians should conduct therapy primarily through the auditory modality and not be concerned with incorporating tactile or visual activities into therapy.

    B. Collaboration with classroom teachers is important in helping children generalize treatment target behaviors.

C. It is helpful, when appropriate, to incorporate reading and writing (literacy) intervention into language therapy.

D. A child's chronological age is not always the best predictor of the kind of treatment that will be appropriate; current skills (developmental level) is a more reliable indicator.

11. A third-grade teacher refers 8-year-old Allyson to you. The teacher is concerned because "Allyson's verbal expression skills just are not what they should be. When she talks, she speaks in real simple sentences. Sometimes, I feel like I'm dealing with a kindergartener, not a third grader." When you speak with Allyson's parents, they say, "Allyson never was much of a talker. She talked late—later than her brothers and sisters. But she was always well behaved, and we never thought she had a problem." You decide that as part of your assessment of Allyson's language skills, you will gather and analyze a language sample using TTR. When you eventually calculate TTR based on her language sample, you find that her TTR is 0.31. You conclude that

A. Allyson is normally developing her syntactic skills.

B. Allyson is delayed in pragmatic skills.

C. Allyson is low in her lexical skills or the number of words she uses expressively.

D. Allyson has receptive morphological problems.

12. A clinician is providing services for a school-age child, Myron, who uses an AAC device. Myron's parents and teacher report that he is having trouble with the device; others frequently do not understand what he is trying to communicate. He is showing increasing signs of frustration, and the clinician has been asked to help reduce his frustration by facilitating his communication with other people. To help Myron communicate more effectively with others so that they understand his messages better, the clinician needs to make sure that the symbols on Myron's AAC device are

A. PECS friendly.

B. transparent.

C. non-iconically opaque.

D. opaque.

13. Justin is a 7-year-old second-grade child who has been diagnosed with Asperger's syndrome. Since he was a toddler, he has had language difficulties. He has just transferred to your school district, and speech–language services have been recommended for him. Justin's parents are anxious for him to begin therapy as soon as possible. You read over the file of reports written by personnel from his previous school district and meet with your school's Student Study Team (SST) to discuss Justin and recommend the best possible program for him in your school district. The report from the previous SLP says, among other things, that Justin's language sample showed that he had difficulty with forms, such as *–er* (e.g., *bigger*) and *–est* (e.g., *biggest*). Problems with these forms reflect poor

A. morphologic skills.

B. pragmatic skills.

C. literacy skills.

D. semantic skills.

14. Because of his diagnosis of Asperger's syndrome, you can assume that Justin will probably have characteristics, such as

A. generally below-average intelligence (IQ 70 or below), a lack of responsiveness to and awareness of other people, and stereotypical body movements, such as constant rocking.

B. a preference for solitude and objects rather than people, a lack of interest in nonverbal and verbal communication, tantrums, head banging, and insistence on routines.

C. a seemingly excellent vocabulary; seemingly normal syntactic skills; and speech that often seems to be a "monologue," in which Justin does not allow his conversational partner to take turns.

D. an IQ of 70 or below, speech characterized by monologues, and head banging.

15. The SST believes that Justin might profit from the SCERTS approach to intervention, which involves

A. an emphasis on improving social communication, implementing ongoing evaluation of regulatory behavior, and training syntactic skills for increased communication success.

B. an emphasis on the importance of targeting goals in social communication and emotional regulation by implementing transactional supports, such as visual supports, environmental arrangements, and communication-style adjustments.

C. an emphasis on improving semantic communicative effectiveness, regulation of emotional state, and transactional environmental supports, such as increased auditory cues.

D. a holistic approach that encourages social communication, effectiveness in regulating transactions, and successful dialogue with others in the environment.

16. Using Brown's morphemes as a reference, which utterance below represents two morphemes?

A. Daddy's
B. Cupcake
C. Choo-choo
D. No no!

17. A school-based SLP is conducting classroom-based intervention with several students diagnosed with specific language impairment. This means that the SLP is

A. conducting pull-out intervention, in which she brings the students to her therapy room and uses classroom materials as part of a small-group therapy session.

B. conducting pull-out intervention, in which she brings a student to her therapy room and uses classroom materials as part of an individual therapy session.

C. teaching language skills to the whole class; the students with SLI are part of this class.

D. going into the classroom and helping language impaired students, individually or in a small-group format, to achieve classroom curriculum goals.

18. In a preschool setting, a typically developing child walks up to a child with SLI and says, "Let's play house. You be the mommy, and I'll be the daddy, and we'll make dinner. Then the grandma will put the baby to bed." The typically developing child is suggesting that they engage in which type of play?

A. Parallel play
B. Associative play
C. Collaborative play
D. Side-by-side symmetrical play

19. The mother of Danny, a 3-year-old who is speaking very little, has been working with an SLP on some language stimulation techniques to build Danny's expressive language skills. One day when they are driving,

Danny points to the sky and says excitedly, "Plane sky!" His mother responds, "Yes, I see that big silver plane flying up in the blue sky! Wow!" She has just used the technique of

A. extension.
B. parallel talk.
C. expansion.
D. recasting.

20. The SLP has noted that when Danny does speak, he appears to have word retrieval difficulties. The SLP decides to target this in therapy. In targeting word retrieval skills, she is working on the area of

A. morphology.
B. semantics.
C. pragmatics.
D. phonology.

21. Jeannette is a 4-year-old girl with specific language impairment. At preschool, the teacher says, "Before you put on your jacket to go outside, be sure to get your snack." Jeannette puts her jacket on first and then tries to get her snack. The teacher becomes angry and believes Jeannette is not following orders. Jeannette is showing difficulty with

A. phonological awareness.
B. pragmatics.
C. syntax.
D. order of mention.

22. Jonathan is a 5-year-old boy with a language impairment. He has a German shepherd at home named Angel. The neighbors have a Rottweiler, and his grandma has a poodle. But Jonathan only calls Angel a "dog;" he does not use the word "dog" to refer to his neighbor's Rottweiler or his grandma's poodle. We can say that Jonathan is demonstrating the pattern of

A. underextension.
B. overextension.
C. restricted semantic categories.
D. overcategorization.

23. Parents bring their son Derek to you. He is 30 months old and only says a few words. The pediatrician has told them to not worry and just give Derek time, saying "He is a boy, after all, and they usually develop language more slowly." But Derek's parents are still concerned. The best recommendation you could give them would be:

A. Do nothing and follow the pediatrician's recommendation to give him time to develop
B. Give them a home language stimulation program, and tell them to come back in a year for a re-evaluation
C. Recommend an immediate, full evaluation of Derek's language skills
D. Send Derek and his parents to a psychologist for an evaluation of his cognitive skills

24. You are working in a school and are told that a new child with an IEP has transferred to your school and will be needing language intervention. On her IEP, it states that she has a "pragmatic language disorder." Which one of the following problems are you MOST likely to see in this student?

A. Difficulties in allowing a conversational partner to have a turn
B. Problems using complex and compound sentences
C. Vocabulary deficits
D. Word retrieval problems

25. Mario is a 4-year-old Head Start preschool child whose teacher has observed some "red flags" in his language development. You decide to interview Mario's parents and observe him in the classroom setting. You also decide to conduct a language sample. You want to conduct a language sample with Mario because

   A. you can use the results to obtain quantitative data, such as percentile ranks and standard deviations, as required by the school district to enroll him in speech–language services.

   B. a language sample's primary diagnostic function is to evaluate the child's language in actual daily settings.

   C. the teacher has requested it, and by law, you need to carry out assessments requested by classroom teachers.

   D. language samples are mandated by the Common Core State Standards.

26. You obtain 50 utterances from Mario. Your analysis of the language sample shows that Mario used 100 words and 120 morphemes. Thus, his average MLU (mean length of utterance in morphemes) is

   A. 5.0.
   B. 4.5.
   C. 2.0.
   D. 2.4.

27. Tonia is a 6-year-old with autism spectrum disorder. As you work with her, you find that she frequently says what you just said. For example, if you say "Tonia, point to the apple," she says "Tonia, point to the apple." What you are observing is Tonia's use of

   A. extrapolated utterances.
   B. immediate echolalia.
   C. delayed echolalia.
   D. semantic replication.

28. You have a new job in a school district where you are serving preschoolers, elementary students, and teens. You will remember that Part C of the Individuals with Disabilities Education Act (IDEA)

   A. is a federal grant program that assists states in operating a comprehensive statewide program of early intervention services for infants and toddlers with disabilities, ages birth through 2 years, and their families.

   B. is a focused early diagnostic program whose goal is to identify language delayed preschool children and refer them to Head Start.

   C. guarantees appropriate augmentative, alternative communication devices for children with cerebral palsy and other medically based conditions.

   D. mandates IEPs that provide for language-based work-study programs for language impaired students in high school.

References and Recommended Readings at www.advancedreviewpractice.com

STUDY AND REVIEW ANSWERS

1. **D.** If parents are using a technique in which they play with their child and describe and comment upon what she is doing and the objects she is interested in (e.g., the parents might say, "You are making the car go fast," or "That pig is pink"), the parents are using the technique of parallel talk.
2. **C.** A 6-year-old child with a language impairment and adequate language comprehension but difficulty initiating interactions with others would best be served by treatment focusing on increasing assertiveness in conversation.
3. **A.** Pragmatics, or social language, is the area in which this student needs the most help.
4. **C.** Adolescence is a time when the use and comprehension of appropriate social language is critical. In addition, collaboration with classroom teachers would yield directions for use of specific classroom materials and ideas that could be used in therapy to target Alyssa's deficient language skills while increasing her academic performance.
5. **D.** A child who shows slow, writhing, involuntary movements has athetoid cerebral palsy.
6. **B.** This item is false because standardized tests do not sample language behaviors adequately. They provide only one or two contexts that sample each behavior.
7. **C.** This utterance would count as 10 words, 11 morphemes.
8. **D.** Increasing use of appropriate discourse skills, turn taking, and conversational repair strategies would be appropriate targets for a child working on pragmatic skills, not semantic skills.
9. **D.** Hypersensitivity to touch, insistence on routines, and lack of interest in human voices are generally characteristic of children with autism, not children with traumatic brain injury.
10. **A.** It is critical to use a multimodal approach to treatment because most children with language disorders will learn more quickly and retain more information this way.
11. **C.** A TTR of 0.31 is low—a TTR of 0.5 is within average range. Thus, this indicates that Allyson is low in her lexical skills or the number of words she uses expressively.
12. **B.** To help Myron communicate more effectively with others so that they understand his messages better, the clinician needs to make sure that the symbols on Myron's AAC device are transparent or easily decipherable by others.
13. **A.** Problems with forms such as *–er* (e.g., *bigger*) and *–est* (e.g., *biggest*) reflect difficulty in the area of morphology.
14. **C.** Because Justin has Asperger's syndrome, the clinician would expect to see seemingly excellent vocabulary skills; seemingly normal syntactic skills; and speech that often appears to be a "monologue," in which Justin does not allow his conversational partner to take turns.
15. **B.** The SCERTS model emphasizes the importance of targeting goals in social communication and emotional regulation by implementing transactional supports, which include visual supports, environmental arrangements, and communication-style adjustments.
16. **A.** The word *Daddy's* has 2 morphemes; the rest of the words contain just one morpheme each.
17. **D.** Classroom-based intervention involves going into the classroom and helping these students, in a small-group format, to achieve classroom curriculum goals.

18. C. The typically developing child is suggesting collaborative play, in which children often adopt roles and play together as a group.
19. A. The mother has used the technique of extension, in which she adds both semantic and grammatical information to Danny's utterance.
20. B. Children who have difficulty with word retrieval need intervention that is focused on increasing their semantic skills.
21. D. Jeannette is having difficulty with order of mention. She is literally following the commands in the sequence given rather than correctly interpreting the teacher's intent.
22. A. Jonathan is specifically demonstrating underextension, because he only thinks his dog is a "dog."
23. C. An immediate, full language evaluation is the best course of action in this case. At 30 months of age, Derek should be saying 200–300 words.
24. A. A student with a pragmatic language disorder is most likely to have difficulties in allowing a conversational partner to have a turn.
25. B. A language sample's primary diagnostic function is to evaluate the child's language in actual daily settings. This is ideal for a young child who might not respond as well to standardized assessment measures.
26. D. Mario's MLU in morphemes is 2.4. The number of words in Mario's language sample is irrelevant to the average MLU in morphemes.
27. B. If you say "Tonia, point to the apple," and she says "Tonia, point to the apple," that is immediate echolalia.
28. A. Part C of the IDEA is a federal grant program that assists states in operating a comprehensive statewide program of early intervention services for infants and toddlers with disabilities, ages birth through age 2 years, and their families.

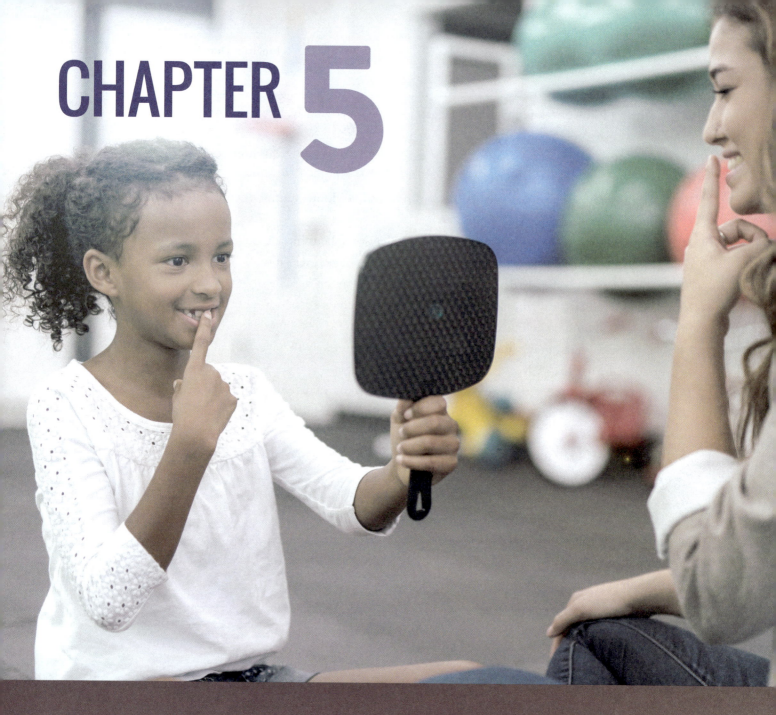

CHAPTER 5

SPEECH SOUND DEVELOPMENT AND DISORDERS

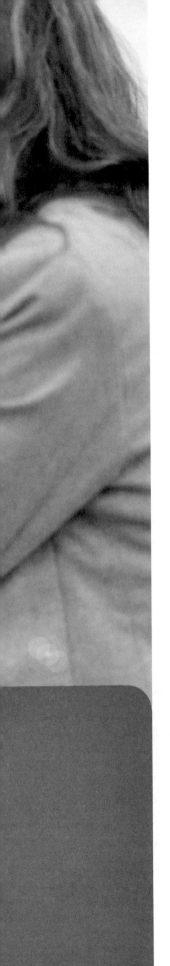

The ability to communicate clearly is a gift that most people take for granted. But sometimes, clear communication with others is disrupted by one or more variables that cause a child to be misunderstood by members of his or her speech community. In some cases, this leads to only minor problems; in other instances, children experience emotional, social, and even academic difficulties related to atypical speech patterns. Today in the U.S., approximately 8–9% of children present with speech difficulties (National Institute on Deafness and Other Communication Disorders, 2017). The World Health Organization's International Classification of Functioning, Disability, and Health—Children and Youth (ICF-CY) advocates a holistic approach to wellness and health for all children in the world. As part of this, it describes speaking and hearing as features of health (World Health Organization, 2007). It is important to keep this overall international perspective in mind when discussing service delivery to children who have difficulties with their speech.

To describe these difficulties, many authors use the term *articulation and phonological disorders*; some prefer either *articulation disorder* or *phonological disorder*. The term *speech sound disorder* is currently the most widely used term. Articulation disorder refers to speech–motor control problems; phonological disorder refers to phonology being a part of the language system. Children with phonological disorders have speech production problems that are specific to deficits in knowledge of phonological rules; they have underlying faulty phonological representations. For purposes of this chapter, the term speech sound disorder (SSD) is used to acknowledge that many children present with reduced intelligibility due to a combination of speech–motor and phonological factors. Foundational principles of articulation and phonology, acquisition and typical development of speech sounds, the nature of SSDs, assessment of SSDs, and, finally, treatment for children who have SSDs are described in this chapter.

FOUNDATIONS OF ARTICULATION AND PHONOLOGY

In order to understand typical development of speech sounds in children, it is necessary to understand the basic definitions used to describe development and disorders. In this section, definitions and concepts from Chapter 2 are reviewed and summarized as part of the foundation for discussion of speech sound development and disorders.

Basic Definitions

- **Language** is an abstract system of symbols used to communicate meaning; it is larger than speech. Speech is the actual motor production of oral language.
- Experts put forth many explanations of the differences between articulation and phonology. Fundamentally, the **articulation** approach looks at children's acquisition of individual phonemes and emphasizes speech–motor control.
- The **phonological** approach studies children's acquisition of sound patterns and the processes underlying such patterns. Phonology focuses on the underlying knowledge of the rules of the sound system of a language (Stoel-Gammon & Menn, 2017).
- Put differently, articulation can be viewed as the surface representation, or what we produce. Phonology is the underlying representation of what we produce.
- In the study of phonology, a topic of great interest is **naturalness**. A natural class, process, property, or rule is one that is preferred or frequently used in phonologic systems. One phonological property is more natural than another if the first is used in a greater number of languages and if it develops before the other property.
- Researchers use the terms **marked** and **unmarked** to describe sounds according to this paradigm. **Unmarked** sounds are those that appear to be natural; they tend to be easier to acquire, and thus are acquired earlier than marked sounds. Unmarked sounds appear in more different languages than marked sounds. **Marked** sounds are less natural and tend to be acquired later.
- For example, /b/ is usually considered an unmarked sound because it is acquired easily and early by most children and because it occurs in many languages of the world. The /th/ sound is considered by some to be marked, because children acquire it later and it is less common in languages around the world.
- A **phoneme** is a class of speech sounds; it is an abstract name given to variations of a speech sound. Because they make a difference in meaning, phonemes are often described as the smallest unit of sound that can affect meaning. For example, *rat* and *fat* have different meanings because of the different initial phonemes /r/ and /f/.
- A phoneme is a group, class, or family of sounds whose variations are called **allophones**. For example, although the phoneme /k/ sounds the same perceptually to the listener, it is produced slightly differently in the words *kitten*, *bucket*, and *cook*. These small differences or variations are called allophones.
- The term **phonemic** refers to the abstract system of sounds, whereas the term **phonetic** refers to concrete productions of specific sounds. Thus, the idealized and abstract description of /t/ is phonemic and is put in slashes. The specific sound production by a speaker would be indicated in brackets: [t].
- The English language has 46 speech sounds, which may be classified as vowels or consonants (see Chapter 2 for a more in-depth description). **Vowels** are always voiced, and the mouth is more open in vowel production than in consonant production.
- Vowels are classified according to the tongue position needed to produce them (front, central, back, high, mid, low). Vowels are also classified according to lip position; for instance, the vowels /o/ and /u/ are produced with lip rounding, while the vowel /i/ is produced with slight lip retraction.

- When two vowels are combined, they form **diphthongs**, which are produced by a continuous change in the vocal tract shape. The /eɪ/ sound in *shake* and *lace* is a dipthong, as is the /aɪ/ sound in words such as *high* and *why*.
- Vowels may be described according to the **distinctive features paradigm**. Consonants may be described according to both the distinctive features paradigm and the **place-voice-manner paradigm**. These paradigms are thoroughly described in Chapter 2.

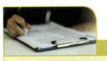

SUMMARY

- Speech is the motor production of oral language. The articulation approach to speech looks at children's acquisition of individual phonemes and emphasizes speech motor control.
- The phonological approach studies children's acquisition of sound patterns within the language system. Consonants and vowels make up the two major categories of speech sounds.

ACQUISITION OF ARTICULATORY AND PHONOLOGICAL SKILLS: TYPICAL DEVELOPMENT

Most people take typical speech sound development for granted. But sometimes, children do not master speech sounds at the expected pace. In order to understand which speech sound errors are age-appropriate and which speech sound errors indicate problematic development, it is necessary to understand theories of development and typical milestones of development in infants and children.

Theories of Development

Early studies of children's articulatory and phonological development consisted mainly of **diary studies**, which described individual children (frequently the children of the researchers). Those early studies focused primarily on environmental influences and on universals of acquisition.

Today's theories and models of development account much more for the child as a learner with unique learning strategies and individual patterns of production. The following is a brief summary of major theories or models of children's speech sound development (McLeod, 2017; Peña-Brooks & Hegde, 2015; Stoel-Gammon & Menn, 2017):

Behavioral Theory

- The behavioral explanation of speech sound acquisition is based on conditioning and learning (Mowrer, 1960; Olmsted, 1971). Behaviorism focuses on describing observable and overt behaviors.
- This explanation treats the acquisition of speech like the acquisition of any other skill. Thus, it is presumed that the acquisition of speech does not require such special phenomena as innate universals. The behavioral theory prevailed from the 1950s to the early 1970s.

- The behavioral theory emphasizes that the child develops the adult-like speech of his or her community through interactions with the caregiver. The theory holds that the child's babbling is gradually shaped into adult forms through principles of classical conditioning that occur primarily during caregiver–child interactions.
- Some experts argue that this theory does not account for an infant's creativity or capacity to produce new patterns. In addition, the evidence is not compelling that caretakers selectively reinforce the child's sounds in the prelinguistic period.

Natural Phonology Theory

- Developed by Stampe (1969), the natural phonology theory proposes that natural phonological processes are innate processes that simplify the adult target word. Some experts believe that natural phonological processes are innate or are acquired early in life and fairly easily.
- According to Stampe, children learn to suppress processes that do not occur in their languages. For example, in German, word-final obstruents (stops, affricates, and fricatives) are devoiced. In German, *hund* (*dog*) is pronounced [hunt]. German-speaking children do not need to suppress the process of word-final obstruent devoicing, because that process is compatible with their community language. English-speaking children do need to suppress that process, however, to match the adult pronunciation of their community. Thus, in English, children need to learn to voice word-final /d/ as in the word *glad*.
- Stampe believed that children represent or store speech forms correctly. What leads to the use of phonological processes is **output constraints**, or constraints on production that lead to simplification of the adult model.
- The concept of the universal or innate status of child phonological processes or rules is controversial. Also, there is no empirical evidence that children have full and accurate perception from the earliest stages of speech production.
- In addition, natural phonology does not account for "nonnatural" simplifications in the speech of children. Many highly unintelligible children produce the sounds of speech in a way that cannot be classified using natural phonology.

Generative Phonology Theory

- Generative phonology is a theory of the sound structure of human languages. There are two major ideas underlying generative phonology.
- First, phonological descriptions are dependent on information from other linguistic levels. Second, phonological rules map underlying representations onto surface pronunciations.
- Generative phonology has been applied to our understanding of children's speech acquisition because it enables a description of the relationship of children's productions to adult pronunciation in terms of phonological rules.
- Some underlying premises of generative phonology have been criticized, and this theory is not broadly applied in the field of speech–language pathology.

Linear Versus Nonlinear Phonology Theories

- The foundational goals of the linear generative phonology theories are to (a) describe phonological patterns that occur in natural languages, (b) create rules that account for these systems, and (c) identify universal principles that apply to various phonological systems.
- Linear generative theories are based on the premise that all speech segments are arranged in a sequential order, that all sound segments have equal value, and that all distinctive features are equal. Thus, no one specific sound segment has control over other segments.
- Basically, linear generative phonology is characterized by rules that operate in a domain of linear strings of segments. Linear phonology theories assume that phonological properties are linear strings of segments and that sound segments are composed of a bundle of independent characteristics or features.
- In the 1980s, nonlinear phonology was developed as an alternative to linear generative phonology and gained attention because linear generative phonology was perceived to have flaws. Linear generative phonology became increasingly viewed as inadequate to account for the effects of stress and other prosodic variables.
- Nonlinear phonology was developed as an alternative to account for the influence of stress and tone features in levels of representation independent of segmental or linear representation. There are various nonlinear phonology theories, and they deemphasize processes or rules and focus on prosodic phenomena. Nonlinear phonological theories assume that there is some sort of hierarchy that helps to organize both segmental and suprasegmental phonological units or properties.
- Nonlinear theories explore the relationships among units of different sizes; for example, they acknowledge the fact that syllable structure could affect the segmental level of a child's production.
- Clinically, one of the biggest contributions of nonlinear phonology has been its attention to multisyllabic words and the way therapy is organized.

Optimality Theory

- This theory was originally used to describe adult languages. Its basic units are constraints, and there are two major types. First, **markedness** constraints denote limitations on output, or what can be produced. Sounds that are difficult to produce are considered marked (e.g., /r/).
- Second, **faithfulness** constraints capture the features that are to be preserved, prohibiting deletion and addition that violate the ambient language (McLeod, 2017).
- According to optimality theory, the aim during children's speech development is for the child's output to match the adult target. This occurs through demoting markedness constraints and promoting faithfulness constraints.

Infant Development: Perception and Production

Perception

- Various types of research methodology have been used to study infant perception. The two major ones are the **high-amplitude sucking paradigm** and the **visually reinforced head turn**. These methodologies observe infants' reactions to changes in their environment.

- It has generally been found that infants under 1 year of age are able to distinguish sounds that are not used in their language; however, this ability begins to decline around 12 months of age. With increasing exposure to the sounds of their own language, babies eventually lose their ability to distinguish sounds that are not used in their language.

Production

- The infant's vocal tract is significantly different from the adult's. Structural differences (e.g., a high larynx, a tongue placed far forward in the oral cavity) constrain an infant's productions, especially during the first 4 months of life.
- Between 4 and 6 months of age, when the epiglottis and velum grow farther apart, the infant becomes capable of producing a much greater variety of sounds. All babies seem to pass through the same stages of vocal development, regardless of what linguistic community they are raised in (Stoel-Gammon & Menn, 2017).
- Oller (1980, 2000) proposed approximate, overlapping stages of development of prelinguistic, nonreflexive vocalizations:

  1. **Phonation stage** (birth–1 month). Speech-like sounds are rare, and most vocalizations are reflexive (e.g., burping, coughing, crying). Some nonreflexive vowels or syllabic consonants may occur.
  2. **Cooing** or **gooing stage** (2–4 months). Most of the infant's productions are acoustically similar to /u/. Some velar consonant-like sounds may occur.
  3. **Expansion stage** (4–6 months). The infant is "playing" with the speech mechanism, exploring his or her capabilities through such productions as growls, squeals, yells, and raspberries (bilabial trills). Some consonant-vowel (CV)–like combinations and vowel-like sounds may be produced.
  4. **Canonical** or **reduplicated babbling stage** (6–8 months). The infant produces strings of CV syllables, such as [mamamama], [dadadada], or [dededede]. Although the infant does not have sound–meaning correspondence, the timing of the CV syllables approximates that of adult speech. By about 8 months, children with hearing losses fall behind hearing peers in language development.
  5. **Variegated** or **nonreduplicated babbling stage** (8 months–1 year). The infant continues to use adult-like syllables in CV sequences, but a variety of consonants and vowels appear in a single vocalization (e.g., [duwabe]).

- Infants make a gradual progression through these stages and into the production of first words. This process is continuous and represents an important transition from the prelinguistic to the linguistic stage of phonological development, which begins around the 1st year, when the first meaningful word is produced.
- During the first 3 years of life, a child's vocal tract anatomy and function change. For example, lip closure improves, the larynx moves farther down the vocal tract, tongue muscle tone increases, and tongue movements become dissociated from jaw movements. With these changes comes improved ability to articulate.

Typical Articulation Development in Children

- The articulation development approach looks at children's development of single phonemes. This approach focuses on the age of mastery for single phonemes of English based on speech–motor control. For example, one might ask, "At what age do most children master the /r/ sound?"
- To assess when mastery of sounds occurs, researchers have generally used cross-sectional and longitudinal methods, which are described in further detail in Chapter 13.
- The results of these cross-sectional and longitudinal studies have sometimes differed due to such variables as different research methodologies and others. The studies have differed in their definitions of "mastery" of sounds, as well. For example, in some studies, a speech sound was considered "mastered" when 75% of the children produced it correctly. In other studies, a sound was viewed as mastered when 90% of the children produced it correctly.
- Table 5.1 summarizes the most commonly reported normative data for mastery of phonemes (these data are based on white, monolingual, English-speaking children).
- Taken together, the results of cross-sectional and longitudinal studies in speech sound acquisition have shown us the following:

  - Vowels are acquired before consonants.
  - The nasal consonants /m/, /n/, and /ŋ/ are among the earliest to be acquired. They are usually mastered between 3 and 4 years of age.
  - Stop sounds are mastered earlier than fricatives. Most stops are mastered between 3 and 4-and-a-half years of age. The stop /p/ may be mastered the earliest.
  - Glides /w/ and /j/ are mastered earlier than fricatives. Glides are mastered between 2 and 4 years.
  - The liquids /r/ and /l/ are mastered relatively late (between 3 and 7 years).
  - Fricatives and affricates are mastered later than stops and nasals. The fricative /f/ is mastered earlier than other fricatives (around age 3). Fricatives /ð/, /θ/, /ʃ/, /s/, and /z/ are mastered last (between 3 and 6 years).
  - Consonant clusters (e.g., *br* in the word *brown*) are acquired later than most other sounds.
  - Typically, two-element consonant clusters (e.g., sk, st, sp) are mastered before three-element clusters (e.g., str, skr, spr). For example, many 4-year-olds can produce the /sp, st, sk/ clusters. Clusters that contain fricatives (e.g., /fl/) are usually harder for children than clusters containing stops (e.g., /kl/) (McLeod, 2017).

Overall Intelligibility

- Intelligibility is defined as understandability. Speech intelligibility is a perceptual judgment made by a listener; it is largely based on the percentage of words in a speech sample that the listener understands (Bankson, Bernthal, & Flipsen, 2017). Intelligibility estimates assume that the listener is an adult who is not familiar with the child.

Table 5.1

Age (Years–Months) at Which Children Mastered Phonemes: Six Studies

Phonemes	Poole (1934)	Wellman et al. (1931)	Templin (1957)	Sander (1972)	Prather et al. (1975)	Arlt & Goodban (1976)
m	3-6	3	3	before 2	2	3
n	4-6	3	3	before 2	2	3
p	3-6	4	3	before 2	2	3
h	3-6	3	3	before 2	2	3
w	3-6	3	3	before 2	2-8	3
b	3-6	3	4	before 2	2-8	3
k	4-6	4	4	2	2-4	3
g	4-6	4	4	2	2-4	3
j	4-6	4	3-6	2	2-4	—
ŋ	4-6	—	3	2	2	3
t	4-6	5	6	2	2-8	3
d	4-6	5	4	2	2-4	3
f	5-6	3	3	3	2-4	3
l	6-6	4	6	3	2-4	4
v	6-6	5	6	4	4+	3-6
ʃ	6-6	—	4-6	4	3-8	4-6
ʒ	6-6	6	7	6	4	4
ð	6-6	—	7	5	4	5
θ	7-6	—	6	5	4+	5
r	7-6	5	4	3	3-4	5
s	7-6	5	4-6	3	3	4
z	7-6	5	7	4	41	4
tʃ	—	5	4-6	4	3-8	4
dʒ	—	—	7	4	4+	4

Note. From *Introduction to Communicative Disorders* (4th ed., p. 149), by M. N. Hegde, 2010, Austin, TX: PRO-ED. Copyright 2010 by PRO-ED, Inc. Reprinted with permission.

- When determining the need for therapy, a general guideline is that the poorer the intelligibility, the more likely the child needs intervention. A child 3 years old or older who is unintelligible to the listener is a candidate for intervention (Bankson et al., 2017).
- Table 5.2 describes intelligibility expectations based on a child's chronological age.

Table 5.2

Quick Reference for Intelligibility Guidelines

Child's chronological age	Intelligibility expectations—percentage understood
2 years	60–70%
3 years	75–80%
4 years	90–100%

Note. Intelligibility refers to the child's understandability to an unfamiliar adult. Based on Gard, Gilman, and Gorman (2012); McLeod, Harrison, McAllister, and McCormack (2013).

Typical Phonological Development in Children

Foundational Concepts

- As stated, the articulation approach to typical development looks at children's acquisition of individual phonemes and emphasizes speech–motor control. The phonological process approach studies children's acquisition of sound **patterns** and the **processes** underlying those patterns. The phonological process approach focuses on language knowledge.
- Researchers who use the phonological process approach believe that children's errors are a way of simplifying the adult model of correct articulation. Such simplifications are called **phonological processes**. Today, the term **phonological patterns** is widely used (McLeod, 2017).
- Phonological patterns are described based on findings of longitudinal as well as large- and small-group studies. The phonological pattern framework helps us describe the error patterns in the speech of young children.

Major Categories of Phonological Patterns

Children may use one or more phonological patterns when producing a given word. For example, in the production of "hou" for "house," a child uses the single pattern of final-consonant deletion. But in saying "Les" instead of "Celeste," a child uses the patterns of weak-syllable deletion, consonant-cluster reduction, and stridency deletion.

Children's phonological patterns can be divided into three categories: substitution, assimilation, and syllable structure. These patterns are described in the following sections.

Substitution Patterns

Substitution patterns are a group of phonological patterns in which one class of sounds is substituted for another:

- In **vocalization**, a vowel (usually /o/ or /u/) is substituted for a syllabic consonant (usually a liquid). For example, a child might say "bado" instead of "bottle," or "noodoo" instead of "noodle."

- In **gliding**, a liquid consonant is produced as a glide. Children frequently make the following substitutions: w/l (wæmp/læmp), j/l (jaɪt/laɪt), w/r (wiŋ/riŋ). Gliding can also occur in consonant clusters (e.g., pwɪti/prɪti).
- In **velar fronting**, an alveolar or a dental replaces a velar; this usually occurs in word-initial position (e.g., ti/ki, doʊt/goʊt).
- In **stopping**, a fricative or affricate is replaced by a stop. For example, a child might make the following substitutions: tu/ʃu, dɪs/ðɪs, bup/butʃ, noʊd/noʊz.
- In **depalatization**, a child substitutes an alveolar affricate for a palatal affricate (e.g., wats/watʃ, dzoʊk/dʒoʊk) or substitutes an alveolar fricative for a palatal fricative (e.g., wɪs/wɪʃ, sip/ʃip).
- In **affrication**, an affricate is produced in place of a fricative or stop (e.g., tʃʌn/sʌn, tʃu/ʃu, butʃ/buʃ).
- In **deaffrication**, a fricative replaces an affricate (e.g., pez/pedʒ, sɪp/tʃɪp, siz/tʃiz).
- In **backing**, a posteriorly placed consonant is produced instead of an anteriorly placed consonant (velars are substituted for alveolars). For example, a child might make the following substitutions: boʊk/boʊt or gæn/dæn.
- In glottal replacement, a glottal stop (ʔ) is produced in place of other consonants (e.g., tuʔ/tuθ, baʔəl/batəl).

Assimilation Patterns

In assimilation patterns, sounds are changed by the influence of neighboring sounds. In the following assimilation patterns, the productions of dissimilar phonemes sound alike:

- **Reduplication**, in which a child repeats a pattern (e.g., wawa/watɚ, baba/batəl)
- **Regressive assimilation** (also called **consonant harmony**), which occurs due to the influence of a later occurring sound on an earlier sound (e.g., gʌk/dʌk, bɪp/zɪp)
- **Progressive assimilation** (also called consonant harmony), in which an earlier occurring sound influences a later occurring sound (e.g., kɪk/kɪs, bup/but)
- **Voicing assimilation**, which can be either **devoicing** (e.g., pɪk/pɪg) or **voicing** (e.g., bad/pad)

Syllable Structure Patterns

The following syllable structure patterns affect the structure of entire syllables, not just certain sounds:

- **Unstressed-** or **weak-syllable deletion**, which involves omission of an unstressed syllable (e.g., -meɪto/tomeɪto, -haɪnd/bihaɪnd, ɛfʌnt/ɛləfʌnt)
- **Final-consonant deletion**, in which the final consonant is omitted (e.g., bɛ-/bɛd, kæ-/kæt)
- **Epenthesis**, in which a schwa vowel is inserted between the consonants in an initial cluster (e.g., təri/tri, bəlæk/blæk) or after a final voiced stop (e.g., stapə/stap, gʊdə/gʊd)
- **Consonant-cluster simplification or reduction**, in which a consonant or consonants in a cluster are deleted (e.g., -pid/spid, sid/spid, bɛs-/bɛst, -pun/spun)
- **Diminutization**, or addition of /i/ to the target form (e.g., dagi/dag, ɛgi/ɛg)
- **Metathesis**, or production of sounds in a word in reversed order; also known as a spoonerism (e.g., pik/kip, lɪkstɪp/lɪpstɪk, pɪsgɛti/spʌgɛti)

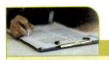

SUMMARY

- Understanding typical speech sound development necessitates an understanding of the theories used to explain this development. These include the behavioral, natural, and generative phonology theories. In addition, it is important to understand the differences between linear and nonlinear theories of phonology.
- It is also important to understand the basics of infant perception and production. In the first year of life, infants go through the stages of cooing and gooing, expansion, canonical or reduplicated babbling, and variegated or nonreduplicated babbling. These stages precede the development of the first word.
- Typical speech sound development can be studied through the articulation or segmental acquisition approach or through the phonological pattern approach. Familiarity with typical development and acquisition of speech sounds is essential to assessing and diagnosing speech sound disorders.

SPEECH SOUND DISORDERS

Typically developing children's difficulty in producing certain speech sounds is often called a functional articulation disorder. A functional disorder (sometimes also described as an idiopathic disorder) cannot be explained on the basis of neurological damage, muscle weakness or paralysis, or structural problems such as cleft palate. The term **functional** does not explain the disorder; it implies only that an organic or underlying physical cause was not found. Thus, many clinicians believe that the origin of functional articulation disorders is unknown. Though this term has been criticized, it is still used in many circles today. As stated previously, a term that is broadly used today is **speech sound disorder** (SSD) (Bankson et al., 2017; Stoel-Gammon & Menn, 2017). This term does not explicitly imply that a person's disordered speech can be attributed to an impairment of articulation or phonology; it is a neutral term that does not describe the cause of the problem.

Frank organic disorders are those that arise from various physical anomalies that affect the function or structure of the speech mechanism. For example, there can be physical damage to the central or peripheral nervous system, the oral mechanism, or all of these. Treatment for organically based disorders usually should be multidisciplinary and involve members of the medical community. In this section, we describe general factors related to SSDs, provide a description of articulatory errors, and discuss organically based disorders that occur secondary to oral structural variables, hearing loss, and neuropathologies.

General Factors Related to Speech Sound Disorders

Researchers have discovered several factors that coexist with SSDs. While these factors cannot be said to be causally related to SSDs, they are correlated with SSDs (Flipsen, Bernthal, & Bankson, 2017a; Peña-Brooks & Hegde, 2015; Stoel-Gammon & Menn, 2017).

Gender
- There is some evidence that female children generally have articulatory skills slightly superior to those of male children. However, the evidence is weak, and the reported sex differences are small or negligible.
- Nonetheless, more boys than girls tend to have SSDs.

Intelligence
- Intelligence has not been shown to be causally related to SSDs. Children of normal intelligence may have difficulty with production of speech sounds.
- Intelligence is associated with SSDs only when it is significantly below normal. Many institutionalized children with intellectual disabilities have SSDs.

Birth Order and Sibling Status
- There is some evidence that firstborn and only children have better articulation skills than those who have older siblings.
- It has also been suggested that the greater the age difference between siblings, the better the articulation of the younger child. This is because if siblings are close to each other in age, the older one may provide a model of inadequate articulation for the younger child.

Socioeconomic Status
- Research has shown that socioeconomic status (SES) is not a strong factor in the etiology of SSDs. There is no evidence that coming from a low-income background causes a child to have articulation disorders.
- However, some studies have shown that children from lower-SES backgrounds make more errors of articulation than children from middle- and upper-class backgrounds.
- One might hypothesize that because families of low-income children tend not to have health insurance, these children cannot be readily treated for factors such as middle-ear infections and dental or orthodontic problems that are associated with SSDs.

Language Development and Academic Performance
- Research has shown that younger children with severe SSDs are more likely to demonstrate language problems than children with mild–moderate language delays.
- Young children with SSDs may be at risk for problems with reading and spelling in the elementary school years.

Auditory Discrimination Skills
- Researchers used to think that children with SSDs had poor auditory discrimination skills, which caused the disorders. However, studies have produced inconsistent results: Some children with SSDs have scored poorly on auditory discrimination tests, whereas others have scored within normal limits.

- Because of these equivocal research findings, it is believed that there is not a strong relationship between articulation and auditory discrimination skills. However, many clinicians still conduct intensive work on auditory discrimination, believing that improved auditory discrimination skills lead to improved articulation skills.

Description of Articulatory Errors

- Earlier in this chapter, **phonological error patterns** were described in detail. It was stated that children may manifest error patterns such as final-consonant deletion, consonant-cluster reduction, assimilation, and others. These error patterns underlie a lack of intelligibility.
- The child is often able to physically produce a sound (e.g., /k/ or /g/), but if she displays the phonological pattern of **fronting** (e.g., tæt/kæt, do/go), she makes an error of the /k/ or /g/ sound despite the motoric ability to produce the sound correctly.
- Children may also make errors that can be categorized as **articulatory errors**. These errors typically involve misproductions of specific phonemes. The child is motorically unable to produce the erred phoneme (e.g., /r/, /s/), so treatment must involve teaching correct production and emphasizing speech–motor control.
- Children may make the following articulation errors:

  - **Substitutions**. An incorrect sound is produced in place of a correct sound (e.g., tink/θink or tæt/kæt/).
  - **Omissions or deletions**. Required sounds are omitted in words (e.g., bo-/bot).
  - **Labialization**. Sounds are produced with excessive lip rounding.
  - **Nasalization**. Oral sounds (especially oral stops like /g/) are produced with inappropriate, usually excessive, nasal resonance.
  - **Pharyngeal fricative**. Fricatives such as /h/ are produced in the pharyngeal area.
  - **Devoicing**. Voiced sounds are produced with limited vocal fold vibrations or without vocal fold vibrations (e.g., dɑk/dɑg).
  - **Frontal lisp**. Sibilant consonants are produced with the tongue tip placed too far forward (between or against the teeth); /s/ and /z/ are the sounds most commonly involved.
  - **Lateral lisp**. Sibilant sounds such as /s/ and /z/ are produced with air flowing inappropriately over the sides of the tongue.
  - **Stridency deletion**. Strident sounds are omitted (e.g., mæ-/mæʃ, -tɑp/stɑp); sometimes stridency deletion is described as a phonological process or pattern.
  - **Initial-, medial-, final-position errors**. These errors occur in the production of a beginning, medial, or final sound of a word.
  - **Prevocalic, intervocalic, postvocalic errors**. Errors occur with reference to consonant position in syllables (e.g., dæbdəlaɪjən/dændəlaɪjən) would involve a postvocalic error; the substitution gɑg/dɑg would involve a prevocalic error.

Organically Based Disorders

Oral Structural Variables

- Some children with deviations of the oral structure have normal speech skills. However, SSDs may also be found in the absence of structural anomalies.
- Thus, there is no demonstrable causal relationship between structural anomalies and SSDs. Nevertheless, the following oral structural abnormalities have been associated with SSDs in some children.

Ankyloglossia (Tongue-Tie)

- Normally, the free tip of the tongue is mobile and permits the production of tip-alveolar sounds, such as /t/, /d/. However, if the **lingual frenum**, which attaches the tongue to the base of the mouth, is too short, tongue tip mobility is reduced.
- When the frenum is thus attached too close to the tip of the tongue, this is diagnosed as a "tongue-tie" or **ankyloglossia**.
- Clipping or cutting the frenum used to be a common surgical procedure; it is rarer nowadays. Research has shown that ankyloglossia is not a frequent cause of misarticulations, and children with short lingual frenums can have normal articulation.

Dental Deviations

- **Malocclusion** refers to deviations in the shape and dimensions of the mandible and maxilla (**skeletal malocclusion**) and the positioning of individual teeth (**dental malocclusion**).
- Most children with malocclusions have a misalignment of the mandible and maxilla and the upper and lower rows of teeth. There are three basic categories of malocclusions, with many more subtypes within categories:

  - In **class I malocclusion**, the arches themselves are generally aligned properly, but some individual teeth are misaligned.
  - In **class II malocclusion**, the upper jaw or maxilla is protruded and the lower jaw or mandible is receded. This is also referred to as an **overbite**. **Overjet** occurs when the child has a class II malocclusion and the upper teeth from the molars forward are positioned excessively anterior to the lower teeth.
  - In **class III malocclusion**, the maxilla is receded and the mandible is protruded.

Oral–Motor Coordination Skills

- Oral–motor coordination skills are frequently evaluated through tests of **diadochokinetic rate** (maximum repetition rate of syllables in rapid succession). For example, a child might be asked to say "pʌtʌkʌ" as fast as possible in succession. The goal is to assess the functional and structural integrity of the lips, jaw, and tongue.

- Some clinicians have observed that children who do poorly on diadochokinetic tests also have difficulty producing some speech sounds accurately. However, not all children with speech sound difficulties do poorly on diadochokinetic tests.
- The relationship between diadochokinesis and speech sound production in conversational speech is unclear. Research has not substantiated the hypothesis that poor oral–motor coordination skills cause articulation problems.

Orofacial Myofunctional Disorders (Tongue Thrust)

- The term **tongue thrust** has recently been expanded to be more inclusive. The current definition of **orofacial myofunctional disorders** (OMD) encompasses any anatomical or physiological characteristic of the orofacial structures (palate, cheeks, tongue, lips, jaw, teeth) that interferes with normal speech or physical, dentofacial, or psychosocial development. This includes swallow, labial and lingual rest, and speech posture differences.
- Usually, a child with OMD exhibits deviant swallows. In a normal swallow, the tongue tip is placed behind the alveolar ridge and the body of the tongue pushes the fluid or solid posteriorly for swallowing.
- In the deviant swallow, the tongue tip pushes against the front teeth (usually the upper central incisors). The tongue tip may protrude between the upper and lower teeth and thus come in contact with the lower lip.
- During speech production, the tongue also may exert some force against the front teeth, and, even at rest, the tongue may be carried more forward in the oral cavity. This can contribute to an anterior open bite.
- It is currently believed that the resting posture of the tongue affects the position of the jaws and teeth more than the tongue function during swallowing.
- According to the American Speech-Language-Hearing Association (ASHA, 2007b), OMD is often related to errors in the production of /s/, /z/, /ʃ/, /ʒ/, /tʃ/, and /dʒ/; in addition, the tip-dental sounds /t/, /d/, /l/, and /n/ may be misarticulated due to weak tongue tip musculature. (*Note*: Some researchers believe that OMD does not *cause* errors of articulation but exists in a correlational relationship with those errors.) Thus, some clinicians perform **oral myofunctional therapy** to correct the deviant swallow.
- ASHA (2007b) has stated that myofunctional therapy is appropriate and within the purview of speech–language pathologists who assess and treat the effects of OMD on swallowing, rest postures, and speech. Speech–language pathologists traditionally work on a team also composed of a dentist, an orthodontist, and a physician (Flipsen et al., 2017a).

Hearing Loss

- Various kinds of speech sound problems are seen in individuals with hearing loss. The degree of hearing loss is frequently related to the severity of the SSD problem.
- Individuals who are born with a profound hearing loss generally have the greatest challenges with articulation, as they cannot monitor their speech production. These individuals may have

difficulties with both consonant and vowel productions, making many substitutions, distortions, and omissions of phonemes.
- Children with mild hearing loss (10–30 dB), especially if the loss is secondary to middle-ear fluid and infections, may have an SSD. Omission of high-frequency voiceless sounds (e.g., /s/, /t/) is common. These children may also use the phonological patterns of final-consonant deletion, stridency deletion, and fronting.

Neuropathologies

Dysarthria

- Dysarthria is a speech–motor disorder caused by peripheral or central nervous system damage. This damage causes paralysis, weakness, or incoordination of the muscles of speech. In children, dysarthria can be caused by cerebral palsy, head injury, degenerative disease, tumor, and stroke.
- All the speech production systems are affected: phonation, resonation, respiration, resonance, and articulation. Thus, assessment and treatment must incorporate all of those systems.
- Dysarthric speech usually is associated with monotonous pitch, deviant voice quality, variable speech rate, and hypernasality. Reduced intelligibility is a key feature of dysarthria, with the child's speech sounding slurred.
- Children with dysarthria have the following common articulatory error patterns:
  - Voicing errors occur, especially those that involve devoicing of voiced sounds.
  - Bilabial and velar sounds are easier than alveolar fricatives and affricates, labiodental fricatives, and palatal liquids.
  - Stops, glides, and nasals are easier than fricatives, affricates, and liquids.
- Treatment for childhood dysarthria is very repetitive and structured. It involves increasing muscle tone and strength, increasing range and rate of motion, and treating other parameters (e.g., respiration) that affect intelligibility.
- Treatment involves intensive and systematic drill, modeling, phonetic placement, and emphasis on accuracy of sound production.
- For children who cannot be 100% intelligible, compensatory strategies (e.g., prosthetic devices) are often used to assist in communication. For very severely involved children, alternative or augmentative communication devices may be used.

Apraxia

- Apraxia of speech is caused by central nervous system damage. There is no weakness or paralysis of the muscles; however, the central nervous system damage makes it difficult to program the precise movements necessary for smoothly articulated speech. Thus, apraxia of speech is described as a **motor programming disorder**.
- Researchers and clinicians have long debated the existence of **developmental apraxia of speech** (DAS) as a clinical entity. More recently, it has been called **childhood apraxia of speech** (CAS).

- For some children, CAS is congenital; these children have not experienced frank, overt damage, such as a stroke. Other children have CAS related to a known neurological impairment (ASHA, 2007a).
- Children who are thought to have CAS demonstrate sensorimotor problems in positioning and sequentially moving muscles for the volitional production of speech. It is hard for them to plan and program the movement sequences necessary for accurate speech production. They frequently show groping behaviors and poor intelligibility due to inconsistent and multiple articulation errors. Inconsistent errors are a hallmark of CAS. It is not a result of neuromuscular weakness.
- Children with CAS usually have the following common characteristics:
  - Slow, effortful speech
  - Prolongation of speech sounds
  - Repetition of sounds and syllables
  - Most difficulty with consonant clusters followed by fricatives, affricates, stops, and nasals
  - More frequent occurrence of omissions and substitutions
  - Voicing and devoicing errors
  - Vowel and diphthong errors
  - Unusual errors of articulation, including metathesis (e.g., dɛks/dɛsk) and addition of phonemes
  - Difficulty with volitional, oral, nonspeech movements
  - Groping and silent posturing of the articulators ("struggling" movements)
  - Deviations in prosody (e.g., rate, stress)
  - Problems with hypernasality and nasal emission (possibly due to poor velopharyngeal control resulting from impaired motor programming)
  - History of feeding problems
  - History of tactile aversions or sensitivities (e.g., very defensive when the clinician attempts to put a tongue depressor into the mouth)
  - Substantially delayed speech production
  - Limited sound inventory
  - Inconsistency in sound productions
- As stated, children with CAS may sound hypernasal and demonstrate inconsistent nasal emission. This is due to impaired motor programming involving the velum. The velum is not weak or too short; rather, motorically it is not able to move in a coordinated and quick enough way to ensure adequate velopharyngeal closure.
- Research indicates that children with CAS may have deficits in phonological awareness; for example, they often have difficulty with rhyming and with identifying syllables. They are also at risk for language, reading, and spelling problems.
- A popular motor–speech assessment used in differential diagnosis for CAS is the *Dynamic Evaluation of Motor Speech Skill* (DEMSS; Strand, McCauley, Weigand, Stoeckel, & Baas, 2013). Recent research reports that this test is reliable and valid as part of a comprehensive protocol for differential diagnosis of children with severe SSDs, including CAS (Strand et al., 2013).

- CAS treatment involves extensive drills that stress sequences of movement involved in speech production; imitation; decreased rate of speech; normal prosody; and increased accuracy in the production of individual consonants, vowels, and consonant clusters.
- Treatment is hierarchical in nature, moving from simple CV and VC sequences into more complex syllable shapes.
- Multimodal cueing is very important in CAS therapy. For example, SLPs should use visual, auditory, and tactile cues to teach treatment targets.
- Children may also need intervention for oral language, spelling, and reading deficits.
- Dynamic Temporal and Tactile Cueing (DTTC) is an intensive, motor-based, drill-like treatment; it is designed for children with severe CAS (Strand, Stoeckel, & Baas, 2006).
- DTTC targets a small number of functional words and phrases. The client practices the target words slowly and, at first, simultaneously with the clinician. Multimodal cues are used, as are daily repetitive practice and systematic feedback. Daily home practice is recommended.
- The overall goal is to have the child produce words correctly spontaneously both inside and outside the clinic. The rationale for practicing a small set of functional words is that it will foster neural maturation of motor planning and programming substrates, which will in turn facilitate future speech motor learning (Strand et al., 2006).
- More recently, a system called Prompts for Restructuring Oral Muscular Phonetic Targets (PROMPT; Hayden, Eigen, Walker, & Olsen, 2010) has been used to treat children with CAS. This approach uses tactile-kinesthetic-proprioceptive cues to support and shape movements of the articulators.
- The gains in CAS therapy are often slow; therefore, treatment should be intensive. Children may need speech therapy for a number of years. Home practice and self-monitoring are essential components of CAS treatment.

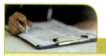

SUMMARY

- Articulatory errors involve misproductions of specific phonemes and are usually functionally or organically based, although the specific etiology is often unclear.
- General factors related to articulation problems include gender, intelligence, birth order, sibling status, socioeconomic status, language development and academic performance, and auditory discrimination skills.
- Organically based disorders have a variety of etiologies that either are correlated with the disorders or cause them. These include tongue-tie, dental deviations, oral–motor coordination problems, orofacial myofunctional disorder (tongue thrust), and hearing loss.
- Children with SSDs based on the neuropathologies of dysarthria and apraxia of speech have unique characteristics that must be addressed in a comprehensive treatment program.

ASSESSMENT OF SPEECH SOUND DISORDERS

When a child is referred for an SSD, the clinician's first job is to determine whether there is a clinically significant problem; this usually begins with a screening. If a clinically significant problem is found, the characteristics of the problem must be described. This process of identifying and describing a clinical problem is **assessment**. In this section, we discuss the components of assessment, which include conducting screenings, carrying out general and related assessment objectives, and conducting in-depth testing. In-depth testing usually involves conversational and evoked speech samples, stimulability assessment, and the administration of standardized tests. Assessment data collected through in-depth testing are scored and analyzed as a foundation for treatment.

Screening

- When it is suspected that a child has an SSD, usually a screening is conducted. A screening is a brief, initial procedure that helps determine whether a child should be assessed further and in more depth.
- Children who pass a screening procedure are judged to have age-appropriate speech sound development. Those who fail a screening are scheduled for a comprehensive assessment.
- Different procedures are available to screen speech sound development. Many clinicians use a brief conversational sample. Sometimes clinicians use pictures to elicit certain sounds. Clinicians may also use standardized screening tests or the screening portions of full-length tests of articulation.

General Assessment Objectives

- In most cases, the clinician's general assessment objectives include gathering a case history, conducting a screening and oral peripheral examination, and conducting a hearing screening. A language assessment may also be necessary.
- Further general assessment objectives include the following:
  - Assessing the child's performance in single-word positions and in conversational speech
  - Assessing the presence of phonological patterns that may help establish patterns in misarticulations
  - Evaluating a child's performance based on developmental norms
  - Evaluating stimulability of speech sounds that are misarticulated
  - Identifying potential treatment targets

Related Assessment Objectives

- In certain cases, clinicians may need to obtain data (if relevant) regarding the following:
  - Audiological assessment
  - Physical or neurological disabilities
  - Dental abnormalities that are negatively affecting intelligibility
  - Possible influences of another language or dialect
  - Concomitant language problems

- Intellectual and behavioral assessment in cases of children with such problems as behavior disorders and intellectual disabilities

Assessment Procedures

Case History

- The first step in a comprehensive evaluation is to gather a case history (see Chapter 13 for a detailed description of the nature and purpose of a case history).
- When a child has an SSD, the clinician may probe more deeply into areas such as the following:
  - What the child and family think the problem is
  - When the problem was first noted
  - Whether the problem is stable or changing
  - The results of any previous treatment
  - The child's general health, with specific attention to the occurrence of ear infections
  - Any accidents, injuries, and diseases that could have caused brain damage
  - The effects of the disorder on the child's academic performance and social life

- The clinician also must assess the child's possible multilingual and multicultural status. If children speak or are exposed to other languages, the influence of such other languages should be evaluated. For a comprehensive description of speech sound differences of children with Asian, Hispanic, and African American–influenced English, see Roseberry-McKibbin (2018), Goldstein and Iglesias (2017), and Stoel-Gammon and Menn (2017).
- Last, many children with SSDs also have concomitant oral and written language problems that can adversely affect academic performance. Therefore, it is important for the clinician to assess a child's language skills as well.

Orofacial Examination

- The clinician examines the client's facial and oral structures to rule out organic problems such as cleft palate.
- The clinician notes the general symmetry of facial structures, the shape and mobility of the client's lips and tongue, and any missing teeth or dental malocclusions.
- The clinician examines the client's hard and soft palates, looking for clefts, fistulas, or structural problems such as a high and vaulted hard palate. The client's soft-palate mobility is evaluated to make sure that the soft palate can move back and up to close the velopharyngeal port during the production of non-nasal sounds (for further details about assessment, see Chapter 13).
- Many clinicians also perform tests of diadochokinetic skill, which evaluate the child's oral–motor coordination, as well as the integrity of oral structures and functions.
- The goal of the orofacial examination is to assess the presence of any structural or functional factors that might be contributing to the SSD. If one or more of these factors is present, the clinician must assess the client's potential for improvement in treatment if the factors are not addressed.

- Despite the presence of abnormal structural or functional factors (e.g., a high and vaulted palate), the child may be stimulable for errored sounds and capable of improving speech.
- However, for some children, abnormal structure, function, or both must be addressed before treatment progress is possible. For example, the first author worked with a second-grade boy who had been in speech therapy for 4 years (with previous clinicians) with minimal progress on the treatment targets of /s/, /z/, /ʃ/, /ʒ/. It was found that due to the boy's thumb-sucking patterns, he had a marked class II malocclusion with substantial overjet. He was physically unable to produce the target phonemes due to the condition of his dentition. It was determined that orthodontia probably would be required before articulation treatment could be successful.

Hearing Screening
- Generally, the child's hearing is screened by a brief audiological procedure. A hearing screening does not determine actual hearing thresholds but only suggests that hearing is or is not within normal limits.
- A child who fails a hearing screening is referred to an audiologist for a complete hearing evaluation. This evaluation may include pure-tone testing, tympanometry, or both. Hearing testing procedures are described in greater detail in Chapter 12.

Specific Components of an Assessment

Conversational Speech Samples
- It is widely held that some children make many more errors at the conversational speech level than at the single-word level (Bankson et al., 2017; Stoel-Gammon & Menn, 2017). Thus, it is optimal to obtain a connected speech sample during assessment.
- Connected speech samples can also enable the clinician to evaluate stress, rate, intonation, and syllable structure. In addition, these samples allow for multiple productions of sounds across a wide variety of words (Bankson et al., 2017).
- It is optimal to collect 50–100 utterances as a representative sample of connected speech. Clinicians can phonetically transcribe all words or just the words that contain errors. It is best to transcribe on the spot if possible.
- It is a good idea to repeat the child's unintelligible words after him or her so that if the sample is recorded, the clinician can understand the speech sample at a later time.
- Samples should be recorded in a quiet environment with high-quality recording equipment such as an up-to-date iPad or smart phone. Noisy toys are not recommended; if they are used, the clinician can use them on the carpet or on a table with a tablecloth to reduce noise.
- Young children might give more representative speech samples if they interact with their family members; in such cases, the clinician can observe the interaction and record notes.
- Clinicians can use toys, games, large pictures, storybooks, and open-ended questions to evoke speech. Especially successful topics include pets, TV shows, siblings, movies, video games, iPad apps, favorite stories, and weekend or vacation activities.

Evoked Speech Samples

- Clinicians can collect speech samples not only through spontaneous conversation, but also through evoked samples. Below are three types of evoked samples that may be used to assess a child's production of sounds in single words:

  - **Imitation**. Typically, the child imitates the clinician's model of single words. Imitation can be **immediate** (e.g., Clinician: "Say 'truck.'" Child: "Truck") or delayed (e.g., Clinician: "Truck. This truck is big and yellow. What is this?" Child: "Truck"). In delayed imitation, a short phrase is placed between the clinician's model and the child's response.
  - **Naming**. The child names objects or pictures, usually after the clinician asks, "What's this?"
  - **Sentence completion**. The child finishes the clinician's sentence. For example, the clinician might say, "Look, here's a big, brown, barking _____." The child would fill in the word "dog" to complete the sentence.

- It is best to evoke single-word productions in conjunction with connected speech samples. As stated, some children make more errors in connected speech samples when sounds are produced in a coarticulated context than they do at the single-word level.

Stimulability Assessment

- **Stimulability** refers to the child's ability to imitate the clinician's model when given auditory and visual cues. Clinicians should select the sounds the child misarticulates and assess the child's stimulability for those sounds. A stimulable child is generally able to imitate the clinician's modeled productions.
- The clinician should ask the child to watch, listen carefully, and "Say what I say." It is best initially to model sounds in isolation. Sounds can later be modeled in words and, if desired, nonsense syllables.
- In terms of prognosis for outgrowing articulation errors, some believe that a stimulable child has a strong possibility of outgrowing errors of articulation without therapy; others believe that a child will make faster improvement with therapy.
- Bankson, Bernthal, and Flipsen (2017) believe that stimulability is a prognostic indicator that shows that individuals with poor stimulability skills should be seen for treatment because it is unlikely that they will self-correct their speech sound errors.
- Many clinicians believe that stimulable sounds are easier to teach than nonstimulable sounds. Therefore, many clinicians use stimulable sounds as a starting point for treatment.
- It is recommended that clinicians assess a child's ability to produce sounds (a) through imitation, (b) in one or more phonetic environments, (c) in key words, (d) through phonetic placement and shaping, or (e) in a combination of these contexts. In therapy, a child's frustration can be reduced if he has at least some capacity to approximate a target sound.

Standardized Tests

- Many standardized tests of speech sound skills are available. For many clinicians, standardized tests are convenient to give because the target words are clearly identified. When used to test highly

unintelligible children, standardized tests may be more reliable than spontaneous, connected samples.
- Standardized tests also satisfy the requirements of many school districts, which require formal test scores. In such cases, clinicians can supplement standardized test results with conversational speech samples.
- Most standardized tests of articulation skills assess the child's production of all phonemes in the initial, medial, and final positions of words at the single-word level. Usually, each phoneme is sampled only once in each position. Such tests yield information, such as, "Johnny made th/s substitutions in the initial, medial, and final positions of words."
- Instruments that measure phonological patterns assess a child's production of words in isolation and in connected speech. However, instead of focusing on individual sounds that are misarticulated, phonological pattern measures assess the child's use of phonological patterns and the percentage of time he or she uses those phonological patterns. For example, a test might yield the information that "Johnny used the phonological pattern of final-consonant deletion in 80% of all tested contexts."
- Most tests of speech skills use picture stimuli. In addition, computerized measures are increasingly being used.

Scoring and Analysis of Assessment Data

Independent Versus Relational Analysis

- Clinicians can score and analyze assessment data in two ways: independent analysis or relational analysis. A more complete picture of a child's speech skills emerges when both types of analyses are performed.
- In **independent analysis**, a child's speech patterns are described without reference to the adult model of the language of the child's community. For example, an independent analysis might state that a child's speech contains /f/, /b/, /s/, and /k/ but would not state if these sounds were produced correctly in comparison to the adult community's standard form.
- Independent analyses can include all vocalizations or only those vocalizations that are recognized as words. Independent analyses provide important information about the phonology of young children who make many errors in sound productions and who may or may not have an extensive repertoire of phonemes.
- Typically, an independent analysis is used with very young children or speakers with limited phonological repertoires. Once the child has a vocabulary of around 50 words, a relational analysis is used.
- In a **relational analysis**, which is more commonly used in clinical settings, a child's speech is compared to the adult model of his or her speech community. For example, a statement based on a relational analysis might say, "The child produced a w/r substitution." This statement involves an evaluation of the child's production in relation to acceptable speech in the wider community.

Standard Procedures

- The following procedures should be followed when scoring and analyzing assessment data:

- Use the International Phonetic Alphabet to transcribe the child's speech. Use diacritics, if possible, to make a more detailed analysis of errors. This is especially critical for children from bilingual backgrounds and children with organically based problems, such as cleft palate.
- Note how consistently the errors are produced, and calculate the percentage of misarticulation for each phoneme in error (e.g., /k/ is misarticulated in 80% of contexts).
- List the phonetic contexts in which any of the misarticulated sounds were produced correctly (e.g., /r/ is produced correctly in word-initial *gr*– blends).
- Calculate the percentage of correctly imitated productions on stimulability trials.
- Analyze the results of any standardized test according to the manual's prescribed procedures.
- List the sounds in error and classify them according to an acceptable format (e.g., omissions–substitutions–distortions; errors in the pre-, inter-, and postvocalic positions of words).
- If the child has multiple misarticulations and it appears that a pattern analysis would be worthwhile, carry out a phonological analysis. List the phonological patterns the child uses and the percentage of time those patterns are used (e.g., "Susie used the phonological pattern of consonant-cluster reduction in 60% of the possible contexts").
- Use published guidelines to decide whether the child is using phonological patterns that should have disappeared by his or her age. For example, a 4-year-old should not be using the pattern of reduplication. Table 5.3 summarizes guidelines given by Stoel-Gammon and Dunn (1985).
- Calculate the child's intelligibility (in percentage) based on the number of utterances or words that are understood with or without knowledge of the context. For example, the clinician could say, "In the known context of discussing a current movie, Mario's connected speech was 60% intelligible to the examiner."
- Calculate the severity of the child's speech problem by calculating percentage of consonants correct (PCC). PCC is the ratio of the number of consonants produced correctly to the total number of consonants:

$$\frac{\text{Total number of correct consonants produced} \times 100}{\text{Total number of consonants produced}}$$

The overall PCC score is interpreted according to the following scale, described by Shriberg and Kwiatkowski (1982):

>85%	Mild
65–85%	Mild to moderate
50–65%	Moderate to severe
<50%	Severe

- Decide whether the child should receive treatment based on the following factors:
  - The child is making speech sound errors at an age when he or she should be producing those patterns and sounds correctly.
  - The child's production differs markedly from that of peers of a similar cultural and linguistic background.

Table 5.3

Phonological Patterns That Disappear Before and Persist After Age 3

Disappear by age 3	Persist after age 3
Reduplication	Final-consonant devoicing
Weak/unstressed syllable deletion	Consonant-cluster reduction
Consonant assimilation	Stopping
Prevocalic voicing	Epenthesis
Fronting of velars	Gliding
Final-consonant deletion	Depalatization
Diminutization	Vocalization

- The child's speech is so unintelligible that it represents a clinically significant problem (e.g., there are social penalties for the child).
- The number of phonemes in error indicates that the child qualifies for treatment in a given clinical setting such as a public school.

- Distinguish SSDs from hearing impairment, CAS, and dysarthria associated with a known neurological condition such as cerebral palsy.
- Distinguish SSDs from typical, predictable errors manifested by a child who speaks a language other than English or is exposed to models who speak a language other than English.
- Describe associated conditions such as autism, fetal alcohol syndrome, or cleft palate, and suggest additional or more intensive evaluation if necessary.
- Make a statement of prognosis, considering whether variables such as hearing impairment, environmental factors, physical disabilities, and intellectual disabilities may affect treatment outcomes.

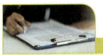

SUMMARY

- Assessment serves two primary purposes. The first is to determine whether the child manifests a clinically significant SSD. The second is to identify and describe the problem if it exists.
- Clinicians usually begin by screening to rule out children who do not need in-depth assessments. An in-depth assessment usually begins with a case history, an orofacial examination, and a hearing screening.
- Specific assessment components include conversational and evoked speech samples, stimulability assessment, and the administration of standardized tests. Assessment data are then scored and analyzed to provide directions for treatment.

TREATMENT OF SPEECH SOUND DISORDERS

Treatment for SSDs may be organized under two major categories: motor approaches and linguistic approaches. This dichotomy is somewhat artificial because motor and linguistic skills are intertwined; thus, these categories are not mutually exclusive. Yet these two broad categories help clinicians conceptualize the foundation for treatment of children who are unintelligible. Treatment depends very much upon whether the child's errors reflect a lack of linguistic knowledge (phonological errors), a lack of motor skills (articulation errors), or both (Flipsen et al., 2017a). Flipsen et al. state that normal speech sound production involves both the production of sounds at a motor level and their use in accordance with the underlying rules of language; thus, these skills are two sides of the same coin.

It is generally believed that motor-based approaches are best for children with several sounds in error (e.g., /r/, /s/, /l/), and linguistic approaches are most appropriate for highly unintelligible children with multiple sound errors. But because many children have difficulties in both areas, clinicians frequently use a combination of motor and linguistic approaches for remediation. In this section, we describe general considerations in the treatment of children with SSDs. We then elaborate upon motor and linguistic approaches and briefly discuss the phenomenon of phonological awareness.

General Considerations in Treatment

- No matter what specific treatment program or combination of programs is used, most clinicians use certain basic procedures in providing treatment for children with SSDs. These steps usually consist of the following:

  - Thorough assessment and analysis of the child's speech sound system
  - Determination of any existing patterns
  - Selection and prioritization of intervention targets
  - Establishment of baselines of target sounds in all contexts: words, phrases, sentences, and conversational speech
  - Specific training for target patterns, sounds, or both
  - Preparation of generalization and maintenance activities

- Most clinicians use a multimodal approach to treatment. This involves use of auditory, visual, and kinesthetic cues.
- Because the primary goal of treatment is effective communication, clinicians are increasingly using language- and meaning-based activities in therapy for SSDs. While some approaches to treatment necessarily involve drills, and sometimes drills on nonsense syllables, it is important to make activities meaningful to the child's communication in his or her daily environment.
- The concept of **communicative potency** looks at how functional words are within an individual child's communication environment. Words and phrases such as *stop*, *yes*, *give me*, and *some more* allow children greater control over their environments.
- Therefore, treatment should use communicatively potent words as much as possible. Children should be taught that correct production of sounds and patterns results in improved communication with others and increased control over their environments.

- Early intervention is a high priority, especially for highly unintelligible children. Some of these children may express distress at an early age if they are difficult to understand.
- If a child has a language impairment that accompanies the SSD, the clinician must integrate language activities into therapy. This can be accomplished in many ways, including increasing morphosyntactic skills, as well as narrative skills, if the child has deficits in these areas.
- It is very important to involve caregivers in therapy, especially in the generalization and maintenance stages. In addition, children must be taught self-monitoring skills.
- Clinicians commonly use standardized tests to assess treatment progress, but this is usually ineffective because tests include only a small number of items to sample each sound or pattern. For example, most standardized tests of articulation test each phoneme only once in each word position. Using a standardized test as a measure of pretreatment skills and posttreatment gains usually fails to show treatment gains.
- Clinicians must always take the child's cultural and linguistic background into account. It is important to distinguish between speech sound **differences** and speech sound **disorders**. Differences usually arise from the influence of the child's first language. Disorders exist when the child makes errors that are not typical for his or her cultural and linguistic speech community (Roseberry-McKibbin, 2018).
- For example, a Spanish-speaking child typically makes b/v and d/ð substitutions. These differences involve interference (also called transfer) from Spanish and do not constitute a disorder and should not be treated as such. A child has a disorder only when his or her speech sound patterns in the primary language or in English differ from those of peers from a similar cultural and linguistic background (Goldstein & Iglesias, 2017; Roseberry-McKibbin, 2018).
- A **developmental approach** to treatment is based on selection of early-developing targets that follow a developmental sequence and are assumed to be easier for children to produce.
- For example, the sounds /p, b, m/ develop early in life and are usually easy for children to produce. With a highly unintelligible young child who produces these phonemes correctly in some contexts, the speech–language pathologist (SLP) who uses a developmental approach would select these sounds for treatment. The underlying premise is that learning speech sounds has a motoric basis and should follow a sequential order based on ease of sound acquisition.
- Proponents of the **complexity approach** (also called the **least knowledge approach**) recommend targeting sounds that are nonstimulable, always incorrect, and later developing.
- The underlying assumption is that presenting more complex input to the child will accomplish two aims: (a) lead to the child's learning simpler, untrained sounds and (b) force the child to learn the complex target (Geirut, 2007; Geirut, Morrisette, Hughes, & Rowland, 1996; Williams, 2014). Put differently, the complexity approach assumes that use of the approach will create a systemwide change (McLeod, 2017).
- For example, a highly unintelligible 5-year-old may have difficulty with many early-developing sounds but produce some of them correctly some of the time (e.g., /k, g, d, t/). She may never produce later-developing sounds such as /s, z, r/ correctly.

- In the complexity approach, the SLP would target these later-developing sounds, assuming that teaching the child to produce /s, z, r/ correctly would lead to correct production of simpler, untrained sounds such as /k, g, d, t/.
- The caveat to this approach is that even though it is considered more efficient than other approaches, it may initially take longer to teach children to produce more complex speech targets. Thus, children may initially remain unintelligible for longer and become frustrated with their continued lack of communicative effectiveness.
- Because of this, when considering whether to use this approach, the SLP must take into account the child's ability to handle frustration, as well as the overall goals of intervention (e.g., immediate intelligibility vs. promoting significant changes in the child's overall speech system).
- Some SLPs use nonspeech oral–motor training as a precursor to teaching sounds or as a supplement to teaching those sounds. These training activities can include blowing horns or whistles, wagging the tongue, sucking liquid through straws, and others (no speech sounds are made). Researchers have questioned the efficacy of these activities, believing that in order to improve speech, SLPs need to focus directly on speech (Peña-Brooks & Hegde, 2015; Flipsen et al., 2017a).
- However, nonspeech oral motor exercises can be part of intervention when SLPs are working with clients who have tongue thrust, dysarthria, and swallowing disorders (Kent, 2015).

Motor-Based Approaches

Van Riper's Traditional Approach

- **Van Riper's traditional approach**, first published in the mid-1930s, is the foundation for motor approaches to articulation therapy (Flipsen et al., 2017a). Van Riper (1978) focused on **auditory discrimination/perceptual training**, **phonetic placement**, and **drill-like repetition and practice** at increasingly complex motor levels until target phonemes were automatized.
- This approach as a bottom-up drill approach that focuses on discrete skills. The progression of therapy goes from the simplest to the most complex movements, and isolated speech sounds are targeted.
- Clinicians who use the traditional approach to remediation of SSDs view articulation errors as resulting from **motor difficulties**, in which the child is physically unable to produce the sound, and from **faulty perceptual skills**.
- **Auditory discrimination/perceptual training** is designed to teach clients to distinguish between correct and incorrect productions of speech sounds. For example, the clinician may say, "Listen. Which is the right way to say this word? *Wabbit* or *rabbit*?" Or the clinician might have the client begin by correctly distinguishing the /w/ from the /r/ sound.
- This type of training is based on the assumption that auditory discrimination training is a precursor to speech sound production training. That assumption is questioned by many researchers and clinicians who believe that production training induces correct discrimination.
- **Phonetic placement** is used when the client cannot imitate the modeled production of a phoneme such as /r/. Phonetic placement begins with having the child produce a sound in isolation. The clinician uses verbal instructions, modeling, physical guidance (e.g., manipulating the client's tongue

with a tongue depressor), and visual feedback (e.g., mirrors, drawings) to show the client how target sounds are produced.
- The assumption underlying production training is that motor practice leads to automatization and thus to generalization of correct productions to untrained contexts. Practice and drill are critical components of treatment.
- Drill occurs at increasingly complex motor levels that are hierarchical in nature. Thus, clinicians who use the traditional approach to therapy to teach /s/, for example, would teach this sound at the following levels of complexity:

    isolation → syllables → words → phrases → sentences reading (if the child reads) → conversation

- Motor-based approaches are most successful with children who have only a few phonemes in error (e.g., /r/, /s/, /l/) and are not highly unintelligible. Motor-based approaches work well for children who have physical difficulty producing target phonemes, because these approaches address the mechanics of sound production.
- In sum, Van Riper's (1978) traditional approach to articulation therapy focuses on (a) establishing correct auditory perception of target phonemes and (b) training accurate motor production of individual phonemes (e.g., separate work on /r/, /s/, /l/). The goal is for the client to accurately use the target phonemes in conversation.
- Today, more clinicians, especially in school districts, are beginning to provide early intervention for these children instead of waiting until they are older and the speech sound errors more firmly entrenched and more difficult to treat.
- Early intervention is highly effective; it takes less time and is much more efficient in remediating errors than intervention that occurs when children are older.
- Motor-based approaches can be incorporated into programs that are based on linguistic principles (e.g., the phonological pattern approach) for clients who have a combination of motor-based and linguistic-based errors.

Context Utilization Approaches
- These approaches recognize that speech sounds are not produced in isolation but rather in syllable-based contexts. Certain phonetic contexts can facilitate correct sound usage (Flipsen et al., 2017a). The most widely-known context utilization approach was developed by McDonald (1964).
- McDonald's sensorimotor approach is based on the assumption that the **syllable**, not the isolated phoneme, is the basic unit of speech production. Principles of **coarticulation** are important in this approach (McDonald, 1964).
- Like Van Riper's approach, McDonald's approach is a bottom-up drill approach to therapy. This system was unique in the mid-1960s because it disagreed with the established assumptions that (a) perceptual training should precede production training and (b) treatment should begin with sounds in isolation.
- According to McDonald (1964), **phonetic environment** is very important in treatment; thus, training should begin at the syllable level. The clinician should administer a deep test

(e.g., McDonald's *Deep Test of Articulation*) to find phonetic contexts where an otherwise misarticulated sound was produced correctly. For example, a child with an /s/ distortion might produce /s/ correctly in the context of *watch–sun*.

- McDonald's (1964) approach includes several basic steps (each step has smaller, more detailed increments; only the basics are presented here):

  1. Heighten the client's responsiveness to connected motor productions; begin with non-error sounds in a variety of bi- and trisyllabic contexts (in nonsense syllables) with differing stress patterns.
  2. Train correct production of misarticulated sounds; find a context in which /s/, for example, is produced correctly (e.g., *watch–sun*), and have the child produce the sound in that context in various syllable stress and phrase and sentence patterns.
  3. Vary the phonetic contexts (e.g., *watch–sit*, *watch–saw*) and have the child practice correct production of the targets in different contexts.
  4. Generalize by facilitating transfer to other phonetic contexts and then to natural communication activities.

McDonald's (1964) sensorimotor approach may be helpful for children with oral–motor coordination difficulties. However, research does not support the assumption that syllabic production of nonerror productions will facilitate the correction of errored productions (Flipsen et al., 2017a).

Linguistic Approaches

- As previously mentioned, linguistic approaches are sometimes used in combination with motor approaches when a child has difficulties with both the motoric and the linguistic aspects of speech sound production.
- Linguistic approaches assume that the child has a rule-governed system with specific patterns, but that this system differs from the adult system in the child's community. Thus, therapy is geared toward modifying the child's underlying rule system so that it matches the adult standard (Flipsen, Bankson, & Bernthal, 2017b).
- The primary goal of linguistic approaches is to establish phonological rules in a client's repertoire. Instead of focusing on individual sounds in treatment, therapy focuses on relationships among sounds. Treatment focuses on building and reorganizing children's phonological representations rather than just addressing surface production of specific sounds.
- Thus, the clinician is attempting to remediate **underlying patterns or rules** instead of discrete phonemes. For example, the clinician might treat the underlying pattern of **stridency deletion** instead of focusing on treating "omission of /s/, /f/, and /ʃ/," as one would if using a motor-based approach.
- The clinician selects sounds or target behaviors called **exemplars**. The assumption is that treatment of these exemplars will facilitate generalization to a whole class of sounds or other sounds in the same word position. In other words, the goal is to speed remediation through generalization of treatment results from a treated sound to untreated sounds.

- Most linguistic treatment programs use **minimal pairs**, or pairs of words that differ by one feature (e.g., *shine–pine*; *bee–beach*). The goal is to show the child that sound production affects meaning.
- The most commonly used linguistic approaches are the minimal pair contrast approaches and the phonological pattern approach (PPA).

Minimal Pair Contrast Therapy

- Contrast approaches vary in terms of how the sound contrasts are used in treatment. Different kinds of contrasts lead to different pairs of treatment stimulus words (Flipsen et al., 2017b).
- In **minimal pair** contrast therapy, the clinician uses pairs of words that differ by only one feature—the feature the clinician is trying to help the child to conceptualize. Of the paired words, one is the target word in which the sound is produced correctly; the other word contains the child's incorrect production.
- For example, if a child substitutes /t/ for /s/, the clinician might contrast the words *sea* and *tea*. The clinician focuses on these word pairs so that the child learns the **semantic** as well as the **motoric** differences between the phonemes. In other words, the child is taught that different sounds signal different meanings.
- In another example, the clinician might remediate the phonological pattern of final-consonant deletion by using pictures contrasting *boat* and *bow*, *bee* and *bead*, and *tea* and *teeth*. Through use of these minimal pair contrasts, the child learns that the final consonant makes a difference in word meaning.
- In **maximal contrast** therapy, also known as the **maximal opposition** approach, the selected word pairs contain maximum numbers of phonemic contrasts.
- For example, contrasts in a minimal pair may involve only one contrast of either place, manner, or voicing; however, in a maximal contrast approach, all three features (place, manner, voicing) may be involved.
- Suppose a child substitutes /t/ for /sh/, resulting in productions such as *top/shop* and *tip/ship*. In the minimal pairs approach, *top* (error) and *shop* (correct target production) would be a training stimulus pair.
- In the maximal contrast therapy approach, /t/ and /sh/ would not be contrasted. The error sound would be contrasted with a sound that is maximally different—for example, /m/. The resulting maximally opposed pairs used in therapy might be *me–she*, *Mack–shack*, and so forth.

Phonological Pattern Approach

- The PPA is based on the assumption that a child's multiple errors reflect the operation of certain phonological rules and that the problem is essentially phonemic, not phonetic (Flahive & Hodson, 2014).
- A child's errors are grouped and described as **phonological patterns** (e.g., "Johnny manifests the use of consonant-cluster reduction and weak-syllable deletion"), not as **discrete sounds** (e.g., "Johnny makes w/r, θ/s, and w/l substitutions").
- Hodson and Paden's (1991) cycles approach (see below) is a widely used phonological pattern approach.

Hodson and Paden's Cycles Approach

- In this phonological pattern approach designed to treat children with multiple misarticulations and highly unintelligible speech, error patterns are targeted for remediation based on stimulability, intelligibility, and percentage of occurrence (40% or greater).
- Because they believe that phonological acquisition is a gradual process, Hodson and Paden (1991) recommend that error patterns not be drilled to a criterion of mastery (e.g., 90% accuracy). Rather, the clinician introduces correct patterns, gives the child limited practice with them, and returns to them at a later date.
- A cycle runs 5–16 weeks, and each child usually requires three to six cycles (30–40 hours at 40–60 minutes per week). Each sound in an error pattern receives 1 hour of treatment per cycle before the clinician proceeds to the next sound in the error pattern. Only one error pattern is treated in each therapy session, but all error patterns are treated in each cycle.
- Thus, for example, cycle 1 might target the phonological patterns of final-consonant deletion and fronting. During the first treatment session, the clinician would spend the whole hour targeting /p/ in word-final position; during session two, the whole hour would be spent targeting /t/ in word-final position; in session three, the clinician would spend the whole hour targeting /k/ (to address the process of fronting); and so forth. During cycles 2 and 3 (if the child needs three cycles), the clinician would repeat the treatment in the above-described manner.
- Each treatment session consists of the following activities (Flahive & Hodson, 2014; Hodson & Paden, 1991): (a) review of the previous session's target words, (b) auditory bombardment (listening to target words that are amplified), (c) activities involving new target words, (d) play break, (e) more activities involving new target words, and (f) repeating auditory bombardment and dismissal. Families are also given activities for home practice.
- Research has shown that the primary strength of the cycles approach is its efficiency. Within a year, after 30–40 hours of therapy, many preschoolers become much more intelligible (Flahive & Hodson, 2014).
- Because many highly unintelligible children have phonological awareness deficits, therapy should address these deficits as well as addressing sound production problems.

Core Vocabulary (Consistency) Approach

- This approach, developed by Dodd and colleagues, is designed to meet the needs of the approximately 10% of children with functional SSDs who have inconsistent errors on the same words in the absence of CAS (Broomfield & Dodd, 2005; Dodd, Holm, Crosbie, & McIntosh, 2010).
- The Core Vocabulary Approach does not fit neatly into motor- or linguistic-based approaches (Flipsen et al., 2017b). Rather, it contains elements of both.
- Some children have impaired ability to phonologically (not motorically) program the sequence of phonemes that make up a word. This difficulty exists despite the presence of average neuromotor abilities and is called inconsistent speech sound disorder (ISSD).
- Successful with children as young as 2 years of age, the core vocabulary approach begins with the assessment of a child's multiple productions of the same word in the same phonetic context. The

child's total score for all words is converted to a percentage; a score of 40% meets the diagnostic criterion for ISSD.
- Therapy revolves around 70 core vocabulary words that are selected (ideally) with the help of parents and teachers. Ecologically valid, functional words, used in the child's environment, are selected for training.
- Children are seen for therapy individually, twice a week, for 30 minutes for 8 weeks. The long-term, 8-week goal is for the child to produce at least 70 pragmatically powerful words consistently, or in the same way. If the child makes developmental errors on the words, this is considered acceptable.
- The overall goals of this approach are increased intelligibility and consistency in the production of at least 70 words that are ecologically valid, or key, in the child's environment.
- When the child has become consistent in word productions, another treatment approach (e.g., the minimal contrast approach) can build upon the foundation that has been laid.

Phonological Awareness Treatment

- Phonological awareness (PA) refers to the explicit awareness of the sound structure of a language, or attention to the internal structure of words (McNeill, Justice, Gillon, & Schuele, 2017).
- Phonological awareness is viewed as a subcategory of **metalinguistic awareness**, which refers to the child's ability to manipulate and think about the structure of language.
- Typically-developing children have emerging PA skills between 3–4 years of age. By 5 years of age, they will have established the following PA skills: syllable segmentation, rhyme awareness, alliteration awareness, letter knowledge, and phoneme isolation (McLeod, 2017). Phoneme segmentation is one of the latest skills to develop, usually becoming established when children are 6–7 years old.
- Deficits in PA skills have been linked with later problems in reading and spelling. It is suggested that young children with severe phonological disorders lack, among other things, PA and that these children are at risk for reading and spelling problems later in their childhood (Goldstein et al., 2017).
- Research shows that children with SSDs that are articulatory rather than phonological in nature may not have difficulties mastering PA skills.
- However, children whose SSDs are phonological in nature and accompanied by difficulties in language are at the greatest risk for failing to achieve PA and eventual literacy skills. By some estimates, almost 50% of these children will not be good readers by third or fourth grade.
- It is recommended that in early childhood, these children receive explicit training to increase their PA. It is believed that this training may prevent later problems with reading and writing (Goldstein et al., 2017).
- Treatment activities are generally designed to increase children's awareness of the sound structure of language. Thus, treatment can include a variety of activities such as sound blending, rhyming, alliteration, and others that focus specifically on sound-structure awareness.
- McNeill, Justice, Gillon, and Schuele (2017) give a detailed description of how to embed PA activities into therapy for children with SSDs; these suggestions are summarized here:
  - Write words clearly and in a large font underneath stimulus pictures for speech production. When practicing speech target words, draw the child's attention to the printed word.

- Use alliteration activities that ask the child to attend to the initial sound in target words. For example, if /s/ and /r/ are target phonemes, the child can be asked to sort cards into piles depending on whether the words start with /s/ or /r/.
- Read storybooks (with the child's target sounds) that feature alliteration and that also feature rhyming; bring the child's attention to these patterns. For example, if the child is working on reducing use of the phonological process of fronting of velars, the SLP could use the Dr. Seuss book *Green Eggs and Ham* and discuss rhyming and alliteration in this story.
- Take target speech words with several phonemes and model segmentation. For example, for the child who fronts velars, the SLP can take the word *green* and say, "Let's break the word *green* into four sounds: g-r-ee-n. Now you say it just the way I did."
- Make cards that have the child's target sounds printed on them and explicitly refer to the printed sound when working on its production. For example, if a child is working on the /v/ sound, the clinician can have a 3 × 5 index card with a large V written on it. During therapy, the clinician can say things like "We are going to practice this sound now [showing card]. What sound does this make?"

■ Many times, SLPs believe that PA activities must stand apart from activities involving speech production. In fact, the first author of this book (who works part time in public schools) often asks students to bring their language arts books from their classrooms into speech sessions. The story the class is currently reading is then used to build PA skills and practice target sounds, as well.

■ For example, the first author was recently providing therapy to a third grader who had difficulty producing /ʃ/. Using a story from the classroom language arts book about Sir Ernest *Sh*ackleton, the first author targeted production of /ʃ/, as well as PA skills.

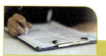

SUMMARY

- Clinicians take certain foundational steps in treating any child with an SSD. Then, based upon the needs of the individual child, they may use a motor-based approach, a linguistic approach, or a combination of those approaches in treatment.
- Motor-based approaches, which focus on improving the child's perceptual and motor skills, treat sounds as isolated segments (e.g., treating /l/, /r/, /s/, etc.). Commonly used motor-based approaches include Van Riper's (1978) traditional approach and McDonald's (1964) sensorimotor approach.
- Linguistic approaches are geared toward finding a highly unintelligible child's underlying patterns and rule system and modifying that rule system to match the adult standard. Common linguistic approaches include the contrast approaches and the phonological pattern approach.
- The core vocabulary approach, used for children with inconsistent speech sound disorder, contains elements of both the motor-based and linguistic approaches.
- Last, many researchers and clinicians advocate for conducting phonological awareness treatment for young children who, it is suspected, have phonological awareness deficiencies that may cause reading, writing, and spelling problems in later childhood.

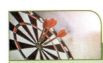

CHAPTER HIGHLIGHTS

- The term *articulation disorder* generally refers to speech–motor control problems: physical difficulty producing sounds. The term *phonological disorder* is usually used to describe an underlying difficulty with the phonological aspect of language knowledge displayed by a highly unintelligible child. Acknowledging that many children have a combination of motor and language knowledge difficulties, many professionals use the term *speech sound disorder*.
- Various theories of phonological development have been proposed. These theories attempt to explain how children acquire phonological rules and the sounds of their speech communities. Most theories fall under the categories of linear and nonlinear phonology theories.
- In order to diagnose speech delays in infants and children, many clinicians turn to developmental norms. Oller (1980) proposed five stages of typical infant speech sound development. Cross-sectional and longitudinal studies have yielded data about the speech sound acquisition of typically developing children. Some researchers have proposed time frames in which typically developing children use certain phonological processes for a time and then stop using those processes as they mature.
- Sometimes children do not develop speech skills in a typical fashion. Such children are said to have a speech sound disorder. This disorder is generally viewed in one of two categories: *functional*, or *idiopathic* (no observable organic cause, unknown etiology), and *organic* (caused by physical damage to the peripheral or central nervous system, the oral mechanism, or all of these).
- Some general factors have been associated with speech sound disorders but have not been proven to be causal in nature. These factors include gender, intelligence, birth order and sibling status, socioeconomic status, language development and academic performance, and auditory discrimination skills.
- Organically based speech sound disorders have been associated with oral structural variables such as ankyloglossia (tongue-tie), dental deviations such as malocclusions, poor oral–motor coordination skills, orofacial myofunctional disorders (tongue thrust), and hearing loss. Neuropathologies such as apraxia of speech and dysarthria directly cause speech sound disorders in children.
- Clinicians assess children for speech sound disorders using a general set of procedures. This includes, at a minimum, gathering a case history, conducting an orofacial examination, and conducting a hearing screening. If relevant, clinicians may also obtain information about other variables (e.g., hearing problems, dental abnormalities, intellectual disabilities) that co-occur with the speech sound disorder.
- When conducting a formal, in-depth assessment, clinicians may use conversational speech samples, evoked speech samples, stimulability assessments, and standardized tests. The results are scored and analyzed, and then a statement of prognosis is made. Treatment goals are created.
- Treatment of speech sound disorders can be artificially dichotomized into motor approaches and linguistic approaches. Often a combination of the two approaches is used. Motor approaches are usually appropriate for a child with several discrete sounds in error (e.g., /s/, /r/, /θ/) who has physical difficulty producing those sounds correctly. Motor approaches, which focus generally on

remediating motor difficulties and faulty perceptual abilities, include Van Riper's (1978) traditional approach and McDonald's (1964) sensorimotor approach.

- Linguistic approaches are generally appropriate for highly unintelligible children who are assumed to have underlying phonological systems that differ from those of the adult speech community. Linguistic approaches attempt to establish phonological rules in children's repertoires and treat underlying patterns or rules instead of discrete phonemes. Commonly known linguistic approaches include the contrast approaches, the core vocabulary approach (which also contains elements of motor approaches), and the phonological pattern approach (especially that of Hodson and Paden [1991]). Many children with phonological disorders benefit from phonological awareness therapy.

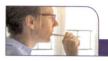

STUDY AND REVIEW QUESTIONS

1. You are working as a clinician in a private clinic. A father brings his son, Johnny, age 4-and-a-half years, for an evaluation. According to his father, Johnny is "hard to understand, and sometimes the kids at preschool make fun of him." The pediatrician has told Johnny's father that Johnny will "outgrow this speech problem on his own," but the father wants to make sure that this advice is correct. Johnny will be starting kindergarten in 6 months, when he turns 5 years of age, and his father wants to be sure that Johnny speaks as intelligibly as possible so that he will not be teased in elementary school. When you evaluate Johnny, you find that he has θ/s, t/f, w/r, d/ð, and j/l substitutions. You decide to place him in therapy. You would begin therapy by addressing the

   A. θ/s substitution.
   B. t/f substitution.
   C. w/r substitution.
   D. d/ð substitution.

2. In Oller's stages of infant phonological development, reduplicated babbling precedes

   A. nonreduplicated or variegated babbling.
   B. expansion.
   C. cooing.
   D. phonation.

3. A clinician evaluates the speech of a 5-year-old child with a phonological delay. The child is not intelligible to her kindergarten teacher or her peers and is placed in therapy to improve her intelligibility. Assuming that this child uses the phonological process of consonant-cluster reduction, which of the following is the word you would most likely put on a word list used for treatment?

   A. Bus
   B. Stopped
   C. Rich
   D. Lassie

4. The therapy technique of *phonetic placement* is used to teach or establish

   A. auditory discrimination.
   B. stimulability.
   C. production of a phoneme in isolation.
   D. minimal pair contrasts.

5. You are serving a preschool attended by 50 children. Most of them are 4 years old, and their parents are highly involved because they are trying to prepare their children for kindergarten. A father is concerned about Justin, his 4-and-a-half-year-old son. Justin is highly intelligible, but his father reports that he has difficulty with consonant clusters in words like *spring*, *street*, and *squirrel*. You tell the father that at 4-and-a-half, it is natural for Justin to have difficulties with words with consonant clusters. However, according to developmental norms, he should have little difficulty with which of the following consonant clusters because many 4-year-olds have mastered them?

   A. Clusters gl, fl, pl
   B. Clusters pr, br, tr
   C. Clusters kst, lk, nd
   D. Clusters sp, st, sk

6. A child comes to you for an evaluation. According to her mother, Sharma has a history of middle ear infections. Her mother reports that Sharma is quite difficult to understand. For example, according to her mother, she says things like gʌk/dʌk and koʊ/toʊ. This child is manifesting the phonological pattern of

   A. fronting.
   B. stridency deletion.
   C. backing.
   D. glottal replacement.

7. The articulation therapy approach that emphasizes the syllable as the basic unit of speech production and heavily uses the concept of phonetic environment is

   A. McDonald's sensorimotor approach.
   B. the maximal contrast approach.
   C. the metaphon approach.
   D. Van Riper's traditional approach.

8. A child is referred to you by his preschool teacher. This child, Damien, is 4 years 3 months old and has transferred from out of state. In his previous state, he was reportedly assessed by an SLP who recommended that he receive intervention before kindergarten. According to the report from the previous clinician, Damien uses the phonological patterns of gliding, consonant-cluster reduction, stopping, reduplication, and final-consonant deletion. Your assessment confirms the presence of these phonological patterns. You would begin treatment by addressing

   A. final-consonant deletion.
   B. gliding.
   C. consonant-cluster reduction.
   D. reduplication.

9. Which one of the following is *false* regarding dental deviations?

   A. *Skeletal malocclusion* refers to deviations in the shape and dimensions of the mandible and maxilla.
   B. *Dental malocclusion* refers to deviations in the positioning of individual teeth.

C. In *class I malocclusion*, the arches themselves are generally aligned properly; however, some individual teeth are misaligned.

D. In *class II malocclusion*, the maxilla is receded and the mandible is protruded.

10. Which one of the following is *false* regarding treatment of children with SSDs?

A. In *maximal contrast* therapy, also known as the *maximal opposition* approach, the selected word pairs contain maximum numbers of phonemic contrasts (e.g., pack-stack).

B. *Hodson and Paden's cycles approach* involves treating children with phonological disorders in cycles in which the child is trained to a criterion of mastery for error patterns such as final-consonant deletion and fronting.

C. *Van Riper's approach* focuses on phonetic placement, auditory discrimination/perceptual training, and drill-like repetition and practice at increasingly complex motor levels until target phonemes are produced correctly in spontaneous conversation.

D. In *minimal pair contrast therapy*, the clinician uses pairs of words that differ by only one feature; of the paired words, one is the target word in which the sound is produced correctly and the other is the child's incorrect production.

Questions 11–13 refer to the following scenario:

A 5-year-old child, Crystal S., is brought to you for an evaluation of her speech. The family speaks only English in the home. According to Crystal's mother, Crystal "loves to talk but most people have trouble understanding her." As you play with Crystal informally, you estimate that she is approximately 50–60% intelligible. You conduct an oral peripheral evaluation, which reveals that she does not have any anatomical or physiological anomalies that would explain why she is so unintelligible. You also conduct in-depth assessment in other areas to determine the nature of her unintelligibility and to determine therapy goals.

11. You discover through your assessment that there are some sounds that Crystal consistently misarticulates. For example, she usually makes a t/k substitution (e.g., *tea/key*). You want to know if she can produce /k/ in isolation. You show her how to produce /k/ by giving her a model, and you tell her, "Watch me make the /k/ sound. Then you do it just like I did." When you are doing this, you are assessing Crystal's

A. phonological knowledge.
B. receptive phonology skills.
C. overall intelligibility.
D. stimulability.

12. You find that Crystal uses a number of phonological patterns. One of those patterns is stopping. You know this when you hear her make such substitutions as

A. bae/baet.
B. to/so.
C. rʌz/rʌʃ.
D. pɛt/pɛst.

13. You are conducting therapy with a highly unintelligible 5-year-old and are targeting phonological awareness skills (among other things). Two target sounds in therapy are /k/ and /g/. You carry out activities that focus on helping the child attend to the initial sound in target words. For example, you have her play a "fishing" game where she catches "fish" with words that begin with /k/ or /g/. After she catches a fish, she puts it into the appropriate "pond." You are targeting which specific phonological awareness skills?

- **A.** Rhyming
- **B.** Syllable segmentation
- **C.** Alliteration
- **D.** Syllabication

14. Lynne is a 6-year-old child with dysarthria of speech secondary to cerebral palsy. You can expect that

- **A.** labiodental fricatives will be the easiest sounds for her to produce.
- **B.** stops, glides, and nasals will be easier for her to produce than fricatives, affricates, and liquids.
- **C.** there is a strong possibility that her intelligibility will be impacted by hoarseness.
- **D.** she will not show voicing errors when she produces sounds.

15. A 3-year-old child is receiving therapy for remediation of several phonological patterns. She very frequently says things like *tar/kar, do/go,* and *ti/ki*. These productions show that she is using the phonological pattern of

- **A.** fronting.
- **B.** glottal replacement.
- **C.** stopping.
- **D.** prevocalic voicing.

16. You are evaluating Ronnie, a 3-year-old boy who is moderately unintelligible. His phonetic inventory includes the phonemes /t, d, m, n, p, b/. He manifests the phonological pattern of final consonant deletion. In therapy, the most appropriate target word to focus on would be

- **A.** path.
- **B.** horse.
- **C.** map.
- **D.** whistle.

Questions 17–19 refer to the following scenario:

Amanda is a 7-year-old with childhood apraxia of speech (CAS). She is frustrated in school because it is hard for her to be understood in class and on the playground; you estimate that she is approximately 60% intelligible. You have just finished graduate school, and Amanda is your first client with CAS.

17. When conducting therapy with her, it will be important to remember to

- **A.** use multimodal cueing and tasks that move up in a hierarchical manner.
- **B.** focus primarily on phonological awareness and auditory discrimination skills.
- **C.** teach her sign language to supplement speech.
- **D.** focus most of intervention on listening skills.

18. When you are listening to Amanda speak, you notice the presence of intermittent hypernasality that is somewhat unpredictable. There is also nasal emission on some consonants. These phenomena occur because

   A. Amanda probably has a shortened velum secondary to CAS.
   B. Amanda's velum is weak and you will need to conduct oral motor exercises to strengthen it.
   C. Amanda has impaired motor programming of the velum resulting in incompetent velar movement.
   D. Amanda may have a partial submucous cleft palate.

19. Amanda has come back from a beach vacation with her parents, and excitedly tells you that she built a "thand castle" on the beach. Amanda has just manifested which type of articulation error?

   A. Addition
   B. Distortion
   C. Coalescence
   D. Substitution

References and Recommended Readings at www.advancedreviewpractice.com

STUDY AND REVIEW ANSWERS

1. **B.** The /f/ sound is developed earlier than the /s/, /r/, /θ/, and /l/ sounds. Thus, beginning therapy by addressing the t/f substitution would be the best approach.
2. **A.** In Oller's stages of infant phonological development, reduplicated babbling precedes nonreduplicated or variegated babbling.
3. **B.** *Stopped* is the only word in the list that contains a consonant cluster.
4. **C.** Phonetic placement is used when a client cannot imitate the modeled production of a phoneme such as /s/ or /r/. The clinician uses a combination of verbal instructions and physical guidance to show the client how to produce the phoneme in isolation.
5. **D.** Clusters sp, st, sk. Developmental norms indicate that these clusters have been mastered by most 4-year-old children. Other, more complex clusters, especially those containing three consonants (e.g., spr, skr), tend to be mastered at later ages.
6. **C.** A child who says things like gʌk/dʌk and koʊ/toʊ is manifesting the phonological pattern of backing.
7. **A.** The articulation therapy approach that emphasizes the syllable as the basic unit of speech production and heavily uses the concept of phonetic environment is McDonald's sensorimotor approach.
8. **D.** Reduplication is the earliest of the listed phonological patterns to be phased out. In typically developing children, reduplication is usually phased out by approximately 2 years 4 months of age.
9. **D.** The maxilla is receded and the mandible protruded in class III malocclusion. In class II malocclusion, the maxilla is protruded and the mandible receded.

10. **B.** In Hodson and Paden's cycles approach, children are *not* trained to a criterion of mastery for error patterns. Rather, the clinician introduces correct patterns, gives the child limited practice with production of those patterns, and moves on to other error patterns.
11. **D.** You are assessing Crystal's stimulability for the /k/ sound by evaluating whether she can imitate your model.
12. **B.** If Crystal says *to/so*, she is demonstrating the phonological pattern of stopping.
13. **C.** Activities that focus on helping the child attend to the initial sound in target words are targeting alliteration skills.
14. **B.** Stops, glides, and nasals will be easier for her to produce than fricatives, affricates, and liquids.
15. **A.** *tar/kar*, *do/go*, and *ti/ki* all reflect the child's use of the phonological pattern of fronting of velars.
16. **C.** The child's phonetic inventory includes the phonemes /t, d, m, n, p, b/, so if he is deleting final consonants, you want the target word to end with a sound that is in his phonetic inventory. The words *path*, *horse*, and *whistle* end in consonants that are not in the child's phonetic inventory, so they are inappropriate treatment targets.
17. **A.** Use multimodal cueing and tasks that move up in a hierarchical manner. Although students with CAS can benefit from intervention focusing on listening and phonological awareness skills, the most important priority is to use multimodal cueing and hierarchical tasks.
18. **C.** Amanda has impaired motor programming of the velum resulting in incompetent velar movement. This results in intermittent hypernasality and nasal emission on some consonants.
19. **D.** Saying "thand" instead of "sand" represents a sound substitution.

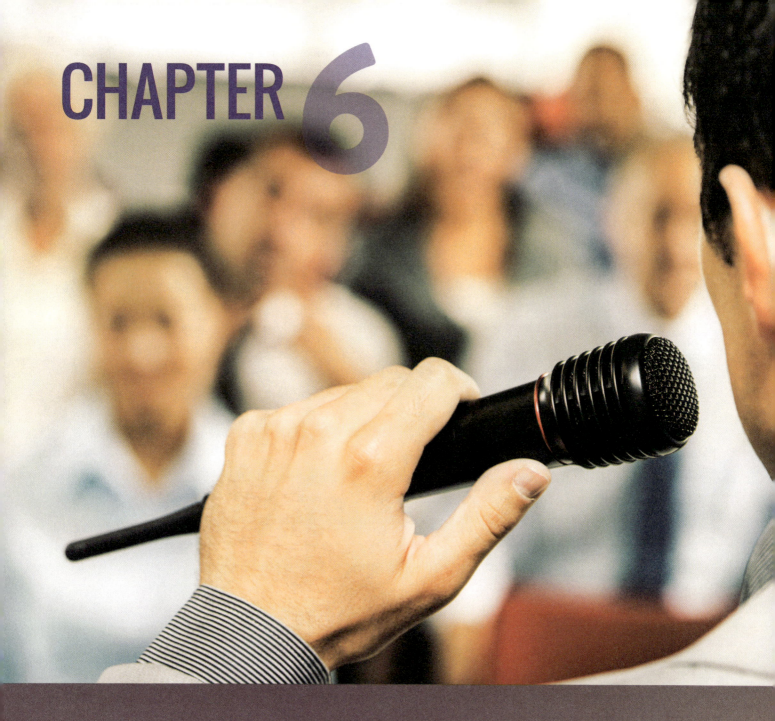

CHAPTER 6

FLUENCY AND ITS DISORDERS

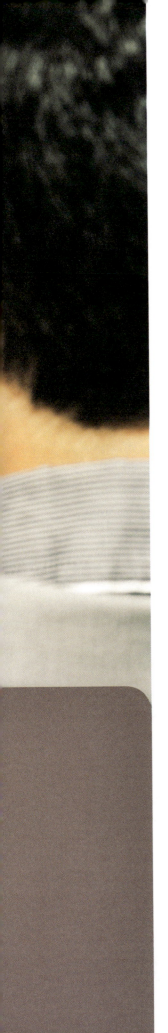

Fluency disorders are speech disorders characterized by a variety of dysfluencies that interrupt the typical flow of speech. Stuttering, cluttering, and neurogenic stuttering are the three main types of fluency disorders, although the most researched among them is stuttering. Fluency may be impaired in such clinical conditions as aphasia, although a diagnosis of stuttering or neurogenic stuttering may not be made in such cases. (Fluency problems associated with aphasia are described in Chapter 8.) In this chapter, we review research and clinical information on stuttering, cluttering, and neurogenic stuttering. (See Bloodstein & Ratner, 2008; Guitar, 2014; Hegde, 2007, 2018a, 2018b, 2018c; Myers & St. Louis, 1992; Yairi & Seery, 2015).

FLUENCY AND STUTTERING: AN OVERVIEW

Stuttering is a disorder of fluency. Fluent speech is smooth, relatively easy, and flowing. Dysfluent or stuttered speech is halting and interrupted. Various forms of dysfluencies disrupt the easy and effortless flow of speech. Familial factors, gender, and ethnocultural variables affect the incidence and prevalence of stuttering. Stuttering onset can be more or less gradual but typically takes place in early childhood. Eventually, stuttering is associated with various types of abnormal motor behaviors, muscular tension, breathing abnormalities, negative emotions, and avoidance behaviors. Theories of stuttering have been built on environmental, genetic, and neurophysiological observations; none are universally accepted, although each line of investigation has contributed to a more comprehensive understanding of stuttering. Many treatment procedures are advocated for adults and children who stutter, but only a few are based on research evidence. The characteristics of stuttering of early onset, neurogenic stuttering, and cluttering also will be described in their respective sections.

Definition and Description of Fluency

Fluency has not been studied as extensively as stuttering. For the most part, only some rudimentary characteristics of fluency have been described as follows:

- For example, fluent speech is flowing, smooth, continuous, relatively rapid, normal in rhythm, produced with less effort and tension, and free from an excessive amount or duration of dysfluencies.
- On the contrary, stuttered speech is halting, abnormal in rhythm, discontinuous, and produced with increased effort; may be slow because of multiple dysfluencies (Bloodstein & Ratner, 2008; Starkweather, 1987).

Definition and Description of Stuttering

Stuttering is the most researched of the fluency disorders. Clinicians have further defined it in diverse ways. Much of this variation is due to theoretical orientation, not clinical approach. Below, a few sample definitions illustrate this variety.

Definition in Terms of Nonspeech Behaviors

- Historically, some experts have defined stuttering in terms of variables that are not specific to speech characteristics. The following three definitions emphasize some of the personal and social consequences of dysfluent speech; instead of dysfluencies that interrupt fluency, these definitions highlight avoidance of speaking or social role conflicts.

  - First, stuttering is defined as an anticipatory, apprehensive, and hypertonic avoidance reaction (Johnson & Associates, 1959); stuttering is not the same as dysfluency. Stuttering is what a person does to avoid stuttering. The problem begins when children, who are punished for their normal nonfluencies, learns to avoid speech, speaking situations, and certain kinds of audiences (listeners, conversational partners). Anticipating trouble in speaking situations, children become apprehensive about the prospect of speaking, experience tension, and, finally, avoid the speaking situation. A diagnosis of stuttering is made not on the basis of dysfluencies but on the basis of consistent avoidance of speaking situations.
  - Second, stuttering is defined as a social role conflict. Sheehan (1970), who offered this definition, believed that the primary problem of stuttering is that the person who stutters cannot play certain social roles normally. For example, people who stutter typically speak with improved fluency when they talk to young children and pets and when they play theatrical roles. However, the same people may have difficulty talking to their bosses, ordering in restaurants, and speaking to strangers. To Sheehan, this indicated a problem in efficiently playing different social roles.

Definition in Terms of Unspecified Behaviors

- Some definitions do not specify any behaviors. They simply refer to stuttering in molar or global terms. The central notion in these definitions is an expert judgment. In essence, an expert's judgment that stuttering has occurred is the definition of stuttering; accordingly, stuttering is what a person says it is. The following two definitions fall into this category:

  - Some define stuttering as a **moment** an expert so judges in a time duration. Accordingly, a time duration during which something believed to be stuttering has occurred is indeed stuttering; it does not specify the behavior that is observed. Although it is widely used, this definition does not specify what stuttering is and thus does not help measure the behavior objectively.
  - Stuttering is an **event**, so recognized by an expert. This definition, also widely used, does not specify the behavior or action that constitutes stuttering. It is similar to the notion of a **stuttering moment** in that it is both nonspecific and unhelpful in objective measurement.

Definition Limited to Certain Types of Dysfluencies
- There are many types of dysfluencies, and they play a major role in the varied definitions of stuttering and its diagnostic criteria. Some classic definitions of stuttering include only part-word repetitions and speech–sound prolongations. Van Riper (1982) restricted stuttering to prolongations of speech sounds and repetitions of sound, syllable, or word.
- The American Speech-Language-Hearing Association adds phrase repetitions to sound, syllable, and word repetitions but makes no mention of sound prolongations (asha.org/definition of communication disorders and variations). All other forms of dysfluencies (e.g., interjections, pauses) may be considered normal kinds of nonfluencies.
- Some distinguish between stuttering-like dysfluencies and normal dysfluencies (Yairi & Seery, 2015). Stuttering-like dysfluencies include repetitions of sounds, syllables, and monosyllabic words and sound prolongations. All other dysfluencies are normal.

Definition Based on All Types of Dysfluencies
- Many experts describe stuttering in terms of the frequency and duration of dysfluencies. In such descriptions, all types of dysfluencies are considered important in defining stuttering. According to this view, all forms of dysfluencies disrupt fluency, and if their frequency or duration is excessive, then a fluency disorder is created. The basis for this view is that listeners tend to classify speech as dysfluent or stuttered even if it contains only word repetitions or interjections (Bloodstein & Ratner, 2008; Hegde & Hartman, 1979a, 1979b).
- Accordingly, stuttering is the production of any or all forms of dysfluencies of excessive frequency, excessive durations, or both. It is important to note that dysfluencies that exceed certain levels of frequency and duration may be grounds for a diagnosis of stuttering.

Forms of Dysfluencies

Regardless of definitional orientations, it is important to understand the different forms of dysfluencies, as they all interrupt fluency. The following are the major types of dysfluencies and their examples:

- **Repetitions**. Saying the same element of speech more than once.
  - **Part-word repetitions** (sound or syllable repetitions). Repetition of a part of a word or a sound or syllable (e.g., "S-S-S-Saturday" or "Sa-Sa-Sa-Saturday").
  - **Whole-word repetitions**. Repetition of an entire word more than once; word repeated may be of single or multiple syllables (e.g., "I-I-I am fine" or "could-could-could not do it").
  - **Phrase repetitions**. Repetition of more than one word (e.g., "I am–I am–I am fine" or "could not–could not–could not do it").
- **Prolongations**. Typically, extension of syllables and silent postures; some call them arrhythmic phonation.
  - **Sound prolongations**. Sounds produced for a duration longer than typical (e.g., "lllllike it" or "Mmmmommy").

- **Silent prolongations**. An articulatory posture held for a duration longer than average but with no vocalization (e.g., the articulatory position for producing the *p* sound in the word *pot* may be held too long; such postures are usually associated with increased muscular tension).

- **Interjections**. Extraneous elements introduced into the speech sequence. These may be one of the following:
  - Sound or syllable interjections (e.g., the common *um* and the schwa interjections);
  - Word interjections (e.g., interjections of *like, okay, well*);
  - Phrase interjections (e.g., interjections of *you know, I mean*).

- **Pauses**. Silent intervals in the speech sequence at inappropriate junctures or of unusually long duration.
- **Broken words**. Silent intervals within words, also known as **intralexical pauses** (e.g., "Be-[pause] -fore you say it").
- **Incomplete sentences**. Often described as incomplete phrases, these are grammatically incomplete productions (e.g., "Last summer I was . . . last summer . . . we went to Paris.").
- **Revisions**. Changes in wording that do not change the overall meaning of an utterance (e.g., "Let me have coffee, maybe tea.").

Theoretical and Clinical Significance of Dysfluencies

Experts do not agree on how to clinically evaluate various forms of dysfluencies. Some think that only certain forms of dysfluencies are stutterings; others think that all forms of dysfluencies, if they exceed certain quantitative limits of duration and frequency, are stutterings (or at least disorders of fluency, even if not diagnosed as stuttering).

- There is evidence that forms of dysfluency that are traditionally not considered indicative of stuttering (e.g., whole-word repetitions or schwa interjections) may still evoke judgments of stuttering from listeners if the frequency exceeds certain limits, typically 5% of the words produced in a given occasion (Hegde & Hartman, 1979a, 1979b). Yairi and Ambrose (2013) summarized past and recent evidence that most parents believe that word repetitions in their young child suggest stuttering.
- Generally, speech that contains 5% or more dysfluencies may be judged dysfluent or stuttered by most listeners. Several clinicians (Bloodstein & Ratner, 2008; Van Riper, 1982), have suggested that along with other characteristics, dysfluencies that exceed certain quantitative limits may be grounds for diagnosing stuttering.
- Research also has shown that listeners may have different tolerance thresholds for different forms of dysfluencies. Part-word repetitions (e.g., "buh-buh-baby") and sound prolongations are judged abnormal at lower frequencies (as low as 2% of words spoken), whereas whole-word repetitions and schwa interjections must reach at least 5% to evoke judgments of **dysfluent** or **stuttered** speech (Hegde & Dansby, 1988; Hegde & Stone, 1991). This may be one of the reasons why there has been such a historical emphasis on part-word repetitions and speech-sound prolongations in the diagnosis of stuttering.

- There is evidence that the frequency of dysfluencies (e.g., 2 in 100 words as against 5) as well as the number of iterations (e.g., and-and—two iterations—versus and-and-and-and—four iterations) are significant variables that prompt a judgment of stuttering (Yairi, 2013). Duration of dysfluencies (a prolongation that last a fraction of a second versus the one that last several seconds) may be another significant variable. Thus, all forms of dysfluencies that exceed certain limits of frequency, iteration, or duration may be judged abnormal, but some forms may be judged abnormal at lower levels of frequency or duration, and perhaps the number of iteration.

Incidence and Prevalence of Stuttering

Incidence and prevalence are related but different concepts established through different procedures.

- The **incidence** of a given disorder or disease is its rate of occurrence in a specified group of people. Incidence is studied by a longitudinal method, starting with a healthy or normal group of subjects and repeatedly observes those individuals over a period of time, counting the number who begin to show a particular disease or disorder. Incidence is a predictive statement. Incidence studies are more expensive and time consuming than prevalence studies.
- **Prevalence** of a particular disorder or disease is determined by cross-sectional method in which the number of individuals who currently have it is counted. The study's investigators collect information from various sources (e.g., clinics and hospitals) and add up the number of patients who are receiving clinical services or have received such services in a given population. Prevalence does not make a predictive statement; it simply gives the current number of people who exhibit a given disorder. Prevalence studies are less expensive and less time consuming than incidence studies. However, head counting often underestimates the prevalence of a disorder by missing those who have not been diagnosed or enrolled in clinical services.
- Most available studies of stuttering are prevalence studies; most are rough estimates. There are only a few studies of the incidence of stuttering. However, incidence and prevalence can be derived from each other.
- Reported incidence and prevalence studies do not agree fully partly because of methodological reasons and partly because of how stuttering is defined, by both the professionals and the parents who report stuttering in their children. Studies that include only part-word repetitions and speech-sound prolongations may report a lower incidence and prevalence rate than those that include all kinds of dysfluencies.

Incidence and Prevalence in the General Population
- A classic study of incidence was conducted in England and reported by Andrews and Harris in 1964. They studied more than 1,000 newborn babies and followed them for 15 years. This is the only longitudinal study of stuttering of such a long duration involving such a large number of subjects. This and other less extensive studies on the incidence and prevalence of stuttering have made the following observations:

- The lifetime expectancy of stuttering is about 5% according to the classic studies; more recent studies suggest as high as 8–11% . One recent study reported an 11.2% incidence rate by age 4 (Reilly et al., 2013; see Yairi & Ambrose, 2013 for a review). This means that 5–11% of the population has a probability of ever stuttering, even if stuttering lasts only a few days, weeks, or months.
- Prevalence of stuttering is about 1% in the general U.S. population; it could be less, around 0.72% according to some studies (Yairi & Ambrose, 2013). Obviously, the prevalence during early childhood is much higher. Somewhat higher incidence rates have been reported for European countries. Some early investigations have shown that the prevalence of stuttering is higher in African Americans than in other ethnic groups in the U.S. (Boyle et al., 2011; Cooper & Cooper, 1998; Robinson & Crowe, 2002), but some later studies show no difference between the European and African American groups of children (e.g., Proctor, Yairi, & Duff, 2008). The issue is not resolved and needs more research. In spite of variations, no society is completely free from stuttering.
- The risk of developing a stutter varies by age, but stuttering typically begins during early childhood. In the majority, stuttering begins between the ages of 3 and 6 years; more recent studies suggest that the risk is over by age 5.
- Adult onset of stuttering is rare. In some cases, a reemergence may occur of early childhood stuttering, from which the individual had recovered. In most cases, adult onset of stuttering is associated with neurological damage or disease; in a few other cases, it may be psychogenic. For example, some adults begin to stutter after a stroke or as a result of Alzheimer's dementia; a few others may begin to stutter under conditions of extreme stress or psychological trauma.
- A review of epidemiological research on stuttering (Yairi & Ambrose, 2013) suggests that (a) by age 5, the risk for developing stuttering is over, earlier than previously thought; (b) the male-to-female ratio near onset is smaller than previously thought; (c) the life-span incidence in the general population may be as high as 8–10%, higher than the 5% reported previously; (d) the general incidence may be lower than the reported 1%; and (e) the effects of race, ethnicity, socioeconomic status, and bilingualism are still unclear.

Prevalence and Gender Ratio

- It is well documented that stuttering is far more common in males than in females. As high as 5:1 male:female ratios have been reported. The most frequently cited ratio is 3:1 (male:female) for children in early elementary grades. More recent studies (Yairi & Ambrose, 2013) suggest a closer male:female ratio at the time of onset (2:1).
- The ratio is larger (perhaps 4:1) in higher grades. This may be because of a slightly higher spontaneous recovery of stuttering in girls or because of a greater number of new cases in boys.
- The documented gender ratio has given rise to hypotheses about possible genetic factors in the etiology of stuttering.

Familial Prevalence

- **Familial prevalence** is the frequency with which a given condition appears in successive generations of blood relatives. It is estimated that the prevalence of stuttering in the families is at least three times higher than that in the general population.
- Familial prevalence is higher in families of a female who stutters than in families of a male who stutters. Familial prevalence and gender ratio interact: sons of mothers who stutter run a greater risk of stuttering than sons of fathers who stutter; daughters generally have a lower risk, but daughters of mothers who stutter have a higher risk than daughters of fathers who stutter.
- Familial incidence may be explained on the basis of genetic or environmental factors; most experts tend to emphasize genetic factors, although the influence of the environmental factors cannot be ruled out and generally are not effectively ruled out in genetic studies.

Prevalence and Concordance Rates in Twins

- **Concordance** is the occurrence of the same clinical condition (or normal trait) in both members of a twin pair. If both members of a twin pair have the same condition, they are **concordant** for that condition; if only one member of a twin pair has a particular condition, the pair is **discordant** for that condition.
- A **concordance rate** for stuttering is based on the number of twin pairs studied and the number in whom stuttering is evident in both members. For instance, if in 100 pairs of twins studied, stuttering is found in both members of 50 pairs, the concordance rate would be 50%; the remaining 50% would be discordant (one twin stutters; the other does not).
- Differential concordance rates in ordinary siblings, identical (monozygotic) twins, and fraternal (dizygotic) twins suggest the importance of genetic variables in stuttering.
- The concordance rate of stuttering for identical (monozygotic) twins is higher than that for fraternal (dizygotic) twins; the rates reported vary across studies with a range of 30–80% of identical twin pairs; in 9 out of 10 pairs, both may stutter.
- The concordance rate for fraternal twins is higher than that for ordinary siblings, though lower than that in identical twins; in 1 out of 15 pairs of fraternal twins, both may stutter. Purely from a genetic standpoint, incidence in dizygotic twins should be the same as that in ordinary siblings; but the reported higher concordance rate for the fraternal twins suggests that at least a *portion* of the concordance rate for identical twins may be due to their common environment.
- Studies of monozygotic twins who have been separated and brought up in different environments and of children who have been adopted by families with and without stuttering members might be more definitive, but well-designed studies of this kind are nonexistent. A few observations have reported ambiguous or inconclusive results.
- Differential prevalence data suggest that both genetic factors (which predispose the individual to stutter) and environmental events (which may trigger the disorder) play a part in the etiology of stuttering. In one large twin study (Felsenfeld, Kirk, Zhu, Stantham, Neale, & Martin, 2000), the authors suggested that 70% of variance may be due to genetic factors and the rest to environmental variables (see a later section entitled "Genetic Hypothesis" on genetic research on stuttering).

Prevalence or Incidence in Other Selected Populations

- The reported prevalence of stuttering is higher than that of the general population for the following:

  - People with developmental or intellectual disabilities (especially children and adults with Down syndrome). The prevalence in this population may be three times higher than in the general population. Some data suggest that many in this group may clutter (see "Cluttering" section later in chapter) or clutter and stutter.
  - People with brain injuries. The incidence in this population may be as high as 19%; incidence in people with epilepsy may be 3% or higher.

- At one time, it was claimed that hearing loss somehow prevents stuttering in children. However, stuttering in people with hearing loss who have oral skills has been documented (Arenas, Walker, & Oleson, 2017); the reported lower prevalence in some earlier studies may be due to the limited oral-language skills in many individuals who are deaf; some deaf persons may repeat or hesitate in their manual communication, suggesting a phenomenon similar to stuttering in oral speech.

Prevalence and Socioeconomic and Ethnocultural Variables

- Some experts have claimed that stuttering is a culturally determined disorder. According to Johnson and Associates (1959), parents who are critical of their children's normal nonfluencies tend to encourage apprehension and avoidance reactions, which he called stuttering. Johnson further claimed that societies and cultures that place a heavy emphasis on verbal skills have a higher prevalence of stuttering; presumably due to lack of such an emphasis in their culture, Native Americans, for example, do not stutter, Johnson believed. This theory has been contradicted by data. Some Native Americans do stutter; as previously noted, stuttering is found in almost all societies and ethnocultural groups (Bloodstein & Ratner, 2008).
- The prevalence rates appear to be somewhat different across ethnocultural groups, but those differences are hard to explain and may even be due to methodological variations across studies.
- Data on the prevalence of stuttering in different socioeconomic classes are contradictory or inconclusive. While one recent study (Reilly et al., 2009) reported higher prevalence of stuttering in children from higher socioeconomic classes than from lower classes, another study (Boyle et al., 2011) reported the opposite. The issue is not resolved, and more research is needed.

Natural Recovery and Persistence

- **Natural recovery from stuttering,** also known as **spontaneous recovery,** refers to its disappearance without professional help. The term may be a misnomer, because such recovery may be associated with an inadvertent use of certain techniques. For instance, a person who stutters may accidentally discover that a slower rate of speech reduces stuttering and adopt such a rate. That is not "natural" recovery.
- The recovery of stuttering of some children and adolescents without professional help has been documented, but the percentage of such recovery has remained controversial. Some early studies have suggested a 45% natural recovery, while others reported as high as 80%.

- The longer the duration of a longitudinal study, the greater the rate of natural recovery. A study that longitudinally observes children for a few months is likely to report a lower rate of natural recovery than the one that observes them for several years. A study that observed children for only 12 months, for example, reported a 6.3% recovery rate, one of the lowest ever (Reilly, et al., 2013). In other words, stuttering may persist for years before natural recovery occurs. The effect on the stuttering itself of repeated speech sampling over years to measure stuttering is not clear. Furthermore, many studies are based on questionnaires, not direct observation or analysis of speech samples.
- Based on available studies, Yairi and Ambrose (2013) conclude that stuttering persists in 11.7% of those who begin to stutter and disappears in 88.3%. However, no study has carefully analyzed the events that take place between the onset and natural recovery. Parent counseling, direct treatment for stuttering, and information parents find after the initial diagnosis that may affect stuttering in children have not been systematically analyzed. If these variables are considered, natural recovery rates may be less than commonly and recently reported. A prospective community cohort study has reported a recovery rate of 65% by age 7 (Kefalianos, Onslow, Packman et al., 2017). Whatever the rate, it applies to groups of stuttering children, not to individual children. It is difficult to predict whether a given child will recover without professional help; therefore, the phenomenon of natural recovery is not a basis for postponing treatment for a child diagnosed with stuttering.
- Two different types of stuttering, **recovered** and **persistent**, have been researched and debated. In one study, children who had better language skills were more likely to recover later (Kefalianos, Onslow, Packman et al., 2017). More research is needed to identify reliable variables that distinguish the recovered and persistent stuttering.

Onset and Development of Stuttering

- Stuttering begins as an increase in the frequency of dysfluencies. At the time of onset, repetitions of monosyllabic whole words may be common. Syllable repetitions also are frequently reported. The number of times a word or a syllable is repeated (called **iteration**) may be high. Repetitions are more common at the beginning of sentences or phrases. Children at the time of stuttering onset may be dysfluent on function words (e.g., pronouns, conjunctions, articles) and content words as well (e.g., nouns, verbs, adjectives, adverbs). Adults, however, are typically dysfluent on content words. The children in the earliest stage may not be concerned about their dysfluencies (Bloodstein & Ratner, 2008).
- The increase may be sudden or gradual, but the dysfluency rate remains highly variable for some time, resulting in periods of normal or near-normal fluency alternating with periods of excessive dysfluency (Bloodstein & Ratner, 2008; Yairi & Seery, 2015).
- Stuttering that persists becomes chronic over time. The child stutters mostly on content words—a change from the earliest stage of stuttering in which the function words also are stuttered. Stuttering increases when the child is excited. The child thinks of himself or herself as a stutterer while still showing little concern. Dysfluencies may be associated with muscular tension and rapid rate in some children.

- When fully established, specific word and situational fears, avoidance of certain words and speaking situations, increased muscular tension during dysfluent speech, and anticipation of stuttering become part of the symptom complex by the late adolescent years or early adulthood.
- In many cases, parents report nothing unusual about the time of onset. Most parents have no specific explanations for the onset, and the explanations some parents may have may not be valid.
- The frequency of dysfluencies may stabilize and become more consistent across situations and time, although some degree of variability is a basic characteristic of stuttering, even in adults with many years of stuttering history.

Associated Motor Behaviors

- Motor behaviors associated with stuttering were historically described as **secondary stutterings**. Stuttering may be associated with various abnormal motor behaviors, including the following:

  - Excessive muscular effort
  - Various facial grimaces
  - Various hand and foot movements (e.g., wringing the hands, tapping the foot)
  - Rapid eye blinking
  - Knitting of the eyebrows
  - Lip pursing
  - Rapid opening and closing of the mouth
  - Tongue clicking

- The number and severity of associated motor behaviors vary across individuals. Whereas some children who stutter show several notable associated motor behaviors, others may show none or show a few that are almost undetectable. Adults who stutter generally show at least a few associated motor behaviors; some show many and severe forms of such behaviors.
- Associated motor behaviors may have been accidentally reinforced. For instance, just when a person who stutters experienced a release from stuttering, he or she may have jerked an arm. From then on, an arm jerk may be associated with stuttering. Such accidentally reinforced associated motor behaviors rarely help the stuttering persons speak fluently.
- Associated motor behaviors are not crucial for a diagnosis of stuttering; excessive frequency and duration of dysfluencies are sufficient. However, the presence of severe forms of motor behaviors associated with increased frequency or duration of dysfluencies virtually assures a diagnosis of stuttering.

Associated Breathing Abnormalities

- In many people, stuttered speech is associated with certain breathing abnormalities. Although not crucial for a diagnosis of stuttering, it is important to consider the following kinds of associated breathing abnormalities:

  - Attempts to speak on inhalation
  - Holding breath before talking

- Continued attempts to speak even when the air supply is exhausted
- Interruption of inhalations by exhalations and vice versa
- Speaking without first inhaling a sufficient amount of air
- Rapid and jerky breathing during speech
- Exhaling puffs of air during stuttered speech
- Generally tensed breathing

- The noted breathing abnormalities do not suggest an inherent respiratory disorder; they are a part of the stuttering symptom complex (Bloodstein & Ratner, 2008). Fluent speech in people who stutter is not characterized by severe forms of breathing abnormalities.

Negative Emotions and Avoidance Behaviors

- When stuttering persists, negative emotions and avoidance of words and speaking situations tend to develop. Avoidance and negative emotions are not crucial to a diagnosis of stuttering, but they are important to consider in a comprehensive program of assessment and treatment. Avoidance of listeners and speaking situations is typically client-specific.
- Negative emotions associated with stuttering include anxiety and apprehension about stuttering, fear of certain speaking situations, frustration in efforts to communicate, and, possibly, a sense of humiliation in certain difficult speaking situations or some hostility toward certain speakers.
- Difficult speaking situations include speaking with strangers and before formal audiences, speaking with people at counters where services or products are bought, speaking on the telephone, ordering in restaurants, speaking to authority figures, and self-introductions or introductions of other people.
- Avoidance of frequently stuttered sounds and words result in circumlocution and use of nonspecific words (e.g., *this* and *that*). However, sounds and words avoided are typically client-specific. For example, a man might avoid words beginning with *b* because he stutters more when saying such words. A woman may avoid saying her boss's name because she stutters whenever she tries to say it.
- Avoidance of eye contact, difficult speaking situations, and so forth may be **safety behaviors**, some researchers speculate (Lowe et al., 2017). But in a behavioral analysis, avoidance is negatively reinforced behavior because it terminates an aversive situation.
- People who stutter may anticipate or expect to have more or fewer problems in certain speaking situations. A majority of people who stutter can predict a certain amount of their stuttering; however, there is no one-to-one correspondence between the anticipated (predicted) stuttering and actual stuttering. Words not expected to be stuttered may be, and those that are expected to be stuttered may not be.
- Children who stutter may experience bullying to a greater extent than those who do not stutter. Bullying may lead to low self-esteem and avoidance of social situations (Blood, Blood, Tramontana, Sylvia, Boyle, & Motzko, 2011).

The Loci of Stuttering

- The **loci of stuttering** refers to the locations in a speech (or oral reading) sequence where stutterings are typically observed. Certain classes of sounds, words in certain positions in a sentence, and certain kinds of words have a high probability of being stuttered. Based on such observations, it is possible to predict the loci of stuttering.

- In the speech of **adults and school-age children** who stutter, stuttering is most likely to occur on:

  - **Consonants rather than vowels**, although some speakers stutter predominantly on vowels. This is explained partly by the greater complexity of consonantal productions than vowel productions.
  - **The "first" factor.** The first sound or syllable of a word, the first word in a phrase, sentence, or grammatical class tend to be stuttered more than those in other places.
  - **Longer and less frequently used words.** Longer words may be more difficult to produce than shorter words and less frequently used words tend to be longer and otherwise complex as well.
  - **Content words** (nouns, verbs, adjectives, and adverbs), more often than on function words (articles, conjunctions, prepositions, and pronouns). This tendency, more pronounced in adults than in children who stutter, may partly be due to the word position. Content words initiate more sentences and phrases than do function words.

- The loci of stuttering in preschool children are the same as those for adults and school-age children except for one factor: Preschool children's stuttering tends to occur on **function words** (especially pronouns, conjunctions, and prepositions). This contrasts with the school-age children and adults who tend to stutter more often on content words than on function words (Bloodstein & Ratner, 2008).

- Preschool children's tendency to stutter more on function words than on content words is partly explained on the basis that such children tend to initiate their phrases and sentences with certain function words, especially pronouns and conjunctions. Therefore, the position of words in a sentence (especially the first position), rather than the grammatical class of words, may be the real variable.

- Preschool children also tend to exhibit many whole-word repetitions. Thus, an early characteristic of stuttering is an increase in whole-word repetitions (along with other forms of dysfluencies).

- Generally, dysfluencies tend to occur at the same loci in the speech of people who stutter and those who speak with normal fluency. Dysfluencies in the speech of people who do not stutter also tend to occur on initial consonants, initial words, longer words, less frequently used words, and content words.

Stimulus Control in Stuttering

There are recognizable external stimuli that trigger stuttering. There are also well-known conditions under which fluency is enhanced. Most of the variations found in the frequency of stuttering are due to variations in external stimuli, called here **stimulus control**. Research has shown that stuttering varies systematically when certain stimulus variables are manipulated. A few important phenomena that suggest a strong stimulus control of stuttering include adaptation, consistency, adjacency, and audience size (Bloodstein & Ratner, 2008).

- **Adaptation** is reduction in stuttering and is greatest during the first few oral readings of a passage; by about the fifth reading, the most reduction will have occurred. There is no transfer of adaptation from one passage to another; it is a temporary phenomenon. To experience adaptation, one has to read the passage aloud; individuals differ in the degree of adaptation exhibited.
- **Consistency effect** may be evident on about 65% of stuttering in given individuals; consistency remains when the study participants reread the same passage after weeks of interval. The effect is presumed to be an indicator of the strength of the stimuli that evoke stuttering. Thus, the adaptation and consistency are opposite phenomena.
- **Adjacency effect**, measured in oral reading, is the occurrence of new stuttering on words that surround previously stuttered words; this effect is studied by having a subject read a passage multiple times, blotting out or otherwise concealing the words on which stuttering occurs, and then having the subject read the passage again to note the occurrence of new stuttering on words adjacent to previously stuttered words. Words that were fluently read during earlier readings may be eventually stuttered if the words were adjacent to previously stuttered words.
- **Audience size effect** refers to the observation that the frequency of stuttering increases with an increase in audience size; stuttering may be nearly absent when the person talks to himself or herself, but may increase markedly with a systematic increase in the number of listeners.

People Who Stutter and Their Families

- Various theories and viewpoints in the past held that certain "personality" variables might be the underlying cause of stuttering. This idea is especially inherent to psychoneurotic conceptions of stuttering, in which people who stutter are thought to exhibit psychoneurotic tendencies.
- Other conceptions, such as those of Johnson and Associates (1959), implied that parents of some children, holding unusually and unrealistically high standards of fluency may place undue pressure on their children or may misdiagnose stuttering based on normal nonfluency. Such views have led to an investigation of the personality of individuals who stutter and their families, especially their parents.
- Personality variables that include level of aspiration, obsessive–compulsive behaviors, oral and anal eroticism, passive dependency, hostility and aggression, self-concept, social adjustment, body image, and so forth, have been investigated over several decades. Various kinds of questionnaires and such projective tests as the Rorschach have been used. This kind of research has shown that those who stutter
  - do not have a distinct personality that may be causally related to their stuttering.
  - are not clinically maladjusted.
  - may have low self-esteem, possibly due to their stuttering.
- Social anxiety, or speech phobia, has been a topic of much research in recent past. The results suggest that (Alm, 2014; Smith et al., 2017)
  - persons who stutter are not clinically or chronically anxious, requiring the diagnosis of anxiety disorders; school-age children who stutter are not more anxious than their peers who do not stutter. This finding suggests that anxiety about speaking situations may develop as a result of stuttering itself.

- many who stutter may have slightly elevated levels of anxiety in speaking situations, often described as speech phobia.
- anxiety in speaking situations may be an effect, not a cause, of stuttering.

- **Temperament** of people who stutter has been another topic of much research interest in recent past (Kefalianos, Onslow, Ukoumunne, Block, & Reily, 2017); research generally suggests that
  - stuttering in children is not significantly related to temperament.
  - nonetheless, children who stutter may score lower than those who do not stutter on such temperamental variables as adaptability, attention span/persistence; they may score higher on negative quality of mood and activity levels.
  - clinical and theoretical significance of temperamental variables are unclear and perhaps questionable.

- Research on parents of people who stutter has shown that the following is true of them:
  - They do not exhibit unique personality patterns that may be causally related to stuttering in their children.
  - They are not clinically maladjusted or neurotic.
  - They may exhibit a somewhat higher standard of behavior and be somewhat more critical of their children than are parents of children who do not stutter; however, the clinical significance of this finding is unclear, and a general conclusion about its importance is unwarranted.

- In essence, neither the personality of people who stutter nor that of their parents seems to provide strong clues to the etiology of stuttering.

Theories of Stuttering

There are environmental (learning), genetic, interactional, neurophysiological, and psychological theories of stuttering. Some theorists consider multiple but by no means all relevant variables (Smith & Weber, 2017). However, no theory explains all aspects of stuttering.

- **Genetic hypotheses** state that stuttering has a genetic basis; higher familial prevalence of persistent stuttering, the well-established gender ratio in the prevalence of stuttering, and a higher concordance rate among monozygotic twins than among the ordinary siblings and dizygotic twins suggest a genetic basis; molecular genetic analysis has implicated multiple loci, including chromosomes 1, 2, 3, 5, 7, 9, 10, 11, 12, 13, 14, 15, 16, and 18 (see Yairi & Ambrose, 2013, for a summary); recovered and persistent stuttering may be two subtypes of the disorder; modified recessive inheritance pattern (Raza, Ali, Riazuddin, & Drayna, 2012), inheritance due to a single gene, and multiple genes (polygenic) inheritance have all been hypothesized. Currently, no genetic transmission theory is universally accepted.
- **Neurophysiological hypotheses** state that the neurophysiological organization involved in speech production may be impaired; include a variety of hypothesis; the **laryngeal dysfunction hypothesis** blames stuttering on slightly delayed voice onset time (VOT); stuttering may be associated with increased tension in the laryngeal muscles, simultaneous activation of laryngeal abductors and

adductors, which are normally active reciprocally, and excessive laryngeal muscle activity during stuttered speech, also measured by such techniques as electromyography.

- **Brain dysfunction hypotheses** include lack of a **dominant hemisphere** to process language (cerebral dominance theory); impaired cerebral blood flow; aberrant brain waves; central auditory dysfunction; and auditory feedback problems. Although brain imaging studies (including functional magnetic resonance imaging [fMRI]) have not revealed much consistency across individuals (Ingham, Grafton, Bothe, & Ingham, 2012), several areas of the brain, including the primary and supplementary motor areas, cingulate motor area, and cerebral vermis are thought to be involved; compensatory activation in the right cortical motor areas and deactivation in the left perisylvian region have been reported (Bhatnagar & Buckingham, 2010). Any abnormal activation patterns may be reversed to normal pattern following successful treatment of stuttering. No hypothesis is entirely supported by evidence; the meaning of brain imaging studies is unclear (Chang, 2014).

- **Learning, conditioning, and related hypotheses** include the claim that stuttering is a learned operant behavior, as operant contingencies can increase or decrease it because stuttering is most effectively decreased under time-out and response cost; other hypotheses suggest that stuttering is an avoidance behavior due to the parental punishment of normal nonfluencies and that stuttering is a cultural phenomenon that exists in some societies and not in others (Johnson & Associates, 1959). The latter hypothesis has no support as stuttering is reported in almost all societies. Stuttering is a social role conflict (Sheehan, 1970). Learning-based hypotheses may explain maintenance of stuttering but have not identified the original learning of the disorder.

- The **mismatch hypotheses** state that the environmental demands placed on a child exceed that child's capacity for fluency (the demands and capacities model; Starkweather, 1987). In the **dual diathesis stressor** model, the mismatch is between emotional and cognitive abilities of the child and the excessive fluent speech demands the child faces. In this model, causes of stuttering are not necessarily the external demands themselves (called stressors) but the inadequate coping with those demands because of diathesis—which is inherited predisposition to have various problems (Hollister, Van Horne, & Zebrowski, 2016). In the **leading-edge hypothesis**, speech disruptions of typically developing children tend to occur on more advanced sentence structures the child is about to learn—the leading-edge skills that place greater demand (Rispoli & Hadley, 2001).

Existing theories are at best limited hypotheses that require the support of additional research. None are universally accepted as an explanation of stuttering.

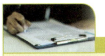

SUMMARY

- Fluent speech is generally rhythmic, smooth, and produced with ease. Stuttered speech contains excessive amounts of dysfluencies, durations of dysfluencies, or both.
- The incidence and prevalence of stuttering have been studied in relation to the general population.

> Studies have looked at spontaneous recovery, prevalence and gender ratio, familial prevalence, and prevalence and concordance rates in twins and other selected populations.
> - Stuttering onset may be gradual or sudden. It is usually characterized by abnormal associated motor behaviors, breathing abnormalities, negative emotions, and avoidance behaviors.
> - Several phenomena such as adaptation, consistency, adjacency, and audience size suggest that various stimuli in the environment affect the frequency of stuttering (stimulus control).
> - There are environmental, genetic, interactive, neurophysiological, and psychological theories of stuttering. No theory explains all aspects of stuttering, and none are universally accepted.

ASSESSMENT AND TREATMENT OF STUTTERING

Assessment of stuttering includes standard procedures such as conducting a hearing screening, gathering a detailed case history from the client or family members, measuring defined stuttering or dysfluencies, and establishing their variability. Information is also recorded on associated motor behaviors, avoidance reactions, negative emotions, and rate of speech. There are several approaches to treating stuttering, including counseling, the fluent stuttering method, the fluency shaping method, the fluency reinforcement method, masking and delayed auditory feedback techniques, and direct stuttering reduction methods.

Assessment of Stuttering

Assessment includes procedures designed to evaluate stuttering and related behaviors. In addition to such standard procedures as hearing screening and orofacial examination, the following are essential considerations (Hegde, 2018b; Hegde & Freed, 2017; Hegde & Pomaville, 2017).

- Case history and interview will help gather information on specific behaviors at the onset of stuttering and its development over the years, as well as variability, familial prevalence, prior clinical services, current education and occupation or future educational and occupational plans, general health, language and speech development, and educational performance in school (in the case of children who stutter).
- Frequency and types of dysfluencies or stuttering may be evaluated by recording an extended conversational speech sample with the clinician and with a member of the family (e.g., the child's mother or father engaged in conversation with the child) and recording an oral reading sample with reading material appropriate for the client's age, interest, reading skill level, and ethnocultural background.
- Variability in stuttering may be assessed by procedures that include the client or the caretaker ratings of stuttering in different situations; verbal reports from family members; or a tape-recorded sample of speech produced at home, at school, or in an occupational setting.
- Relative dysfluency rates in reading and conversation may be determined by recorded oral reading and conversational speech samples.

- Associated motor behaviors may be assessed by taking note of the associated motor behaviors exhibited during assessment, having a family member describe them, asking the adult client to list his or her associated motor behaviors, or administering one of the **behavior assessment batteries** soon to be described.
- Avoidance behaviors may be assessed by having the client list the sounds, words, situations, and audiences typically avoided; taking note of words and sounds avoided during the interview; having family members describe a child's avoidance reactions; and administering one of the **behavior assessment batteries** soon to be described.
- Speech rate and articulatory rate may be assessed by counting the number of words or syllables spoken per minute in at least three 2-minute samples of continuous speech (for speech rate); counting the number of syllables produced while discounting all stutterings and pauses that exceed 2 seconds (for articulatory rate).
- Negative emotional reactions may be assessed by having the client describe his or her negative emotions about speech, particular speaking situations, specific audiences, and so forth; asking family members or friends about negative emotions the client typically expresses; or administering the *Behavior Assessment Battery for Adults who Stutter* (Vanryckeghem & Brutten, 2017) or the *Behavior Assessment Battery for School-Age Children Who Stutter* (Brutten & Vanryckeghem, 2006a) or *Communication Attitude Test for Preschool and Kindergarten Children Who Stutter* (Brutten & Vanryckeghem, 2006b), all of which help assess negative attitudes and emotions associated with speech as well as avoidance behaviors of adults and children who stutter.
- Stuttering severity may be assessed by calculating the percent dysfluency rate (the higher the percentage of words spoken or read stuttered, the greater the severity) or administering an assessment instrument such as the *Stuttering Severity Instrument–Fourth Edition* (SSI-4; Riley, 2009).
- Effects of stuttering on a person who stutters may be assessed by interview or by administering the *Overall Assessment of the Speaker's Experience of Stuttering* (OASES; Yaruss & Quesal, 2010) along with the **behavior assessment batteries** previously described.
- Issues in the diagnosis of stuttering:
  - Some clinicians claim that it is difficult to distinguish stuttering from normal dysfluency; stuttering, however, is reliably diagnosed by the parents; an excessive amount of all dysfluency types or an increased frequency of sound and syllable and single-syllable word repetitions, multiple iterations of those repetitions, sound prolongations, and increased tension and effort in producing those dysfluencies makes stuttering relatively easy to diagnose.
  - Some researchers have listed multiple iterations of repetitions, speech sound prolongations, and tension and effort as warning signs of stuttering (incipient stuttering), but this makes very little clinical sense because the same behaviors are also listed as stuttering; there are no warning signs other than stuttering itself.
  - If a child's dysfluency rate or other behaviors taken to mean stuttering do not meet the criterion adopted by the clinician, the only course open is to re-evaluate the child at a later time.

- Diagnosis of stuttering may be made by using one of several diagnostic criteria:
  - A dysfluency rate that exceeds 5% of spoken words when all kinds of dysfluencies are counted
  - A certain frequency of part-word repetitions, speech-sound prolongations, and broken words (at least 2% of the words spoken)
  - Excessive duration of dysfluencies (1 second or longer)
  - Presence of stuttering-like dysfluencies, at least at 3% of syllables produced (multiple repetitions of syllables and words, prolongations of sounds, presence of schwa vowel in syllable repetitions, tension associated with dysfluencies)

Treatment of Stuttering

There are several approaches to stuttering treatment, described in various sources (Bloodstein & Ratner, 2008; Bothe, 2004; Guitar, 2014; Hegde, 2007, 2018c; Van Riper, 1973). Specific procedures of treating stuttering include psychological methods including counseling, the fluent stuttering method, the fluency shaping method, the fluency reinforcement method, masking and delayed auditory feedback techniques, and direct stuttering reduction methods.

- Some typical controversies raised in the treatment of stuttering in preschool children include the following:
  - Some clinicians argue that preschoolers may go through a phase of stuttering that is best ignored. But there is no research that supports this assertion.
  - Other clinicians argue that when stuttering is diagnosed, it is best to take a wait-and-see approach. Because many children recover naturally, treatment may be unnecessary.
  - Still others argue that it is not possible to predict who will recover, in spite of continued research efforts, and therefore it is best to offer treatment when a diagnosis is made.
  - Natural recovery may take 18 months to several years; most parents would not like to let their children stutter for that duration.
  - Early treatment of stuttering is effective; those who receive treatment during their preschool years are 7.7 times more likely to experience resolution of stuttering than those who do not receive treatment (Onslow & O'Brian, 2013).

General Treatment Goals

Regardless of the specific treatment approaches, clinicians must keep in perspective certain general goals for their clients who stutter, including the following:

- Achieving a reduction in the amount of stuttering; if possible, reducing all dysfluencies to within normal limits
- Establishing normal-sounding fluency that is naturally produced, without special techniques, strategies, or unsustainable attention to certain ways of talking (e.g., excessively slow speech)
- Reducing associated motor behaviors that make the stuttering even worse, because of their abnormality

- Reducing avoidance and negative feelings about speech, speaking situations, self, and others. Some treatment techniques spend more time on this aspect of treatment; those that do not do this achieve the same goal by inducing fluency in natural settings. Clients who are fluent in varied settings have no reason to avoid speech or feel negatively about it.
- Counseling the client, family members, or both about stuttering in general; answering their questions about stuttering and its personal, social, emotional, and occupational effects; and describing how the clinician plans to manage them within the treatment framework planned for the client
- Counseling the client and family members about the treatment goals and procedures and their responsibilities in conducting home treatment sessions, reinforcing fluency in natural settings, and generally promoting maintenance of fluency over time and across situations

Psychological Methods of Treatment

Psychological methods of treatment include psychotherapy and counseling. Psychiatrists and psychologists offer psychotherapy. Various forms of counseling may be offered by qualified speech–language pathologists.

- The somewhat varied methods of psychological treatment include the following:
  - Discussion of psychological problems associated with stuttering
  - Discussion of feelings, emotions, and attitudes associated with stuttering
  - Discussion and resolution of potential psychological conflicts, unconscious psychosexual conflicts, and various kinds of negative reactions
  - Re-education of the client about a more realistic and rational approach to the stuttering problem
- There is no strong evidence that psychotherapy or counseling, offered exclusively, is effective in treating stuttering.
- Speech–language pathologists who offer counseling do so in conjunction with other methods designed to enhance fluency and reduce stuttering. In such cases, it is difficult to claim effectiveness for any one method used. There is independent evidence that direct behavioral treatment of stuttering is effective, however.

Fluent Stuttering Method

- An older method of treating stuttering is Van Riper's (1973) fluent stuttering approach, also called the **stutter-more-fluently** approach. The method modifies the severity and the visible abnormality of stuttering. The goal is not necessarily normal fluency, but more fluent (less abnormal) stuttering. This method involves the following steps:

  - **Teaching stuttering identification.** The client is taught to identify his or her stuttering and associated problems (e.g., feelings and attitudes) in both clinical and everyday situations.

- **Desensitizing the client to his or her stuttering.** The client is encouraged to be open and honest about his or her stuttering and voluntarily stutter in many speaking situations to get desensitized.
- **Modifying stuttering.** The client is taught to produce more fluent, easier, and less abnormal stuttering by the clinician, encouraging the client to
  - face difficult speaking situations and use feared words without avoidance;
  - use **cancellations** (pausing after a stuttered word and saying the word again with more relaxed stuttering);
  - use **pull-outs**, or change stuttering in mid-course (e.g., by slowing down and using soft articulatory contacts instead of blocking on sounds or words); and
  - use **preparatory sets** (e.g., changing the manner of stuttering so that the stuttering is less abnormal).
- **Stabilizing the treatment gains.** The client is encouraged to use the techniques of stuttering modification (cancellations, pull-outs, and preparatory sets) in all speaking situations.
- **Counseling the client.** The client is encouraged to discuss the emotions and attitudes he or she associates with stuttering to gain a more realistic and accepting view of the difficulties.

■ A limitation of the fluent stuttering method is rare establishment of normal fluency, as only modified stuttering is the goal. Relapse of stuttering may also be a problem, as its evidential base is weak.

Fluency Shaping Method

■ The goal of fluency shaping (also called the **speak-more-fluently** approach) is to establish normal fluency (not fluent stuttering). Teaching the various skills of fluency (e.g., appropriate management of airflow to produce and sustain fluent speech, slower rate of speech through syllable prolongation, and gentle onset of phonation) is the main treatment task (Guitar, 2014; Hegde, 2007, 2018c).

■ In different treatment programs, one or more of such fluency skills may be emphasized or deemphasized; for instance, in some programs, airflow management may not be as important as prolonged speech. Different clinicians may target different combinations of fluency skills. Treatment targets and procedures include the following:

- Teach airflow management (i.e., inhalation of air and immediate slight exhalation before phonation; maintenance of an even airflow throughout an utterance).
- Teach gentle, soft, relaxed, and easy onset of phonation, beginning after the initiation of exhalation.
- Teach a reduced rate of speech through syllable prolongation, with no pauses (break in phonation) between words, with continuous phonation and without breaks in between words. Typically, the vowel following the initial consonant is prolonged. If preferred, delayed auditory feedback can be used to reduce the rate of speech.
- In teaching all skills, use instructions, modeling, shaping, corrective feedback for errors, and positive reinforcement for correct responses.

- Note that fluency shaping induces stutter-free speech, not normal-sounding fluency. Explicit airflow management and rate reduction through syllable prolongation reduce stuttering while inducing a monotonous and unnatural-sounding speech. Therefore, clinicians should shape normal prosodic features (e.g., increased rate, normal vocal intensity, and normal intonation) after stutter-free speech is stabilized.
- Implement maintenance strategies (e.g., teaching self-monitoring skills and training family and friends to monitor and reinforce fluency in natural settings and over time). For more information, see under the section "Generalization, Maintenance, and Working With Families."

■ An abbreviated fluency shaping program that includes only prolonged speech (reduced rate of speech) as its target behavior is called the Camperdown Program, which was developed by O'Brian, Onslow, Cream, and Packman (2003). Clients practice prolonged speech with a model video supplied to them. The speech rate is gradually increased, and a maintenance phase is introduced with periodic clinic meetings.

■ As noted, a limitation of the fluency shaping method is that it generates slow, deliberate, and somewhat unnatural-sounding fluency. This limitation is the main reason a relapse of stuttering is common in clients who have been treated with the fluency shaping method. Clients tend not to maintain the slower rate needed to sustain that fluency, as such a rate is socially and personally unacceptable. When they increase their speech rate, stuttering tends to return.

Fluency Reinforcement Method

A simple method that works with many young children is to positively reinforce fluent speech in naturalistic conversational contexts. In this method, the clinician

- arranges a pleasant and relaxed therapeutic setting;
- evokes speech with the help of picture books, toys, and other play materials;
- positively reinforces the child for fluent utterances with verbal praise, tokens, or both;
- frequently models a slow, relaxed speaking rate that assures stutter-free speech; and
- reshapes normal prosody if a slower rate is an added target.

■ Fluency reinforcement alone may be effective with young children, whereas with older children and adult clients, adding a slower speech rate as a target may increase the effectiveness of the technique.

■ Fluency reinforcement techniques may include the highly researched Lidcombe Program (Onslow et al., 2003). Arnott, Onslow, O'Brian, Packman, Jones, and Block (2014) have reported the effectiveness of the Lidcombe Program in group setting. The technique is also being researched for its effectiveness when delivered through an Internet webcam (telepractice or telehealth model) with no clinical attendance.

Masking and Delayed Auditory Feedback Techniques

Both delayed auditory feedback (DAF) and masking noise reduce stuttering, possibly because the speech rate is slowed down; speech tends to be monotonous.

- In using the DAF technique, the clinician uses a DAF machine that allows for variable delays; determines a client-specific duration of delay that assures stutter-free speech; has the client practice stutter-free speech for varying lengths of time to eliminate stuttering; and fades the delay in gradual steps to reshape normal prosody while maintaining fluency. Speech may be slowed by instruction and modeling. There is no compelling reason to use a DAF machine; maintenance of fluency has been problematic.
- In using the masking noise, the clinician determines a minimum level of auditory masking that induces stutter-free speech; has the client practice stutter-free speech; and fades the masking noise to reshape normal prosody while maintaining fluency. Relapse of stuttering is common.

Direct Stuttering Reduction Methods

Direct stuttering reduction methods seek to reduce stuttering directly, without teaching specific fluency skills or modifying stuttering into less abnormal forms. To reduce stuttering directly, behavioral methods of pause-and-talk (time-out) or response cost may be used (Hegde, 2007; 2018c) as follows:

- **Pause-and-talk (time-out).** In this method, the person who stutters is taught to pause after each dysfluency and then resume talking. The clinician
  - says "stop" or gives other signals (e.g., turning a light on) as soon as a dysfluency is observed and makes sure that the client completely ceases talking;
  - avoids eye contact with the client for about 5 seconds;
  - re-establishes eye contact after the time-out duration and lets the client continue his or her speech; and
  - maintains eye contact, smiles, and employs other social reinforcers for fluent speech.

- **Response cost.** In this method, for every instance of stuttering, the clinician takes away a token, which is awarded for every fluent production. In a variation of this procedure, a bunch of tokens are initially given to the client, and a single token is withdrawn for each dysfluent production; this variation is not recommended. Most of the positive evidence is related to the classic procedure of giving tokens for fluency and taking it away for dysfluency (Hegde, 2018c). The specific procedure includes
  - reinforcing the client for every fluently spoken word, phrase, or sentence with a token that is backed up with other kinds of reinforcers for which the client exchanges the tokens at the end of the session;
  - taking a token away in a matter-of-fact manner immediately following a stuttering or at the earliest sign of it;
  - progressing from words and phrases to conversational speech; and
  - fading the tokens when fluency is sustained at 98% or better across three or four sessions and maintaining fluency with verbal praise alone.

- Both time-out and response cost can help establish more natural-sounding fluency. The methods do not achieve fluency by slowing the rate of speech or explicitly managing the airflow. In fact, if a client begins to use any of these strategies (e.g., begins to speak slowly), the clinician discourages their use. Consequently, there is no need to add such additional treatment targets as natural-sounding fluency.

- Of the two techniques, time-out is the better researched, although evidence on the effectiveness of response cost in treating young children, including preschoolers, is accumulating (Hegde, 2004).
- Response cost is preferred for preschoolers and children in the early elementary grades; time-out is preferred for older children and adults. Many young children do not stop talking when told to stop after a dysfluency; therefore, time-out is not as effective as response cost with them.

Some Special Considerations Based on the Client's Age

In treating preschool and early school-age children, the clinician considers the following:

- Parent counseling and closely working with the parents is the most crucial element in treating young children; training parents in treatment procedures that they can implement at home is the other critical element of successful treatment.
- Counseling the parents and the child on handling not only bullying from other children, but all negative reactions from others is important.
- When confronted with negative reactions or bullying from others, the child may be taught to say, "You know, sometimes I have difficulty saying certain words but I am working on it" (Guitar, 2014). If the child can't say that, perhaps parents or siblings or teachers might help; parents may be counseled to discuss frankly their child's problem with others who show negative reactions. Such discussions may reduce negative reactions and actually promote sympathetic and supportive reactions.
- Selecting effective reinforcers for the child needs careful planning and some experimentation.
- Simple fluency reinforcement in naturalistic play and conversational settings may be quite effective with preschoolers; response cost is another effective procedure for preschoolers.
- The child should enjoy therapy; this means that the clinician should generously reinforce fluency, minimize stuttering and corrective feedback, and select an effective reinforcer.

In treating older students and adolescents, the clinician may consider the following:

- Teaching self-monitoring skills; older children can "count" their stutterings, may be taught to stop soon after an instance of stuttering, and can ask parents and others to pay attention to their fluency (reinforcement priming).
- Fluency shaping and pause-and-talk are two good choices for this group.
- Slower reading rate and resulting fluency may be reinforced in oral reading.
- Older students may be taught to talk frankly about their stuttering to reduce teasing and bullying.
- Fear and avoidance may be reduced by instilling fluency in everyday situations; students may be taken to natural settings to reinforce fluency there.
- Parent counseling and parent training will be just as important as at the previous age level.
- Training teachers to prompt and reinforce fluency, to be patient listeners, and generally to support the clinician's effort will be essential.

In treating adults, the clinician may consider the following:

- Teaching self-monitoring skills will be important and may be achieved to the maximum extent.
- Discussing their ideas about stuttering and explaining the treatment and the evidence for it will be essential.
- Fluency shaping and pause-and-talk (time-out) are two excellent choices for this group.
- Spousal counseling and training spouses to evoke and reinforce fluency will be important.

Generalization, Maintenance, and Working With Families

Regardless of the treatment procedure used, the clinician works on getting the clinically established fluency comprehensive for everyday situations by taking the following steps:

- When fluency reaches the targeted level in three to five clinical sessions, the clinician invites unfamiliar people into the sessions and has the client engage in conversation with the visitors
- Inviting parents, siblings, and friends take part in the treatment sessions and get trained on prompting fluency skills and reinforcing fluent productions
- Taking the client out of the clinic room and into more natural settings to reinforce fluency in natural conversation
- Reinforcing fluency in varied natural situations so that the client will learn to approach rather than avoid speech and speaking situations
- Teaching self-monitoring skills to the client; the client may stop at the earliest sign of a stutter, may stop when a fluency skill is mismanaged (e.g., forgetting to slow down), and may learn to measure his or her own stutterings and fluency skills
- Training parents, spouses, or other family members to hold informal treatment sessions at home and generously reinforces fluency in all naturalistic settings
- Periodically conducting follow-ups to assess maintenance and provide additional support in the form of brief treatment sessions to help maintain fluency across time

Pharmacological Treatment

No pharmacological treatment has replaced the behavioral methods of treating stuttering; all are still experimental.

- Tranquilizers and sedatives may reduce the severity of stuttering, but their side effects (drowsiness, sexual dysfunction, and risk of permanent and serious movement disorders) contradict their use.
- Drugs (especially olanzapine and pagoclone) that interfere with the uptake of dopamine have been used.
- No drug has been shown to establish normal-sounding fluency that lasts. At the most a 30–40% reduction in stuttering may be expected; the person would still be considered to be stuttering.
- It should be noted that the same drugs that reduce stuttering (e.g., olanzapine) may induce stuttering in patients without a history of stuttering but with certain neuropathology (Bar, Hager, & Sauer, 2014).

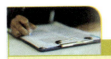

SUMMARY

- Assessment of stuttering includes standard assessment procedures and a detailed interview of the client, family, or both.
- Detailed assessment of stuttering includes measurement of the frequency, types, and variability of dysfluencies, associated motor behaviors, avoidance behaviors, speech rate, and negative emotional reactions.
- Traditional approaches to the treatment of stuttering include psychological methods, the fluent stuttering method associated with Van Riper (1973), masking and delayed auditory feedback techniques, and the fluency shaping method.
- More behaviorally oriented approaches to treatment include the fluency reinforcement method and the direct stuttering reduction methods (time-out and response cost).
- Current evidence does not support pharmacological treatment.

NEUROGENIC STUTTERING

Neurogenic stuttering (also called acquired stuttering) resembles stuttering of early childhood onset, but it is associated with diagnosed neurological disorder or disorders. Up to 5% of patients with stroke may experience neurogenic stuttering for varying durations of time (Theys, van Wieringen, Sunaert, Thijs, & De Nil, 2011). Several characteristics of neurogenic stuttering are unique and help distinguish it from stuttering of childhood onset. Neurogenic stuttering may be persistent or transient and may be associated with aphasia or apraxia of speech; occasionally, it may be seen in the absence of aphasia in people who have had a stroke. Different neuropathological conditions may produce the same symptom complex (Hegde, 2018a, 2018b, 2018c).

Definition and Etiology of Neurogenic Stuttering

Neurogenic stuttering (NS) is a form of fluency disorder associated with documented neuropathology, often in older individuals; other neurogenic speech disorder (e.g., apraxia or dysarthria) or language disorder (e.g., aphasia) may or may not be evident. The age of onset of NS is 67 years. Etiologic factors of NS include the following:

- Cerebral vascular disorders that cause strokes are the most frequent causes; the cortico-basal ganglia network may be affected, including such multiple areas as inferior frontal cortex, superior temporal cortex, intraparietal cortex, basal ganglia, and their white matter interconnections (Theys, De Nil, Thijs, van Wieringen, & Sunaert, 2013)
- Right hemisphere disorder
- Extrapyramidal diseases, especially Parkinson's disease; progressive supranuclear palsy; brain tumors; brain surgery, including bilateral thalamotomy; seizure disorders; dementia, especially dialysis dementia
- Drug toxicity, especially from drugs prescribed for asthma, depression, schizophrenia, and anxiety

- Bilateral brain damage, causing more persistent NS; multiple lesions of a single hemisphere or some drug toxicity, causing transient NS
- Left hemisphere strokes, Parkinson's disease, Alzheimer's disease, or olivopontocerebellar atrophy that rekindles stuttering of early onset that was remediated or spontaneously reduced
- Traumatic brain injury, multiple sclerosis with cerebellar lesions, bilateral thalamic strokes, seizures, and neurosurgery for tumors or vascular disorders may reduce or eliminate stuttering in some cases

Description of Neurogenic Stuttering

Stuttering of childhood onset and NS share many common symptoms but differ on a few diagnostic features. Characteristics of neurogenic stuttering include the following:

- Evidence of neuropathology and neurologic symptoms that are consistent with the diagnosed neurological diseases
- Adult onset of stuttering, often in older people with documented neuropathology (e.g., traumatic brain injury, drug toxicity, and neurosurgery may cause neurogenic stuttering at any age)
- A generally increased rate of dysfluencies (including syllable and word repetitions and frozen articulatory postures) common to stuttering of early onset and neurogenic stuttering
- Positive signs or symptoms of NS that contrast with stuttering of childhood onset include repetitions of medial and final syllables in words, dysfluent production of function words, dysfluencies in imitated speech, rapid speech rate, and general symptoms of brain injury
- Negative signs of NS that contrast with the signs of stuttering of early childhood onset include no or minimal adaptation effect; minimal variability in stuttering frequency across different speech tasks; few associated motor behaviors; minimal effects of delayed auditory feedback, masking noise, rhythmic speech, choral reading, shadowing, and singing; no obvious anxiety associated with speech or speaking situations; no specific word fears; and absence of attempts at avoiding speech or speaking situations

Assessment and Treatment of Neurogenic Stuttering

Assessment of NS begins with a review of a client's medical records to establish a neurological basis for suspected fluency disorder. Specific procedures include the following:

- Assessment of potentially coexisting aphasia, apraxia of speech, dysarthria, and dementia
- Stuttering assessment techniques described previously
- Differential evaluation of both positive and negative features of NS to establish diagnosis and rule out stuttering of early childhood onset (Recent investigators have suggested that variations in the positive signs may make it difficult to distinguish early-onset stuttering from NS; a positive neuropathology is needed to make the diagnosis.)
- Most of the research published on NS constitutes case studies describing the symptoms of individual cases.
- Controlled treatment research on NS is limited or nonexistent. A few case studies involving single patients have reported modest improvement in fluency following the administration of drugs

generally prescribed for epilepsy or psychosis; the same drugs may induce stuttering if taken in higher doses.
- Treatment of NS is done in the context of other speech or language disorders that coexist; for instance, procedures appropriate for treating aphasia, apraxia of speech, dysarthria, traumatic brain injury, and dementia are essential in a comprehensive treatment program.
- Most clinicians handle treatment symptomatically, by reducing the rate of speech with instructions, delayed auditory feedback, or a pacing board (for more about diagnosis and treatment of neurologically based disorders, see Chapter 8).
- When a reduced speech rate minimizes dysfluencies, the clinician will fade the slower rate and teach the client to speak with a more normal rate.
- Relaxation and biofeedback may be tried to see if they are beneficial.
- Because no efficacy studies on the treatment of NS have been published, clinicians may have to experiment with procedures that have a significant effect in individual clients.

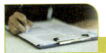

SUMMARY

- Neurogenic stuttering is a form of fluency disorder associated with a variety of neurological diseases or disorders, including vascular disorders that cause strokes, traumatic brain injury, and degenerative neurological disorders that may result in dementia (e.g., Alzheimer's and Parkinson's diseases).
- Neurogenic stuttering is assessed and treated in the context of any existing neurological diseases and associated disorders of communication.

CLUTTERING

Cluttering is a disorder of fluency that often coexists with stuttering. It is characterized by a reduced speech intelligibility, rapid and irregular speech rate, imprecise articulation, dysfluencies, disorganized language, poor prosody, and inefficient management of discourse (Myers & Bakker, 2013). Speakers who clutter do not manifest obvious concern about their speaking patterns. Some may report poor thought organization. Little experimentally controlled research exists on treatment of cluttering, although it has been found that decreasing the rate of speech and increasing the client's awareness of the problem are often effective (Hegde, 2018a, 2018c; Myers & Bakker, 2013; Myers & St. Louis, 1992; St. Louis & Schulte, 2011).

Definition and Description of Cluttering

The prevalence of cluttering in the United States is unknown, but in Germany it is reported to be 1.8% of 7- to 8-year-old children. Like stuttering, cluttering is more common in males than in females. The characteristics of cluttering are as follows:

- Rapid but disordered articulation and resulting indistinct (unintelligible) speech; rate variations
- Impaired prosodic features with frequent pauses
- Impaired fluency with excessive amounts of dysfluencies, especially word and phase repetitions, interjections, and revisions; possible rapid repetition of syllables, along with other forms as well
- Clearer articulation and improved intelligibility at slower rate of speech
- Omission and compression of sounds and syllables
- Jerky or stumbling rhythm
- Monotonous tone
- Spoonerisms (unintentional interchanges of sounds in a sentence; e.g., "Many thinkle peep so" instead of "Many people think so")
- Disorganized language production
- Reportedly, a lack of concern about or reduced awareness of one's speech problem
- Lack of anxiety about or negative reactions to one's speech difficulty
- Disorganized thought processes (a controversial feature of cluttering)

The causes of cluttering are unknown. Genetic transmission and subtle brain damage have been among suggested factors. Some experts think that it is a central language disorder (a disassociation between thought and language) but there is little empirical support for this idea.

Assessment and Treatment of Cluttering

Cluttering is assessed much like stuttering of early childhood onset with an emphasis on its special features (e.g., excessive rate and rate variations, articulatory breakdowns and speech intelligibility, prosodic variations, dysfluencies, lack of concern). A detailed case history and an extended speech sample will help analyze the symptom complex. There is little or no controlled treatment research on cluttering.

- Clinicians may administer the Cluttering Severity Instrument, a computer software program developed by Bakker and Meyers (2011) to assess and rate the overall intelligibility, speech rate regularity, speech rate, articulatory precision, typical disfluency, language organization, discourse management, and prosody.
- Reducing the rate of speech usually improves clarity as well as fluency. If thought problems or language formulation problems are dominant, teaching the client to plan sentences and other forms of expression before actually producing them might be helpful.
- Increasing a client's awareness of his or her speech problems through the use of audio- or video-recordings can be helpful. Some people who clutter are surprised when confronted with recordings of their own speech. Unfortunately, video samples do not always convince people who clutter of their problem, especially the increased speech rate.
- Maintenance of fluent speech with typical articulation is the major problem in treating persons who clutter. Systematic treatment research is needed to develop unique and more effective treatment procedures for cluttering.

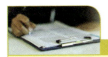

SUMMARY

- Cluttering is a disorder of fluency characterized by rapid, imprecise, jerky, and disorganized speech.
- Little research exists about its treatment. Reducing the speaking rate and increasing self-awareness helps some people who clutter to sound more intelligible.

OTHER TYPES OF FLUENCY DISORDERS

There are a few other unusual types of fluency disorders that are psychiatric in nature (Hegde, 2018a, 2018b, 2018c). The two main forms include:

- **Malingered stuttering.** This is faked stuttering exhibited to gain an advantage from the problem; symptoms are well planned (researched by the individual); the individual knows he or she is faking; gains may be negative reinforcement that occurs when a child, faking stuttering, avoids a difficult oral presentation to the class; diagnostic features include lack of adaptation, absence of reduction in stuttering under delayed auditory feedback, masking noise, and reduced speech rate.
- **Psychogenic stuttering.** Although psychogenic is a vague term, stuttering falling under this controversial term is of adult onset; it is not malingering because it is not consciously fabricated to gain an advantage; the individual may be unaware of the origin of the problem; dysfluencies are similar to those found in stuttering of childhood onset; may be associated with depression, anxiety, post-traumatic stress, and such other psychiatric disorders; triggering factors include stressful life situation including divorce, illness, death of a loved one, loss of job, and so forth; may be associated with neurodegenerative diseases, convulsive disorders, stroke, traumatic brain injury, and so forth in some individuals, complicating a psychogenic diagnosis; dysfluencies may not be affected by adaptation, masking noise, and delayed auditory feedback.

CHAPTER HIGHLIGHTS

- Fluent speech is flowing, smooth, relatively rapid, and effortless. Stuttering, cluttering, and NS are the three main forms of fluency disorders.
- Dysfluencies, including repetitions, prolongations, broken words, interjections, pauses, incomplete sentences, and revisions interrupt the flow of fluency. When dysfluencies exceed 5% of words spoken, listeners tend to judge the speech as dysfluent or stuttered.

- Stuttering may be defined as (a) all types of dysfluencies that exceed a measure such as 5% of words spoken, (b) production of part-word repetitions and speech-sound prolongations, (c) moments or events judged to be stutterings, and (d) anticipatory, apprehensive, hypertonic, and avoidance reaction.
- In early childhood, stuttering begins as an initial increase in the amount of dysfluency. Associated motor behaviors, breathing abnormalities, negative emotions, and avoidance behaviors tend to develop in due course and to varying extents across individuals.
- Stuttering occurs at such predictable loci as initial sounds and words, consonants, longer and unfamiliar words, content words in older children and adults, and function words in younger children.
- Stuttering is under strong stimulus control, as evidenced by such phenomena as adaptation, consistency, adjacency, and dependence on audience size.
- Genetic, neurophysiological, psychological, learning-based, and mismatch theories have tried to explain stuttering. None of the hypotheses are fully supported by experimental evidence.
- Assessment of stuttering includes a detailed case history; measurement of types and frequency of dysfluencies in conversational speech and oral reading; evaluation of the variability of dysfluencies; assessment of negative emotions, avoidance reactions, and associated motor behaviors; measurement of speech and articulatory rates; and application of a chosen diagnostic criterion.
- Treatment of stuttering includes a variety of procedures, including counseling and psychotherapy; delayed auditory feedback and of masking noise; the fluent stuttering method; the fluency shaping method; fluency reinforcement; and direct stuttering reduction techniques (time-outs and response cost).
- Neurogenic stuttering is a fluency disorder associated with various forms of neurological disorders; it may be transient or persistent. It is distinguishable from early-onset stuttering by several features and is assessed and treated in the context of the neurological diseases and associated additional speech disorders (e.g., apraxia of speech, aphasia).
- Cluttering, includes rapid but disordered articulation, prosodic abnormalities, and reduced speech intelligibility, possibly combined with a high rate of dysfluencies and disorganized thought and language. Treatment of cluttering involves teaching a slower speech rate.
- Some atypical types of stuttering include malingered stuttering and psychogenic stuttering with psychiatric connotations.

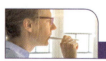

STUDY AND REVIEW QUESTIONS

1. The position that stuttering indicates a social role conflict was taken by

    A. Van Riper.
    B. Wischner.
    C. Sheehan.
    D. Bloodstein.

2. Research on the prevalence of stuttering has shown that

    A. familial incidence is higher than in the general population.

    B. sons of stuttering mothers run a greater risk than sons of stuttering fathers.

    C. blood relatives of a stuttering woman run a greater risk of stuttering themselves than those of a stuttering man.

    D. all of the above.

3. Stuttering in preschool children is more likely on

    A. content words.

    B. function words.

    C. final words in a sentence.

    D. vowels.

4. Which one of the following is a fact about stuttering adaptation?

    A. The greatest reduction in stuttering occurs only on the seventh reading.

    B. There is transfer from one reading passage to the other.

    C. Most of the reduction in stuttering occurs by the fifth reading.

    D. A higher magnitude of adaptation occurs with an increased time interval between readings.

5. Studies on the rates of natural recovery of stuttering suggests that

    A. less than 20% of children who stutter recover naturally.

    B. all children who stutter recover by age 8.

    C. once started, stuttering persists in all children.

    D. the recovery rate may be as low as 45% or as high as 90%.

6. Parents generally report that the onset of stuttering in their children is associated with

    A. nothing unusual.

    B. stressful family situations.

    C. accidental head injury.

    D. severe illness.

7. The fluent stuttering treatment

    A. aims at eliminating stuttering.

    B. seeks normally fluent speech.

    C. was developed by Van Riper.

    D. was developed by Johnson.

8. In treating older students and adults who stutter, a clinician decides to use the direct stuttering treatment (reduction) procedure; specifically, the clinician then selects

    A. time-out.

    B. the fluency shaping approach.

    C. approach-avoidance reduction treatment.

    D. the fluent stuttering approach.

9. Such skills as airflow management, gentle phonatory onset, and reduced rate of speech are targets in

  A. the fluent stuttering technique.
  B. the fluency shaping technique.
  C. counseling to reduce psychological conflicts.
  D. direct stuttering reduction strategies.

10. A mother calls a clinician and shares concerns about her child's speech. According to the mother, her daughter, Rachel, is difficult to understand. The mother describes Rachel's speech as "sort of rushed, and she kind of stutters sometimes." The clinician who tests Rachel concludes that Rachel clutters. Based upon this diagnosis, one would expect to see that Rachel

  A. has a rapid rate of speech but is intelligible and is probably secretly anxious about her speech.
  B. is dysfluent but has clear articulation and no spoonerisms.
  C. has excellent language skills and is highly dysfluent with no speech rate problems.
  D. has a lack of anxiety or concern about her speech; uses spoonerisms; and has rapid, disordered articulation resulting in unintelligible speech.

11. When the speech–language pathologist provides treatment for Rachel to help her become more intelligible, which techniques would probably be ideal for her?

  A. Reducing Rachel's rate of speech and increasing her awareness of her speech through audiotapes or videotapes
  B. Reducing Rachel's rate of speech but not increasing her awareness of her speech through audiotapes or videotapes, because this could create self-consciousness, which could make the cluttering worse
  C. Helping Rachel maintain a rapid rate of speech but working on increasing her intelligibility through emphasizing the final consonants of words
  D. Probing to see if Rachel has negative emotions (that her mother is unaware of) about her speech and spending most of therapy time helping her deal with these emotions

12. The theory that stuttering is caused by lack of a unilateral hemispheric control of language is the

  A. cerebral dominance theory.
  B. approach-avoidance theory.
  C. diagnosogenic theory.
  D. hemispheric domination theory.

13. A researcher wants to study the occurrence of stuttering in a given city. She wants to know how many adults and children in Middletown City have officially been diagnosed with stuttering. She does not necessarily want to give a predictive statement; rather, she just wants to know the number of individuals in Middletown who stutter. The researcher wants to study the

  A. incidence.
  B. prevalence.
  C. matched samples.
  D. population statistics.

14. A 5-year-old child, Marcus, has been identified as needing treatment for his stuttering. His parents report that he has been stuttering since he was 3 years old, and the stuttering has become worse. Now children tease him, and his parents are concerned that, when he enters kindergarten, the teasing will become worse. The clinician decides to use one of the direct stuttering reduction methods with Marcus. Select the appropriate technique.

  A. Delayed auditory feedback and slowed speech
  B. Auditory masking
  C. Response cost
  D. Airflow management and parental counseling

15. A 32-year-old man, Frank, wants to go to law school. He is very bright, but stutters and has been working in minimum-wage jobs where he does not have to do much talking. Frank shares that he has passed the entrance examination to get into law school, but he is afraid to enroll in classes. He feels frustrated by his dilemma and says that he is experiencing a great deal of anxiety about his situation. The clinician decides to use the fluent stuttering method. This would involve

  A. not discussing Frank's feelings and attitudes but rather teaching and establishing skills such as airflow management, reduced rate, and easy onset of phonation.
  B. encouraging Frank to discuss his feelings and attitudes about his stuttering, desensitizing him to his stuttering, and using procedures such as time-out and response cost.
  C. using DAF, masking, and procedures such as time-out and response cost.
  D. allowing Frank to discuss his feelings and attitudes toward his situation, desensitizing Frank to his stuttering, and helping him to modify his stuttering through the use of such techniques as cancellations and pull-outs.

16. You have been asked to assess Rudy, a 65-year-old man, for suspected neurogenic stuttering. In your assessment, you expect to observe

  A. absence of repetitions on medial and final sounds in words.
  B. presence of dysfluencies in imitated speech.
  C. presence of marked adaptation.
  D. a significant number of severe associated motor behaviors.

17. People who stutter and their families

  A. do not have unique personality traits that explain stuttering.
  B. are diagnosed with clinically significant anxiety disorders.
  C. have unique temperament related to stuttering.
  D. have obsessive compulsive traits.

18. The leading-edge hypothesis

  A. suggests that speech disruptions are most likely on the most complex language structures.
  B. discounts the concept of inherent vulnerability to speech problems.
  C. suggests advanced structures about to be learned induce speech disruptions.
  D. is a new model of stuttering treatment.

19. A male child's risk for developing stuttering is the greatest when

    A. his brother stutters.
    B. his father stutters.
    C. his cousin stutters.
    D. his mother stutters.

20. An employee in a tech company was able to routinely excuse himself from making oral presentations to his team because of his stuttering; provided other factors also support it, what would be your likely diagnosis of this client?

    A. Typical stuttering
    B. Psychogenic stuttering
    C. Malingered stuttering
    D. Neurogenic stuttering

References and Recommended Readings at: www.advancedreviewpractice.com

STUDY AND REVIEW ANSWERS

1. **C.** Sheehan believed that stuttering indicates a social role conflict.
2. **D.** Research on the prevalence of stuttering has shown all of the listed findings—that familial incidence is higher than in the general population, that sons of stuttering mothers run a greater risk than sons of stuttering fathers, and that blood relatives of a stuttering woman run a greater risk than those of a stuttering man.
3. **B.** Stuttering in preschool children is more likely on function words.
4. **C.** One fact about stuttering adaptation is that most of the reduction in stuttering occurs by the fifth reading.
5. **D.** The reported natural recovery rates for stuttering ranges between a low of 45% and a high of 90%
6. **A.** Parents generally report that the onset of stuttering in their children is associated with nothing unusual.
7. **C.** Van Riper developed the fluent stuttering treatment to reduce the abnormality of stuttering.
8. **A.** In treating older students and adults who stutter, a clinician decides to use the direct stuttering treatment (reduction) procedure; specifically, the clinician then selects time-out.
9. **B.** Such skills as airflow management, gentle phonatory onset, and reduced rate of speech are targets in the fluency shaping technique.
10. **D.** Because Rachel clutters, one would expect to see a lack of anxiety or concern about her speech; use of spoonerisms; and rapid, disordered articulation resulting in unintelligible speech.
11. **A.** Reducing Rachel's rate of speech and increasing her awareness of her speech through audiotapes or videotapes is the best method of helping her become more intelligible.
12. **A.** The cerebral dominance theory proposed that lack of a unilateral dominant hemisphere is the cause of stuttering.

13. B. In establishing the prevalence of a disorder, the investigator head-counts the number of individuals who currently have a particular disorder.
14. C. One technique of the direct stuttering reduction method is response cost.
15. D. The fluent stuttering approach of Van Riper involves allowing Frank to discuss his feelings and attitudes toward his situation, desensitizing him to his stuttering, and helping him to modify his stuttering through the use of such techniques as cancellations and pull-outs.
16. B. To diagnose neurogenic stuttering, you look for, among other signs, presence of dysfluencies in imitated speech.
17. A. People who stutter and their families do not have unique personality traits that explain stuttering.
18. C. In the leading-edge hypothesis, advanced structures about to be mastered induce speech disruptions.
19. D. A male child's risk for developing stuttering is the greatest when his mother stutters.
20. B. Psychogenic stuttering, in which a clear advantage is gained by the symptoms.

CHAPTER 7

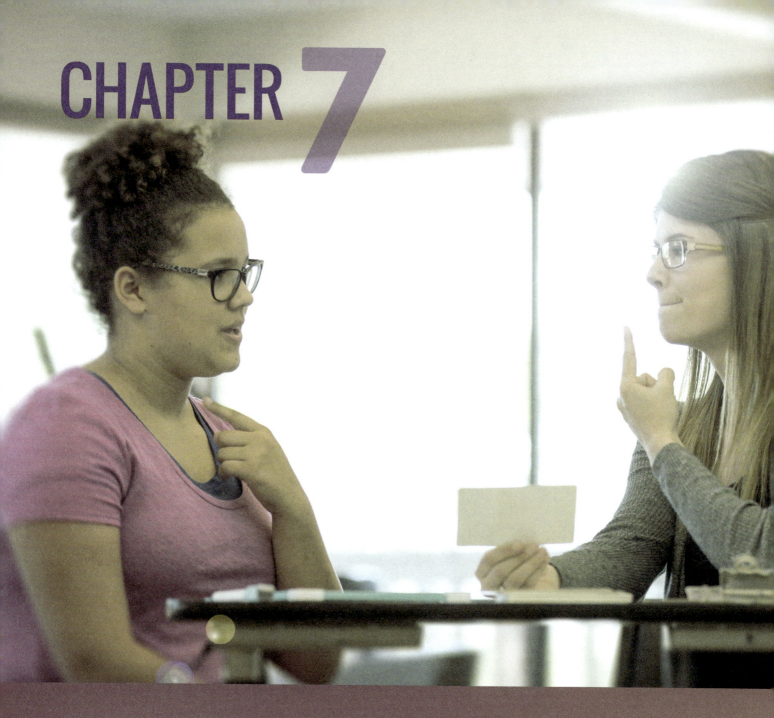

VOICE AND ITS DISORDERS

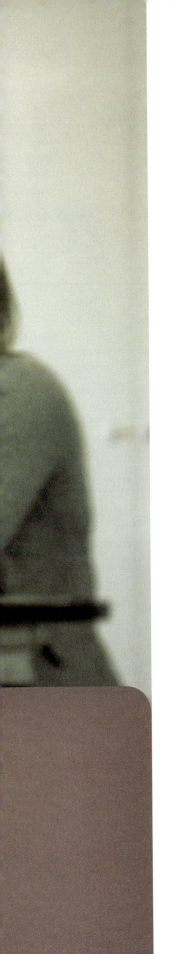

Voice and its disorders are gaining significant attention from communication disorders professionals, as well as the general public. Society is increasingly recognizing the value of a clear, professional-sounding, and pleasing voice for optimal communication. With the advent of television shows like American Idol and The Voice, people are becoming more interested in the voice. Communication disorders professionals, due to their sophisticated training and use of measurement instrumentation, are learning more about how to treat voice disorders and help patients achieve maximally competent voice production. With the incidence of voice disorders estimated to be between 3% and 9% of the U.S. population, it is important for clinicians to learn how to assess and treat voice disorders (Roy, Merrill, Gray, & Smith, 2005). In this chapter, we discuss normal aspects of voice, disorders of voice and resonation, and aspects of assessment and treatment.

VOCAL ANATOMY AND PHYSIOLOGY

In this section, the topics of laryngeal anatomy and physiology and voice changes through the life span are discussed (Chapter 1 contains more detailed information about laryngeal anatomy and physiology and the neurological mechanisms that control vocalization. These concepts are briefly reviewed in this chapter).

The Larynx

Basic Principles

The larynx is a valve located at the top of the trachea and serves several biological functions.

The larynx connects superiorly to the oral cavity and vocal tract and inferiorly to the lungs and trachea. It can be considered a passageway between the upper and lower airways. The larynx has an important function during swallowing as it elevates during the swallow. Housed within a cartilage of the larynx are the vocal folds. The vocal folds act as a valve that **adducts** (closes) or **abducts** (opens) the airway. When the vocal folds close, they block the entrance to the trachea so food, liquids, and other particles do not enter the lungs during swallowing (Hulit, Fahey, & Howard, 2015).

- Vocal fold closure is also necessary for building adequate air pressure to assist in the performance of biological functions such as getting rid of body waste, coughing, heavy lifting, and child bearing.

  - Vocal fold closure is also needed to begin the process of vocal fold vibration. The vocal folds vibrate to produce the source of sound for voice.

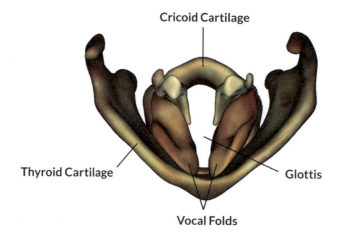

| Figure 7.1 | Thyroarytenoids (vocal folds). Used with permission from Anatomage. |

- The opening between the vocal folds is called the **glottis.**
- The vocal folds have a layered structure that is composed of the epithelium, the thyroarytenoid (TA) muscle, and the layers of the lamina propria (see Chapter 1). According to the **cover-body theory of phonation**, the epithelium and the superficial, intermediate, and deep layers of the lamina propria vibrate as a "cover" on a relatively stationary "body." This body is composed of the remainder of the TA muscle. Figure 7.1 shows the TA muscle.
- During phonation, **mucosal wave action** occurs. This is the movement of the mucous membrane of the vocal folds (*Note*: Vocal surgery can reduce mucosal wave action, resulting in a voice that the listener perceives as rough and gravelly).
- The **ventricular (vestibular)** or **false** vocal folds lie laterally and above the "true" vocal folds. They do not usually vibrate during normal phonation and are used only during activities, such as lifting and coughing.
- The ventricular folds protect the true vocal folds and also protect the airway during swallowing (Sapienza & Hoffman Ruddy, 2017). The ventricle is the space between the true and false vocal folds.

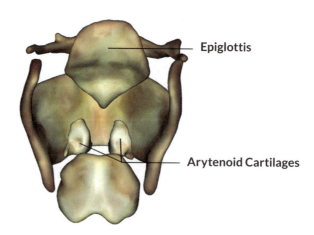

| Figure 7.2 | Arytenoid cartilage and epiglottis. Used with permission from Anatomage. |

- The **aryepiglottic folds** make up the upper part of the quadrangular membrane. They course from the arytenoid cartilage and the lateral portion of the epiglottis on each side and form the lateral borders of the laryngeal inlet.
- The cuneiform cartilages lie within the aryepiglottic folds. Because the pyriform sinus lies between the thyroid cartilage and the aryepiglottic folds, a bolus may be lodged in the pyriform sinuses, causing difficulty with swallowing. Figure 7.2 shows the arytenoid cartilage and epiglottis.
- **Cranial nerve VII** (facial nerve) innervates the posterior belly of the digastric muscle (a suprahyoid muscle).
- The primary cranial nerve involved in laryngeal innervation is **cranial nerve X** (vagus nerve). The primary branches of the vagus nerve that innervate the larynx are the superior laryngeal nerve (SLN) and the recurrent laryngeal nerve (RLN).
  - The SLN has internal and external branches. The internal branch provides all sensory information to the larynx, and the external branch supplies motor innervation solely to the cricothyroid muscle and may affect the ability to modulate frequency.
  - The RLN supplies all motor innervation to the interarytenoid, posterior cricoarytenoid, thyroarytenoid, and lateral cricoarytenoid muscles. This nerve supplies all sensory information below the vocal folds. If there is a lesion of the RLN, the patient may experience (among other problems) difficulty adducting the vocal folds (Boone, McFarlane, von Berg, & Zraik, 2013).
- In terms of vascular supply of the larynx, the three primary "feeding" arteries are the superior laryngeal, cricothyroid, and inferior laryngeal arteries.
- The superior laryngeal and cricothyroid arteries are usually branches of the superior thyroid artery, which is part of the external carotid artery. Figures 7.3a and b show the RLN.

Key Structures and Cartilages

Hyoid Bone
The larynx is suspended from the hyoid bone, a U-shaped bone that sits above the thyroid cartilage. Many extrinsic laryngeal muscles are attached to the hyoid bone, thus supporting the laryngeal framework. Figure 7.4 illustrates the hyoid bone in relation to other key laryngeal structures.

Epiglottis
The epiglottis is a leaf-shaped cartilage attached to the hyoid bone; it is narrow at the base (petiole) and wide at the top. The epiglottis protects the trachea by folding inferiorly and posteriorly over the false and true vocal folds, directing liquids and food into the esophagus during swallowing.

Thyroid Cartilage
The largest of all the laryngeal cartilages, the thyroid cartilage is composed of two lamina, or flat plates of cartilage, that are joined at the midline and form an angle. This angle, or prominence, is sometimes called the Adam's apple. It is particularly prominent in men. The thyroid cartilage also has two superior and two inferior **cornua** (horns); ligaments and muscles attach to the thyroid cartilage at these points. The thyroid

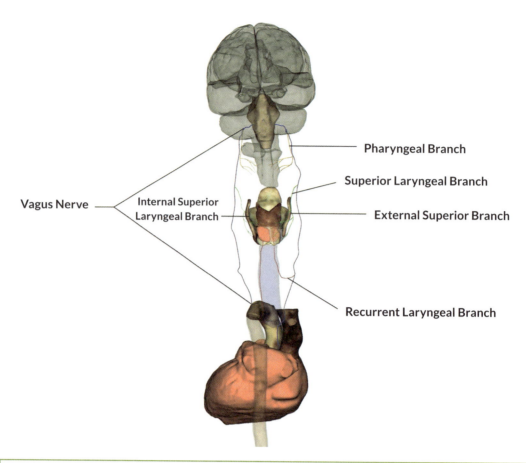

Figure 7.3a Recurrent laryngeal nerve. Used with permission from Anatomage.

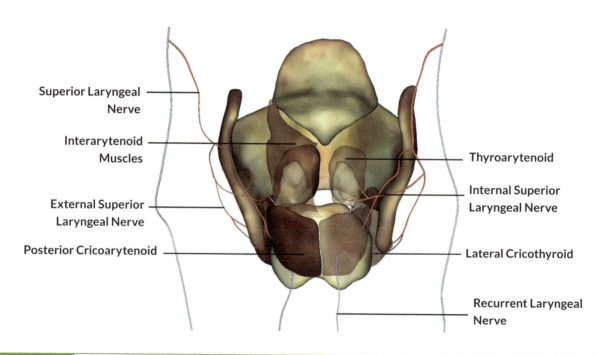

Figure 7.3b Innervation. Used with permission from Anatomage.

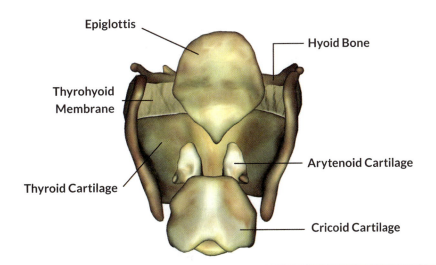

Figure 7.4 Hyoid bone, epiglottis, cricoid cartilage, and the thyroid cartilage. Used with permission from Anatomage.

cartilage also articulates with the cricoid cartilage at the cricothyroid joint; the anterior movement of the thyroid cartilage at this joint allows the vocal folds to lengthen (Sapienza & Hoffman Ruddy, 2017).

- The thyroid cartilage is an unpaired cartilage that houses and shields the vocal folds and other structures of the larynx.

Cricoid Cartilage
This is the second largest laryngeal cartilage. This cartilage is thinner anteriorly and broader posteriorly.

- The cricoid cartilage is unpaired and completely surrounds the trachea. It is linked with the paired arytenoid cartilages and the thyroid cartilage.

Arytenoid Cartilages
The paired arytenoid cartilages are positioned on the supraposterior surface of the cricoid cartilage on either side of the midline, creating the **cricoarytenoid joint**. When the arytenoids move medially and rock at the cricoarytenoid joint, the vocal folds adduct; lateral movement causes abduction. The arytenoids are also connected to the epiglottis by the **aryepiglottic folds**.

- The arytenoid cartilages are shaped like pyramids. The vocal processes are the most anterior angle of the base of the arytenoids. The TA muscle and cover of the true vocal folds attach posteriorly in the larynx at the vocal processes.
- The lateral and posterior cricoarytenoid muscles attach to the muscular processes, and the interarytenoid muscle attaches to the lateral edges of the arytenoid cartilages.

Corniculate Cartilages
The paired corniculate cartilages are small and cone-shaped and sit on the apex of the arytenoids. They play a minor role in vocalization. Figure 7.5 shows the arytenoid cartilages, cricoarytenoid joint, epiglottis, lateral and posterior cricoarytenoid muscles, and the interarytenoid muscle.

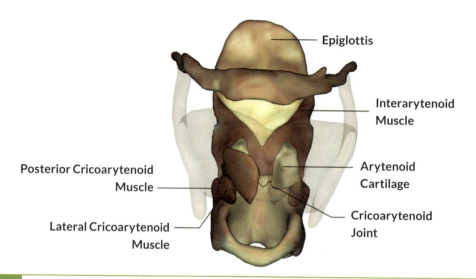

Figure 7.5 Arytenoid cartilages, cricoarytenoid joint, epiglottis, lateral and posterior cricoarytenoid muscles, and the interarytenoid muscle. Used with permission from Anatomage.

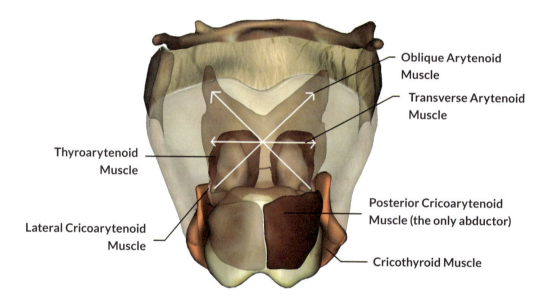

Figure 7.6 Intrinsic laryngeal muscles. Used with permission from Anatomage.

Cuneiform Cartilages

The cuneiform cartilages are tiny, cone-shaped cartilage pieces under the mucous membrane that covers the aryepiglottic folds. They play a minor role in maintaining structure of the aryepiglottic folds.

Intrinsic Laryngeal Muscles

There are five intrinsic laryngeal muscles (see Figure 7.6). Each muscle has both their origin and insertion to structures within the larynx. All of the muscles, except one muscle, are vocal fold adductors. The intrinsic laryngeal muscles are primarily responsible for controlling vocalization.

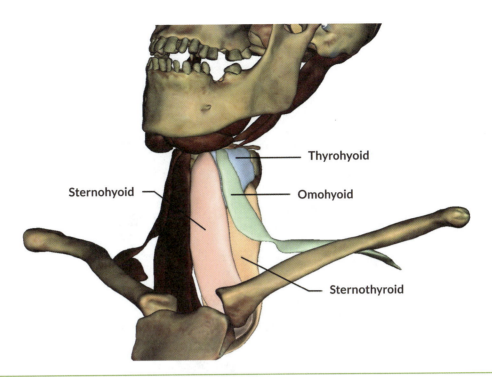

Figure 7.7 Infrahyoid laryngeal muscles. Used with permission from Anatomage.

The following are the intrinsic laryngeal muscles:

- Thyroarytenoid
- Cricothyroid
- Posterior cricoarytenoid (the only abductor)
- Lateral cricoarytenoid
- Interarytenoid (transverse and oblique)

Extrinsic Laryngeal Muscles

The extrinsic laryngeal muscles have one attachment to a structure outside the larynx and one attachment to a structure within the larynx. All extrinsic laryngeal muscles are attached to the hyoid bone.

- These muscles elevate and lower the position of the larynx in the neck. They give the larynx fixed support.
- The **infrahyoid** laryngeal muscles (Figure 7.7) lie below the hyoid bone. Their primary function is to depress the larynx. They are sometimes called the **depressors.** They influence the pitch of the voice; lower frequencies resonate better in a longer tube. A list of the infrahyoid muscles follows (one can remember them by the acronym TOSS):

  - Thyrohyoid
  - Omohyoid
  - Sternothyroid
  - Sternohyoid

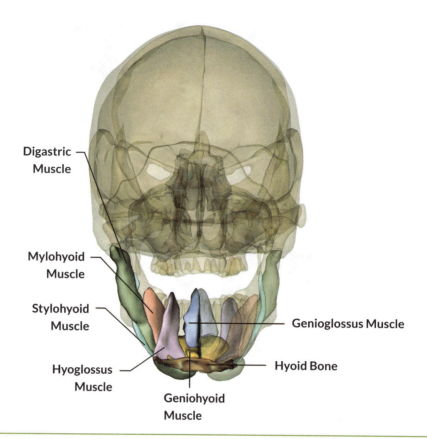

Figure 7.8 Suprahyoid laryngeal muscles. Used with permission from Anatomage.

- The **suprahyoid** laryngeal muscles lie above the hyoid bone (Figure 7.8); their primary function is to elevate the larynx. They are sometimes called **elevators.** They influence pitch by elevating the larynx and creating a smaller resonating tube. Suprahyoids are also responsible for raising the larynx during swallowing. The suprahyoid muscles follow:

- Digastric (anterior and posterior bellies)
- Geniohyoid
- Mylohyoid
- Stylohyoid
- Genioglossus
- Hyoglossus

Voice Changes Through the Life Span

Infancy Through Adolescence

Mean Fundamental Frequency
From birth throughout middle age there is a gradual and discernible decline in mean fundamental frequency (MFF). As people grow older, their voices become lower in pitch, though there are some gender differences later in life.

- Most studies suggest that boys' and girls' voices are similar before adolescence. During adolescence, changes in pitch become noticeable.
- The MFF of 7- and 8-year-old children ranges from 281 to 297 Hz. The MFF of 10- and 11-year-old children ranges from 238 to 270 Hz.
- The MFF of 19-year-old females is 217 Hz; 19-year-old males have an MFF of 117 Hz.

Maximum Phonation Time

Maximum phonation time (MPT) refers to a client's ability to sustain "ah." Usually, the client is asked to breathe deeply and "say ah for as long as you can."

- The MPT of 3- and 4-year-old children ranges from 7.50 to 8.95 seconds. The MPT of 5- to 12-year-old children ranges from 14.97 to 17.74 seconds.

Changes Resulting from Puberty

During puberty, girls' voices may lower by three to four semitones; boys' voices may lower by as much as an octave. Boys may show pitch breaks, huskiness, and hoarseness as their pitch lowers due to laryngeal growth.

Adulthood

Men have an MFF of 100–150 Hz. The typical fundamental frequency for men is approximately 125 Hz. Women have an MFF of 180–250 Hz, and the average fundamental frequency for women is approximately 225 Hz. Men typically have larger vocal folds, which is why their MFF is lower than a woman's MFF.

- Adults aged 18–39 have an MPT ranging from 20.90 to 24.60 seconds.

The Geriatric Voice

Females 70–94 years old have an MFF of 201 Hz; males 70–89 years old have an MFF that ranges from 132 to 146 Hz.

- Adults aged 66–93 years have an MPT ranging from 14.20 to 18.10 seconds.
- The voice can go through many changes throughout later adulthood. Certain diseases (e.g., Parkinson's disease) can have a significant effect on the voice causing weakness, tremors, hoarseness, and breathiness; however, some generalizations can be made about the aging voice.
- Age-related changes in the larynx include hardening of the laryngeal cartilages, degeneration and atrophy of the intrinsic laryngeal muscles, degeneration of glands in the laryngeal mucosa, degenerative changes in the lamina propria, deterioration and decreased flexibility of the cricoarytenoid joint, and degenerative changes in the conus elasticus.
- These changes alter the vibratory pattern of the vocal folds and may cause **presbyphonia** (or **presbylaryngis**), an age-related voice disorder characterized by perceptual changes in quality, range, loudness, and pitch in the older speaker's voice (Boone et al., 2013).
- A person's fundamental frequency appears to lower with each successive decade of life through 50 years of age. A female's voice continues to lower in fundamental frequency as long as she lives, whereas a male's fundamental frequency begins to get slightly higher in his 60s and in every decade after that.

- Some older people speak more slowly and with decreased loudness. The decreased loudness may be related to increases in breathiness.

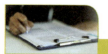

SUMMARY

The larynx is a biological valve that helps humans perform certain functions. It also houses the vocal folds, which vibrate to produce voicing.

- Key structures in the laryngeal area include the hyoid bone, epiglottis, thyroid cartilage, cricoid cartilage, arytenoid cartilages, corniculate cartilages, and cuneiform cartilages. There are two groups of laryngeal muscles: the intrinsic and the extrinsic laryngeal muscles.
- There are three sets of vocal folds: the aryepiglottic folds; the ventricular, or false vocal folds; and the true vocal folds, which vibrate to produce voice.
- Cranial nerve X (vagus nerve), with its superior and recurrent laryngeal nerve branches that innervate the larynx, is the key cranial nerve in laryngeal function.
- The voice changes throughout the life span. Mean fundamental frequency declines from birth on, with more dramatic changes for the male in adolescence. Older males and females differ in fundamental frequency changes. Maximum phonation time grows greater between childhood and adulthood. It usually decreases as people age.

VOCAL PITCH, LOUDNESS, AND QUALITY

Pitch, loudness, and quality are important perceptual characteristics of the voice. People's personality, intelligence, and competence are often judged by these parameters (Isetti, Xuereb, & Eadie, 2014; Justice & Redle, 2014). Recent research has shown that even children can be negatively judged by adults around them if the children are dysphonic (Ma & Yu, 2013). Voice disorders tend to affect vocal pitch, loudness, and quality. Experienced clinicians listen for disturbances in these aspects of voice when evaluating clients with voice disorders.

Pitch

The vocal folds vibrate to make sound for voice. During vibration, vocal folds have a closed phase and an open phase which equals one cycle of vibration. Frequency, the number of cycles per second, is the rate at which the vocal folds vibrate. Higher frequencies have more cycles per second than lower frequencies. Pitch is the perceptual correlate of frequency and is typically described as how high or low the voice sounds. Pitch is largely based on the frequency of vocal fold vibration as is called **fundamental frequency.** Speaking fundamental frequency is generally considered an individual's habitual or typical speaking pitch.

- Pitch is determined by mass, tension, and elasticity of the vocal folds. Higher pitch results when the vocal folds are thinner, more tense, or both; lower pitch results when the folds are thicker, more

relaxed, or both. Frequency can stay constant and pitch can change by changing the size or length of the resonating cavity, the vocal tract. A smaller resonating tube will be perceived as a higher pitch.
- **Frequency perturbation**, or **jitter**, refers to irregularities or cycle-to-cycle variations in vocal fold vibration that are often heard in dysphonic patients.
  - Jitter can be measured instrumentally as a patient sustains a vowel. Patients with voice problems, such as tremor or hoarseness, might show a large amount of jitter. People with no laryngeal pathology are able to sustain a vowel with less than 1% jitter.

Loudness

The perceptual correlate of intensity is loudness, which is determined by the amplitude of the sound signal; the larger the amplitude of vibration, the more intense the sound signal, the greater its perceived loudness.

- Changes in air pressure created during vocal fold vibration displaces air particles. A chain reaction of air particle disturbance creates a sound wave. Force determines the extent to which air particles are displaced from their resting state to a maximum point of displacement. Amplitude is the magnitude of particle displacement. The greater the **amplitude**, the louder the voice.
- **Amplitude perturbation**, or **shimmer**, refers to the cycle-to-cycle variations in vocal fold amplitude. It can be measured instrumentally as a patient sustains a vowel. A speaker with no laryngeal pathology should have a very small amount of amplitude perturbation with each vibratory cycle. Some experts believe that more than 1 dB of variation across cycles makes a patient sound dysphonic. Patients who have difficulties with regularity of vocal fold vibration (e.g., roughness) might show large amounts of shimmer.
- Measures of shimmer and jitter have been used in voice assessment because they can be useful in early detection of vocal pathology, though their utility is often debated.

Quality

Definition

Quality is the perception of the sound of an individual's voice. The determination of voice quality is frequently subjective (Stemple, Roy, & Klaben, 2014) and is often based on the degree of clarity, breathiness, strain, loudness, pitch, and regularity in vibration of the voice.

Types of Vocal Quality

Hoarseness
The hoarse voice shows a combination of breathiness and harshness, which results from irregular vocal fold vibrations. Hoarse voices often sound breathy, low pitched, and husky. There may also be pitch breaks and excessive throat clearing.

Harshness

The harsh voice is described as rough, unpleasant, and "gravelly" sounding. It is associated with excessive muscular tension and effort. The vocal folds are adducted too tightly, and the air is then released too abruptly.

Strain-Strangle

In a strain-strangle voice, phonation is effortful, and the patient sounds as if she is "squeezing" the voice at the glottal level. Initiating and sustaining phonation are both difficult. Talking fatigues such patients, and they experience much tension when they speak.

Breathiness

The breathy voice results from the vocal folds being slightly open, or not firmly approximated, during phonation. Air escapes through the glottis and adds noise to the sound produced by the vocal folds.

- Breathiness may be due to **organic** (physical) or **nonorganic** (nonphysical, or **functional**) causes. Patients often complain that they feel like they are running out of air.
- Breathy voices are often quiet, with little variation in loudness. Patients frequently show restricted vocal range.

Glottal Fry

Also called **vocal fry**, glottal fry is heard when the vocal folds vibrate very slowly with no clear, regular pattern of vibration. The resulting sound occurs in slow but discrete bursts and is of extremely low pitch. The voice sounds "crackly."

- Vocal fry may be the vibratory cycle we use near the bottom of our normal pitch range. Typically, it is produced near the end of a long phrase or sentence when air flow rate and subglottal air pressure are both low and lung volume is less.
- For some patients, use of vocal fry may help modify vocal quality problems, such as stridency. Other patients work to eliminate vocal fry by slightly increasing subglottal air pressure and slightly elevating their pitch level (Boone et al., 2013).

Diplophonia

Diplophonia means "double voice." It occurs when a listener can simultaneously perceive two distinct pitches during phonation.

- Diplophonia usually occurs when the vocal folds vibrate at different frequencies due to differing degrees of mass or tension. A client with a unilateral polyp, for example, might sound diplophonic.

Stridency

A patient with a strident voice sounds shrill, unpleasant, somewhat high pitched, and "tinny."

- Physiologically, stridency is often caused by hypertonicity or tension of the pharyngeal constrictors and elevation of the larynx. Tense patients may sound strident.

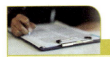

SUMMARY

Pitch (the perceptual correlate of frequency) and loudness (the perceptual correlate of intensity) are important vocal parameters that clinicians must evaluate in all voice patients. Measures of jitter and shimmer can be helpful in evaluating the dysphonic patient.

- Vocal quality is often affected by pathological changes of the vocal folds and the laryngeal mechanism. Patients can manifest such vocal qualities as hoarseness, harshness, strain-strangle, breathiness, glottal fry, and diplophonia.
- Experienced clinicians evaluate patients' pitch, loudness, and quality as factors in determining if a voice disorder exists.

EVALUATION OF VOICE DISORDERS

A thorough voice evaluation is critical to creating an individualized, successful treatment program. When conducting evaluations, clinicians must remember to carry out a thorough oral peripheral examination, a hearing screening, and analysis of a speech–language sample. Gathering a complete case history is important. A team-oriented approach to evaluation is always necessary; the team may consist of specialists from medicine, education, and professional voice pedagogy. Clinicians, depending upon their settings and the availability of technology, typically use both instrumental and perceptual tools to evaluate patients' voices (Owens, Farinella, & Metz, 2015).

Case History: Purposes and Goals

In taking a case history, the clinician needs to do the following:

- Obtain information about variables, such as perceptions of the patient, onset, duration, causes, and variability of the voice problem.
- Obtain information about any associated symptoms or problems, such as slurring of speech, difficulty swallowing, excessive coughing, and so forth.
- Identify any factors (e.g., health, environment, family history) that might be contributing to the problem.
- Gather information regarding previous therapy, medical intervention, or other attempts to deal with the voice problem.
- Obtain patient and significant others' descriptions of daily vocal load and usage patterns.
- Obtain patient's medical history, including any surgeries that required intubation, traumas, hospitalizations, and current medications being taken.
- For culturally and linguistically diverse clients, obtain their specific perceptions of what constitutes a "typical-sounding" voice in their particular culture (Behlau & Murry, 2012).

A Team-Oriented Approach

A multidisciplinary, team-oriented approach is critical to a thorough evaluation of voice disorders. Before beginning therapy, it is always necessary to obtain a medical evaluation of the vocal mechanism; this is performed by a laryngologist (i.e., board-certified otolaryngologist who specializes in the larynx or voice). In some cases, before treatment is initiated, it may also be necessary to refer the patient to a neurologist. The team always includes the speech–language pathologist, but teams may include the following: general practitioner, neurologist, otolaryngologist, classroom teacher, school nurse, psychologist, counselor, voice scientists, and vocal pedagogy teachers.

Instrumental Evaluation

Instrumentation is increasingly being used to provide an objective, data-based description of the dysphonic patient's vocal characteristics (Ikuna, Kunduk, & McWhorter, 2014; Roy et al., 2014). A description of each type of evaluation follows.

Indirect Laryngoscopy (Mirror Laryngoscopy)

In indirect laryngoscopy, the specialist uses a bright light source and a small, round 21–25-mm mirror, angled on a long, slender handle, to lift the velum and press gently against the patient's posterior pharyngeal wall area.

- The specialist maneuvers the mirror to view the laryngeal structures during phonation (usually the patient's production of "eeeee") and during quiet respiration.

Direct Laryngoscopy

Direct laryngoscopy is performed by a surgeon when the patient is under general anesthesia in outpatient surgery. The laryngoscope is introduced through the mouth into the pharynx and positioned above the vocal folds.

- The patient cannot phonate during this procedure; thus, vocal function cannot be determined. However, the surgeon can obtain a direct microscopic view of the larynx.
- Direct laryngoscopy is valuable when a biopsy is required due to the suspicion of laryngeal cancer.

Flexible or Rigid Endoscopy With Videostroboscopy

- When an endoscope is attached to a video camera, it is known as videoendoscopy. If it also utilizes a stroboscopic (flashing) light source, it is known as videostroboscopy.
- Videostroboscopy can be helpful in differentiating between functional and organic voice problems. It can also be used to detect laryngeal neoplasms (tumors). The specialist can perform videostroboscopy by using a *flexible* fiber-optic endoscope, a *rigid* endoscope, or both. The rigid endoscope is introduced orally; the flexible endoscope is introduced nasally, using a 3.6-mm tube (see Figure 7.9). There is a light at the tip of either scope; this light is fiber optic and comes from an external light source. The structures are illuminated by the light and viewed by the specialist at the other end of the endoscope through a window lens.
- Flexible fiber-optic laryngoscopy uses a thin, flexible tube containing a lens and fiber-optic light bundles. The specialist inserts the tube through the patient's nasal passage, passes it over the velum, and maneuvers it into position above the larynx. The fibers transmit the laryngeal image to the

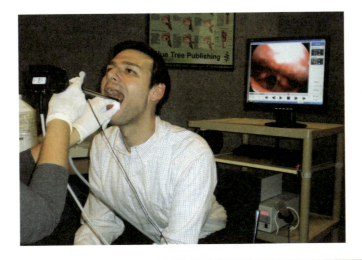

Figure 7.9 Videostroboscopy. Used with permission from Dr. Cari Tellis, Professor, Misericordia University.

specialist's eyepiece. The patient is able to speak and sing during the procedure. The specialist can obtain an excellent, prolonged view of the velopharyngeal and vocal mechanisms. The specialist can also view the false vocal folds to observe if maladaptive compensatory movement of the false vocal folds is present during phonation (Sapienza & Hoffman Ruddy, 2017).

- The strobe light is a pulsing light that is flashed at the same fundamental frequency of the vocal folds and permits the optical illusion of slow-motion viewing of the vocal folds during a variety of tasks. The observer perceives the rapidly presented images as a complete picture of cycle-to-cycle vibration (vibratory pattern of phonation).
- The specialist places a microphone on the patient's neck along the thyroid cartilage to record the voice signal and then introduces the scope, switches on the stroboscopic light, and asks the patient to phonate. The resulting image on the monitor screen is projected through optic devices, such as a digital distal chip, an endoscope, and pixels on the monitor screen.
- The stroboscopic image yields information about the periodicity or regularity of vocal fold vibrations, vocal fold amplitude (horizontal excursion), glottal closure, presence and adequacy of the mucosal wave, and the possible presence of lesions or neoplasms.

Acoustic Analysis

Acoustic measurements of voice are often used as a means of evaluating the effectiveness of voice therapy (Haynes & Pindzola, 2012).

- **Sound spectography** is the graphic representation of a sound wave's intensity and frequency as a function of time. The **spectrogram**, or resulting picture, reflects the resonant characteristics of the vocal tract and the harmonic nature of the glottal sound source (Boone et al., 2013).
- Spectrograms can be represented by a wideband (Figure 7.10) or narrowband (Figure 7.11). Wideband spectrograms provide better time resolution, while narrowband spectrograms have better frequency resolution. Individual harmonics are easily seen using a narrowband spectrogram; therefore,

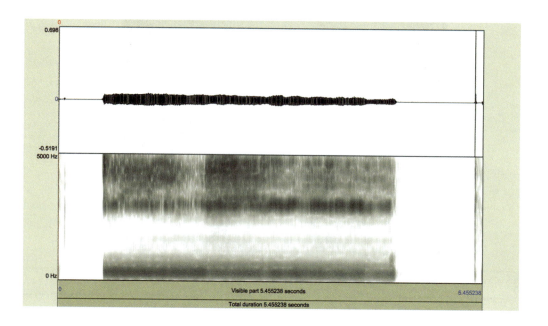

Figure 7.10 Wideband spectrogram. Used with permission from Dr. Cari Tellis, Professor, Misericordia University.

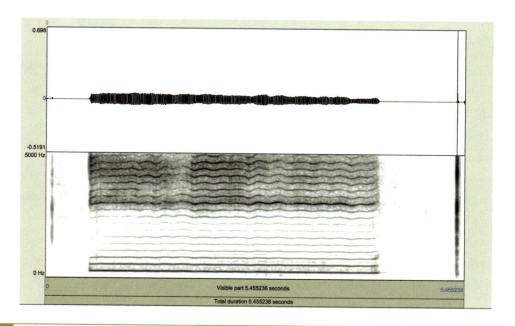

Figure 7.11 Narrowband spectrogram. Used with permission from Dr. Cari Tellis, Professor, Misericordia University.

this type of spectrogram is useful for evaluating clients with voice disorders, because it creates a graphic representation of the stability (or instability) of the harmonic structure (Sapienza & Hoffman Ruddy, 2017).

- The sound or speech spectrograph is extremely useful for quantitative analysis of speech. It produces waveform displays of amplitude and frequency, spectrograms, and other analysis displays in real time.

- The Sona-Graph's memory can store up to 2 megabytes of sampled data; this translates to approximately 50 seconds of speech sampled at 20 kHz. These same analyses can also be made on the Computer Speech Laboratory (CSL; also made by Kay Elemetrics).

■ Clinicians can use the above-described instruments to obtain baseline measurements prior to therapy or surgery. Post-therapy or post-surgery measurements may be obtained and compared to the baseline measurements of a patient's voice to quantitatively document vocal improvement or decline. Surgeons often rely upon these measurements to help with evaluating the success of vocal surgery that has been performed.

Electroglottography

The noninvasive procedure of electroglottography (EGG) yields an indirect measure of vocal fold closure patterns.

■ Surface electrodes are placed on both sides of the thyroid cartilage, and a high-frequency electric current is passed between the electrodes while the patient phonates. The laryngeal and neck tissues conduct the current.

■ A glottal wave form results, and the specialist is able to observe vocal fold vibration. EGG can also detect breathy and abrupt glottal onset of phonation.

■ Researchers and practitioners disagree about the efficacy of EGG as a diagnostic technique. It is currently recommended as a cross-validation tool with other measures of vocal fold functioning.

Laryngeal Electromyography

Laryngeal electromyography (LEMG) is an invasive procedure that directly measures laryngeal function to study the pattern of electrical activity of the vocal folds and to view muscle activity patterns.

■ The specialist inserts needle electrodes into the patient's peripheral laryngeal muscles; the resulting electrical signals are judged as either normal or indicative of pathology.

■ When the specialist interprets the electrical signals, she is looking for (a) reduced or increased speed of muscle activation, (b) extraneous bursts of muscle activity, or (c) onset or termination of muscle activity.

■ LEMG is useful when attempting to determine vocal fold pathology, especially one that is caused by neurological and neuromuscular diseases. It is also useful in verifying excessive muscle activity prior to the injection of Botox (botulinus toxin, described later) for patients with spasmodic dysphonia (SMD).

Videokymography

A recently developed procedure, videokymography is a high-speed medical imaging method used to visualize human vocal fold vibration dynamics (Stemple et al., 2014).

■ Videokymography uses a traditional rigid endoscope and a modified videocamera to work in standard and high-speed modes. In the high-speed mode, the camera selects one active horizontal line (transverse to the glottis) from the whole laryngeal image. The successive line images are shown in real time on a commercial TV monitor.

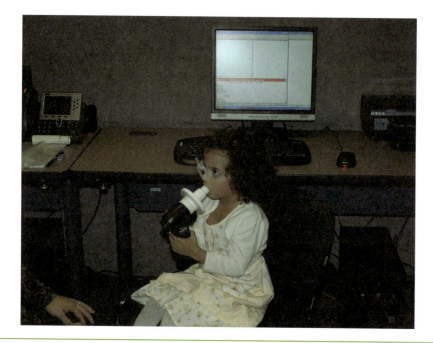

Figure 7.12 Spirometry. Used with permission from Dr. Cari Tellis, Professor, Misericordia University.

- This system allows visualization of left–right vocal fold asymmetries, propagation of mucosal waves, and movement of the upper and lower margins of the vocal folds.

Aerodynamic Measurements

Aerodynamic measurements refer to the airflows, air volumes, and average air pressures produced as part of the peripheral mechanics of the respiratory, laryngeal, and supralaryngeal airways.

- Specialists use aerodynamic measurements to evaluate dysphonia, monitor voice changes and treatment progress, and differentiate between laryngeal and respiratory problems. Many specialists want to assess a patient's lung volume because breath support for optimal voice may be lacking. Specific measures can be made of the following parameters:

  - **Tidal volume**—amount of air inhaled and exhaled during a normal breathing cycle
  - **Vital capacity**—the volume of air that the patient can exhale after a maximal inhalation
  - **Total lung capacity**—total volume of air in the lungs

- Various instruments may be used to obtain aerodynamic measurements. Some of the most common include **wet spirometers**, **dry spirometers**, **manometric devices**, and **plethysmographs**. (For further description of these forms of instrumentation, see Boone et al., 2013 and Stemple et al., 2014; see Figure 7.12 for Spirometry.)
- There are computer-based systems that use a face mask to measure parameters of airflow and air pressure during voice production. The software also contains normative data for comparison. Some key parameters obtained by the instruments include mean sound pressure level (SPL), mean peak air pressure, mean airflow during voicing, and mean pitch.

Acoustic Measurements

Many instruments can be used to measure acoustic characteristics of voice production.

- With the Visi-Pitch, the patient speaks into a microphone, and the Visi-Pitch displays his or her frequencies on a computer monitor. The Visi-Pitch IV (Model 3950, Kay PENTAX Corp.) is a popular clinical tool that measures dynamic range, intensity and frequency variability, pitch and loudness, and other parameters.
- The Visi-Pitch is noninvasive and affordable, and it gives instant visual feedback to both clinician and patient.

Perceptual Evaluation

Basic Principles

In perceptual voice evaluation, the clinician makes subjective judgments of many vocal parameters, including the patient's pitch, volume, vocal quality, resonance, respiration, and ability to sustain phonation.

- Many rating scales are available for making these judgments; Figure 7.13 is an example of a scale that the clinician can use for making subjective judgments.
- The Consensus Auditory–Perceptual Evaluation of Voice (CAPE-V) is a research and clinical tool created to encourage a standardized approach to evaluating and documenting auditory–perceptual judgments of voice quality. It is not intended as a standalone assessment of an individual's voice; rather, it should be used in conjunction with laryngeal examination and instrumental assessments (Sapienza & Hoffman Ruddy, 2017).
  - The clinician uses a nominal rating scale to evaluate various vocal parameters; the clinician's written descriptions may also be included (Kempster, Gerratt, Abbott, Barkmeier-Kraemer, & Hillman, 2009).

Pitch Assessment

To assess pitch, clinicians make subjective judgments about the following:

- The patient's habitual pitch, or typical conversational pitch
- Whether the client is using optimal pitch (judged to be the most appropriate, comfortable pitch for that individual)
- Whether the pitch is appropriate to the client's gender and age, rather than too high or too low
- Whether the patient is **mono-pitched**, that is, lacking appropriate inflections, as judged by members of his or her culture

Loudness Assessment

To assess loudness, clinicians make subjective judgments about the following:

- Parameters such as harshness, hoarseness, breathiness, and vocal tension
- Whether the client's loudness is appropriate to daily situations
- Whether the client's voice is too soft or too loud due to possible physical factors (e.g., asthma, hearing loss)

University Speech and Hearing Center

Client _____ Age _____ Sex _____

Clinician _____ Date/time _____

		Normal	Mild	Moderate	Severe	Profound
1.	Voice quality Breathy/Harsh/Hoarse	1	2	3	**(4)**	5

The voice was judged hoarse on 90% of the utterances produced in conversational speech.

		Normal	Mild	Moderate	Severe	Profound
2.	Pitch Too high/Too low	1	2	3	**(4)**	5

The client's pitch was judged too high on 80% of the utterances produced in conversational speech.

		Normal	Mild	Moderate	Severe	Profound
3.	Loudness Too loud/Too soft	1	2	**(3)**	4	5

The client's voice was judged too loud during most of the assessment time.

		Normal	Mild	Moderate	Severe	Profound
4.	Nasal resonance Hypernasal/Hyponasal	1	2	**(3)**	4	5

The client's voice was judged hypernasal on 45% of the utterances produced in conversational speech.

		Normal	Mild	Moderate	Severe	Profound
5.	Oral resonance Reduced oral resonance	1	**(2)**	3	4	5

The client spoke with limited mouth opening; on most utterances, the oral resonance was reduced.

		Normal	Mild	Moderate	Severe	Profound
6.	Muscle tension Hypertense/Hypotense	1	2	**(3)**	4	5

The client's muscles of the face, neck, and chest were judged hypertense during conversational speech.

		Normal	Mild	Moderate	Severe	Profound
7.	Abusive vocal behaviors	1	2	3	**(4)**	5

Client has a history of vocally abusive behaviors including loud and excessive talking, loud cheering at games, and screaming and yelling while playing with friends.

Comments and Recommendations: *The client speaks with excessive muscular tension and effort; voice is excessively hoarse most of the time; there is a history of frequent and severe abusive vocal behaviors. Voice therapy is recommended to reduce the frequency and severity of such behaviors.*

Figure 7.13 Summary of voice assessment data using a rating scale. The comments are for illustration only; a given client may not exhibit all the problems described. From *Introduction to Communicative Disorders* (5th ed.), by M. N. Hegde, forthcoming, Austin, TX: PRO-ED. Copyright by PRO-ED, Inc. Reprinted with permission.

Resonance Assessment

To assess resonance, clinicians subjectively judge the presence of the following:

- **Hyponasality**—nasal resonance absent on nasal sounds
- **Hypernasality**—too much nasal resonance on non-nasal sounds

Respiration Assessment

To assess respiration, many clinicians look for the following types of breathing:

- **Clavicular breathing.** When the patient inhales, the shoulders elevate. Often there is strain and tension. Clavicular breathing is inefficient.
- **Diaphragmatic–abdominal breathing.** This technique includes the use the abdominal region and the lower thoracic cavity. There is little to no chest or shoulder movement. Diaphragmatic–abdominal breathing is ideal for professional voice users, including singers, teachers, and public speakers.
- **Thoracic breathing.** The patient who uses thoracic breathing uses inhalation to expand the thorax by using the intercostal muscles to raise the ribs.

Phonation Assessment

To assess a patient's ability to sustain phonation, clinicians use simple measures, such as the following:

- **Maximum phonation time.** As mentioned earlier, maximum phonation time (MPT) is a measurement of the patient's ability to sustain phonation (e.g., "ah") during one exhalation. The clinician generally gives the patient three trials and compares the patient's MPT (in seconds) with norms. MPT enables the clinician to observe adequacy of respiration, glottal efficiency, and the possible presence of vocal pathology, such as nodules.
- **s/z ratio.** This procedure is used to help determine whether there is laryngeal pathology present; it indicates the efficiency of glottal closure. The patient is asked to produce two long /s/ phonemes, then two long /z/ phonemes. The clinician divides the longest /s/ by the longest /z/. For example, a patient may sustain /s/ for 15 seconds and /z/ for 9 seconds. This would yield an s/z ratio of 15/9, or 1.6. An s/z ratio of more than 1.4 is indicative of possible laryngeal pathology. Because /z/ is a voiced sound, a vocal fold lesion may interfere with glottal closure and, thus, reduce the length of time /z/ can be sustained.

Quality of Life Evaluation

It is important to determine the effect of the voice disorder on overall quality of life. Several scales and questionnaires exist for clients to fill out with their initial case history.

- One of these measures is the Voice Handicap Index (VHI) (Jacobson, Johnson, Grywalski, Silbergleit, Jacobson, & Benninger, 1997), an 85-item scale that consists of three subscales to assess a client's quality of life: **physical** (aspects of the voice disorder itself), **functional** (how the voice disorder impacts daily activities), and **social** (how the client feels about the voice disorder).

- A shorter version, the VHI-10, is also available. For pediatric clients, caregivers can complete the Pediatric Voice Handicap Index (pVHI) (Zur, Cotton, Kelchner, Baker, Weinrich, & Lee, 2007). The VHI can also be used to track changes before, during, and after voice therapy to assess if the disorder's negative impact on the client's quality of life has diminished.

- A similar scale, the Voice Related Quality of Life (VRQOL) scale (Hogikyan & Sethuraman, 1999), is a 10-item questionnaire for adult clients that assesses social-emotional and physical-functional impacts of a voice disorder.
- The Pediatric Voice Related Quality of Life (PVQROL) scale (Boseley, Cunningham, Volk, & Hartnick, 2006) is available for parents and caregivers to complete for pediatric clients.

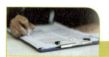

SUMMARY

A comprehensive, multidisciplinary team assessment of the voice patient is necessary as a foundation for appropriate treatment. A key component of assessment is a thorough case history.

- Instrumentation procedures that various specialists can use to assess a patient's voice include indirect or mirror laryngoscopy, direct laryngoscopy, flexible or rigid endoscopy with videostroboscopy, electroglottography, electromyography, and videokymography. Instruments may also be used to obtain aerodynamic and pitch measurements.
- In a perceptual evaluation (which can occur alone or accompany instrumental evaluation), clinicians often use rating scales and informal tasks to assess pitch, loudness, vocal quality, resonance, respiration, and the ability to sustain phonation.
- Quality of life scales provide insight on how a voice disorder impacts several aspects of an individual's life.
- Ideally, each patient is evaluated through a combination of measures that permit both qualitative and quantitative baseline measures and documentation of progress in voice therapy.

DISORDERS OF RESONANCE AND THEIR TREATMENT

Resonance is the modification of sound by the structures through which the sound passes. The resonating structures that lie below and above the larynx (e.g., the oral and nasal cavities) modify the laryngeal tone. Voice disorders of resonance include an absence of a desired resonance (hyponasality), inadequate (cul-de-sac) resonance, or inappropriate (assimilative) resonance. Appropriate resonance or lack thereof is based in part on cultural and linguistic norms. Among some cultural and linguistic groups (e.g., Americans living in the United States), there is little tolerance for hypernasality in conversational speech. Some Asians (speakers of Chinese, for example) may have slightly more hypernasality than Americans perceive as normal or desirable (Roseberry-McKibbin, 2014). Clinicians must always take patients' cultural and linguistic backgrounds into account when judging resonance.

Hypernasality

Hypernasality is the most common resonance disorder presented by patients who come for services. A person who exhibits hypernasality, or excessive nasality, sounds like he or she is speaking through the nose.

- Hypernasality results when the velopharyngeal mechanism does not close the opening to the nasal passage during the production of non-nasal sounds. The air and sound escape through the nose, adding unnecessary nasal resonance to non-nasal speech sounds.
- Hypernasality is especially noticed on vowels because these sounds are voiced, longer than most consonants, and are usually not substituted with different placement. Hypernasality is more prominent on high vowels than low vowels, because a high tongue position reduces space for oral resonance and increases sound pressure through the velum (Kummer, 2014).
- When clients are hypernasal, they often speak with decreased or insufficient intraoral breath pressure, affecting the production of fricatives, affricates, and plosives. These classes of sounds are produced "weakly" due to lack of sufficient intraoral breath pressure.
- Hypernasality can occur due to functional or organic factors. In the case of functional hypernasality, there is no physical reason for the hypernasality; the patient has made a habit of "talking through the nose." Functional nasality is often found in the speech of deaf people; they have adequate velopharyngeal mechanisms but are unable to monitor the sound of their own voices.
- Patients who are hypernasal due to organic factors have a physical problem that may need to be corrected surgically. **Cleft palate** is a major cause of hypernasality. Patients with inadequate cleft repairs are often severely hypernasal.
- Patients may also be hypernasal due to the presence of a **submucous cleft** of the hard or soft palate (described in more detail in Chapter 10), which is often associated with a bifid uvula.
- **Velopharyngeal inadequacy** or **insufficiency** (VPI), another cause of hypernasality, means that the velopharyngeal mechanism is inadequate to achieve closure; as a result, the nasal cavities are not sealed off appropriately from the oral cavity. The etiology of VPI is heterogeneous and may be neurological, structural, or learned. Major causes of VPI are the following:

  - Decreased muscle mass of the velum (not enough velar tissue) to achieve closure
  - Adenoidectomy or tonsillectomy. This occurs especially when a child's velopharyngeal mechanism initially did not have sufficient muscle mass. The adenoids and tonsils are masses that can help compensate for an otherwise inadequate velopharyngeal mechanism. When these masses are surgically removed, the basic velopharyngeal inadequacy may become apparent.
  - Paresis (weakness) or paralysis of the velum, which reduces its mobility, so it is unable to assist in achieving adequate closure. Velar paresis and paralysis frequently occur secondarily to cerebral palsy, stroke, head injury, debilitative diseases, such as Parkinson's disease, and other conditions of neuropathology.

- Assessment of hypernasality can include subjective, perceptual judgments as well as use of instrumentation such as the nasometer (described in the "Treatment Principles" section of this chapter).

Hyponasality

Hyponasality, or **denasality**, is a lack of appropriate nasal resonance on nasal sounds /m/, /n/, and /ng/. Patients often substitute oral sounds for nasal sounds (e.g., "*b*aby" instead of "*m*aybe"). Frequent substitutions are b/m, d/n, and g/ng.

- Hyponasality can be temporary, due to conditions such as colds and allergies. It can also occur due to obstructions in the nasal cavity (e.g., nasal polyps or papilloma), enlarged adenoids or tonsils, or a deviated septum. Hyponasal patients may be mouth breathers.
- Enlargement of the tonsils and adenoids is common in young children and can result in marked hyponasality. Hypertrophy of the tonsils and adenoids can block both the oropharyngeal and nasal pathways; in severe cases, sleep apnea can result. Assessment of the degree of obstruction may be performed using lateral X-ray studies of the nasopharyngeal area.
- Assessment of hyponasality can include subjective, perceptual judgments as well as use of instrumentation, such as the nasometer (described later).

Assimilative Nasality

Assimilative nasality occurs when the sound from a nasal consonant carries over to adjacent vowels. For example, in the word **banana**, the /ə/ and /æ/ sounds appear hypernasal because they are next to the nasal sound /n/.

- In assimilative nasality, the velar openings begin too soon and last too long, thus nasalizing vowels that occur next to nasal phonemes.
- Assimilative nasality can be functionally or organically based; assessment and treatment depend on etiology.

Cul-de-Sac Resonance

Cul-de-sac (bottom of the sack) resonance occurs when sound waves enter the vocal tract but are blocked from exiting. The trapped sound is then absorbed by the soft tissues in the vocal tract, creating speech that sounds muffled or hollow. There are three different types of cul-de-sac resonance, depending on where the obstruction occurs.

- **Oral** cul-de-sac resonance occurs when sound is partially blocked from exiting the oral cavity during speech production. This can be produced by backward retraction of the tongue; the tongue is carried too far posteriorly in the oral cavity. Individuals who are deaf and those with neurological disorders often have difficulty making proper tongue adjustments, resulting in cul-de-sac resonance. People with no organic deviations also may acquire the habit of carrying the tongue too far back in the oral cavity while speaking. A small mouth (microstomia) can also create oral cul-de-sac resonance.
- **Nasal** cul-de-sac resonance occurs when sound is partially obstructed from exiting the nasal cavity during the production of speech. This mostly occurs when an individual has VPI combined with a blockage in the anterior nasal cavity, such as a deviated septum or a narrowing of the nares (stenosis).

- **Pharyngeal** cul-de-sac resonance occurs when sound is blocked from exiting the oropharynx during speech production. Hypertrophied tonsils, adenoids, scarring, or other structural abnormalities of the pharyngeal wall may cause pharyngeal cul-de-sac resonance.
- Regardless of where the blockage occurs, cul-de-sac resonance is always caused by a structural anomaly (Kummer, 2014).

Treatment Principles

Medical Intervention

It is always imperative, as a first step in determining the direction of treatment, to ascertain whether the disorders of resonance are due to functional or organic factors. Organically based resonance problems must be treated medically before therapy can be successful.

- Medical treatment can take the form of surgery, prostheses, or both. For example, a child with a cleft palate may undergo surgery to repair a cleft and then be fitted with a prosthesis. (A more detailed description of medical intervention is presented in the section "Craniofacial Anomalies" in Chapter 10).
- Speech therapy may be warranted when the abnormal resonance is a result of improperly learned articulation placement, such as a high tongue placement for all vowels or the consistent use of a nasal sound for an oral sound. These may have been compensatory strategies as a result of a structural abnormality, so speech therapy may still be needed after surgical intervention (Kummer, 2014).

Treatment of Hypernasality

Biofeedback can be effective in treating hypernasality. Electronic instruments provide instantaneous visual feedback of oral and nasal resonance.

- The **nasometer**, an instrument created by Kay Elemetrics, allows the patient to receive visual feedback through a computer display. Feedback includes the target level of **nasalance** (oral–nasal ratio) and the amount of nasalance the patient is producing. The patient's productions can be shaped so they increasingly reflect an oral–nasal resonance balance that is within normal limits.
- Specific treatment techniques for hypernasality include the following:
  - Employing visual aids, such as a piece of tissue or a mirror, which can be put under a patient's nose so he or she can see appropriate versus inappropriate nasal airflow during phonation
  - Ear training, or helping patients learn to monitor their own productions (instruments such as the nasometer and even recording devices, video or audio, are helpful)
  - Increasing the patient's mouth opening so that oral resonance is enhanced
  - Increasing the patient's loudness, which can be accompanied by respiration training
  - Improving the patient's articulation, which often results in the voice being perceived as less hypernasal (exaggerating consonants can contribute to a perception of less hypernasality)
  - Changing the patient's speaking rate, first assessing whether increasing or decreasing the rate decreases hypernasality

- Decreasing pitch, which can contribute to greater oral resonance, especially if the patient's habitual pitch is too high

Treatment of Hyponasality

As with hypernasality, hyponasality can often be effectively treated through feedback such as that provided by the nasometer and video or audio recordings.

- Specific techniques that can decrease hyponasality involve increasing the patient's awareness of the nasal cavity as a resonator. These techniques include the following:
  - Focusing or directing of the tone into the facial "mask," which is the area above the maxillary sinuses and around the nasal bridge. The clinician demonstrates and then has the patient say words with nasal sounds (e.g., moon, me) in an exaggerated way. This produces vibrations in the mask. The patient is asked to feel the vibrations, focusing his or her attention in the mask area. Appropriate resonance is then shaped from that point of reference.
  - Nasal-glide stimulation. The clinician selects words with many glides and nasals (e.g., lawnmower, many, manners, lemon). The patient practices saying these words in various combinations. The combination of glides and nasals helps direct resonance more appropriately into the nasal cavity and gives the patient auditory and kinesthetic feedback about proper utilization of the nasal cavity.

- Visual aids. A piece of tissue or a mirror may be put under the patient's nose so he or she can see appropriate versus inappropriate nasal airflow during phonation.

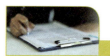

SUMMARY

Resonance is an important component of voice and must be evaluated as part of a thorough voice assessment. Difficulties with resonance include hypernasality, hyponasality, assimilative nasality, and cul-de-sac resonance.

- Treatment may include medical intervention if necessary; the patient with medical–physical needs will not progress until those needs are dealt with.
- When the clinician has ascertained that physical factors have been accounted for and treated appropriately, then he or she can use appropriate treatment techniques to help patients achieve optimal resonance patterns.

DISORDERS OF PHONATION AND THEIR TREATMENT

Many disorders of phonation are associated with physical factors. Some patients have cancer of the larynx; others have progressive diseases of the central nervous system. Some patients present with pathological changes in the vocal folds due to vocally abusive habits, with consequent perceptual sequelae, such as hoarseness, breathiness, harshness, and low pitch; others show no changes in the vocal folds but still have abnormal vocal traits. Other patients may seek assistance to change their voice, speech patterns, and overall communication style after undergoing gender reassignment. In this section, we describe some of the major physical factors associated with voice disorders of phonation. Basic treatment principles are also discussed.

Carcinoma and Laryngectomy

Basic Principles

The larynx is one of the most common sites of cancer, accounting for approximately 1% to 2% of all cancers and 20% of all head and neck cancers. In the United States in 2014, more than 55,000 Americans developed cancer of the head and neck (American Academy of Otolaryngology, 2014).

- Laryngeal cancer is found more frequently in men than in women and is considered a multifactorial disease.
- Variables that can contribute to laryngeal cancer are alcohol, tobacco, exposure to environmental toxins (e.g., radiation, asbestos), gastroesophageal reflux, and a combination of these cofactors. People who are heavy smokers and drinkers of alcohol are especially at risk.
- Cancer of the throat can also occur as a result of infection with the human papilloma virus (HPV).
- Early warning signs of laryngeal cancer include hoarseness, difficulty swallowing, a sore throat that does not go away, ear pain, pitch change (usually lower due to added mass on vocal folds), and a lump in the neck or throat.
- Successful treatment of laryngeal cancer is highly dependent upon early detection and intervention.
- Tests that are used to help detect laryngeal cancer include physical examination, laryngoscopy, endoscopy, CT scan, MRI, PET scan, bone scan, barium swallow, and biopsy (National Cancer Institute, 2014).

Medical Treatment

Medical treatment depends on the site, type, and extent of the cancer. Tumors can be **supraglottic** (above the vocal folds), **glottic** (at the level of the vocal folds), or **subglottic** (below the vocal folds). **Metastasis** (spread of the cancer to other regions) and **node involvement** are also major considerations.

- The head and neck cancer will likely be staged using a system of I to IV, which indicates how the cancer is spreading. This staging system is based on the size of the tumor, how deep it extends into tissues or structures, if it is affecting adjacent organs, if there is lymph node involvement, and whether the cancer has metastasized to nonadjacent organs. Biopsy of the tumor is necessary to correctly stage the cancer. Staging the cancer aids in determining the proper course of treatment and is a strong prognostic factor (Sapienza & Hoffman Ruddy, 2017).
- As a part of this staging system, doctors classify and treat laryngeal cancer based upon three primary categories: **T** (primary site of tumor), **N** (involvement of the lymph nodes), and **M** (metastasis). Thus, the patient's medical chart will probably feature a TNM designation to describe the site(s) and extent of the cancer. There are different criteria to stage supraglottic, glottic, and subglottic cancer.

- A multidisciplinary team is crucial for the treatment and rehabilitation of a patient with head and neck cancer. This team may include, but is not limited to, a head and neck surgeon, radiation and/or medical oncologists, radiologists, pathologists, nurses, the speech-language pathologist, occupational and physical therapists, and a registered dietician (Sapienza & Hoffman Ruddy, 2017).
- There are three basic types of medical treatment for laryngeal cancer: surgery, chemotherapy, and radiation. These options are not exclusive and may be combined to create the best outcome for a patient.

  - A laryngectomy, or surgery to remove the larynx, can consist of a total laryngectomy (in which the entire larynx is removed) or a hemilaryngectomy (in which only the diseased part of the larynx is removed). Patients with advanced laryngeal cancer involving lymph nodes and metastasis may undergo total laryngectomy with radical neck dissection, in which the lymphatic system in the neck is removed. The person who has had his larynx removed is known as a laryngectomee.
  - Chemotherapy may be used alone or in conjunction with other measures to increase the survival of patients with advanced cancer when the original tumor is large and metastasis is a risk. Side effects of chemotherapy include weight and hair loss, nausea, and weakness.
  - Radiation therapy, alone or combined with surgery, may be used for some patients. Doctors often use radiation therapy before surgery is attempted to try to eliminate the cancer. Some patients prefer radiation therapy to laryngectomy if given a choice. Side effects of radiation can include, but is not limited to, skin burns, risk of cavities, edema, swallowing problems, diminished taste, sore throat, fatigue, thick secretions, thrush (type of yeast that excessively grows in moist areas of the oral cavity, pharynx, and larynx), and xerostomia (dry mouth due to trauma to the salivary glands).

General Issues in Rehabilitation of the Laryngectomee

A team approach is critical in rehabilitation after a laryngectomy. Laryngectomees and their families need support from the surgeon, speech–language pathologist, social worker, nurse, vocational counselor, nutritionist, and maybe a counselor or psychologist to deal with accompanying emotional issues.

- The patient and family will most probably need both pre- and postoperative counseling to deal with the substantial emotional issues and life changes that accompany a laryngectomy. The first few days after the surgery often constitute an emotional "low point" for patients.
- Experienced, rehabilitated laryngectomees can be substantially helpful in providing information and support both pre- and postsurgically. Presurgical support may include providing education on how the anatomy and physiology of voice, speech, and swallowing will change due to a total or partial laryngectomy. Potential postoperative roadblocks should be discussed prior to surgery so that the patient is knowledgeable of problems that may occur following surgery.
- Consultation and support, both written and verbal, are needed pre- as well as postsurgery. Patients and families who do not receive presurgical support tend to suffer more depression and isolation than those who receive information and support prior to surgery. Clinicians must remember that spouses and significant others need support just as the patient does.

Types of Alaryngeal Speech

Because the vocal folds are not present after a laryngectomy, normal voicing is not possible and breathing is different. To allow the patient to breathe, the surgeon creates a **stoma**, or opening in the lower part of the neck, and connects it with the trachea. The patient now breathes through that opening.

Figure 7.14 illustrates the anatomy and physiology of the head and neck before and after a total laryngectomy. Because of the altered anatomy and physiology, a new source of sound is needed for voicing.

Laryngectomees produce vocalizations in three ways: with the use of external devices, via esophageal speech, or by having surgical modifications or implanted devices in the laryngeal area.

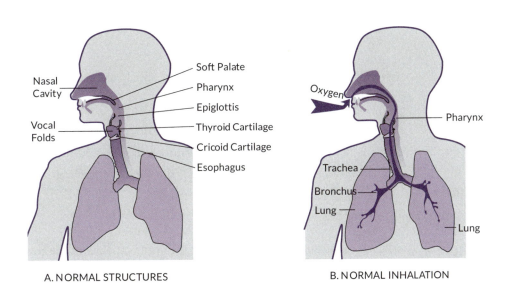
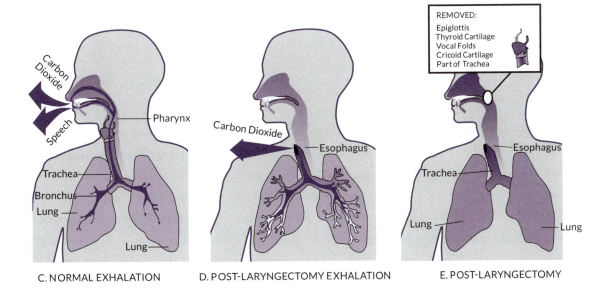

Figure 7.14 Before and after laryngectomy: physiology of the head and neck.

- A widely used external device is the artificial larynx or electrolarynx, a mechanical, handheld device that generates sound.

  - The patient presses the electrolarynx against the neck or within the mouth (intraoral electrolarynx) and turns on the unit with the thumb. The sound generated by the vibrator is transferred to the mouth, and the patient then articulates in a slightly exaggerated manner to increase intelligibility. If the patient speaks more slowly than usual, this is also helpful to intelligibility.
  - The electrolarynx is beneficial because it can be used immediately following surgery and can be kept as a backup means of communication if the patient decides to try esophageal speech or use a prosthesis. The electrolarynx, however, creates speech that is rather robotic in quality and may be distracting to listeners.

- The esophagus is also a source of sound. Patients can be taught esophageal speech in which they literally speak on burps or belches.

  - Successful air intake for esophageal speech depends on appropriate tension of the upper esophageal sphincter. There must be a critical wall tension to permit airflow in and out. Esophageal voice is produced by a pharyngoesophageal segment (PES); the PES is the vibratory source. It can be located in the cricopharyngeus or elsewhere in the larynx.
  - There are two methods of esophageal speech:

    - In the injection (positive pressure) method, the patient impounds the air in the mouth as in saying /t/, /k/, or /p/. The impounded air is pushed back into the esophagus and then expelled, producing vibrations of the soft tissues of the esophagus, particularly the cricopharyngeus muscle. The patient shapes the resulting belch into speech.
    - In the inhalation (negative pressure) method, the patient is taught to inhale rapidly while keeping the esophagus open and relaxed. The inhaled air passes through the esophagus and sets its tissues into vibratory motion. The resulting sound is shaped into speech.

  - Esophageal speech techniques are preferred by some because they are inexpensive, hands-free methods that do not rely on devices or prostheses; however, they are difficult to learn.

- **Surgical modifications and implanted devices** can also serve as sound sources. In the popular **Blom-Singer tracheoesophageal puncture** (TEP), the tracheoesophageal wall, which separates the trachea and the esophagus, is punctured. This puncture can be created during the total laryngectomy operation (primary TEP) or approximately six weeks following the laryngectomy after the tissue has healed (secondary TEP) (Sapienza & Hoffman Ruddy, 2017). A shunt or tunnel is opened to connect the two structures. To keep the tunnel open, the Blom-Singer prosthetic device (see Figure 7.15) is inserted. The configuration of the device, which is a small 1.8–3.6-cm plastic or silicone tube, prevents the passage of fluid and food into the trachea.

  - There are two major types of devices: one that the patient herself can insert and manipulate and an indwelling device that can be inserted and removed only by the physician (Boone et al., 2013).

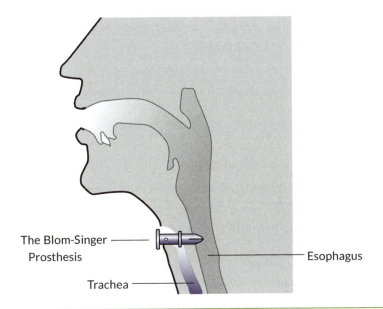

Figure 7.15 The Blom-Singer prosthetic device in place.

Patients who choose the type of device that they themselves can insert and manipulate must have the manual dexterity to remove, clean, and re-insert the device into the tracheoesophageal fistula. Thus, persons with arthritis or other physical issues may need a device that is inserted by the physician (Deem & Hagerman, 2011).

- To speak, the patient exhales and occludes the stoma with a finger; the pulmonary air enters through the anterior opening of the tube, passing from the trachea to the esophagus. This sets the esophagus into vibration, resulting in sound production. The stoma can also be occluded with a hands-free one-way valve, in which air enters the valve and is shunted up to vibrate the esophagus. The patient modifies the sound into speech.
- Compared to other alaryngeal speech options, tracheoesophageal speech is perceived to be the most natural sounding voice quality. However, there may be complications related to the surgery to place the prosthesis, and, over time, the prosthesis may leak and need to be replaced. The prosthesis also requires a high level of daily care and maintenance, may be expensive, and is not always hands-free if occlusion is best achieved with the patient's finger.

Voice Disorders

One way to categorize voice disorders is to group them into **hyperfunctional** and **hypofunctional** categories. **Hyperfunctional** voice disorders are ones that are caused by excessive muscle action of the vocal mechanism. There is not enough airflow, creating a voice that is tense, strained, rough, and hoarse. Most vocal fold lesions, such as, but not limited to, vocal nodules, cysts, and polyps (to be discussed), cause hyperfunctional voice disorders, because the laryngeal muscles and surrounding structures (such as the false vocal folds) overactivate to compensate for the lesion that is obstructing the vocal folds from adducting properly.

- **Hypofunctional** voice disorders are ones that are caused by inefficient muscle action of the vocal mechanism. The vocal folds do not come together fully, causing excessive airflow and creating a

vocal quality that is breathy, hoarse, reduced in loudness, and possibly aphonic. Vocal fold paresis and paralysis are hypofunctional voice disorders.
- One problem with categorizing voice disorders this way is that some voice disorders do not fit into these categories. For example, paradoxical vocal fold motion disorder (to be discussed) is neither hyperfunctional nor hypofunctional.

Physically Based Disorders of Phonation

Physically based disorders of phonation refer to any disorder that compromises the structure or vasculature (blood supply) of the vocal folds or laryngeal cartilage. Some of these disorders may be **congenital** (present at birth). Some may be acquired as a result of laryngeal trauma, damage to the vocal folds, or vocally abusive behaviors.

- Many disorders of voice occur due to vocally abusive behaviors. The sophisticated vocal mechanism works well when used properly, but it is extremely sensitive to abuse, which often causes a variety of voice problems. These problems are sometimes described as resulting from **phonotrauma**, or trauma or injury to the vocal folds.
- **Abusive behaviors** that can damage the vocal mechanism include: excessive shouting; screaming; cheering; excessive talking; coughing; hard glottal attacks; throat clearing; strained and explosive vocalizations; excessive laughing and crying; speaking with inappropriate pitch, loudness, or both; and speaking in noisy environments.
  - Adults in occupations such as teaching or coaching may be more vulnerable to vocal abuse than adults in vocations that do not require a great deal of speaking (especially at a loud volume).
  - The majority of vocally abusive behaviors are associated with excessive muscular effort, tension, and consequent irritation of the vocal folds. Excessive effort and tension can cause physical damage to the vocal folds (phonotrauma) and create physical pathologies.
  - Patients who abuse their voices often demonstrate increased laryngeal airway resistance. The voice problems that result from vocally abusive behaviors are due to such physical damage to and pathological states of the larynx.
- Therapy, medication, surgery, or a combination of those treatments are generally used to correct voice disorders resulting from pathological changes to the vocal folds due to abuse (Stemple & Thomas, 2010). If patients continue the abusive practices and do not change their vocal habits, pathological changes to the vocal folds, with consequent voice problems, are likely to recur.

The following section summarizes different physically based disorders of phonation. Behavioral voice therapy techniques will be described following a review of all voice disorders.

Vocal Nodules

Vocal nodules are small nodes that develop on the superficial layer of the lamina propria of the vocal folds and protrude from surrounding cells (see Figure 7.16). In the beginning, the nodules are reddish or pinkish. As they develop over time, they appear white or grayish because they become fibrous and callous-like.

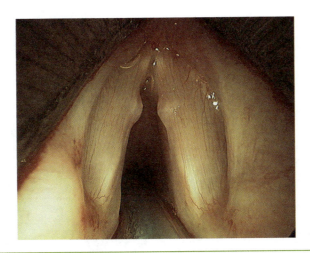

Figure 7.16 Nodules. Used with permission from Thomas L. Carroll, MD.

- Vocal nodules can be unilateral; however, they are typically bilateral and sit opposite each other on the two folds. They typically appear at the junction of the anterior and middle two-thirds of the folds.
- Nodules are well defined in the beginning stages but become more diffuse later because of inflammation of the surrounding tissue. Nodules develop over time as the result of prolonged vocally abusive behaviors.
- Vocal nodules increase the mass and stiffness of the vocal folds. Consequently, the folds vibrate at a slower rate, resulting in lower pitch. The nodules also make smooth vocal fold approximation impossible, contributing to breathiness and hoarseness of voice. Vocal fatigue is also common.
- Vocal nodules are seen most frequently in children who scream and yell on playgrounds and in adults whose career or leisure activities involve vocally abusive practices (e.g., yelling at sports events). Singers are especially susceptible to vocal nodules. Vocal rest can usually reduce swelling of the nodules, but prolonged abuse of the vocal folds will result in larger and more persistent nodules. Unless the patient changes his or her abusive behaviors, the nodules will rarely disappear.
- Persistent nodules are frequently treated in two ways: voice therapy or surgery. Surgery involves tissue excision or removal of the nodules through microdissection or laser.
- Some doctors have been using cold steel lasers or microspot CO_2 (heat) lasers, whose beam is so small that the heat cannot penetrate the surrounding tissues. The goal of laser and microdissection is to remove the nodules while disturbing as little of the mucosa and surrounding tissue as possible.
- Most nodules respond positively to behavioral voice therapy, and it should be the initial method of intervention. When nodules are removed with phonosurgery without vocal hygiene education and behavioral voice therapy, the nodules may reoccur (Sapienza & Hoffman Ruddy, 2017).

Polyps

Polyps, like nodules, are masses that grow and bulge out from surrounding tissue. Polyps are softer than nodules, originate in the middle one-third of the superficial lamina propria, and may be filled with fluid

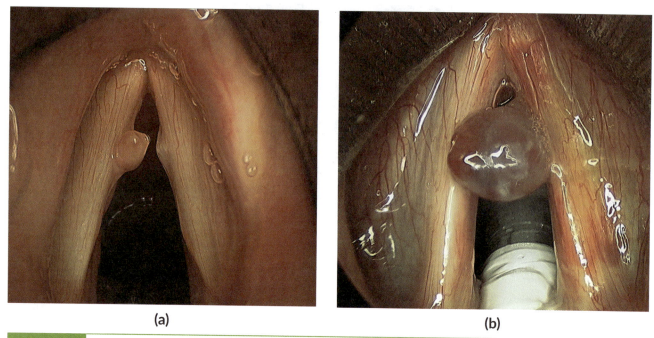

Figure 7.17 Polyp. Used with permission from Thomas L. Carroll, MD.

or have vascular tissue. They tend to be unilateral as opposed to the typically bilateral nodules. Figures 7.17 a and b shows vocal polyps.

- **Sessile polyps** have a broad base on the vocal fold and are blister-like; **pedunculated polyps** are attached to the vocal folds by a stalk.
- It is believed that traumatic use of the vocal folds results in submucosal hemorrhage (bleeding within the folds), which leads to the formation of tumor-like polyps. Polyps can grow over time or can be created after just one instance of severe vocal abuse (e.g., screaming when attacked).
- Polyps are more frequently seen in adults than in children, who are more susceptible to developing vocal nodules. Patients with polyps usually sound breathy and hoarse. They may also have **diplophonia** ("double voice," in which two different pitches are heard simultaneously), because the healthy fold vibrates at a different rate than the fold with the polyp.
- Polyps may disappear with voice rest and changes in vocal habits, or they may persist and become worse with time and no treatment. Techniques for treating patients with vocal polyps are described in the later section.

Cysts

A cyst appears on the membranous portion of the vocal fold. It is unilateral, benign, and filled with a mucus-like fluid. If left untreated, a cyst can create a reactive lesion on the opposite vocal fold. Cysts are a result of vocal abuse. Figure 7.18 shows a picture of a cyst.

- The effect of voice quality depends on the size and shape of the cyst and how much it impacts vocal fold vibration. Hoarseness can range from mild to severe.

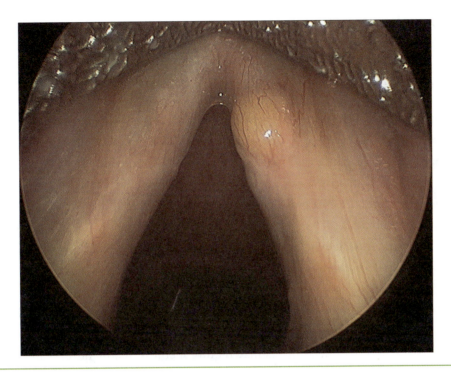

Figure 7.18 Cyst. Used with permission from Thomas L. Carroll, MD.

- Unlike treatment for vocal nodules, voice therapy is often not the preferred treatment method for a vocal fold cyst. Surgical removal of the cyst is often the most effective. However, it is imperative that the patient is educated on proper vocal hygiene to prevent another cyst from forming (Sapienza & Hoffman Ruddy, 2017).

Granuloma

A **granuloma** is a localized, inflammatory, vascular lesion that is usually composed of granular tissue in a firm, rounded sac. Granulomas frequently develop on the vocal processes of the arytenoid cartilages in the posterior laryngeal area. They can be unilateral or bilateral.

- Granulomas may be caused by vocal strain, intubation during surgery, injury to the larynx, and laryngopharyngeal reflux (LPR). Granulomas are most often associated with contact ulcers.
- Patients with granulomas often sound breathy and hoarse; they feel the need to frequently clear their throat due to a globus sensation. However, throat clearing only makes the irritation worse. The degree of dysphonia depends on the granuloma size and how much it interferes with glottal efficiency. A small, unilateral granuloma may not affect the vocal quality at all due to minimal interference with glottal efficiency.
- Granulomas are treated by surgery, voice therapy, or both. If the granuloma is associated with LPR, lifestyle changes may be recommended, such as diet modification and/or prescription medications (Sapienza & Hoffman Ruddy, 2017).

Contact Ulcers

Contact ulcers are sores or craterlike areas of ulcerated, granulated tissue that develop (usually bilaterally) along the posterior third of the glottal margin.

The causes of contact ulcers include the following:

- The slamming together of the arytenoid cartilages that occurs during low-pitched phonation accompanied by hard glottal attack and sometimes by increased loudness. Frequently, contact ulcers are seen in hard-driving patients who speak forcefully and talk excessively.
- Gastroesophageal reflux (discussed earlier), in which stomach acid is forced into the esophagus. The acid pools in and irritates the area between the arytenoid cartilages; this can occur especially at night when one is sleeping.
- Intubation for surgery, especially if intubation is prolonged or the tube is too large for the patient's larynx. Seventy percent of children who are intubated have a lacerated glottal area; this can cause permanent scarring and dysphonia.
- Patients with contact ulcers may complain of vocal fatigue and pain in the laryngeal area. They frequently sound hoarse and often clear their throats.
- Depending on the etiology, contact ulcers may require medical treatment (e.g., medication for gastroesophageal reflux). Surgery is not recommended; because the area is already ulcerated and highly irritated, healing after surgery is usually poor. Voice therapy techniques (described later in the chapter) are geared toward taking the extra effort out of phonation.

Vocal Fold Thickening

Prolonged use of vocally abusive behaviors, such as throat clearing, screaming, and others, can cause the vocal folds to thicken slowly and gradually. The vocal folds usually thicken along the anterior two-thirds of the glottal margin.

- Vocal fold thickening results in a breathy voice with lowered pitch. It is often a precursor to nodules or polyps. When these appear, the voice becomes increasingly hoarse. Vocal fold thickening can be reduced through elimination of the vocally abusive behaviors.

Traumatic Laryngitis

Traumatic laryngitis differs from infectious laryngitis, which occurs due to infections, colds, or allergies (of bacterial or viral origin). Traumatic laryngitis is created when the patient engages in vocally abusive behaviors, such as continual yelling.

- Vocally abusive behaviors irritate the vocal folds, which get swollen. Consequently, the voice is hoarse and may be low pitched with pitch breaks.
- Voice therapy usually consists of vocal rest and strategies for changing the vocally abusive behaviors.

Hemangioma

Hemangiomas are similar to granulomas but are soft, pliable, and filled with blood. Hemangiomas are usually caused by intubation or hyperacidity due to gastroesophageal reflux. They can also be congenital.

Acquired hemangiomas occur in the posterior glottal area and primarily create a hoarse vocal quality. Congenital hemangiomas occur in the subglottic region and create difficulty breathing and stridor (Iriz et al., 2009).

- Usually hemangiomas are surgically excised. Follow-up voice therapy is often necessary to improve vocal quality.

Reinke's Edema

Reinke's edema is also known as **polypoid corditis, diffuse polyposis,** or **polypoid degeneration,** and it occurs when fluid builds up in the superficial lamina propria (Reinke's space) of both vocal folds, causing excessive swelling. It is a result of continuous abuse, such as exposure to cigarette smoke and LPR. If the swelling progresses significantly without intervention, it can potentially compromise the airway. An example is shown in Figure 7.19.

The significant increase in the mass of the vocal folds creates a voice that is low pitched and perceived as gravelly. Reinke's edema is more noticeable in women because of the deep voice it creates.

- A key component of treatment of Reinke's edema is the reduction or elimination of exposure to toxins and irritants. It is imperative that the patient quits smoking, which is obviously not as easy as it sounds.

  - If the edema is detected relatively early and harmful exposure is decreased, surgical intervention is often not needed.
  - If the edema is more advanced and does not respond, surgical removal of the fluid with suction is used. However, if the patient continues to smoke or is exposed to other irritants following surgery, there is a significant likelihood of recurrence.
  - Proper education and counseling strategies are often needed for clients with Reinke's edema (Sapienza & Hoffman Ruddy, 2017).

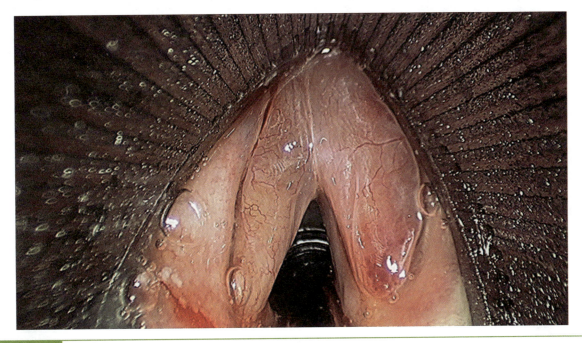

Figure 7.19 Reinke's. Used with permission from Thomas L. Carroll, MD.

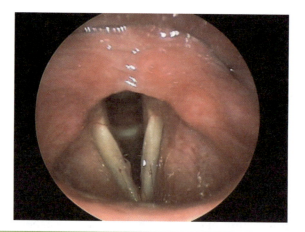

Figure 7.20 Varices. Used with permission from Dr. Cari Tellis, Professor, Misericordia University.

Varices

Varices are distended and prominent veins, usually at the mid portion of the superficial lamina propria, that are a result of phonotrauma, such as shouting and over use during singing. An example is shown in Figure 7.20. Women are more susceptible to varices during their menstrual cycle.

- Varices may be minor and not create any perceptual difference, but some individuals may be hoarse and have a loss of their upper range. The clinician should advise voice rest and provide vocal hygiene education. Surgery may be needed, in which case, cold instrument dissection is recommended (Sapienza & Hoffman Ruddy, 2017).

Vocal Fold Hemorrhage

When a blood vessel bursts within the vocal folds, the tissues are exposed to blood; this is known as a **vocal fold hemorrhage**. An example is shown in Figure 7.21. Phonotrauma is the most common cause of hemorrhage. The use of blood thinners and presence of varices increase the risk for hemorrhaging.

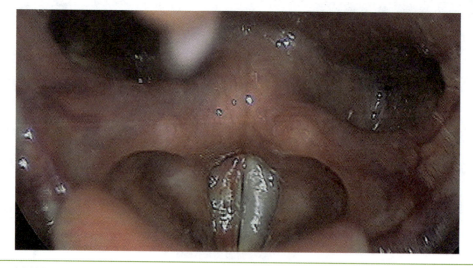

Figure 7.21 Vocal fold hemorrhage. Used with permission from Thomas L. Carroll, MD.

- Depending on the severity of the bleeding, the voice will sound hoarse and can range from mildly dysphonic to completely aphonic.
- Phonosurgery of varices can prevent hemorrhaging. Total voice rest is recommended if the vocal fold is currently hemorrhaging (considered the **acute** phase).
- After the hemorrhage has healed, any remaining voice issues that are a result of scar tissue can be treated through vocal fold augmentation techniques, such as fat or collagen injection (Sapienza & Hoffman Ruddy, 2017).

Hyperkeratosis

Hyperkeratosis refers to a rough, pinkish lesion that can appear in the oral cavity, larynx, or pharynx. Hyperkeratosis of the vocal folds may involve the epithelial cover of the folds as well as the superficial layer of the lamina propria. These lesions are often benign but may be precursors to malignancy.

- Hyperkeratotic growths occur due to tissue irritation and may arise in response to such causes as smoking, gastroesophageal reflux, and vocal abuse.
- The voice symptoms presented by patients range from mild to severe hoarseness or harshness, reduced loudness, and low pitch. Treatment involves eliminating the tissue irritants, possible ablative surgery, and voice therapy.

Leukoplakia

Leukoplakia are benign growths of thick, whitish patches on the surface membrane of the mucosa. Examples are shown in Figure 7.22. These growths may extend into the subepithelial space.

- Leukoplakia occur due to tissue irritation, especially that caused by smoking, alcohol, or vocal abuse. They may appear on the anterior third of the vocal folds and under the tongue.

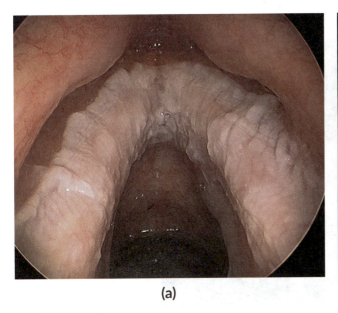
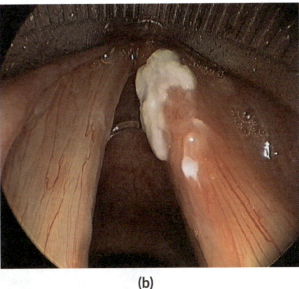

(a)   (b)

Figure 7.22 Leukoplakia. Used with permission from Thomas L. Carroll, MD.

- Though benign, leukoplakia is considered precancerous and must be monitored to ensure that it does not develop into squamous cell carcinoma.
- Patients with leukoplakia may sound rough, hoarse, low-pitched, breathy, and soft in volume. Diplophonia may also be present.
- Treatment usually involves a combination of surgery, voice therapy, and eliminating exposure to tissue irritants. It is highly recommended that the client understand the relationship between chronic irritation and the risk of the leukoplakia recurring, potentially leading to cancer.

Laryngomalacia

A congenital condition also known as **congenital laryngeal stridor**, **laryngomalacia** involves soft, "floppy" laryngeal cartilages. The epiglottis is particularly affected. Laryngomalacia is the most common cause of stridor in infants (Sapienza & Hoffman Ruddy, 2017).

- The epiglottis is very soft and pliable due to abnormal development. When the child breathes, the epiglottis resists the airstream, causing **stridor**, or rough, breathy noise upon inhalation.
- Because this condition usually resolves spontaneously by the time the child is 2 or 3 years old, no treatment is normally required after the initial diagnosis. However, in severe cases, the child may have substantial breathing problems, which will require treatment.

Subglottal Stenosis

Subglottal stenosis is the narrowing of the subglottic space, and it is a condition that can be acquired or congenital (Figure 7.23). It is the third most common congenital condition (Sapienza & Hoffman Ruddy, 2017).

- Congenital subglottal stenosis is the result of arrested development of the conus elasticus or interruption of the cricoid cartilage during embryological development. It is defined as a lumen 4.0 mm in diameter or less at the level of the cricoid (Boone et al., 2013).

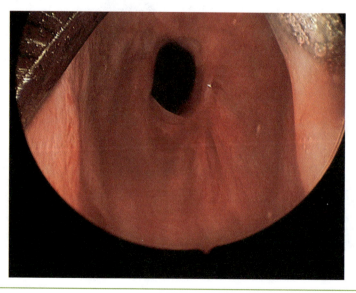

Figure 7.23 Subglottal stenosis. Used with permission from Thomas L. Carroll, MD.

- Acquired subglottal stenosis can occur as a result of endotracheal intubation that occurs as part of surgery or lifesaving procedures. Prolonged intubation can result in stenosis, scarring, or hypertrophy in children. If stenosis is severe and there is no exchange of air, a tracheostomy may be necessary.
- If stenosis is moderately severe, children will often display exercise intolerance and stridor. Vocal fold paralysis may also be present if mechanical trauma was the cause of the stenosis (Sapienza & Hoffman Ruddy, 2017). Patients may need surgical or endoscopic intervention, followed by voice intervention.

Papilloma

Papillomas are sometimes called **juvenile papillomas** because they tend to occur primarily in children (although they can occur in adults, as well). Juvenile papillomas are a result of perinatal infection transmitted by the mother. When children reach puberty, papillomas often cease to be a problem.

- Papillomas are wart-like growths caused by the HPV. They are pink, white, or both and may be found anywhere in the airway (including but not limited to the larynx) (see Figure 7.24).
- The true vocal folds are the most common site for papillomas (Sapienza & Hoffman Ruddy, 2017).
- Hoarseness, breathiness, and low pitch are the most frequent perceptual symptoms of papilloma. Airway obstruction is a major and potentially life-threatening concern.
- At present, most patients with papilloma are treated through multiple surgeries; some patients have had 30–100 surgeries for papilloma removal.
  - Repeated surgeries strip the mucosa and create vocal fold scar tissue, which affects vocal quality. After surgery, children often sound even more hoarse and low pitched than before. Laryngeal webbing (discussed later in this section) can also occur. However, doctors are most concerned about airway preservation; thus, sequelae like hoarseness and laryngeal webbing are not considered high-priority problems.

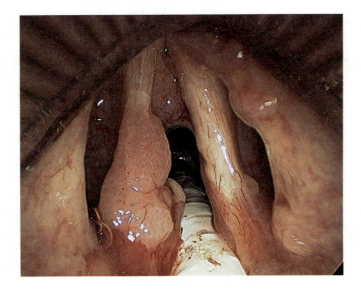

Figure 7.24 Papilloma. Used with permission from Thomas L. Carroll, MD.

- Treatments include **cup forceps surgery** (diminishing in popularity), **interferon** medication, and **CO_2 laser surgery** (widely used). Carefully performed, CO_2 laser surgery helps preserve mucosa and surrounding tissue while ablating the papillomas. Interferon can be effective but has potentially serious side effects, including induced autoimmune diseases.
- Indole-3-carbinol has been used to treat recurrent respiratory papillomatosis (Rosen, Woodson, Thompson, Hengesteg, & Bradlow, 1998). This Food and Drug Administration–approved nutritional supplement is highly concentrated in broccoli, cabbage, cauliflower, and brussels sprouts. Eighteen months after treatment with indole-3-carbinol, one-third of the subjects in this study had not responded to the treatment, one-third of the subjects had reduced growth of the papillomas, and one-third of the subjects had complete cessation of the papilloma growth.
- Voice therapy can be helpful after surgical treatment. Therapy can involve using relaxation exercises, teaching the patient to use amplification devices, and helping the patient decrease supraglottic hyperfunction. Therapy does not prevent recurrence of the papilloma, but it can help patients make the best use of their weakened and scarred vocal mechanism.

Laryngeal Web

A **laryngeal web** is a membrane that grows across the anterior portion of the glottis (Figure 7.25). There are two basic types of laryngeal webs: **congenital**, or present at birth, and **acquired**, due to trauma to the inner edges of the vocal folds. The vocal folds may be traumatized by forceful or prolonged intubation, surgery, severe laryngeal infection, or accidental injury.

- A laryngeal web will most likely cause difficulty breathing and inspiratory stridor. The voice will sound hoarse and the patient will have difficulty sustaining phonation; the severity of symptoms depends on the degree of webbing (Sapienza & Hoffman Ruddy, 2017).
- Treatment for infants with congenital webs involves immediate surgery followed by tracheostomy.

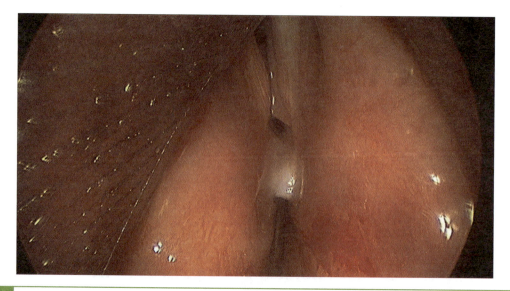

Figure 7.25 Laryngeal web. Used with permission from Thomas L. Carroll, MD.

- Treatment for webbing in adults involves surgery to remove the web. After surgery, the surgeon places a **laryngeal keel** (a fingernail-size, rudder-shaped stent device) between the vocal folds to prevent the web from growing back. The patient generally undergoes 6–8 weeks of voice rest while the keel is in place. After the keel is removed, voice therapy may be required to assist in return of normal phonation.

Laryngeal Trauma

Seen more frequently in children than in adults, **laryngeal trauma** refers to many kinds of injury to the larynx. Causes of laryngeal trauma include burns (thermal or chemical), motor vehicle accidents, sports-related accidents, attempted strangulations, and gunshot wounds. Young children may suffer trauma by swallowing sharp objects. The voice will usually sound hoarse and the patient will most likely exhibit stridor upon inhalation and exhalation (Sapienza & Hoffman Ruddy, 2017).

- Patients generally undergo surgery designed to reconstruct the vocal mechanism. The success of surgery depends on several factors, including the health of the overall vocal tissue prior to surgery.
- Patients who smoke or have gastroesophageal reflux disease (GERD), for example, must cease smoking or have treatment for the GERD before surgery occurs so that the vocal tissue will be as optimal as possible. If vocal tissue is compromised before surgery, more scarring from surgery can occur.
- Most patients undergo voice therapy after surgery. The postsurgical necessity of voice therapy varies from patient to patient, depending on the degree of dysphonia displayed. Voice therapy success depends largely on the proficiency of the remaining or surgically reconstructed laryngeal mechanism.

Sulcus Vocalis

Sulcus vocalis is the thinning and bowing of the superficial lamina propria of the vocal folds; it can be unilateral or bilateral (Figure 7.26). Its exact cause is unknown; however, it is believed to be related to a

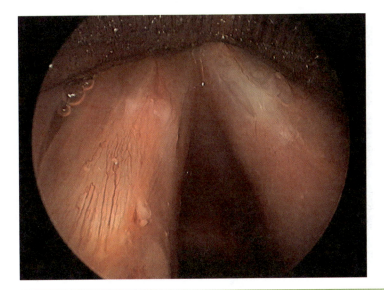

Figure 7.26 Sulcus vocalis. Used with permission from Thomas L. Carroll, MD.

smoking history among certain ethnicities. Other theories hold that sulcus vocalis is congenital or is the result of trauma or infection.

- Sulci are classified based on how deep the depression extends. The effect on vocal quality depends on the depth of the sulcus, but overall, individuals with sulcus vocalis may sound hoarse, experience fatigue, and need to use increased effort for phonation.
- Sulcus vocalis can be managed with surgical augmentation using fat or fascia; other techniques include medialization and augmentation using collagen injectables (Sapienza & Hoffman Ruddy, 2017).

Gastroesophageal Reflux Disease and Laryngopharyngeal Reflux

Gastroesophageal reflux disease (GERD), mentioned earlier, occurs when gastric contents spontaneously empty into the esophagus when the person has not vomited or belched (see Figure 7.27). Reflux is referred to as **laryngopharyngeal reflux** (LPR) when the gastric contents spill into the upper pharynx and upper airway, causing irritation in the mucosa of these areas (Sapienza & Hoffman Ruddy, 2017). Patients may experience heartburn, acid indigestion, sore throat, and hoarseness. Consequent pathological vocal fold changes, such as **contact ulcers** (bilateral ulcerations on the medial surfaces of the vocal processes of the arytenoid cartilages), may also occur.

- Manometric evaluation (a form of aerodynamic evaluation) for patients with GERD can be very effective. When a team of professionals is planning for anti-reflux surgery, esophageal manometric evaluation is critical.
- Treatment options include antacids, propping up the head at night, use of prescription medications, not exercising directly after eating, and changes in dietary habits. Some patients may need to decrease the amount of coffee they drink, because coffee drinking has been associated with GERD.
- Medical personnel should usually be involved in treatment of patients with GERD. Treatment plans for these patients usually include behavioral, medical, and surgical therapies, as well as voice therapy.

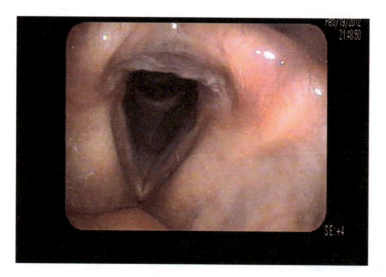

Figure 7.27 Laryngopharyngeal reflux. Used with permission from Thomas L. Carroll, MD.

Ankylosis

In **ankylosis**, or stiffening of the joint(s), the movement of the arytenoids is restricted because of a bone-joint disease, such as arthritis. Cancer can also cause ankylosis. The vocal folds are attached to the arytenoids; when the arytenoids are stiff, the vocal folds do not close fully.

Idiopathic Voice Disorders

Paradoxical Vocal Fold Motion Disorder

In paradoxical vocal fold motion (PVFM) disorder, also called **laryngeal dyskinesia** and **episodic paroxysmal laryngospasm**, there is an inappropriate closure or adduction of the true vocal folds during inhalation, exhalation, or both. The term **paroxysmal** indicates that the symptoms occur in periodic attacks.

- Patients with PVFM often appear asthmatic. Sometimes they undergo a tracheotomy to relieve their symptoms. Some patients display stridor and dysphonia; others display only stridor.
- PVFM has been attributed to both psychological and physiological causes. Some experts view it as a conversion disorder in patients with psychological problems. Others believe it may be due to pharmacological, neurological, and other variables.
- Some persons with PVFM have upper-airway sensitivity to laryngeal irritants. Irritants in the airway are likely to contribute to PVFM in children. These irritants include sinus drainage or postnasal drip; laryngopharyngeal reflex; and exposure to irritating smoke, fumes, gas, dust, mist, or vapors.
- Identification of PVFM has increased a great deal in recent years and has been documented in both males and females of all ages. Most clients with PVFM fall between 10 and 40 years of age, but the condition has been identified in children as young as 4 months old.
- Treatment may include a combination of psychological, medical, and behavioral approaches. Some patients respond well to voice therapy involving endoscopy and direct feedback, in which they learn the nature of the disorder as well as how to relax the entire vocal mechanism. Some clients also benefit from respiratory training. Children and adolescents may respond well to visual biofeedback techniques and relaxation exercises.

Neurologically Based Voice Disorders

Paralysis

Because the vocal folds are composed primarily of muscle, they can be paralyzed when their nerve supply is cut off. Muscles that are not stimulated by the nerves do not move, resulting in paralysis.

Vocal folds can become paralyzed due to the following:

- Accidental injury of the RLN during certain **surgical procedures** (e.g., a thyroidectomy, in which a cancerous thyroid gland is surgically removed)
- Progressive, debilitative **neurological diseases**, such as amyotrophic lateral sclerosis

- **Malignant diseases**, causing tumors outside the larynx to affect vocal fold mobility
- **Intubation trauma**, causing compression of the recurrent laryngeal nerve, dislocation of the arytenoids, and other difficulties
- **Laryngeal trauma** that is so severe it is irreparable (e.g., gunshot wound)
- Stroke
- Vagus nerve deficits

Even in patients who can achieve a near normal-sounding voice despite vocal fold paralysis, coughing is not vigorous because of the difficulty in achieving the necessary amount of subglottal pressure for the vocal folds to close firmly. Some patients demonstrate dysphagia, breathiness, and reduced pitch and volume.

- In **unilateral paralysis**, only one vocal fold is paralyzed and assumes a static position (Figure 7.28). In some cases, the normal fold may move toward the paralyzed fold to make contact; the voice in such cases may sound almost normal. In other cases, the paralyzed fold may be so far away from midline that the healthy fold cannot make contact to achieve closure. This causes aphonia.
- **Bilateral paralysis**, or paralysis of both vocal folds, may lead to a wide-open glottis, causing aphonia. When the vocal folds are paralyzed in an abducted position, aspiration can occur. If the vocal folds are paralyzed in an adducted position, the patient struggles for breath, but the voice is not significantly dysphonic. If both vocal folds are paralyzed in the paramedian position (close to the midline), it can be life threatening because the airway is obstructed. In these severe cases, a patient may need a tracheotomy to create a more direct airway and prevent respiratory failure.
  - A number of treatment techniques are available for patients with vocal fold paralysis. In cases of unilateral paralysis, doctors create a bulge in the paralyzed fold so that the healthy fold meets it more readily. Substances used to create the bulge include collagen, calcium hydroxyapatite Radiesse® fillers, and autologous fat (the patient's own fat).

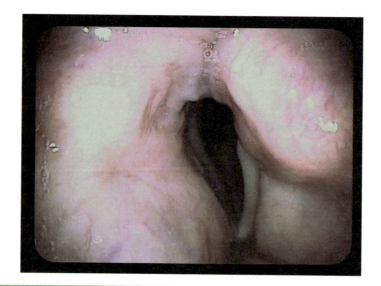

Figure 7.28 Unilateral paralysis. Used with permission from Dr. Cari Tellis, Professor, Misericordia University.

- One popular technique used to achieve vocal fold medialization is medialization laryngoplasty. The surgeon creates a small window in the thyroid cartilage, medializes the vocal fold, and places a small silastic implant to keep the paralyzed fold medialized.
- Another surgical procedure used to achieve vocal fold medialization is arytenoid adduction, which is recommended if there is a large glottic gap posteriorly (Sapienza & Hoffman Ruddy, 2017). When the arytenoid cartilage is surgically adducted, the paralyzed fold is moved closer to the midline so the patient can produce better voicing.
- In nerve–muscle pedicle reinnervation, the surgeon takes a pedicle of a neck strap muscle with innervation and sutures it either into the adductors for medialization purposes or into the posterior cricoarytenoids to promote abduction.
- Paralysis may also be treated with behavioral voice therapy techniques. Refer to the "Behavioral Voice Therapy" section for techniques.

Spasmodic Dysphonia

Spasmodic dysphonia (SMD) is a focal laryngeal dystonia. Although it has traditionally been considered psychologically based, most experts today believe that SMD has neurogenic causes with possible emotional side effects. Currently, it is thought to be caused by abnormal functioning of the basal ganglia (National Institute on Deafness and Other Communication Disorders [NIDCD], 2014). The average age of onset is between 40 and 50 years. Nearly 80% of individuals diagnosed with SMD are female (Adler, Edwards, & Bansberg, 1997). There are two types of SMD:

- **Abductor spasmodic dysphonia** (ABSD) is created by intermittent, involuntary, fleeting vocal fold abduction when the patient tries to phonate. Loudness is reduced, and the patient is occasionally aphonic, with breathy or whispered speech. Treatment options include Botox (botulinus toxin) injections, speech therapy involving relaxation techniques and continuous voicing, and pharmacological intervention.
- **Adductor spasmodic dysphonia** (ADSD), the most common type, is characterized by overpressure due to prolonged overadduction or tight closure of the vocal folds. The voice may sound choked and strangled. Popular current treatment techniques include:
  - *CO_2 laser surgery.* Here the paralyzed fold is thinned with a CO_2 laser beam. This creates a 2-mm-wide groove, whose healing and scarring action pulls the vocal fold away from the midline, widening the glottis. Repeated surgeries may be necessary.
  - *Recurrent laryngeal nerve (RLN) resection.* Here the RLN is cut to paralyze the vocal fold on that side. This reduces vocal fold hyperadduction. RLN resection has met with mixed success. It is currently considered to be a viable option for patients with severe SMD who do not wish to have repeated, frequent Botox injections.
  - *Botox injections.* Botox, a neurotoxin injected directly by needle into the vocal folds, creates a flaccid paralysis, and hyperadduction ceases. Injections are usually repeated every 3–6 months. Botox is currently the treatment of choice among many specialists.

- *Augmentative and alternative devices.* These devices can be helpful. For example, some can amplify a person's voice over the phone. Special software can be added to a computer or handheld device such as a cell phone or personal digital assistant to translate text into synthetic speech (NIDCD, 2014).
- *Voice therapy.* Voice therapy can include inhalation phonation; increased pitch; relaxation; head turning; counseling; the yawn–sigh approach; and soft, breathy phonation onset using /h/ (*Note*: Pushing techniques are counterproductive for patients who have RLN resection; spasticity can recur).

- Though not as common, individuals may also have mixed SMD, which is characterized by both involuntary adduction and abduction of the vocal folds.

Neurological Diseases

Because patients with neurological diseases tend to manifest dysarthria, with some exceptions, treatment techniques often follow principles based upon therapy for dysarthria. Described in this section are the most common neurological diseases that cause voice disorders.

Multiple Sclerosis

Patients with multiple sclerosis (MS) experience progressive and diffuse demyelination of white matter, with corresponding preservation of axons, at the brainstem, cerebellum, and spinal cord.

- Patients may have impaired prosody, pitch, and loudness control; harshness; breathiness; hypernasality; articulation breakdown; and nasal air escape.
- There are currently no treatments to cure MS or directly modify the progression of the disease; however, there are treatments available to treat the symptoms of MS. Pharmacological intervention may include adrenocorticotrophic hormone to reduce acute symptoms. Corticosteroids, such as prednisone, may also be used.

Myasthenia Gravis

- This neuromuscular autoimmune disease produces fatigue and muscle weakness. There is a decreased amount of acetylcholine at the myoneuronal junction, so muscles have difficulty contracting.
- Patients often sound hypernasal, breathy, hoarse, monotonous, and soft in volume. Dysphagia and distorted articulation may also be present.
- Myasthenia gravis is often treated with corticosteroids, which improve strength and endurance of the bulbar musculature. One other treatment option for myasthenia gravis is a **thymectomy**, the removal of the thymus gland. In individuals with myasthenia gravis, this gland is often abnormal; this procedure rebalances the immune system and can decrease symptoms in approximately 70% of patients (Sapienza & Hoffman Ruddy, 2017).

Amyotrophic Lateral Sclerosis

Amyotrophic lateral sclerosis (ALS), or **Lou Gehrig's disease**, is a progressive, fatal disease involving degeneration of the upper and lower motor neuron systems.

- Patients with ALS often sound breathy, low pitched, and monotonous. They have poor respiratory control. Individuals with ALS will present with a combination of dysarthria, dysphonia, and dysphagia.
- Patients with ALS do not respond well to medications, but riluzole has been shown to slow muscle deterioration in some people.
- Because ALS is progressive, many clinicians focus treatment efforts on augmentative/alternative forms of communication that can be used even in the later stages of the disease.

Parkinson's Disease

Parkinson's is caused by a lack of dopamine (a neurotransmitter) in the substantia nigra of the basal ganglia. It can be idiopathic (occurring in isolation or primary form) or secondary to other conditions, such as dementia.

- Patients with Parkinson's disease often sound breathy, low in pitch and loudness, and monotonous.
- Treatment includes **L-dopa** (levodopa) to increase dopamine in the substantia nigra; voice treatment may also be indicated. The popular **Lee Silverman Voice Treatment** (LSVT) program emphasizes stimulating patients to increase respiratory and phonatory efforts and to sustain those efforts over time. LSVT is an intensive treatment, which is provided for 4 weeks, 4 sessions a week, for 60 minutes per session.

Psychogenic Voice Disorders

Psychogenic, or "functional," voice disorders occur when the voice is abnormal in the presence of normal laryngeal structures. A laryngoscopic examination reveals essentially normal vocal structures, but during attempted phonation, the vocal folds may remain fully or partially abducted. Aphonia in the absence of any organic cause has been treated with either counseling or psychotherapy, or behavior therapy.

- For counseling or psychotherapy, clinicians often refer the patient to a professional psychologist, psychiatrist, or marriage and family counselor. During therapy sessions, clients are encouraged to speak freely about themselves and their problems. With the support of a sympathetic listener, clients are expected to resolve their psychological conflicts and return to normal phonation.
- Clinicians who employ **behavior therapy** treat conversion aphonia by modifying the client's behaviors. Refer to the upcoming section ("Behavioral Voice Therapy") for specific voice therapy techniques. A summary of the most common psychogenic voice disorders is discussed in this section.

Hysterical (Conversion) Aphonia

In **hysterical**, or **conversion**, **aphonia**, there is usually no evidence of a structural pathology. There is no known physiological or neurological basis for the patient's voice loss. The loss can be sudden or gradual.

- Patients with conversion aphonia often experience voice loss after an emotionally traumatic event, such as a violent crime. The voice loss may represent an unconscious attempt to avoid dealing with the traumatic event. The voice problem is thus viewed as a conversion reaction, or translation of the emotional trauma into another set of symptoms.
- Conversion aphonia considerably impacts all aspects of an individual's life, especially occupationally and socially. For many patients with conversion aphonia, the prognosis for return to normal voice is quite good. Clinicians must, after gathering an extensive case history and viewing the overall situation, make accurate decisions about the most effective course of treatment for conversion aphonia patients.

Muscle Tension Dysphonia

Another functional voice disorder, **muscle tension dysphonia** (MTD) occurs when there is significant over activity of the head and neck muscles during phonation. In some cases, the intrinsic laryngeal muscles are also uncoordinated. MTD can be attributed to high levels of stress and depression, although other speculated causes include vocal abuse and GERD. The voice is high-pitched and strained because of the increased tension (Sapienza & Hoffman Ruddy, 2017).

- Voice therapy is often used to treat MTD (refer to behavioral voice therapy techniques in the next section). The most common treatment method for MTD is circumlaryngeal massage, in which pressure is applied to the hyoid bone, thyrohyoid space, and posterior aspect of the thyroid cartilage to create a more normal laryngeal posture (Sapienza & Hoffman Ruddy, 2017).

Mutational Falsetto (Puberphonia)

In **mutational falsetto**, or **puberphonia**, a young man speaks with a high pitch, although the larynx has grown normally and puberty is completed. This can occur due to psychosocial factors (e.g., embarrassment about the newly developing low voice), endocrine disorders, neurologic diseases, or physical causes (e.g., hearing impairment or immature maturation of the larynx). Though puberphonia can occur as a result of physiological and neurological causes, it is included in the **psychogenic** section of the text due to its psychogenic nature.

- For patients with puberphonia, it is optimal for treatment to be initiated in the teens or early 20s. Some atrophy of the vocal muscles may occur if the mutational falsetto persists untreated.
- In patients with a pitch that is too high, especially young men with puberphonia, the larynx is often elevated, with accompanying tension of the laryngeal musculature. Patients with puberphonia can especially benefit from digital manipulation of the thyroid cartilage. In this technique, during vowel production, the patient is taught to apply a gentle inward push on the anterior aspect of the thyroid cartilage while sustaining a vowel (Desai & Mishra, 2012).

Behavioral Voice Therapy

When choosing a voice therapy technique, it is important that the clinician understand *why* the voice disorder is occurring (structural, neurological, etc.) and *how* the vibration of the vocal folds is impaired (too much/not enough closure, too much/not enough airflow, partial/absent mucosal wave, increased mass, etc.). If applicable, the clinician can consider whether the voice disorder is hyper- or hypofunctional. To choose the best technique based on the signs and symptoms present, it is also important to understand how each voice therapy technique impacts the physiology of the vocal mechanism. For example, it would be counterintuitive to choose a voice therapy technique that facilitates forceful vocal fold adduction in a patient with a hyperfunctional voice disorder because there is already too much maladaptive muscle action.

- If the voice disorder is the result of poor vocal hygiene, it is crucial that the patient reduces or eliminates vocal abuses (e.g., stop smoking cigarettes).
- Clinicians can also help clients, especially adults, to ascertain whether environmental modifications within their workplaces (e.g., using a microphone for voice amplification in a noisy classroom) can help decrease the need for using vocally abusive behaviors, such as shouting.
- Before delving into specific voice therapy techniques, refer to the list below for general tips and guidelines to keep in mind prior to beginning and throughout the course of therapy:
  - Always ensure that a medical evaluation is completed before starting voice therapy. Do not begin treating clients without clearance from their medical doctor (ideally, a laryngologist or ear-nose-throat [ENT] doctor).
  - Maintain a cooperative working relationship with a laryngologist; be knowledgeable about laryngeal surgical procedures and medications and their effects on and interactions with voice treatment methods.
  - Ensure that periodic medical examinations are completed during the course of voice therapy.
  - Combine, in most cases, techniques designed to reduce vocally abusive behaviors with those that facilitate efficient and normal voice production.
  - Help patients understand the nature of the disorder, what habits are maintaining the disorder, and the harmful results of the vocally abusive behaviors.
  - Work with illustrations of vocal anatomy and physiology, and explanations, as some adults may benefit from readings.
  - Offer computer games to children to motivate them to change their vocally abusive behaviors and improve their voices. For example, Kay Elemetrics (2004) has voice-game software.
  - Design a program to help patients reduce abusive behaviors and establish vocally appropriate behaviors.
  - Work closely with the patient's significant others (e.g., parents, siblings, spouses) to help reduce vocally abusive behaviors and to reinforce healthy vocal behaviors.
  - Establish baselines of vocally abusive behaviors and the frequency of abnormal voice productions in and outside the clinic.
  - Ask patients (or parents of young children) to measure their vocally abusive behaviors for a few days and graph their frequency on a daily basis to establish the baselines of vocally abusive behaviors in natural settings.
  - Consistently use audio recordings for feedback, ear training, and development of patients' ability to self-monitor; video recordings are even better.

- Support patients, especially adults, in identifying and making needed lifestyle changes, such as avoiding smoke (including secondhand smoke) and alcohol, taking appropriate allergy medications, and drinking enough water.

Summarized in this section are the most commonly used behavioral voice therapy techniques. It should be noted that this list is not exhaustive; as interest and research in voice therapy continues to expand, techniques will be refined and new protocols will surface. Some of these techniques can be used in conjunction with others; they are not mutually exclusive.

Lessac-Madsen Resonant Voice Therapy

Lessac-Madsen Resonant Voice Therapy (LMRVT) was developed by Verdolini-Abbott (2008), who has published a clinician's manual detailing exactly how to adhere to this voice therapy protocol. LMRVT is most commonly used with hyperfunctional voice disorders because it increases airflow and decreases muscle action for phonation.

- The principle of LMRVT is to eliminate vocal fold injury by configuring the larynx and surrounding structures to reduce the level of respiratory effort and impact stress on the vocal folds.
- LMRVT emphasizes a **forward focus** and **easy phonation**, and sensory processing is a key component; the client is encouraged to feel the vibrations resonating in the front of the face and mouth, particularly on the alveolar ridge and surrounding facial plates (Verdolini, Druker, Palmer, & Samawi, 1998). Rather than explicitly teaching how the larynx is mechanically configured to produce a more resonant voice, LMRVT relies on implicitly learning the configuration by imitating the clinician's models and attending to sensory information.

Chest Resonance

The concept of chest resonance is similar to that of the head and facial resonance described previously in LMRVT, but the feelings of vibration are forward focus and are placed in the chest.

- Chest resonance can be used for clients who have maladaptive high laryngeal positioning.
- Chest resonance can also be used for clients with Reinke's edema who are not candidates for surgery because they will not change their smoking habits.
- The clinician should instruct clients to let the voice "fall" to the chest; clients should not be pushing or forcing their voice down. Clients can start by humming to feel the vibrations in their chest and shape the hums into /h/ initial words and phrases, vary rate and pitch, and generalize into different conversational situations and environments.

Yawn–Sigh

The yawn–sigh method is used for hyperfunctional voice disorders because its goal is to increase airflow. The client is instructed to yawn and then sigh.

- The clinician instructs patients to drop their tongues when they sigh; this helps to drop the larynx and retract the false vocal folds, reducing the tension in the larynx. The yawn–sigh can be incorporated into resonant voice therapy.

Vocal Function Exercises

Vocal function exercises (VFEs) are a systematic protocol developed by Stemple (2006), who has published a manual for clinicians to follow. VFE increases the flexibility of the vocal folds through structured practice and can be used with hyper- or hypofunctional voice disorders.

- Stemple (2005) describes VFE as "physical therapy for the vocal folds" but states that VFEs are not just for those with voice disorders; like healthy individuals who exercise to maintain their physical health, VFE can be used by anyone to maintain vocal health. The importance of the relationship between respiration, phonation, and articulation is also emphasized. The VFE protocol consists of four exercises that should be practiced twice daily (morning and evening), two times each, and are to be completed as softly as possible and without tension.
- Stemple notes that it is important that the client understand that maximum phonation time will improve with the improvement of vocal fold vibration, not by increased lung volumes and forceful breaths.

Stretch and Flow

Originally developed by Stone and Casteel (1982), stretch and flow is a hierarchical voice therapy technique with a focus on airflow management. It can be used with individuals with hyperfunctional voice disorders. Stretch and flow emphasizes the coordination between respiration and phonation as well as reducing the tension and effort of phonation.

Twang

Lombard and Steinhauer (2007) report the use of **twang** with clients with hypofunctional voice disorders; however, it can also be used with hyperfunctional voice disorders, such as vocal nodules.

- Twang is a vocal quality similar to that of the singing style of country music.
- Anatomically, twang is created by the narrowing of the aryepiglottic sphincter, which forms a resonating cavity that matches that of the ear canal.
- Twang is perceived by the listener as louder but requires less effort and fatigue.
- Twang can be facilitated with implicit models of the non-linguistic phrase, "nya-nya," (/njæ, njæ/) or by prompting the client to cackle like a witch.
- A client may be encouraged to place the voice in the back of the mouth and to feel relaxed; twang should not be forced. Once clients get accustomed to the facilitator, they can imitate the clinician's models of words with the /æ/ sound, such as "maybe" and "back."
- Words with bilabial sounds (/m, b, p/) may also be used because when produced, bilabials create pressure at the lips and velopharyngeal port, which opens up the vocal folds (known as **transglottal pressure equalization**).
- Clients should be able to switch between their baseline voice and the twang quality (negative practice). Once they can do this, clients are encouraged to generalize twang into their conversational speech.

Integrated Implicit–Explicit Approach to Voice Training

Traditional voice therapy models typically rely on implicit, auditory–perceptual cues to teach novel vocal qualities (Verdolini-Marston, Burke, Lessac, Glaze, & Caldwell, 1995). Based on a theory derived from toddler acquisition of speech, implicit, auditory-perceptual voice therapy typically uses a model produced by the clinician that a client mimics (Stemple, Glaze, & Klaban, 2010; Verdolini-Marston et al., 1995). Once the client correctly mimics this implicit model, the auditory stimulus is taken through a behavioral hierarchy of voice production. This approach is based on the theory that intensive repetition and habitual use will allow for the integration of the auditory stimulus and generalization of voice production due to implicit memory and control of the vocal mechanism (Guenther, 2006; Verdolini, 1997).

- An integrated implicit–explicit approach to voice therapy consists of five steps, combining auditory–perceptual cues with knowledge of anatomy and physiology and outlined by Tellis (2018).
- The integration of implicit and explicit instruction to assist learning, generalization, and retention of a novel motor skill is promoted by current motor learning theory (Sanchez & Reber, 2013; Shmuelof et al., 2012; Taylor & Ivry, 2011; Taylor, Krakauer, & Ivry, 2014; Tellis, 2018; Toner & Moran, 2014).
- This voice therapy approach combines auditory-perceptual cues with higher cortical understanding of the vocal mechanism (unlike exclusive implicit learning approaches) and incorporates new motor learning theory into the approach including intentionality (Breivik, 2007); motor imagery (Eaves, Riach, Holmes, & Wright, 2016); action observation (Buccino, 2014; Rizzolatti & Sinigaglia, 2010); and varied brain processing during performance (Bertollo et al., 2016).
- Clinicians who are interested in using an integrated implicit-explicit approach to voice therapy can utilize any model based in the anatomy and physiology of the vocal mechanism. One that is recommended is the Estill voice training model (Steinhauer, Klimek, & Estill, 2017).

Singhale

Singhale (or **inhalation phonation**) is an exercise in which voice is produced on an inhalation rather than an exhalation.

- Singhale can be used in conjunction with other voice therapy techniques to reduce ventricular phonation (Sapienza & Hoffman Ruddy, 2017).
- Singhale serves to naturally humidify the vocal folds.
- Clients can be instructed to siren up and down in pitch on a singhale; this increases the flexibility of the vocal folds.

Hard Glottal Attack (and Decreasing It)

Some speech–language pathologists may use pushing or valsalva maneuvers to facilitate vocal fold closure in hypofunctional voice disorders. While this may help a patient achieve voice, some clinicians believe this technique is maladaptive because hard glottal onsets used repeatedly may cause lesions (such as vocal nodules) to form.

- Teaching clients stiff or smooth true vocal fold onset can help them transition out of using hard glottal attack if it is becoming a maladaptive behavior.

Coughing and Throat Clearing

Coughing and throat clearing can be used as a way to get vocal fold closure through a natural biological function. They can be used with hypofunctional voice disorders, puberphonia, and muscle tension dysphonia.

- The cough is facilitated first into a vowel and then to a lip trill. The client is then instructed to lip trill on a pitch, which will facilitate voice.

Rhythmic Breathing

This type of respiratory training can be used with clients with paradoxical vocal fold motion disorder (PVFMD) because it coordinates breathing with the opening of the vocal folds.

- The client is instructed to sniff in and exhale with pursed lips.
- Next, the false vocal folds are retracted (tell the client to pretend to yawn to facilitate false vocal fold retraction).
- Then the client should quietly inhale through the nose and exhale through the mouth, doing two counts of each in an "in in, out" pattern.
- Clients may also choose to do this pattern of inhalation and exhalation on the /f/ sound or through pursed lips.
- Once clients are independent in using rhythmic breathing, they can try to use it in different contexts, such as while walking and while walking and counting.

Lombard Effect

Speech-range masking can be an effective treatment technique for individuals (especially men) who wish to lower their vocal pitch.

- The clinician asks the patient to begin oral reading and records the patient's reading.
- Near the tenth word, masking is introduced.
- Utilizing the **Lombard effect** (in which the patient's voice becomes louder in the presence of background noise) with the introduction of masking noise, the voice usually spontaneously becomes louder and lower.
- Patients can then listen back to their lower voice and be encouraged that they are capable of producing this type of voice (Boone et al., 2013).

Gender Issues and the Voice

Basic Principles

Sometimes, clinicians serve clients who are experiencing gender reassignment. Some clients go from female to male, but more typically clients go from male to female. In these types of cases, the term **transsexual** has been used; however, today, the term **transgender** is most commonly used.

- The World Professional Association for Transgender Health (WPATH; 2014) estimates that there are 1.5 million transgender persons in the United States. The WPATH has introduced guidelines for service delivery to and care of persons who are undergoing gender identity changes. The guidelines recognize that these clients can be supported by receiving assistance in changing their voice, speech patterns, and overall communication style.
- For most transgender clients, the primary voice concern is achieving appropriate pitch. Vocal pitch factors that need to be modified include intonational variability, fundamental frequency, lower and

upper limits of the frequency range, and others (Gelfer & Schofield, 2000). Fundamental frequency of speech is used to measure the success of voice therapy in male-to-female transgender clients (McNeill, Wilson, Clark, & Deakin, 2009).

- Pitch disorders due to **hormonal changes** may affect some patients, especially women. Menstruation, menopause, use of oral contraceptives, and virilization (increased masculinity) of the female voice have all been associated with pitch changes.
- Pitch changes before and during menstruation are not usually a major problem. However, such changes are troublesome to professional singers. Lowered levels of estrogen and progesterone before menses can cause vocal fold thickening, with consequent hoarseness and lowered pitch.

Treatment

The female-to-male transgender client can often achieve lowered vocal pitch through hormonal therapy. Testosterone thickens the vocal folds, thus helping produce a lower pitch. Testosterone also increases muscle definition and increases facial and body hair.

- Male-to-female clients generally take estrogen, which successfully produces some physical changes, such as the softening of overall muscle definition. However, estrogen does not affect the vocal folds; the vocal folds remain the same as they always were, and the client's pitch remains masculine sounding.
- Some male-to-female clients undergo vocal surgery to achieve a higher pitched voice. For example, thyroplasty and longitudinal incision of the vocal folds can help the male-to-female client talk with a higher pitched voice. Even with surgery, however, experts recommend that these clients undergo voice therapy (Boone et al., 2013).
- Many clients experiencing gender reassignment experience vocal fatigue; it is important, in therapy, to build their vocal stamina and build up their endurance gradually so that they do not harm their vocal folds.
- Voice therapy for male-to-female clients includes several components (Adler, Hirsch, & Mordaunt, 2006; Case, 2002; Hooper, 2000; Stemple et al., 2014). One is teaching the client to use a greater number of rising pitch inflections at the ends of utterances. Other techniques to help the client sound more feminine include teaching the client to use greater articulatory precision, a softer voice, and more modals (*can, may, will, shall, must*). Clinicians can teach clients how to place their tongues more anteriorly in their mouths during speech; this helps clients achieve a more "forward" resonance, which is believed to be characteristic of the female voice (Hancock & Helenius, 2012).
- The clinician can also help the client learn to adopt more feminine body language, including gestures and facial expressions. Nonverbal communication is an important aspect of treatment.
- Transgender clients often need psychological support and counseling, as well as voice therapy. Clinicians must recognize that the issues experienced by transgender clients are complex and affect every area of the clients' lives—social, professional, personal, and others (Sue & Sue, 2013). These clients often find that support groups of other transgender clients are extremely helpful in dealing with issues surrounding gender reassignment (McCready, Campbell, Crutchley, & Edwards, 2011).

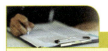

SUMMARY

Patients often seek evaluation and treatment for voice disorders that have been caused by physical changes to the larynx. One major physical change, for some patients, involves laryngeal cancer.

- Patients who have surgery for total removal of the larynx need specific rehabilitation to learn alaryngeal speech. Other patients present voice disorders that result from physical changes caused by abusive vocal habits, neurological problems, or irritation by environmental agents.
- Disorders of loudness and pitch can be caused by organic or functional factors. Treatment will depend upon the etiology of the problem, as well as the patient's cultural perception of what constitutes a normal voice.
- Patients who have psychogenic voice disorders have frequently undergone emotional trauma with consequent loss of voice. For many of these patients, behavioral therapy, counseling or psychotherapy, or a combination is quite successful in voice restoration.
- Clinicians sometimes see transgender patients who are going from female to male; more typically, transgender clients are going from male to female. For the latter group, surgery combined with voice therapy to help the client sound more feminine appears to be an optimal situation.

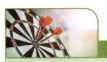

CHAPTER HIGHLIGHTS

- Having a normal, optimal-sounding voice depends on the health and intactness of the larynx and its structures. Key structures include the major laryngeal cartilages: thyroid cartilage, cricoid cartilage, arytenoid cartilages, and the corniculate and cuneiform cartilages. Cranial nerve X, the vagus nerve, is the nerve primarily responsible for innervation of the larynx.
- Key laryngeal muscles include the intrinsic laryngeal muscles: thyroarytenoids, cricothyroids, posterior cricoarytenoids, lateral cricoarytenoids, and interarytenoids. The extrinsic laryngeal muscles include (a) the infrahyoids or laryngeal depressors—thyrohyoids, omohyoids, sternothyroids, and sternohyoids—and (b) the suprahyoids or laryngeal elevators—digastrics, geniohyoids, mylohyoids, stylohyoids, genioglossus, and hyoglossus.
- Each individual's voice undergoes changes during his or her life span. These changes involve mean fundamental frequency and maximum phonation time.
- Vocal pitch (frequency) and volume (intensity) are important parameters of the voice. Vocal quality is greatly affected by patients' daily vocal habits.
- Evaluation of voice disorders should be comprehensive and based on a multidisciplinary team approach. A medical evaluation should be conducted before any therapy is initiated.
- Optimally, a voice evaluation should include (a) gathering a thorough case history, (b) conducting additional assessments, such as an oral peripheral examination and hearing screening, (c) performing instrumental analysis, and (d) conducting perceptual analysis of vocal characteristics.

- Disorders of resonance include hypernasality, hyponasality, assimilative nasality, and cul-de-sac resonance. For the patient with resonance problems, it is critical to rule out organic causes, such as velopharyngeal inadequacy. Therapy will not succeed unless any physical basis for the resonance problem is resolved.
- Disorders of voice are often associated with physical factors involving pathological changes of the laryngeal mechanism. These factors include carcinoma, physical changes due to vocal abuse, neurological problems, and vocal fold irritation created by environmental agents. Treatment often involves medication, surgery, therapy, or a combination of these approaches.
- Psychogenic voice disorders occur when the voice is abnormal in the presence of normal laryngeal structures. Hysterical or conversion aphonia is often attributed to an underlying emotional etiology. Patients with psychogenic voice disorders can often be successfully treated with a variety of behavioral strategies. However, some patients may require psychotherapy or counseling.
- Transgender patients who are going from male-to-female status or female-to-male status have unique needs that must be sensitively and thoroughly addressed.

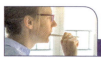

STUDY AND REVIEW QUESTIONS

1. You are evaluating a girl who has been referred because of difficulties associated with partial submucous cleft palate accompanied by a bifid uvula. During your evaluation, you can probably expect to find

    A. hypernasality, leading to difficulty producing nasals adequately.
    B. hypernasality, accompanied by decreased intraoral breath pressure, leading to difficulties with adequate production of fricatives, affricates, and plosives.
    C. hyponasality, accompanied by increased intraoral breath pressure, leading to difficulties with adequate production of liquids and glides.
    D. hypernasality, accompanied by difficulty producing vowels and nasals adequately.

2. The suprahyoid laryngeal muscles lie above the hyoid bone; they are sometimes called **elevators.** The suprahyoid muscles are the

    A. digastrics, geniohyoids, thyrohyoids, stylohyoids, genioglossus, and sternothyroids.
    B. thyrohyoids, digastrics, stylohyoids, and hyoglossus.
    C. geniohyoids, mylohyoids, stylohyoids, and genioglossus.
    D. digastrics, geniohyoids, mylohyoids, stylohyoids, genioglossus, and hyoglossus.

3. Sometimes specialists assess the lung volume of voice patients because breath support is inadequate. Specialists can measure _____ or the total volume of air in the lungs; other measurements can include _____

or the amount of air inhaled and exhaled during a normal breathing cycle and _____ or the volume of air that the patient can exhale after a maximal exhalation.

   A. Total lung capacity, tidal volume, vital capacity
   B. Vital capacity, tidal capacity, total lung volume
   C. Vital capacity, total lung capacity, tidal volume
   D. Tidal volume, total lung capacity, vital volume

4. You have been asked to counsel with Doug, a 45-year-old man who has smoked and drank alcohol since he was a teenager. He now has laryngeal cancer, and before surgery, the surgeon asks you to talk with Doug about esophageal speech. You explain to Doug that there are two basic types of esophageal speech. In one method, the patient is taught to keep the esophagus open and relaxed while inhaling rapidly. In the other method, the patient impounds the air in the oral cavity, pushes it back into the esophagus, and vibrates the cricopharyngeus muscle. The second method is called the

   A. inhalation method.
   B. injection method.
   C. inspiratory injection method.
   D. laryngeal airway resistance method.

5. A singer comes to you for therapy. She has had bypass surgery, and in the process, there was damage to her recurrent laryngeal nerve. In the course of intervention, you will most likely focus on

   A. blowing exercises for more precise direction of her airstream.
   B. abdominal exercises to strengthen the foundation for respiration.
   C. chewing exercises to improve overall oral coordination.
   D. strategies to improve vocal fold adduction.

6. A 67-year-old man comes to you for a voice evaluation. He was referred by his primary care doctor. He states that his voice has been getting "weaker" for the past 5–6 months. Upon oral peripheral examination, you find that he has fasciculations (tremors) of the tongue and some general facial weakness. The first thing you would do is

   A. refer him to a psychologist for an evaluation.
   B. take detailed notes and tell him to come back in 6 months.
   C. begin voice therapy, focusing on strengthening exercises.
   D. refer him to a neurologist for an evaluation.

7. You are asked to see an 8-year-old boy, Jason, for potential therapy because he is very hoarse. Jason has been hoarse for approximately 8 months. He is an active, happy third grader who loves sports and is engaged in various types of sports (soccer, baseball, etc.) year-round. Reportedly, Jason frequently screams at games. At the school, there is a 15-minute recess in the morning and a 30-minute recess after lunch. You observe Jason on the playground at recess several times over a period of 2 weeks and see that he loves to run, play, and yell loudly with his friends. Jason's parents have given you a letter from the ENT that definitively states that Jason has vocal nodules. After an evaluation, the first thing you would do is

   A. prescribe 2–3 weeks of almost total voice rest, telling Jason and his parents that he can speak only when he absolutely has to—no yelling at recess or when he plays sports.

   B. monitor Jason's vocal status by seeing him once every 2 months for the next year to observe whether his hoarseness gets better or worse.

   C. focus on identification and reduction of vocally abusive behavior, such as yelling and screaming, using computer games to help motivate Jason to use better vocal habits.

   D. give Jason and his parents reading materials that discuss vocal abuse and tell the parents that if the hoarseness does not resolve in 1–2 months, you will probably see Jason for voice therapy.

8. Vivian, a 72-year-old woman, has just had surgery for laryngeal cancer. The clinician is trying to support Vivian in many ways, including asking several laryngectomy patients from a local support group to come and talk with Vivian about her options for speech. The support group members strongly recommend the Blom-Singer prosthetic device. They explain that the device is used by laryngectomees to

   A. shunt air from the esophagus to the trachea so that the salpingopharyngeus muscle will vibrate during inhalation.

   B. assist in the development of competent esophageal speech.

   C. prevent particles of food from entering the trachea.

   D. shunt the air from the trachea to the esophagus so that the patient can speak on pulmonary air entering the esophagus.

9. Patients who might be treated with CO_2 laser surgery, recurrent laryngeal nerve resection, Botox, voice therapy, or a combination would probably have

   A. contact ulcers.   C. hemangioma.
   B. paradoxical vocal fold motion. D. spasmodic dysphonia.

10. A client comes to a clinician seeking voice therapy. Chris is a 25-year-old male-to-female transgender client who has undergone several procedures to become more feminine. She tells you that she is also taking estrogen. She shares that she needs help to speak in a more feminine way, but she does not know how to go about this. She is also dealing with emotional issues surrounding her gender reassignment. In this case, the clinician should ideally

   A. tell Chris that various surgical procedures, such as thyroplasty, are available and that having surgical procedures will be sufficient to help her change her voice to sound more feminine.

   B. advise Chris that surgical procedures are unnecessary, but that voice therapy will help her to sound more feminine by teaching her new communication patterns, such as higher pitch and more feminine intonation patterns.

C. advise Chris that a combination of voice therapy and counseling will be the best way for her to sound more feminine and also receive emotional support as she deals with gender reassignment issues.

D. advise Chris that a combination of counseling, surgery, and voice therapy to teach her more feminine pitch levels and communication patterns would best serve her needs.

11. The cover-body theory of phonation states that

A. the epithelium and the superficial, intermediate, and deep layers of the lamina propria vibrate as a "cover" on a relatively stationary "body." This body is composed of the remainder of the TA muscle.

B. the epithelium, the deep layer of the lamina propria, and much of the superficial layer of the lamina propria vibrate as a "cover" on a relatively stationary "body," which is made up of the remainder of the superficial layer, the deep layer, and the TA muscle.

C. the superficial layer of the lamina propria and much of the intermediate layer of the lamina propria vibrate as a "cover" on a relatively stationary "body," which is made up of the remainder of the intermediate layer, the deep layer, and the TA muscle.

D. the epithelium and much of the intermediate layer of the lamina propria vibrate as a "cover" on a relatively stationary "body," which is made up of the remainder of the intermediate layer and the TA muscle.

Questions 12–16 refer to the following scenario:

As a clinician in a medically based private practice, you receive a referral of 22-year-old Juanita, a college cheerleader. Juanita has been a cheerleader since her freshman year at Freeport College; she is now a senior. She works part-time as a telemarketer, and, according to her boyfriend, she is always "glued to her cell phone." She also sings in the college chorus. She has been hoarse for several years and tells you during the case history, "I've ignored the way I sound—it's just me. I haven't felt like I've needed to change anything." However, she shares that lately, she has been feeling a lot of pain and the hoarseness is substantially worse. She says, "Sometimes when I talk, it's almost like there's a 'double voice.'" She tells you that she is worried because she will graduate from college in 3 months and will be looking for a job. She is worried that employers will not want to hire someone who "sounds like a frog." You immediately refer Juanita to an otolaryngologist for a thorough examination of her vocal folds. You then proceed to do your own instrumental and perceptual evaluation. You come up with a number of findings, including the fact that Juanita has increased laryngeal airway resistance, a maximum phonation time of 6 seconds, and dysphonia. You think that she is a probable candidate for phonosurgery but will wait for the otolaryngologist's diagnosis and recommendations.

12. When you assess Juanita, you indeed find the presence of "double voice." The perception of two distinct simultaneous pitches during phonation is

A. glottal fry.
B. diplophonia.
C. strain-strangle.
D. cul-de-sac resonance.

13. You need to view Juanita's vocal folds. You know that the otolaryngologist will do this also, but you are fortunate to have instrumentation available to you. You decide to use a procedure that uses a pulsing light to permit the optical illusion of slow-motion viewing of the vocal folds. This is called

    A. electroglottography.

    B. videostroboscopy.

    C. electromyography.

    D. videofluoroscopy.

14. Measures of jitter and shimmer are becoming more common in use with voice patients because they can be useful in early detection of vocal pathology. Although you suspect that the otolaryngologist will find obvious vocal pathology, given Juanita's history of prolonged hoarseness, you still want to obtain measures of jitter and shimmer because these can serve as an excellent baseline—especially if Juanita has phonosurgery. When you take these measures, you might expect to see

    A. a small amount of shimmer and a large amount of jitter.

    B. a large amount of jitter with only a small or moderate amount of shimmer.

    C. large amounts of both jitter and shimmer, with more than 1 dB of variation across vibratory cycles when jitter is measured.

    D. large amounts of both jitter and shimmer, with more than 1 dB of variation across vibratory cycles when shimmer is measured.

15. You receive a phone call and a report from the otolaryngologist that Juanita will indeed need phonosurgery for the presence of bilateral vocal fold polyps (the right polyp is larger than the left). The otolaryngologist wants you to obtain quantitative measurements of Juanita's voice before phonosurgery; he wants to use these baseline measures as a comparison with measures taken after phonosurgery to evaluate whether the phonosurgery was successful. To obtain these quantitative measurements, you will probably use

    A. esophageal manometry.

    B. indirect laryngoscopy.

    C. a sound spectrograph.

    D. a plethysmograph.

16. As part of counseling Juanita, you share with her that phonosurgery will be necessary. You emphasize that if she continues to abuse her voice, she may have to have repeated surgeries. These repeated surgeries can cause her voice to sound gravelly and rough, which is primarily a result of

    A. reduced mucosal wave action.

    B. insufficient air supply for optimal phonation.

    C. resonance problems.

    D. papillomas.

References and Recommended Readings at www.advancedreviewpractice.com

STUDY AND REVIEW ANSWERS

1. **B.** A client with a partial submucous cleft palate and bifid uvula will most likely manifest hypernasality, accompanied by decreased intraoral breath pressure, leading to difficulties with adequate production of fricatives, affricates, and plosives.
2. **D.** The suprahyoid muscles or elevators are the digastrics, geniohyoids, mylohyoids, stylohyoids, genioglossus, and hyoglossus.
3. **A.** Sometimes specialists assess the lung volume of voice patients because breath support is inadequate. Specialists can measure total lung capacity, or the total volume of air in the lungs; other measurements can include tidal volume, or the amount of air inhaled and exhaled during a normal breathing cycle, and vital capacity, or the volume of air that the patient can exhale after a maximal exhalation.
4. **B.** In the injection method, the patient impounds the air in the oral cavity, pushes it back into the esophagus, and vibrates the cricopharyngeus muscle.
5. **D.** The singer who had damage to her recurrent laryngeal nerve would benefit from strategies to improve vocal fold adduction.
6. **D.** The first thing a clinician must do with a patient who exhibits potential signs of a neurological problem is refer the patient to a neurologist.
7. **C.** Voice rest for an 8-year-old boy is somewhat unrealistic. There is no indication that he needs a counselor. He is old enough to identify and reduce vocally abusive behaviors.
8. **D.** The Blom-Singer device is used to shunt air from the trachea to the esophagus so that the patient can speak on that air.
9. **D.** The above-listed treatment techniques are commonly used with patients who have spasmodic dysphonia.
10. **D.** It would be best for the clinician to advise Chris that a combination of counseling, surgery, and voice therapy to teach more feminine pitch levels and communication patterns would best serve her needs.
11. **A.** The cover-body theory of phonation states that the epithelium and the superficial, intermediate, and deep layers of the lamina propria vibrate as a "cover" on a relatively stationary "body." This body is composed of the remainder of the TA muscle.
12. **B.** The term *diplophonia* refers to the perception of a "double voice."
13. **B.** Videostroboscopy is the only procedure that uses a pulsing "strobe" light for perceived slow-motion viewing of the vocal folds.
14. **D.** Measurements of jitter, or frequency perturbation, indicate that in a normal speaker with no vocal pathology, jitter should be less than 1% as the speaker sustains a vowel. Measurements of shimmer, or amplitude perturbation, evaluate the cycle-to-cycle variation of vocal intensity. Some experts believe that more than 1 dB of variation across cycles when shimmer is measured causes a patient to sound dysphonic.
15. **C.** The sound or speech spectrograph is very useful for quantitative analysis of speech and is often used to obtain baseline measurements of a patient's vocal characteristics prior to phonosurgery. Post-surgery measures could be obtained and compared to the baseline measurements of Juanita's voice to quantitatively document vocal improvement or decline.
16. **A.** If a patient experiences repeated vocal surgeries, reduced mucosal wave action of the vocal folds is a real possibility. Reduced mucosal wave action can make the voice sound rough and gravelly to the listener.

CHAPTER 8

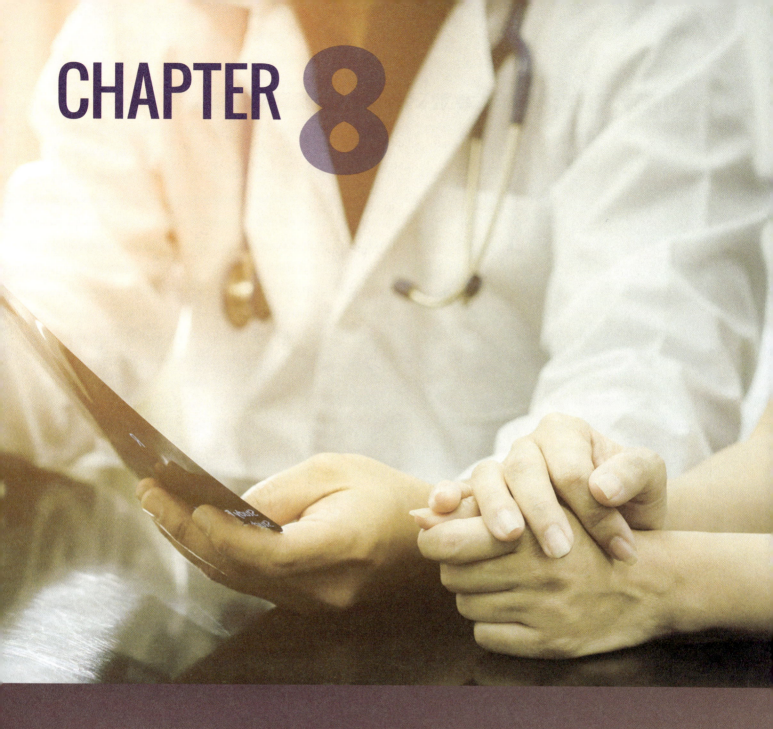

NEUROLOGICALLY BASED COMMUNICATIVE DISORDERS

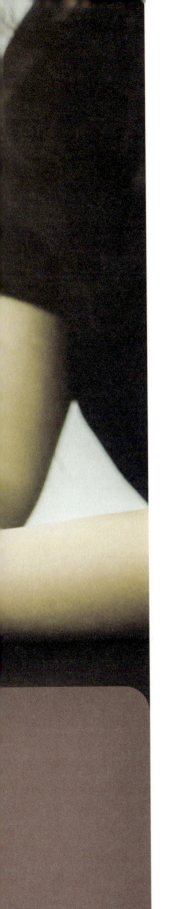

This chapter provides an overview of the nature, assessment, and treatment of aphasia, dementia, right hemisphere disorder, and traumatic brain injury, all associated with neuropathology. Motor speech disorders and dysphagia, also associated with neurological problems, are discussed in the next chapter.

To understand the communication disorders described in this chapter, an adequate knowledge of neuroanatomy and basic neuroscience is essential. For more information, see Chapter 1 and consult other sources (Bhatnagar, 2017; Love & Webb, 2016; Nolte, 2009; Seikel, King, & Drumright, 2016; Webb & Adler, 2016).

APHASIA

Aphasia, a neurologically based language disorder, is caused by various types of neuropathologies (most commonly, stroke). It can be classified as fluent, nonfluent, or subcortical. It may or may not be accompanied by alexia, agraphia, or agnosia. Assessment of patients with aphasia may involve standardized tests and functional assessment tools. Treatment of aphasia is concerned with verbal expression, auditory comprehension, reading, writing, and nonverbal modes of communication (Chapey, 2008; Davis, 2014; Hegde, 2018a, 2018b, 2018c, 2018d; Hegde & Freed, 2017; Helm-Estabrooks, Albert, & Nicholas, 2014; LaPointe & Stierwalt, 2018).

Incidence and Prevalence of Aphasia

Clinicians should get the latest available updates to the demographic statistics summarized below because statistics frequently change. For the latest information, visit the websites of the National Stroke Association, American Stroke Association, National Aphasia Association, National Institute of Neurological Diseases and Stroke, and Centers for Disease Control and Prevention (CDC). Current demographic statistics are as follows:

- About 795,000 new cases of stroke are reported each year; about a quarter of all strokes are repeat events.
- In the United States, a stroke occurs about every 40 seconds (Benjamin et al., 2017).
- Annually, more than 130,000 deaths occur due to strokes, equivalent to one every 4 minutes (Benjamin et al., 2017).
- More than 50% of those who survive a stroke have aphasia.
- Strokes cause permanent disability in more than 300,000 people per year.

- The incidence of strokes increases with advancing age; two-thirds of stroke patients are age 65 and older.
- Men are more prone to strokes than women, although more women experience strokes, because of their longevity.
- African-American men and women have a higher incidence (nearly 2 times higher) of strokes than White men and women (Benjamin et al., 2017).
- South Asians also have a high prevalence of strokes.
- Hispanics and African Americans tend to have strokes at an earlier age than Whites.
- About 87% of all strokes are ischemic; Whites are more prone to this type of stroke than people of other racial backgrounds; African Americans, Hispanics, Native Americans, and Asians are more prone to hemorrhagic strokes than Whites.

Neuropathology of Aphasia

Aphasia is caused by various kinds of neuropathologies. A leading cause of death in the United States, cerebrovascular accidents (CVA), commonly known as **strokes**, often lead to aphasia. Strokes may be ischemic or hemorrhagic.

- **Ischemic strokes**

  - are caused by a blocked or interrupted blood supply to the brain. Thrombosis or embolism, two kinds of arterial diseases that cause problems in blood circulation. A collection of material that blocks the flow of blood, a **thrombus**, is usually due to **atherosclerosis**, a condition in which cholesterol and other fatty substances build up in the blood, narrowing arteries and obstructing blood flow. An **embolus** is a mass of arterial debris or a clump of tissue from a tumor that originates somewhere else in the body, travels to the brain, and gets lodged in a smaller artery and, thus, blocks the flow of blood.
  - deprive a focal area of brain tissue of the blood supply, causing an **ischemic core** or **infarct**, which is an irreversible cell death that occurs within an hour. During ischemia, a surrounding area of tissue that is not totally deprived of blood flow also exists, known as the **ischemic penumbra**; while tissue function is compromised, the penumbra still receives enough blood flow to prevent necrosis (cell death). With immediate and proper medical attention, the penumbra can be saved from lasting damage, creating a more positive prognosis for the patient. Figure 8.1 shows the core and penumbra.
  - may also be **transient ischemic attacks** (TIAs), which are smaller ischemic events that are typically broken down by the body within 24 hours. Single TIAs may not cause permanent deficits, but repeated attacks may. A TIA may also predict a larger, more detrimental ischemia in the future (Manasco, 2014).

- **Hemorrhagic strokes**

  - are caused by bleeding in the brain due to ruptured blood vessels, with **hypertension** (high blood pressure) being a major risk factor. Blood vessel ruptures may be **intracerebral** (within the brain) or **extracerebral** (within the meninges, resulting in subarachnoid, subdural, and epidural varieties of stroke). Hemorrhagic strokes tend to have a sudden onset characterized by a severe "thunderclap" headache.

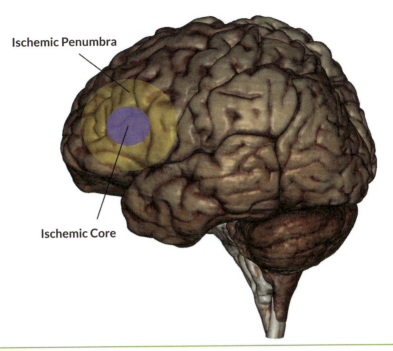

Figure 8.1 Core and penumbra. Used with permission from Anatomage.

- interrupt the blood flow to the brain, thus causing tissue damage.
- damage the cells when the blood pools in the brain.
- increase intracranial pressure caused by the increased bleeding within the cortex or between the skull and cortex, resulting in further tissue damage.

■ Individuals have a greater chance of surviving an ischemic stroke than a hemorrhagic stroke; emergency surgery is necessary to stop the bleeding from a hemorrhage. Individuals who receive prompt medical attention and survive the hemorrhagic stroke are likely to have fewer long-lasting deficits than someone who survives an ischemic stroke.

Key Terms

A few key terms are used in describing aphasia symptoms:

■ **Paraphasia**—an expressive language error that is not the result of a motor deficit; types include:

- **Semantic paraphasia**—substitution of one word for another; may be *related* in meaning (e.g., "marker" for "pencil") or *unrelated* (e.g., "cup" for "pencil")
- **Phonemic** (or **literal**) **paraphasia**—errors at the sound level; phonemes in the intended word may be substituted, omitted, or transposed (e.g., "tup" for "cup")
- **Neologistic paraphasia** (or **neologism**)—nonwords a person creates; they are unintelligible, unrelated to the intended word, and 50% or more of the words are meaningless (Goodglass, Kaplan, & Barresi, 2001b) (e.g., saying "skeen" instead of "pencil")

■ **Perseveration**—a word that is repeated inappropriately instead of an intended word. For example, during a naming task, a patient may correctly name a pencil but can then perseverate on the word "pencil" when naming the next items; perseveration may also occur on paraphasic speech (**perseverative paraphasia**)

- **Logorrhea**—excessive and inappropriate production of speech, often tangential and meaningless
- **Empty speech**—substitution of such general words as *this*, *that*, *stuff*, and *thing* in place of more specific words
- **Agrammatic speech**—omission of grammatic features in speech; speech that consists mostly of **content words** (nouns, verbs, etc.) and lacks **function words** (articles, conjunctions, prepositions, etc.)
- **Anomia**—naming difficulty or word-finding deficit with varying severity
- **Circumlocution**—production of nonspecific words and "beating around the bush," often due to word finding problems
- **Automatic language** (**preserved language**)—language that is rote or overlearned and thus spared (e.g., reciting the alphabet, counting numbers, singing a familiar song)

Definition and Classification of Aphasia

Among the available definitions, some are nontypological, suggest a single disorder; others are typological that classify aphasia into types. Other definitions are based on cognitive functions (Hegde, 2018a).

- **Nontypological definition**. A basic nontypological definition is that aphasia is a language disorder due to recent brain injury (Benson & Ardila, 1996). Language comprehension and expression, along with reading and writing, may be impaired to varying extents.
- **Typological definition**. Goodglass, Kaplan, and Barresi (2001a) define *aphasia* as the "disturbance of any or all of the skills, associations, and habits of spoken or written language, produced by injury to certain brain areas that are specialized for these functions" (p. 5). Fluent, nonfluent, and subcortical aphasias are among the major types.
- **Cognitive definitions**. Impaired cognition is an element in these definitions of aphasia. For example, Davis (2014) defines *aphasia* as "a selective impairment of the cognitive system specialized for comprehending and formulating language, leaving other cognitive capacities relatively intact" (p. 1).

Progressive communication disorders that are due to such neurological diseases as Alzheimer's disease and Parkinson's disease are *not* aphasia. Also, confused or abnormal language with generally intact grammar but often describing unreal events (e.g., hallucinations and delusions associated with such psychiatric disorders as schizophrenia) is not aphasia.

Nonfluent Aphasias

Nonfluent aphasias are characterized by limited, agrammatic, effortful, halting, and slow speech with impaired prosody.

Broca's Aphasia

The classic nonfluent variety, Broca's aphasia (BA) is historically considered to involve Broca's area (Brodmann's areas 44 and 45) in the posterior inferior frontal gyrus of the left hemisphere (LH) of the brain. Broca's area is supplied by the upper division of the middle cerebral artery. Damage to Broca's area is not always necessary to produce BA, because symptoms characteristic of it may be observed in some patients whose Broca's area is *intact*. Damage limited to Broca's area results in faster recovery than damage that is extensive. The anterior segment of the left arcuate fasciculus (a white matter tract lying deep in the posterior part of Broca's area) and the sensory motor area reliably predict nonfluent aphasia (Fridriksson, Guo, Fillmore, Holland, & Rorden, 2013). BA is characterized by the following:

- Impaired naming, especially confrontation naming (anomia)
- Nonfluent, effortful, slow, halting, and uneven speech
- Limited word output; short phrases and sentences
- Misarticulated or distorted speech sounds
- Agrammatic or telegraphic speech (often limited to content words, with omission of function words)
- Impaired repetition of words and sentences, especially the grammatical elements of a sentence
- Rarely normal but better auditory comprehension of spoken language than production
- Difficulty in understanding syntactic structures
- Poor oral reading and poor comprehension of material that has been read
- Writing problems (slow and laborious writing that is full of spelling errors and letter omissions, possibly because patients are forced to use their nonpreferred left hand due to paralysis of the right hand)
- Monotonous speech
- Awareness of expressive language deficits often manifested as frustration
- Such neurological symptoms as right-sided paralysis or weakness (paresis)
- Emotional reactions when frustrated, along with depression, may be additional symptoms
- Coexisting motor speech disorders (apraxia and dysarthria)

A lesion in the area of the brain shown in Figure 8.2 would create symptoms characteristic of BA.

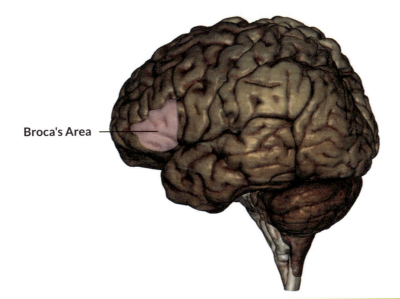

Figure 8.2 Broca's area. Used with permission from Anatomage.

Transcortical Motor Aphasia

Transcortical motor aphasia (TMA) is a nonfluent variety caused by lesions in the supplementary motor cortex and/or the area anterior to Broca's area, which is not affected. The areas supplied by the anterior cerebral artery and the anterior branch of the middle cerebral artery are affected in TMA. The name is misleading because no form of aphasia is a motor problem (Hallowell, 2017). TMA is characterized by the following:

- Absent or reduced spontaneous speech (presumably due to damage to the anterior superior frontal lobe, involved in speech initiation)
- Nonfluent, paraphasic, agrammatic, and telegraphic speech
- Intact repetition skill, a distinguishing characteristic of TMA; possibly repeating long and complex sentences without errors
- Echolalia and perseveration
- Awareness of grammaticality (patients may correct a grammatically incorrect model)
- Refusal to repeat nonsense syllables
- Unfinished sentence productions
- Limited word fluency
- Use of simple and imprecise syntactic structures
- Attempts to initiate speech with the help of such motor activities as clapping, vigorous head nodding, and hand waving
- Generally good comprehension of simple conversation (generally intact Wernicke's area); comprehension possibly impaired for complex speech
- Slow and difficult reading aloud
- Seriously impaired writing
- Motor disorders including rigidity of upper extremities; absence or poverty of movement (akinesia); slowness of movement (bradykinesia); buccofacial apraxia; and right hemiparesis, which may be more commonly observed than right hemiplegia
- Apathy, withdrawal, and little interest in communication

Overall, characteristics of TMA tend to resemble those of BA but with intact repetition skill.

A lesion to the supplementary cortex and/or anterior to Broca's area shown in Figure 8.3 would create symptoms characteristic of TMA.

Mixed Transcortical Aphasia

Mixed transcortical aphasia (MTA) is a somewhat rare variety of nonfluent aphasia caused by lesions in the watershed area or the arterial border zone of the brain (between the areas supplied by the middle cerebral arteries and the anterior and posterior arteries, described in Chapter 1); the damage spares and isolates Broca's area, Wernicke's area, and the arcuate fasciculus. MTA is characterized by the following:

- Limited spontaneous speech
- Automatic, unintentional, and involuntary nature of communication
- Severe echolalia (parrotlike repetition of what is heard), a distinguishing feature in the context of severe communication deficits; possible repetition of whatever the examiner says

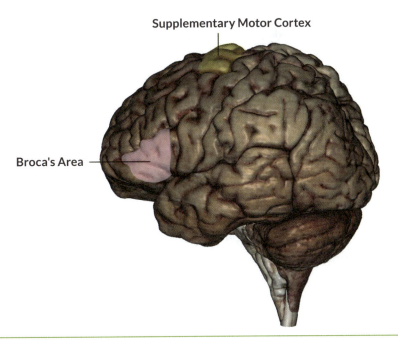

Figure 8.3 Supplementary motor cortex. Used with permission from Anatomage.

- Severely impaired fluency
- Severely impaired auditory comprehension for even simple conversation
- Marked naming difficulty and neologism; impaired confrontation naming
- Mostly unimpaired automatic speech (e.g., possible recitation of months in a year or a number series) if somehow initiated and not interrupted
- Severely impaired reading, reading comprehension, and writing

Neurologic symptoms include bilateral upper motor neuron paralysis (spastic paralysis that affects the volitional muscles), weakness of all limbs (quadriparesis), and visual field defects.

Global Aphasia

Global aphasia (GA) is the most severe form of nonfluent aphasia. It is caused by extensive lesions affecting all language areas (the perisylvian region), usually due to occlusion of the left middle cerebral artery. Widespread destruction of the frontotemporoparietal regions of the brain is common, though in rare cases Broca's and Wernicke's areas may be spared or the subcortical structures of the thalamus and basal ganglia may be involved. The more common sites of damage are supplied by the middle cerebral artery. GA is characterized by the following:

- Profoundly impaired receptive and expressive language skills and no significant profile of differential skills
- Greatly reduced fluency, expressions limited to a few words, exclamations, and serial utterances
- Impaired repetition, naming, and auditory comprehension
- Perseveration

- Impaired reading and writing
- Intact response to whole-body commands (e.g., stand up, lie down) in a few cases
- Coexisting verbal and nonverbal apraxia
- A right-sided paresis or paralysis, right-sided sensory loss, and neglect of the left side of the body may be observed in many patients, although GA without hemiparesis has been reported.

Fluent Aphasias

Varieties of fluent aphasias are characterized by relatively intact fluency but generally less meaningful, or even meaningless, speech. The speech is generally flowing, abundant, easily initiated, and well articulated with good prosody and phrase length. Lesions producing fluent aphasias are farther away from the areas of the brain responsible for motor control; thus, individuals with fluent aphasia usually will not have hemiparesis or other gross motor impairments (Manasco, 2014).

Wernicke's Aphasia

Wernicke's aphasia (WA) is the classic variety of fluent aphasia caused by lesions in Wernicke's area. Figure 8.4 illustrates Wernicke's area. Generally, the lesions are limited to the posterior one third of the superior temporal gyrus in the LH of the brain; occasionally, the lesions may extend throughout the temporal region and into the inferior parietal region. Wernicke's area is supplied by the inferior/posterior branch of the left middle cerebral artery. WA is characterized by the following:

- Incessant, effortlessly produced, flowing speech with normal, or even abnormal, fluency (**logorrhea**) with normal phrase length
- Rapid rate of speech with normal prosodic features and good articulation
- Intact grammatical structures
- Severe anomia
- Paraphasic speech containing semantic and literal paraphasias, extra syllables in words, and neologisms
- Circumlocution
- Empty speech
- Poor auditory comprehension, especially for sentences and names of common objects; much worse comprehension of speech when there is background noise, movement, or conversation
- Impaired conversational turn taking
- Impaired repetition skill
- Reading and writing problems, especially if the lesions extend to the inferior parietal region toward the visual association cortex, the angular gyrus, or both; difficulty recognizing sounds associated with written words and meanings of printed words; excessive but meaningless writing, frequent misspellings, and neologistic writing
- Generally poor communication in spite of fluent speech
- **Anosognosia**, an inability to recognize and acknowledge deficits (lack of insight). Individuals may not recognize their communication breakdowns and may not attempt to correct themselves. Persons with WA may confabulate an excuse for their errors (Manasco, 2014). They may sound confused but are less frustrated with their failed attempts at communication.

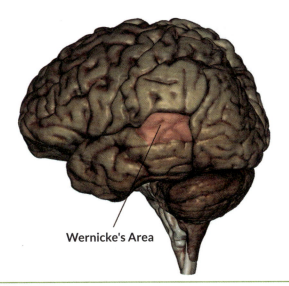

Figure 8.4 Wernicke's area. Used with permission from Anatomage.

- Paranoia, homicidal and suicidal thoughts, and depression may be additional features.
- Individuals with Wernicke's aphasia are generally free from obvious neurological symptoms; paresis and paralysis are uncommon.

Transcortical Sensory Aphasia

Transcortical sensory aphasia (TSA) is a variety of fluent aphasia caused by lesions in the temporoparietal region of the brain, especially in the posterior portion of the middle temporal gyrus; Broca's area, Wernicke's area, and the arcuate fasciculus may be largely unaffected, but parts of the occipital lobe may be affected. The name is misleading, because no form of aphasia is a sensory problem (Hallowell, 2017). The affected region is supplied by the posterior branches of the left middle cerebral artery. TSA is characterized by the following:

- Fluent speech with normal phrase length, good prosody, normal articulation, and apparently appropriate grammar and syntax
- Paraphasic and empty speech
- Severe naming problems and pauses in speech due to the naming difficulties
- Good repetition skills but poor comprehension of repeated words
- Echolalia of grammatically incorrect forms, nonsense syllables, and words from foreign languages (unlike patients with TMA)
- Impaired auditory comprehension of spoken language
- Difficulty in pointing, obeying commands, or answering simple yes–no questions
- Normal automatic speech (e.g., counting)
- Tendency to complete poems and sentences started by the clinician
- Good reading (aloud) but poor comprehension of material that has been read
- Generally better oral reading skills than other language skills
- Writing problems that parallel those in expressive speech

- An initial hemiparesis that may disappear, leaving the patient with no obvious neurologic impairment.
- Neglect of one side of the body may be common.

Patients with TSA sound similar to those with WA; however, repetition is intact in patients with TSA, whereas it is impaired in patients with WA.

Figure 8.5 shows the posterior middle temporal gyrus, a common lesion site (but not the only one) that creates TSA.

Conduction Aphasia

Conduction aphasia (CA) is a rare and controversial variety of fluent aphasia caused by lesions in the region between Broca's area and Wernicke's area, especially in the supramarginal gyrus in the inferior parietal lobe and the arcuate fasciculus (Berthler, Lambon Ralph, Pujol, & Green, 2012; Davis, 2014). Other affected areas include the upper portions of the temporal lobe and the insula. CA is characterized by the following:

- Disproportionate impairment in repetition (a distinguishing characteristic); especially impaired repetition of longer words, function words, and longer phrases and sentences
- Variable speech fluency across patients; generally less fluent than patients with Wernicke's aphasia
- Paraphasic speech (phonemic paraphasias)
- Marked word-finding problems, especially for content words
- Empty speech because of omitted content words
- Efforts to correct errors in speech, though not always successful
- Good syntax, prosody, and articulation

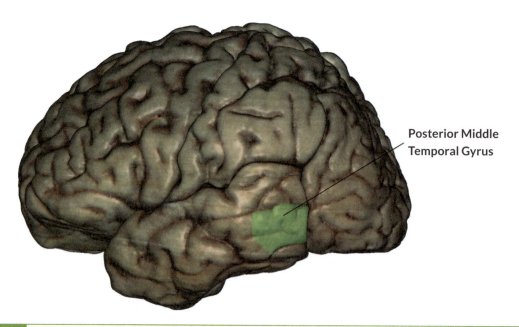

Figure 8.5 Posterior middle temporal gyrus. Used with permission from Anatomage.

- Severe to mild naming problems
- Near-normal auditory comprehension, especially for routine conversational speech
- Being better at pointing to a named stimulus than at confrontation naming
- Highly variable reading problems; better comprehension of silently read material
- Writing problems in most cases
- Buccofacial apraxia (difficulty in performing buccofacial movements when requested) in most patients
- Absence of neurological symptoms in some, paresis of the right side of the face and limb in others; oral apraxia and right sensory impairment may be present; recovery from most of these impairments is common

Symptoms of CA are similar to those of WA. The main difference is that unlike patients with Wernicke's, those with CA have good to normal auditory comprehension.

Figures 8.6 and 8.7 show the arcuate fasciculus and the supramarginal gyrus, lesion sites hypothesized to be associated with CA.

Anomic Aphasia

Anomic aphasia (AA), a fluent type, is controversial, mostly because it may be caused by lesions in different regions of the brain, including the angular gyrus, the second temporal gyrus, and the juncture of the temporoparietal lobes.

AA is a type of aphasia, whereas **anomia** is a naming difficulty (a symptom) common to most forms of aphasia, as well as many forms of nonfocal brain disease. AA is characterized by the following:

- A most debilitating and pervasive word-finding difficulty, which is its distinguishing feature; no impairment of pointing to named objects
- Generally fluent speech; normal syntax except for pauses (possibly due to word-finding problems)
- Use of vague and nonspecific words, resulting in empty speech
- Semantic paraphasias
- Circumlocution
- Good auditory comprehension of spoken language
- Intact repetition, unimpaired articulation
- Normal oral reading skills, good reading comprehension, and normal writing skills

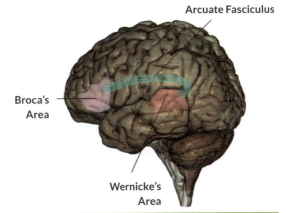

Figure 8.6 Arcuate fasciculus. Used with permission from Anatomage.

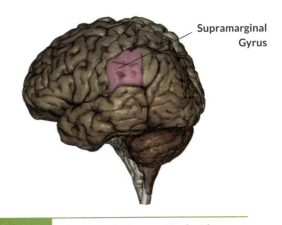

Figure 8.7 Supramarginal gyrus. Used with permission from Anatomage.

The distinguishing feature of AA is that, generally, most language functions, except for naming, are relatively unimpaired.

In patients who recover from any type of aphasia, a persistent naming difficulty may be a residual symptom.

Subcortical Aphasia

Aphasia is typically produced by cortical damage; however, extensive subcortical damage, with or without the involvement of the cortical areas of the brain, may cause aphasia, hence **subcortical aphasia** (SA) (Hallowell, 2017). The effects of the subcortical lesions may extend to the cortical regions, however.

Lesions in such subcortical regions as the basal ganglia, cerebellum, and the thalamus have been linked to SA (Payne, 2014).

- Basal ganglia lesions may produce anomic, global, Broca's, Wernicke's, or transcortical motor aphasia.
- Thalamic lesions may cause fluent aphasia with paraphasia and comprehension deficits; generally, thalamic lesions are associated with word-finding and naming problems, limited verbal output, and neologisms; auditory comprehension and repetition skills may be acceptable (Manasco, 2014).
- Cerebellar lesions tend to produce aphasia symptoms that are more subtle than those found in cortical forms of aphasia; limited fluency, mild anomia, agrammatism, and mild speech comprehension problems may be the dominant symptoms.

Subcortical lesions may affect blood flow to the cerebral language regions and thus explain some of the symptoms of SA.

Crossed Aphasia

Crossed aphasia (CA) is aphasia that occurs due to a right hemisphere (RH) brain lesion in right-handed individuals (Kim, Yang, & Paik, 2013). The right hand remains unaffected, and therefore, the individual's writing skills are intact. Symptoms of CA may include those of MTA, in some cases, and transient fluent aphasias in others.

Aphasia in Bilingual Populations

Globally, 50–80% of speakers are bilingual. Therefore, aphasia in bilingual speakers is more common than generally realized (Amberber & Cohen, 2012; Lorenzen & Murray, 2008; Paradis, 1998).

- In the United States, about 150,000 bilingual individuals have aphasia in any given year. About 45,000 new cases of bilingual aphasia are reported every year, and that number is expected to increase as the number of bilingual persons increases.
- In both the bilingual and the unilingual speakers, language is represented in the LH. Nonetheless, some specific regions may be more concerned with one or the other language. This "amalgamated hypothesis" of cerebral representation of two or more languages can better account for the differential recovery of languages following strokes in bilingual speakers (Lorenzen & Murray, 2008).
- In bilingual individuals with aphasia, there is a differential pattern of language impairment, as well as language recovery. In some, the first language (L1) may be more impaired than the second (L2);

in others, the reverse is true. Most (about 65%) may recover both languages, some only one language, and some only the dominant language. Some patients may recover one language first and the other after months. Some patients may lose the first recovered language as they begin to recover the other language. The extent of "recovery" may vary, regardless of the language in which it occurs.

- No particular variable (e.g., the age of L2 acquisition, current use) predicts the patterns of deficits or their recovery.
- Translational skills (between the two languages) also may be differentially impaired and recovered (see Lorenzen & Murray, 2008, for a review).
- Some patients may mix languages or automatically translate their own or heard utterances into one of their languages.
- In persons who are bilingual and have aphasia, clinicians should analyze individual patterns, not just known patterns, as individual differences predominate.

Assessment of Aphasia

Specific speech and language skills along with reading and writing skills are assessed in aphasia. Related cognitive functions also may be assessed, depending on the clinician's theoretical view and treatment goals. Both standardized and client-specific procedures may be used. Other standard assessment procedures, including a detailed case history, interview of the family and the client, review of the medical records, and hearing and diadochokinetic evaluations are completed before administering standardized tests and client-specific, clinician-prepared skill-oriented procedures. The main goals of assessment are to determine (a) whether the client has aphasia; (b) if so, the type of aphasia; and (c) whether the client has any coexisting disorder.

- A quick bedside examination in which the clinician asks a few personal questions (e.g., the client's name), requests nonverbal responses (e.g., "Point to the window"), asks questions related to orientation (e.g., "Is California a state in Canada?"), and requests a brief reading and writing sample (Davis, 2014) will help understand the current status of the individual. The clinician also may administer one of the several **screening tests**. Screening test examples include *Aphasia Rapid Test* (Azuar et al., 2013), *Bedside Western Aphasia Battery* (Kertesz, 2006), *Boston Diagnostic Aphasia Examination–Third Edition* (BDAE-3, the short form) (Goodglass et al., 2001b), and *Mississippi Aphasia Screening Test* (Nakase-Thompson, 2004).

- Standardized tests include:

  - The *Minnesota Test for Differential Diagnosis of Aphasia* (MTDDA; Schuell, 1973) evaluates auditory, visual, and reading impairments; speech and language deficits; and visuomotor, writing, numerical, and arithmetic problems. Dated, but its subtests are still in use.
  - The *Boston Diagnostic Aphasia Examination–Third Edition* (BDAE-3; Goodglass et al., 2001b) evaluates articulation, fluency, word finding, repetition, serial speech, grammar, paraphasias, auditory comprehension, oral reading, reading comprehension, writing, and musical skills (e.g., singing); helps classify aphasia into types.

- The *Western Aphasia Battery–Revised* (WAB-R; Kertesz, 2006) evaluates speech content, fluency, auditory comprehension, repetition, naming, reading, writing, calculation, drawing, nonverbal thinking, and block design; helps classify aphasia into types.
- The *Neurosensory Center Comprehensive Examination for Aphasia* (NCCEA; Spreen & Benton, 1977) evaluates language comprehension and production; reading and writing; word fluency and sentence construction, digit and sentence repetition; visual object naming; articulation; visual and tactile functions.
- The *Porch Index of Communicative Ability–Revised* (PICA-R; Porch, 2001) evaluates auditory comprehension, reading, oral expressive language, pantomime, visual matching, writing, and copying; requires intensive training to administer and score.
- The *Aphasia Diagnostic Profiles* (ADP; Helm-Estabrooks, 1992) evaluate overall severity of aphasia, along with comprehension, word retrieval, repetition, and alternative communication; helps classify aphasia.
- The *Comprehensive Aphasia Test* (CAT; Swiburn, Porter, & Howard, 2004) evaluates expressive and receptive language, aphasia's social, psychological, and practical effects on the individual; helps plan therapy; includes a screen for cognition.

- **Functional communication** assessment targets daily living skills and communication in everyday settings. These skills may be assessed by observing how a client communicates his or her basic needs in natural contexts. These skills also may be assessed by specific tests. Functional communication tests include:

  - The *Assessment of Living with Aphasia* (Simmons-Mackie et al., 2014) evaluates the effects of aphasia on everyday living; a self-reported quality-of-living assessment.
  - The *Communicative Abilities in Daily Living–Third Edition* (CADL-3; Holland, Frattali, & Fromm, 2018) rates reading, writing, estimation of time, use of verbal and nonverbal contexts in communication, role playing, social conventions, nonverbal symbolic communication, humor, absurdity, and metaphor.
  - The *Burden of Stroke Scale* (BOSS; Doyle, McNeil, Hula, & Mikolic, 2003) evaluates limitations in mobility, self-care, sleep, cognition, and social relations, along with psychological distress associated with stroke.
  - The *Communicative Effectiveness Index* (CETI; Lomas et al., 1989) rates functional communication skills related to social needs, life skills, basic needs, and health threats; giving yes–no answers, expressing physical pain or discomfort, and starting a conversation are rated.
  - The *Functional Independence Measure* (FIM; State University of New York, 1990) evaluates severity of disability ("burden of care"); an advantage of this test is that it is integrated into Medicare and Medicaid's reimbursement for clinical services.
  - The *Functional Assessment of Communication Skills for Adults* (FACS; Frattali, Thompson, Holland, Wohl, & Ferketic, 1995) helps rate social communication; communication of basic needs; reading, writing, and number concepts; and daily planning. Clinicians or others familiar with the client may make the observations and complete the rating form.

- The *Amsterdam-Nijmegen Everyday Language Test* (ANELT; Blomert, Kean, Koster, & Schokker, 1994) with two parallel forms, each containing 10 items, helps assess pragmatic language skills related to familiar daily-living activities.
- Examples of specific skills tests include *Revised Token Test* (McNeil & Prescott, 1978) with a computerized version (Sung et al., 2011), which helps assess auditory comprehension; *Auditory Comprehension Test for Sentences* (ACTS; Shewan, 1979); *Functional Auditory Comprehension Task* (FACT; LaPointe & Horner, 1978); *Reading Comprehension Battery for Aphasia–Second Edition* (RCBA-2; LaPointe & Horner, 1998); *Nelson-Denny Reading Test* (NDRT; Brown, Fishco, & Hanna, 1993); and *Gates-MacGinitie Reading Test* (GMRT; MacGinitie, MacGinitie, Maria, & Dreyer, 2000).

An Outline of Aphasia Assessment

Going beyond such standard procedures as case history, orofacial examination, and a hearing screening, the clinician needs to assess specific speech and language skills relevant for a diagnosis of aphasia (Brookshire, 2015; Chapey, 2008; Davis, 2014; Hallowell, 2017; Hegde, 2018a, 2008c; Hegde & Freed, 2017; Helm-Estabrooks et al., 2014). Standardized tests include subtests to assess most, if not all, of the skills. The clinician also may administer client-specific and task-specific procedures given in the following outline.

Assessment of Repetition Skills
- Repetition of single words (single-syllable words with visible voiced consonants [e.g., *bed*] and blends and multisyllable words)
- Repetition of object names, verbs, numbers, letters, and function words
- Repetition of sentences (short and commonly used sentences, e.g., "Sit down"; progressively longer sentences next)
- Repetition of a few short but infrequently used sentences

Assessment of Naming Skills
- Responsive naming (naming with contextual cues, e.g., the clinician asks, "What do you use to write?" or "What color is snow?")
- Confrontation naming (e.g., while showing a picture, the clinician asks, "What is this?")
- Word fluency (recalling names that belong to a specific category; e.g., the clinician tells the client, "Name all the animals you can think of")

Assessment of Sentence Production, Narration, and Discourse
- Production of single sentences when a word is supplied (e.g., the clinician asks, "Please make a sentence with the word *sun*")
- Production of multiple sentences (e.g., the clinician says, "Tell me about your favorite sports team," or "Tell me about your favorite book")
- Narrative skills (e.g., the clinician tells a story to the client and asks to retell it; asks the client to tell a story he or she knows)

- Discourse (the clinician asks the client to talk about a topic of interest; may suggest such topics as travel to foreign lands or current sociopolitical topics)
- More spontaneous discourse (the clinician asks the client to describe what he or she does on weekends, or how he or she performs a specific task, such as making a sandwich or posting a letter)

Assessment of Speech Fluency
- Speech dysfluencies (the clinician counts the number of dysfluencies per 100 words)
- Speech tempo (the clinician calculates words spoken per minute and the mean length of utterance)

Assessment of Functional Communication Skills
- Making simple requests (e.g., "Pencil, please" when asked to write something)
- Engaging in telephone conversation
- Participating in conversation
- Recognizing faces and voices
- Keeping appointments
- Understanding environmental signs
- Writing own name
- Making a grocery list

Assessment of Auditory Comprehension of Spoken Language
- Hearing evaluation
- Visual evaluation
- Appropriateness of nonverbal response to clinician's verbal commands
- Comprehension of natural commands given without gestures (e.g., "Move your chair a little closer" or "Close your eyes")
- Comprehension of multistep commands (e.g., "Pick up the pencil and the comb and place them in the box")

Assessment of Comprehension of Single Words
- Comprehension of single items (e.g., "Point to your *nose*") and semantic groups of items (e.g., colors or animals)
- Comprehension of words that vary semantic class and phonemic similarity

Assessment of Comprehension of Sentences, Paragraphs, and Discourse
- Comprehension of simple sentences given as commands (e.g., "Point to the *book*, *pen*, and *cat*") or of requests to perform actions (e.g., "Give me the *pencil*")
- Comprehension of a brief and simple story that is told and follow-up questions asked
- Comprehension of more complex stories
- Understanding conversational speech during informal assessment (evaluation of correct and incorrect verbal and nonverbal responses)

Assessment of Reading Skills
- Comprehension of silently or orally read material (e.g., matching single printed words to pictures, matching printed words with spoken words, crossing out words that do not belong in a list)
- Verbal completion of printed sentences (e.g., reading the printed incomplete sentence "We wear hats on our . . . " and completing it with the verbal response "head")

Assessment of Writing Skills
- Graphomotor skills (letter formation)
- General writing skills
- Automatic writing
- Confrontation writing (e.g., the clinician says, "Write the names of these pictures")
- Writing to dictation
- Narrative writing (e.g., the clinician says, "Write a story about this picture")
- Premorbid writing samples for comparison

Assessment of Gestures and Pantomime
- Expression through gestures and pantomime
- Comprehension of gestures and pantomime

Assessment of Automated Speech and Singing
- Recitation of the alphabet, days of the week, months of the year, and numbers
- Recitation of prayers, poems, and nursery rhymes
- Singing
- Humming a tune

Assessment of Bilingual Speakers With Aphasia
- A detailed history of learning two languages and their usage
- Basic functional communication (as in monolingual speakers) as initial assessment targets
- More detailed assessment of differential impairment and recovery in the two languages
- A well-trained interpreter who is competent in the two involved languages may be essential
- Some bilingual tests to consider include the following, but translated tests should be used with caution:
  - The *Bilingual Aphasia Test* (Paradis & Libben, 1987) has been used frequently and researched extensively; it can help assess aphasia in several languages (Fabbro, 2001). It is available online
  - The *Multilingual Aphasia Examination–Revised Edition* (Benton & Hamsher, 1994) helps evaluate aphasia in English, French, German, Italian, and Spanish
  - *Boston Diagnostic Aphasia Examination* (Translated) (Goodglass et al., 2001b)
  - *Communication Abilities in Daily Living* (Translated) (Holland et al., 1998)

Treatment of Aphasia

Single-subject design studies have produced impressive evidence supporting aphasia treatment, although some reviewers who inappropriately exclude such studies and consider only randomized group clinical trials may draw questionable conclusions of limited effectiveness (Brady et al., 2012). There is still, however, a great need to show that aphasia therapy improves communication skills in everyday life and improves the quality of life (Brookshire, 2015). Both individual and group treatment approaches are available (Basso, 2003; Brookshire, 2015; Chapey, 2008; Davis, 2014; Dobkin & Dorsch, 2013; Elman, 2007, 2011; Hegde, 2018a, 2018d; Helm-Estabrooks et al., 2014; Marshall, 1999).

Treatment must take into account the client's cultural and linguistic background. For example, in many minority groups, family and extended family members may be helpful in assisting with home carryover of treatment targets.

- Aphasia treatment may be:

  - **Restorative**. Such therapies aim to help a patient regain skills that were lost by reducing the severity of the deficits.
  - **Compensatory**. This kind of therapies help individuals increase their ability to function despite their deficits by teaching compensatory behaviors (e.g., use of alternative and augmentative communication devices).
  - **Social**. Social approach to treatment minimizes an individual's communication barriers; training communication partners on the most effective ways to communicate with an individual with aphasia is a commonly used social approach (Manasco, 2014).

- Prognosis for treatment is better if the individuals

  - are younger and healthier.
  - are better educated and in verbally demanding occupations.
  - have smaller lesions.
  - have no other medical or behavioral disorders.
  - have good hearing acuity.
  - have normal or adequately corrected vision.
  - have better motor skills.
  - have better preserved language skills.
  - have less severe aphasia.
  - receive treatment soon after onset.
  - receive effective treatment techniques in an accurate manner for a long enough duration.
  - receive support from family members who get involved in treatment.
  - maintain their health during the course of treatment.

Treatment of Auditory Comprehension

Lesions within the posterior superior temporal (PST) lobe suggest a better prognosis in the treatment of auditory comprehension than those outside the PST lobe. Comprehension is generally better for frequently used words, nouns, picturable words, shorter sentences, syntactically simpler sentences, active sentences, personally relevant sentences, slower speech, words that are stressed, speech in quiet surroundings, redundant messages, repeated phrases, and speech preceded by alerting stimuli (e.g., "Ready?" "Listen!"). Louder speech and video presentation of stimuli are ineffective.

Auditory comprehension therapy is frequently used, but there is little or no experimental evidence supporting it.

Auditory comprehension therapy is sequenced as follows:

- **Comprehension of single words**—understanding nouns and verbs (e.g., the clinician asks the patient to point to named body parts and objects, or to choose pictures representing specific named actions); the difficulty level of this task may be increased by increasing the field size to choose from or by prompting the client to match words to line drawings, realistic pictures, and physical objects (Chapey, 2008).
- **Comprehension of spoken sentences**—understanding questions (e.g., the clinician asks yes–no questions and open-ended questions), following spoken directions (e.g., the clinician asks the client to follow simple and then more complex directions), and sentence verification (e.g., clinician asks the client to verify the meaning of sentences by matching a sentence to a picture that represents it).
- **Discourse comprehension**—understanding narratives and questions (e.g., the clinician asks the client to retell a story the clinician narrates and respond to such personally relevant questions as "Do you like to watch football games?").

Treatment of Verbal Expression: Naming

Naming is the most frequently targeted expressive verbal skill. Naming skills are subsequently expanded into longer and grammatically more correct and communicatively more functional utterances.

In treating naming, most effective words are client-specific (e.g., names of family members, activities the client engages in) and functional (to enhance communication in a variety of settings).

Naming treatment techniques include initially modeling the target responses and subsequently cuing to evoke a response without modeling the actual response. The clinician promptly reinforces all correct or approximate responses to the modeled or cued stimulus. Some of the commonly used cues include the following:

- Incomplete sentences (e.g., the clinician says, "You write with a _____")
- Phonetic cues (e.g., the clinician says, "The word starts with a *p*")
- Syllabic cues (e.g., the clinician says, "The word starts with *spoo*_____")
- Silent phonetic cues (e.g., the clinician exhibits a silent articulatory posture for /p/ for *pen*)
- Personalized verbal cues (a cue that is specific to the experience of the patient; e.g., instead of prompting "It starts with an *m*" for the word *mechanic*, the clinician may say "He works on your Toyota") (Freed, Celery, & Marshall, 2004)
- Functional descriptions of objects (e.g., the clinician says, "It is something you roll or kick")
- Descriptions and demonstrations of actions (e.g., the clinician says, "You use this to write like this," followed by writing)

- Patient's description as stimulus for naming (e.g., the clinician says, "Tell me what you do with this and then say its name")
- Patient's demonstration of function as stimulus for naming (e.g., the clinician says, "Show me how to use this and tell me its name")
- Paired objects or pictures with their printed name as stimuli for naming (e.g., the clinician shows a book and the printed word *book* and asks, "What is this?")
- Patient's spelling as stimulus for naming (e.g., the clinician says, "Spell this word first and then say it")
- Patient's spelling and writing as stimuli for naming (e.g., the clinician says, "Spell this word, write the word, and then say it")
- Associated sounds as stimulus (e.g., the clinician says, "It makes an *arf-arf* sound")
- Rhyme as stimulus (e.g., the clinician says, "What is this? It rhymes with _____")
- Synonyms (e.g., "dwelling" to evoke "house"); antonyms (e.g., "woman" to evoke "man"); associated words (e.g., "plate" to evoke "cup"); generic words (e.g., "man" to evoke "husband"); superordinates (e.g., "flower" to evoke "rose")

The clinician may use the **semantic feature analysis (SFA)** to reduce naming difficulties.

- SFA selects words that belong to a particular family because of their shared meanings; for instance, the word *ball* may be evoked by its physical properties of shape, color, and activity (round, small, big, red, bounce, kick, etc.)
- For each stimulus picture, specific semantic features that include **group**, **description**, and **function** are used to have the stimulus named and described. The client is not only asked to name a stimulus, but also to answer questions related to such semantic features as follows: "What category does it belong to?" "Where can you find it?" "How would you describe it?" "What is it used for?" "What makes it special or different?" Such questions promote more elaborate responses than just naming. (See Boyle, 2004 and Wambaugh, Mauszycki, Cameron, Wright, & Nessler, 2013 for procedural details; see Efstratiadou, Papathanasiou, Holland, Archonti, & Hilari, 2018 for a review of procedures and evidence.)

Instead of teaching isolated names of objects, the clinician may teach the naming skills in the context of **narration**, **discourse**, and **conversation**. This will help teach the dual targets of naming and more elaborate speech.

- The clinician engages the client in narration, discourse, or conversation and may provide phonetic, semantic, or other kinds of cues for the naming response.
- The clinician reinforces not just naming, but also narrative, discourse, or conversation around the stimulus. (See Boyle, 2011 for a critical review of studies on this method.)

Treatment of Verbal Expression: Expanded Utterances

Expansion of verbal expression involves systematically increasing the length and complexity of target responses.

- Names taught may be expanded into phrases and sentences that are functional and effective in naturalistic communication; modeling, initially used, is faded out.

- Action-filled pictures and stories may be used to teach narratives and discourse; sequenced pictures help evoke narratives with temporal sequences.
- Conversational speech is the final treatment target; description of daily activities (e.g., cooking) and special events (e.g., planning a vacation) that are of interest to the client may be used to promote conversational speech.

Clinicians also may consider using published treatment programs to expand verbal productions of persons with aphasia:

- *Promoting Aphasics' Communicative Effectiveness* (*PACE*) **(Davis & Wilcox, 1981).** This program helps teach conversational exchanges between two persons, with an emphasis on effective communication, not necessarily grammaticality. The clinician and the client exchange the roles of listener and speaker.
- The *Helm Elicited Language Program for Syntax Stimulation* (Helm-Estabrooks, 1981; Helm-Estabrooks et al., 2014). The clinician tells a short story and asks questions about it. The clinician may tell an incomplete story and lets the client complete it. *What*, *who*, *when*, and *where* questions, declaratives, comparatives, and yes–no questions may be taught.
- The *Response Elaboration Training* (*RET*). This method helps teach the production of expanded sentences that contain progressively increased amount of information. Instead of naming or describing the treatment stimuli, the client is encouraged to talk about them in a more naturalistic and elaborate manner, drawing upon personal experiences and world knowledge. The method, as modified by Wambaugh, Nessler, and Wright (2013) may be used to teach procedural discourse (e.g., "Tell me in detail how you would go about moving to a new house") and personal recounts ("Please talk for five minutes about anything you like").

Treatment of Reading Skills

Target reading skills are selected based on an assessment of premorbid reading skills and the current need for reading. Functional reading skills may be sequenced as follows:

- Survival reading skills (e.g., reading letters, menus, bank statements, and maps)
- Reading newspapers, books, and letters
- Reading and comprehension of printed words
- Reading and comprehension of phrases and sentences
- Reading and comprehension of paragraphs and extended material

Treatment of Writing Skills

Target writing skills also are selected based on an assessment of premorbid reading skills and the current need for writing. Functional writing skills may be sequenced as follows:

- Initially writing functional words (e.g., one's own name, names of family members)
- Writing functional lists (e.g., a grocery list)
- Writing short notes, reminders, addresses, and so forth
- Filling out forms
- Writing letters

Depending on the client's current writing skills, teaching procedures include the following:

- Pointing to the correct printed letter the clinician names
- Pointing to printed words and phrases
- Saying the sound of a printed letter shown
- Saying a printed word shown
- Tracing printed letters
- Copying printed words and phrases
- Spelling words correctly
- Writing to dictation
- Spontaneous writing of phrases and sentences
- Spontaneous extended writing (e.g., making a grocery list, writing a note to a spouse, writing a letter to a friend)

Group Treatment for Aphasia

Group treatment of aphasia, common before it gave way to individual therapy, can be more efficient than individual treatment (Elman, 2007, 2011; Marshall, 1999), although more research and evidence are needed to establish its effects (Lanyon, Rose, & Worrall, 2013). "Aphasia groups" are now common in many clinics.

- These groups create a comfortable environment for a client to interact with others who are going through a similar experience. Group treatment typically follows a period of individual treatment, and sessions are held less frequently than individual sessions.
- The emphasis in group sessions depends on the members' skill level. For the more basic groups, total communication via any means may be a good target; for the more advanced group, conversation, narrative skills, and problem solving may be the targets.

Social Approaches to Treating Aphasia

Critical of an undue emphasis on linguistic structures, including grammatical accuracy, that may not necessarily promote social and functional communication, some clinicians emphasize the importance of social communication as the target of aphasia therapy (Elman, 2011; Simmons-Mackie, 2008). In the social approaches:

- The main treatment goal is natural interaction, conversation, functional communication, and enhancement of life participation (Elman, 2011)—all designed to reduce social isolation. It is important to teach compensatory (adaptive) strategies to minimize the effects of aphasia.
- Treatment sessions are held in more naturalistic settings (e.g., the client's home, a restaurant, a health care facility).
- The person with aphasia, the family members, and significant others help set the treatment goals. Training communication partners from the community is a part of the treatment (Lyon, 1992).

Some Experimental Approaches to Treating Aphasia

Several experimental treatment approaches are being researched. Clinicians should watch for additional research on the following:

- Non-invasive brain stimulation (Shaw, Szaflarski, Allendorfer, & Hamilton, 2013). Repetitive transcranial magnetic stimulation (rTMS) and transcranial direct current stimulation (tDCS) have shown some beneficial effects in clients with chronic aphasia.
- Drug treatment is another experimental approach that needs to be researched further. Dopamine agnostics, piracetam, amphetamines, and donepezil have been tried in both the acute and chronic stages of aphasia (Bakheit, 2004); results have been unimpressive (Elsner, Kugler, Pohl, & Mehrnholz, 2013).
- Physical exercises to improve fitness, balance, and strength might be an adjunct to speech–language therapy (Dobkin & Dorsch, 2013).
- Digital devices, such as iPods, may be useful in speech–language therapy because of their ability to provide audio and video feedback of a client's performance (Fridriksson et al., 2012).

Treatment of Bilingual Speakers With Aphasia

Generally, the same treatment principles and procedures may be effective in treatment of bilingual speakers with aphasia, though more treatment research is needed on these clients.

- The treatment targets are similar for the monolingual and bilingual clients (naming, functional communication skills, and reading and writing in the dominant language).
- Treatment in the weaker language may produce beneficial generalized effects on the stronger language.
- Treatment is tailored to individual needs and patterns of social communication involving the dominant language of the client.

Alexia and Agraphia

Alexia is loss of previously acquired reading skills due to recent brain damage. **Dyslexia** is children's difficulty learning to read, possibly genetically based.

- **Pure alexia** is reading problem when writing and other language skills are intact. This disorder is often due to a lesion in the inferior occipitotemporal region, which is thought to contain the visual word form area (Turkeltaub et al., 2014). Visual cortices and Wernicke's area may be separated in pure alexia (Starrfelt, Olafsdottir, & Arndt, 2013). Alexia may be associated with aphasia (Brookshire, 2015; Hegde, 2018a; Helm-Estabrooks et al., 2014).
- **Agraphia** is the loss or impairment of normally acquired writing skills due to lesions in the foot of the medial frontal gyrus of the brain, sometimes referred to as **Exner's writing area** (Keller & Meister, 2014). Various kinds of writing problems are evident in most patients with aphasia and dementia.

Agnosia

Agnosia is impaired understanding of the meaning of certain stimuli, without peripheral sensory impairment. Because the patients can see, feel, and hear stimuli but cannot understand their meaning, agnosia is a disorder of recognition (Bhatnagar, 2017). Impairment often is limited to one sensory modality; the meaning of stimuli may be grasped in another modality. There are several forms of agnosia (Benson & Ardila, 1996):

- **Auditory agnosia** is associated with bilateral damage to the auditory association area and is characterized by impaired understanding of the meaning of auditory stimuli, normal peripheral hearing, difficulty in matching objects with their sound, and normal visual recognition of objects.
- **Auditory verbal agnosia** (pure word deafness) is associated with bilateral temporal lobe lesions that isolate Wernicke's area; results in impaired understanding of spoken words, normal peripheral hearing, normal recognition of nonverbal sounds, normal recognition of printed words, and normal or near-normal verbal expression and reading.
- **Visual agnosia** is a rare disorder often associated with bilateral occipital lobe damage or posterior parietal lobe damage; they cause impaired visual recognition of objects, which may be intermittent (auditory or tactile recognition of objects may be normal).
- **Tactile agnosia** is associated with lesions in the parietal lobe, and they cause impaired tactile recognition of objects when visual feedback is blocked (as with a blindfold) and impaired naming and description of objects clients can feel in their hands.

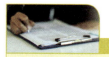

SUMMARY

- Aphasia, a neurologically based language disorder, is most frequently caused by stroke and may be fluent, nonfluent, or subcortical. Clinicians must take into account individual issues, such as the presence of bilingualism or left-handedness when assessing persons with aphasia.
- Aphasia may be assessed through standardized aphasia tests. Clinicians may also design their own functional assessment tools, which target the patient's communication skills in everyday settings.
- Treatment of patients with aphasia generally involves the following skill areas: auditory comprehension, verbal expression (naming), verbal expression (expanded utterances), reading, and writing.
- Aphasia may be accompanied by alexia and agraphia (reading and writing problems) or agnosia (auditory, auditory verbal, visual, and tactile).

DEMENTIA

Dementia is a major health problem primarily found in people 65 years of age and older. It is an acquired neurological syndrome associated with persistent or progressive deterioration in intellectual functions, emotions, and behavior. Assessment of dementia includes informal procedures and standardized tests. In treating dementia, the clinician helps clients manage their daily routines and helps families cope (Bayles & Tomoeda, 2014; Bourgeois, 2011; Hallowell, 2017; Hegde, 2018a, 2018b; Hopper et al., 2013; Kimbarow, 2016; Payne, 2014; Wilson, Rochon, Mihailidis, & Leonard, 2012).

Definition and Classification of Dementia

Clinicians should search online to get the most current demographic data available on dementia and the diseases that cause it. Published data are usually a few years old and are subject to change. Useful sites include those of the National Institute of Neurological Diseases and Stroke, Alzheimer's Association, National Institute on Aging, Alzheimer's Disease Education and Referral Center, and Centers for Disease Control and Prevention (CDC).

- The prevalence of dementia may be as high as 25% in people age 65 years and older. After the age of 65, prevalence doubles every 5 years.
- The American Psychiatric Association (APA) (2013) describes **dementia** as a significant decline in one or more areas of the following cognitive domains: complex attention, executive function, learning and memory, language, perceptual-motor, or social cognition. Decline in one or more such functions affects everyday living activities. Cognitive decline is not due to delirium or other mental disorders. Unlike in previous definitions, memory impairment is not essential to diagnose dementia as it may not be evident in the early stages.
- APA classifies dementia as major (more severe) or minor (mild). In **mild cognitive impairment** (MCI), the deficits are more severe than those produced by normal aging but are not severe enough to significantly affect activity participation (Bayles & Tomoeda, 2013; Bourgeois, 2011).
- Dementia is progressive in most cases but reversible in about 20%. Reversible dementia is a temporary intellectual impairment due to such treatable conditions as metabolic disturbances, nutritional deficiencies, chronic renal failure, persistent anemia, drug toxicity, and lung and heart diseases. Reversible dementia is similar to **delirium**.

Dementia of the Alzheimer Type

Alzheimer's disease (AD) is associated with the most common form of dementia. It is considered a **cortical** dementia and accounts for approximately 60–70% of irreversible dementia (Bayles & Tomoeda, 2013; Bourgeois, 2011; Davis, 2014).

- There are two subtypes of AD: early-onset AD (EOAD) and late-onset AD (LOAD). EOAD (onset up to age 60 or 65) accounts for only up to 6% of all AD. The rest are LOAD; in the majority of cases, onset occurs during the 70s and 80s.
- More women than men are affected. DAT is associated with a family history of Down syndrome, a prior brain injury, and low level of education.
- Genetic inheritance accounts for some cases of DAT; 60% of those with EOAD have a positive family history; of those, autosomal dominant inheritance is seen in 13%. In most cases, multiple-gene environmental interactions are suspected. Three single genes have been identified in autosomal dominant inheritance associated with EOAD: (1) APP on 21q21.2, (2) PSEN1 on 14q24.3, and (3) PSEN2 on 1q31-q42. A fourth gene, APOE on 19q13.2, is thought to be a risk factor for LOAD

(Alonso Vilatela, Lopez-Lopez, & Yescas-Gomez, 2012). Several other genes have been tentatively identified for LOAD, but none have been confirmed.

- Neuropathology of DAT involves the following:

  - **Neurofibrillary tangles.** Neurofibrils are filamentous structures in the nerve cells, dendrites, and axons; these structures are thickened, twisted, tangled, forming unusual loops and triangles.
  - **Neuritic plaques**. Also known as **amyloid plaques**, these are abnormal deposits of amyloid protein that cause cortical and subcortical tissue degeneration. The cerebral cortex and hippocampus (concerned with memory) are especially vulnerable to plaques, resulting in destroyed cortical and subcortical synaptic connections.
  - **Granulovacuolar degeneration.** The neurons within the hippocampus are especially susceptible to this atypical formation of membranous fluid-filled cavities containing granular debris.
  - **Neuronal loss.** The loss of neurons, also known as **general neuronal atrophy,** secondary to the changes described previously, results in a shrunken brain. The shrinkage is most obvious in the cerebral hemispheres, especially in temporal and parietal lobes.
  - **Neurochemical changes.** Depletion of neurochemicals that help transmit messages across brain structures is a hallmark of dementia. Such neurochemicals as acetylcholine, somatostatin, vasopressin, and corticotropin, are severely depleted in AD.

- Symptoms of early-stage DAT (the early stage typically lasts about two years following the diagnosis) include the following:

  - Subtle memory problems (especially for recent events)
  - Somewhat pronounced difficulty with new learning and visuospatial problems (e.g., copying three-dimensional figures)
  - Behavior changes, including self-neglect and avoidance of routine tasks (e.g., avoiding cooking, asking a partner to keep the score while playing tennis), indifference, and irritability
  - Other potential symptoms include depression, slight disorientation in new surroundings, and subtle language changes that may not be evident to family members; motor functions are normal

- Symptoms of mid to late-stage DAT include the following:

  - Intensified early-stage symptoms
  - Severe problems recalling remote and recent events
  - Intensified visuospatial problems
  - Widespread intellectual deterioration
  - Hyperactivity, restlessness, agitation, meaningless handling of objects
  - Problems with arithmetic calculations
  - Profound disorientation to place, time, and person; prone to restlessness and wander
  - Problems with self-care (e.g., difficulty dressing and/or bathing)
  - Difficulty managing daily routines
  - Lack of affect, tact, and judgment
  - Loss of initiative; indifference

- Paranoid delusions and hallucinations
- Aggressive or disruptive behaviors
- Inappropriate humor and laughter
- Worsening of the symptoms in the evening (**sundowner syndrome**)
- Seizures, myoclonic jerks (sudden muscular contractions), incontinence, dysphagia, physical deterioration, and severe decline in motor function—all in the very late stage

■ Language problems associated with DAT include the following:

- General word-finding problems
- Naming problems, verbal and literal paraphasias, and circumlocution
- Problems comprehending abstract meanings
- Impaired picture description
- Difficulty generating a list of words that begin with a specific letter
- Echolalia (repeating what others say), palilalia (repeating one's own utterances), and logoclonia (repeating the final syllable of words)
- Empty (meaningless) speech, jargon, and hyperfluency
- Incoherent, slurred, and rapid speech
- Pragmatic language problems, including inattention to social conventions (e.g., greetings); difficulty initiating and maintaining conversation; decreased speech output; inappropriate speech
- Reading and writing problems
- No meaningful speech, mutism, and complete disorientation to time, place, people, and self in the final stages

Frontotemporal Dementia

Frontotemporal dementia (FTD) is due to degeneration of the frontal and temporal lobes. Also known as **frontotemporal lobar degeneration**, it is a group of heterogeneous diseases that includes a behavioral variant of FTD (bvFTD) and primary progressive aphasia (PPA). The classic Pick's disease (PiD) and the resulting dementia is a part of FTD, which constitutes up to 10% of dementia cases (third most common form of dementia, after DAT and dementia due to Lewy bodies). In patients younger than 65 years of age, it is the second most common (after DAT). The typical onset of PiD takes place between ages 40 and 60.

■ Neuropathology of FTD includes the following:

- Degeneration of nerve cells in the left and right frontal lobes, temporal lobe, or both lobes in the two hemispheres
- In the classic Pick's disease, possibly focal atrophy, involving the anterior frontal and temporal lobes, the orbital frontal lobe, and the medial temporal lobe
- The presence of Pick bodies (dense intracellular formation in the neuronal cytoplasm) and the presence of Pick cells (ballooned and inflated neurons) in the cortical layers
- The absence of Pick bodies and Pick cells in some variants of FTD, but the presence of atrophied, gliosed, and swollen brain cells

- Symptoms of the behavioral variant of FTD, which accounts for 70% of patients with FTD, include the following:

  - Notable behavioral changes as initial symptoms in patients with marked right-sided atrophy; notable language changes in those with marked left atrophy
  - Behavior disorders, including uninhibited and inappropriate social behaviors (hugging people in the street); compulsive behaviors, including excessive eating (and weight gain); and delusions, more pronounced in patients with right-sided atrophy
  - Emotional disturbances, including depression, apathy (lack of motivation), withdrawal, irritability, mood fluctuations, occasional euphoria, excessive jocularity, and exaggerated self-esteem
  - Impaired judgment and reasoning and lack of insight

- Language problems associated with FTD include the following:

  - Dominant language problems with somewhat better-preserved memory and orientation, contrasted with patients who have DAT
  - Anomia (word finding problems), more pronounced with temporal lobe atrophy
  - Progressive loss of vocabulary and consequent paraphasia and circumlocution
  - Difficulty defining common words and problems reciting category-specific words (e.g., animals)
  - Limited spontaneous speech, echolalia, and nonfluent speech
  - Impaired comprehension of speech and printed material

Primary Progressive Aphasia

- Primary progressive aphasia (PPA), another form of FTD, has a nonfluent (nfvPPA), a semantic (svPPA), and a logopenic (lvPPA) variants. It is aphasia in the initial stages with predominantly language impairment and intact cognitive skills until at least 2 years post-onset (Kirschner, 2014). Unlike aphasia due to stroke, it has a progressive neuropathology, eventually leading to dementia. Some investigators consider all three varieties of PPA as varieties of FTD (e.g., Chare et al., 2014; Kirschner, 2014), whereas others include only the nonfluent and semantic varieties and exclude the more recently identified logopenic variant (e.g., Karageorgiou & Miller, 2014). Up to 69% of patients with PPA may be classified into one of the three variants (Gomo-Tempini et al., 2011; Kertesz & Harciarek, 2014); 31% of patients with PPA cannot be classified.
- NfvPPA and svPPA can be differentiated from CVA-based aphasia by the slow and gradual onset of symptoms, whereas CVAs produce sudden, acute deficits.
- The nfvPPA (nonfluent variant) is associated with structural and metabolic changes limited to the left perisylvian language area, which includes Broca's area. Pathology typical of Pick's disease and Alzheimer's disease may be evident. The nfvPPA accounts for 27% of PPA (Wicklund et al., 2014); about one fifth of the patients in this category also may present Parkinsonian features.
- The nfvPPA is characterized by the following:

- Earliest signs of anomia, phonemic paraphasias, word-finding difficulties, and apraxia of speech; subsequently, reduced fluency; articulation problems; agrammatism, resembling BA; impaired repetition; slower rate and prosodic impairments
- Memory and cognition relatively preserved until about 2 years post-onset; daily living skills unaffected; holding a job possible
- Behavioral changes typical of the behavioral variant of frontotemporal dementia (bvFTD), including apathy, disorganization, inappropriateness, and aggression, within two years
- Slow progress of the disease, with an 8–10-year survival rate

■ The svPPA (semantic variant) is also associated with FTD, though the initial symptoms are those of aphasia; atrophy of the temporal lobe, especially in the left, is evident; accounts for 7% of PPA (Wicklund et al., 2014). The frontal lobe later atrophies. Symptoms of svPPA appear in one third of all cases with FTD (Kertesz & Harciarek, 2014).

■ Characteristics of svPPA include the following:

- Progressive loss of word meaning (hence, the name)
- Anomia
- Semantic paraphasias
- Initially intact fluency and repetition skills; repetition of words not named or comprehended; intact phonological skills, motor skills, and orientation to time and space
- Excessive and disinhibited speech; logorrhea
- Impaired turn taking in discourse
- Visual agnosia and prosopagnosia as the right temporal lobe gets involved
- Progressively shorter sentences and phrases; eventual mutism
- Behavior changes (disinhibition, irritability, bizarre food choices, compulsive behavior) in the later stages, especially when the atrophy spreads to the right temporal lobe and frontal lobes

■ The lvPPA (logopenic variant) is associated with neuropathology typical of Alzheimer's disease and frontotemporal dementia. Damage to the left posterior superior temporal and middle temporal gyri and the inferior parietal lobule constitutes the main neuropathology in lvPPA. This variant accounts for 35% of PPA (Wicklund et al., 2014).

■ The lvPPA is characterized by the following:

- Slow speech, with word-finding pauses (similar to nfvPPA); unlike nfvPPA, no agrammatism, speech–motor control problems, telegraphic speech, or prosodic deficiencies
- Only moderate naming difficulties in the early stages
- Severe difficulty repeating phrases and sentences; intact repetition of short single words in initial stages; impaired subsequently
- Impaired sentence comprehension
- Behavioral changes (apathy, anxiety, irritability, and agitation)

PPA is not without controversy, because not all patients fit into one of its three varieties (Wicklund et al., 2014). The presence of apraxia of speech in the nonfluent variety (Rascovsky & Grossman, 2013), and the newer variety of lvPPA add to this controversy. Figure 8.8 displays information about FTD.

Not all professionals agree on the classification of Pick's disease shown in the figure. This chart depicts it as its own disease/synonymous with bvFTD, while others consider it the same as semantic dementia.

Dementia Associated With Parkinson's Disease

Parkinson's disease (PD) is a single neurodegenerative disease entity; **parkinsonism** refers to a group of neurological disorders that include hypokinesia, tremor, and muscular rigidity. PD is possibly due to both genetic and environmental factors.

PD is more common in males than in females, and onset is typically between 50 and 56 years of age.

Only about 35–55% of patients with PD have dementia. Some experts classify dementia associated with PD as **subcortical** (motor symptoms precede intellectual deterioration).

- Neuropathology of PD includes the following:

  - Basal ganglia and brainstem degeneration
  - Presence of abnormal structures called Lewy bodies, small pathologic spots typically found in the substantia nigra (a structure at the top of the brainstem)
  - Frontal lobe atrophy resulting in widened sulci
  - Reduced inhibitory dopamine due to loss of cells in the substantia nigra (a midbrain structure)
  - Neurofibrillary tangles and plaques of the kind found in Alzheimer's disease

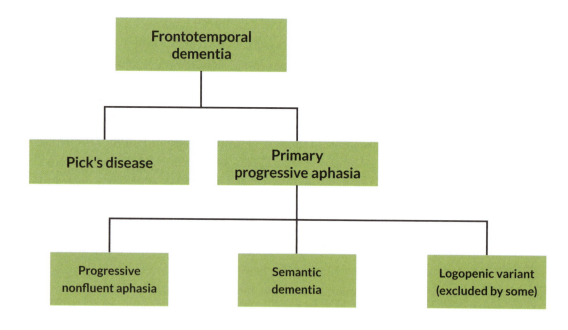

Figure 8.8 Frontotemporal dementia.

- Neurologic symptoms of PD include the following:
  - Slow voluntary movements (bradykinesia)
  - Tremors in resting muscles, starting in hand or foot and spreading; tremors exacerbated during stress
  - Muscle rigidity (increased tone and resistance to movement)
  - A mask-like face
  - Reduced eye blinking, festinating gait (also called festination), disturbed posture, frequent falls, and freezing during movement
  - Swallowing disorders
  - Sleep disturbances
  - Cogwheel rigidity, or tension in a muscle that gives way in little jerks when the muscle is passively stretched

- Speech, language, and related problems associated with PD (Brin, Velickovic, Ramig, & Fox, 2004) include the following:
  - Reduced speech volume
  - Voice problems that include monopitch and monoloudness
  - Long and frequent pauses in speech
  - Slow, fast, or festinating speech rate
  - Dysarthric speech
  - Serious memory problems, problems in abstract reasoning and problem solving
  - Impaired visuospatial perception
  - Impaired word-list generation
  - Severe naming and language comprehension problems in later stages of the disease
  - Apathy, confusion, hallucination, and delirium
  - Micrographia (writing in extremely small letters)

Dementia Associated With Huntington's Disease

Huntington's disease (HD) affects about 40–70 persons in a million; the typical age of onset is 35–40 years. It affects males and females equally. The estimated lifespan is about 20 years post-diagnosis. Genetic etiology is supported; mutation on the short arm of chromosome 4 has been documented. Half the offspring of a patient may have the disease. A malformed protein called **huntingtin** kills the brain cells that control movement. Because the behavior/personality changes and movement disorders like rigidity and bradykinesia are usually the earliest signs of HD, it may be misdiagnosed as PD until choreiform movements become evident. This type of dementia may be classified as **subcortical**, as the structures of the basal ganglia are some of the areas affected by the mutant huntingtin protein.

- Neuropathology of HD includes the following:
  - A loss of neurons in the basal ganglia; significant loss of neurons in the caudate nucleus, putamen, and substantia nigra

- Possible atrophy in the prefrontal, temporal, and parietal lobes, as well
- Reduced levels of inhibitory neurotransmitters, especially GABA (gamma-amino butyric acid) and acetylcholine

■ Symptoms of HD disease include the following:

- Chorea (irregular, spasmodic, involuntary movement of the neck, head, and face)
- Increasingly uncontrollable tic-like movement disorders
- Gait disturbances and progressively reduced voluntary movements
- Slow movement in the advanced stages of the disease, leading to little or no voluntary movement
- Behavioral disorders that include excessive complaining, nagging, eccentricity, irritability, emotional outbursts, a false sense of superiority, depression or euphoria, schizophrenic-like behaviors (delusions and hallucinations), and suicide attempts

■ Speech, language, and cognitive–linguistic problems associated with HD include the following:

- Deterioration in intellectual functions, including memory, attention, concentration, and executive functioning skills
- Impaired word-list generation
- Naming problems
- Dysarthria
- Incontinence, sleep disturbances, sleep reversal, and dysphagia
- Muteness in the final stages

■ Table 8.1 compares Alzheimer's disease, Parkinson's disease, and Huntington's disease.

Infectious Dementia

Certain infectious diseases cause dementia. Dementia due to human immunodeficiency virus (HIV) infection and Creutzfeldt-Jakob disease are well known.

■ Dementia due to HIV infection is subcortical and is known as **AIDS dementia complex** or **human immunodeficiency virus encephalopathy**; it has the following features:

- Opportunistic brain infections in people infected with the AIDS virus (e.g., cryptococcal meningitis) can lead to dementia.
- HIV infection itself can cause dementia.
- Dementia is of slow onset, but deterioration is rapid in the final stages.
- Neurologic symptoms include disturbed gait, tremor, headache, seizures, ataxia, rigidity, motor weakness, facial nerve paralysis, and incontinence.
- Dementia symptoms include forgetfulness, poor concentration, slow or impaired thinking, apathy and loss of interest in work, depression, mania, confusion, hallucinations, delusions, and memory loss.
- Language problems are less prominent until mutism settles in the final stage.

■ Creutzfeldt-Jakob disease causes another form of infectious dementia. Although no virus has been microscopically found, it is thought to be caused by an unconventional infectious agent called a

Table 8.1

A Comparison of Alzheimer's Disease, Parkinson's Disease, and Huntington's Disease

Dementia	Alzheimer's disease	Parkinson's disease	Huntington's disease
Onset (age)	Typically 70–80 years, but early onset type can occur up to age 60–65	Typically 50–56 years	35–40 years
Progression	10 years post-diagnosis	20 years post-diagnosis but can progress more quickly	20 years post-diagnosis
Neurological basis	Neurofibrillary tangles, amyloid plaques, granulovacuolar degeneration, neuronal loss, neurochemical changes; highly evident in temporal lobes	Basal ganglia and brainstem degeneration, presence of Lewy bodies in the substantia nigra, frontal lobe atrophy, reduced inhibitory dopamine, neurofibrillary tangles and plaques	Mutant huntingtin protein, loss of neurons in basal ganglia, caudate nucleus, putamen, and substantia nigra; possible atrophy in prefrontal, temporal, and parietal lobes; reduced levels of inhibitory neurotransmitters, especially GABA
Earliest symptoms	Short-term/recent memory, visuospatial deficits, behavior changes. Changes are often initially mistaken as normal aging	Motor deficits, especially pill-rolling tremor	Movement disorders (rigidity, bradykinesia), then personality changes
Motor skills	Remain intact until **very late stage in disease progression,** during which the individual becomes non-ambulatory	**Early in disease (precede cognitive deficits):** bradykinesia, tremors in resting muscles, rigidity, reduced eye blinking, festination, disturbed posture, frequent falls, impaired initiation; individuals may be able to execute motor plans if obstacle is placed in front of them	**Earliest signs:** rigidity, bradykinesia, then chorea. **Other motor deficits:** tic-like movements, gait disturbances, progressively reduced voluntary movements; ambulation may still be possible in **mid to late stages,** but fall risk is increased. **Advanced stages:** slow movement, non-ambulatory leading to little or no voluntary movement
Behavior changes	**Early stages** of disease: including self-neglect, avoidance of routine, indifference, irritability, depression, disorientation in new surroundings. **Mid stage:** behavior/cognitive deficits may worsen at nighttime. **Later stages:** aggressive and disruptive behavior, inappropriate humor/laughter	Apathy, confusion	First personality changes occur **early in disease.** Can include excessive complaining, nagging, eccentricity, irritability, emotional outbursts, false sense of superiority, depression or euphoria, schizophrenic-like behaviors, suicide attempts
Memory deficits	**Early stages:** short-term memory affected; Mid to late stages: Short- and long-term deficits	Serious memory problems	Severe memory deficits in **later stages**

(continues)

Table 8.1 (continued)

Dementia	Alzheimer's disease	Parkinson's disease	Huntington's disease
Visual–perceptual deficits	Present **at early stages** of disease (e.g., difficulty copying shapes/figures); Intensified in **mid–later stages**, including difficulties with visuoconstructive tasks, paranoid delusions and hallucinations also present	**As disease progresses**, individuals develop hallucinations, delirium, impaired visuospatial perception	Delusions and hallucinations
Speech and voice characteristics	**Early stages**: unimpaired/within functional limits **Toward end of disease progression** speech becomes incoherent, rapid, slurred; decreased speech output	Reduced volume, mono-pitch, monoloud, long and frequent pauses; slow, fast, or festinating speech rate; dysarthric speech (hypokinetic)	Dysarthria (hyperkinetic)
Expressive language	**Early stages**: word finding deficits and circumlocution **As disease progresses**, deficits in: naming, picture description, hyperfluency; verbal and literal paraphasias present; echolalia, palilalia, and logoclonia; empty speech; jargon; writing impairment Mutism may occur in **final stages**	**Later in disease**: severe naming deficits; deficits in word–list generation	**Later stages**: impaired word-list generation, naming problems Mutism in **at end of disease progression**; alternative and augmentive communication techniques can be used to communicate basic wants/needs
Receptive language	**Early stages**: difficulty with auditory comprehension of language **Later stages**: Difficulty understanding abstract meaning and reading	**Later in disease**: severe language comprehension problems	Remains mostly intact even into final stages of disease
Cognition/problem-solving skills	Deficits in **mid–late** stages: disorientation, impaired attention, loss of tact, judgment, initiative, management of routine, and self-care; difficulties with math	**As disease progresses**, deficits in abstract reasoning and problem solving	**Early stages**: deficits in attention, concentration, and executive functioning By **later stages**, physical/motor deficits outweigh cognitive ones

prion (the word stands for **proteinaceous infectious particle**, a form of abnormal protein found in the brains of people with the disease); the features of this disease include the following:

- Neuropathology of Creutzfeldt-Jakob disease is a widespread spongiform state in the brain; neuron loss may be found in cortical areas, the basal ganglia, the thalamus, the brainstem, and the spinal cord.

- Physical symptoms include fatigue and sleep disturbances.
- Neurological symptoms include cerebellar ataxia, tremor, rigidity, chorea, athetosis, and visual problems.
- Symptoms of dementia include memory problems and reasoning impairments.
- Psychiatric symptoms include depression, anxiety, euphoria, hallucinations, and delusions.
- The final stage is characterized by stupor, mutism, seizures, and pneumonia that often leads to death.

Other Forms of Dementia

There are many other forms of dementia that space does not allow us to describe (Brookshire, 2015; Hegde, 2018b; Lubinski, 1995; Toner, Shadden, & Gluth, 2011). Notable among them are the following:

- **Vascular dementia.** Vascular diseases may cause bilateral cortical, subcortical, or mixed damage resulting in dementia. Small, cortical ischemic strokes are a common etiology of vascular dementia. More common in men than in women, and more common in African Americans than in Whites, vascular dementia is associated with chronic hypertension. A distinguishing feature of vascular dementia is its sudden onset.
- **Dementia associated with multiple cerebrovascular accidents**, infarctions within the deep structures of the brain, and atrophy of subcortical white matter caused by repeated infarcts are also associated with a long-standing hypertension.
- **Lewy body dementia.** This common form of dementia is caused by **Lewy bodies**, which are excessive protein deposits in neuronal cell bodies, causing pathologies similar to those found in Parkinson's and Alzheimer's diseases (hence, sometimes described as **mixed dementia**). Lewy bodies also may be found in the brains of patients with DAT and PD. Early forms may be confused with DAT. As opposed to PD, in which degeneration begins in the subcortex, Lewy body dementia is caused by degeneration of the cortex *and* subcortex due to deposits of Lewy bodies in these locations. Hallucinations and delusions are vivid and present early in the progression of Lewy body dementia, which distinguishes it from DAT and PD. Another key factor in differential diagnosis from PD is that individuals with Lewy body dementia will have a negative reaction to the drug L-Dopa, which is used to treat motor symptoms of PD.
- **Dementia associated with traumatic brain injury.** Repeated brain injuries, especially those that cause prolonged periods of unconsciousness, are a cause of dementia. Cortical, subcortical, and mixed types of damage may be associated with this type of dementia.
- **Wernicke-Korsakoff syndrome.** Wernicke's encephalopathy and the Korsakoff syndrome may be separate diseases but tend to be different stages of the same set of cognitive impairments, hence, called **Wernicke-Korsakoff syndrome**. Both diseases are caused by vitamin B1 (thiamine) deficiency, often related to chronic alcohol abuse. Other causes include dietary deficiencies, eating disorders, and chemotherapy. Confusion, vision problems, coma, hypothermia, and ataxia are the initial symptoms of Wernicke's encephalopathy. Subsequent Korsakoff symptoms include amnesia, disorientation, tremor, coma, with predominant memory problems.

Assessment of Dementia

A thorough case history, clinical examination, interview of the family and other caregivers, neurological assessment (including brain imaging and laboratory tests), communication assessment, and assessment of intellectual (cognitive) functions are essential to diagnose dementia (Bayles & Tomoeda, 2014; Bourgeois, 2011; Hallowell, 2017; Hegde, 2018c; Hegde & Freed, 2017; Payne, 2014; Weiner & Lipton, 2012). A definitive diagnosis of dementia is possible only after an autopsy, as there are no definitive blood or other laboratory tests for dementia.

- Asking the person to point to stimuli or administering automatic speech tasks are not useful in diagnosing mild forms of dementia. It is best diagnosed on the basis of verbal description, storytelling of both immediate and delayed variety, and word fluency (saying words that belong to a class, such as forms of transportation).
- In assessing dementia, the following skills or domains are typically sampled:
  - Awareness and orientation to surroundings
  - Mood and affect, to assess depression or lack of emotional responses
  - Speech and language
  - Memory, executive functions, and other cognitive variables
  - Abnormal thinking (e.g., hallucinations or delusions)
  - Visuospatial skills

- The clinician may use one of the several available screening and diagnostic tests for dementia. Dementia screening tests include the *Mini-Mental State Examination–Second Edition* (Folstein & Folstein, 2001), which screens naming, attention, and calculation; the *Saint-Louis University Mental Status Examination* (Tariq, Tumosa, Chibnall, Perry, & Morley, 2006), which screens orientation, recall, calculation, backward number recitation, and answering questions about a story told to the persons; and the *Montreal Cognitive Assessment, Version 3* (Nasreddine, 2011), which screens several skills including naming, memory, attention, verbal fluency, and sentence repetition.
- Dementia diagnostic tests include:
  - The *Arizona Battery for Communication Disorders of Dementia* (ABCD; Bayles & Tomoeda, 1993) helps assess mild to moderate impairments in speech discrimination, visual perception and literacy, visual fields, visual agnosia, mental status, linguistic expression, linguistic comprehension, and visual–spatial construction associated with Alzheimer's disease.
  - The *Functional Linguistic Communication Inventory* (Bayles & Tomoeda, 1994) helps assess various communication skills in individuals in middle to late stages of DAT.
  - The *Addenbrooke's Cognitive Function–Revised* (Mioshi, Dawson, Mitchell, Arnold, & Hodges, 2006) targets attention and orientation, memory, fluency, language, and visuospatial skills for assessment.
  - The *Global Deterioration Scale* (Reisberg, Ferris, de Leon, & Crook, 1982) evaluates levels of functioning ranging from *no cognitive impairment* to *very severe cognitive decline*. Information is gathered from a variety of sources.
  - The *Repeatable Battery for the Assessment of Neuropsychological Status Update* (Randolph, 2012) evaluates memory, visuospatial/constructional, language, attention, and delayed memory.

- The *Progressive Aphasia Severity Scale* (Sapolsky, Domato-Reilly, & Dickerson, 2014) evaluates articulation, fluency, comprehension, repetition, reading, writing, and functional communication in primary progressive aphasia, a form of dementia.
- The *Functional Communication Profile–Revised* (Keilman, 2003) evaluates basic communication skills, including verbal, nonverbal, sign, and augmented modes of communication exhibited in natural settings.

■ Various tests of aphasia may be helpful in assessing functional communication problems associated with dementia.

■ Intellectual skills may be assessed by administering selected tests of memory and general intelligence.

■ The clinician may use such client-specific tasks as picture description to help assess various intellectual and language skills, including temporal sequencing, logical connections, grammaticality of sentences, topic maintenance, and so forth.

Clinical Management of Dementia

The main clinical concern is to offer intervention that will help slow the progression of dementia, sustain communication and other skills to the extent possible, and improve daily communication and living skills. Helping family members and caregivers cope with the progressively deteriorating dementia, for which there is no cure, is also a major concern. There is evidence that behavioral communication intervention is helpful to most patients with dementia (Hopper et al., 2013). Physical activity and exercise are also known to be helpful (Mahendra, 2016; Stubbs et al., 2014). In the early and intermediate stages, communication, memory, and behavioral management are targeted.

■ Management of daily activities, memory, and communication skills may include teaching the following strategies to the client (Bourgeois, 2007; Bourgeois & Hickey, 2009):

- Establishing a simple routine
- Keeping phone numbers and possessions in a specific place
- Carrying a card or wearing a bracelet with the names, addresses, and phone numbers of caregivers
- Using external cues to improve memory and behavior (e.g., using such graphic aids as **memory wallets** (a collection of written and picture cues; see Bourgeois, 2007); writing a list of things to do every morning; using various reminders of activities and their times, including sticky notes, alarms, written instructions, staff reminders, self-monitoring devices, and various signs; writing a checklist of things to do before leaving the house, and so forth
- Writing down important information when memory begins to fail

■ Communication training may be a part of a general intervention strategy, which might include the following (Hopper et al., 2013):

- Improving or sustaining basic, functional communication skills as long as possible is a goal of communication intervention
- Caregiver and family involvement in communication training is crucial

- Attempts to minimize the effects of deficits by compensatory behaviors are worthwhile (e.g., written notes to remind oneself of appointments)
- Behavioral interventions may be combined with such drugs as donepezil, an acetylcholinesterase inhibitor

■ Family members and caregivers need counseling and support. The family members should be (a) educated about dementia, (b) urged to monitor their emotional reactions, including depression, (c) offered counseling and other support services, and (d) offered respite care of patients. In addition, family members may be trained to use effective communicative strategies to better manage daily-living skills (Small, Gutman, Makela, & Hillhouse, 2003). Caregivers may be trained to do the following:

- Approach the patient slowly, touch the patient gently, establish eye contact, and engage attention
- Use gestures, smiling, posture, and other cues
- Eliminate or limit environmental distractions
- Talk about simple and concrete events
- Simplify speech, use short sentences, paraphrase, restate, and rephrase
- Ask yes–no questions
- Avoid slow speech, as it may lead to communication breakdowns
- Point out the topic, person, or thing before speaking about it
- Structure the client's room and the living environment to establish a routine
- Always say goodbye or give other departing signals
- Reduce emotional outbursts by analyzing the conditions under which they occur and eliminating those conditions
- Minimize demands made on the client

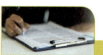

SUMMARY

- Dementia is progressive deterioration in cognition and behavior; it is usually found in people over 65 years of age.
- Dementia takes various forms; some are reversible, but most are progressive. Alzheimer's dementia is the most common type. Other types include frontotemporal dementia and dementias that are associated with Parkinson's disease and Huntington's disease. Various forms of infections cause dementia. The most prominent of this variety is the AIDS dementia complex and dementia associated with Creutzfeldt-Jakob disease.
- Assessment of patients with dementia includes administration of informal tasks and standardized tests.
- Treatment of patients with dementia is concerned with helping them manage their daily routines, including communication, as effectively as possible and helping families cope with the dementia.

RIGHT HEMISPHERE DISORDER

The symptoms of **right hemisphere disorder (RHD)**, also called **right hemisphere brain damage** and **right hemisphere syndrome**, vary depending upon the site of lesion. Typically, however, symptoms include attentional (perceptual) and affective symptoms; communicative deficits are found in 50–78% of the cases. Assessment of patients with RHD is mostly client-specific, although a few standardized tests are available. Treatment often addresses such problems as impaired attention, impulsive behavior, pragmatic communication impairments, and visual neglect (Blake, 2018; Blake, Frymark, & Venedictov, 2013; Blake, Tompkins, Scharp, Meigh, & Wambaugh, 2014; Davis, 2014; Tompkins, 2012).

The Right and the Left Hemispheres

- The left hemisphere (LH) and the right hemisphere (RH) of the brain have subtle structural differences (Nolte, 2009):

  - The LH is slightly larger in diameter
  - The lateral sulcus in the LH is slightly longer than that in the RH
  - The left planum temporale (a part of the superior surface of the superior temporal gyrus) is also larger than the right

- The LH controls most aspects of language, but the RH controls the following:

  - Understanding holistic gestalt stimuli, visual perception, geometric, mathematical, and spatial information (e.g., figure–ground relationship)
  - Facial recognition, drawing, and copying
  - Arousal, attention, and orientation
  - Emotional experience and expression
  - Perception of musical harmony, pitch, and melody
  - Language comprehension in general and meanings of related words in particular; prosodic features of communication; understanding ambiguous meanings; expressing and understanding the emotional tone of speech; understanding discourse; and pragmatic language skills (e.g., socially appropriate communication, turn taking, topic maintenance)
  - More diffusely organized functions compared to those of the LH functions

Symptoms of Right Hemisphere Disorder

The two hemispheres are susceptible to the same kinds of neuropathology, including cerebrovascular accidents, tumors, head trauma, and various neurological diseases. Posterior lesions do not produce motor problems. Frontal lobe injuries cause motor problems as well as longer hospitalization.

Perceptual and attentional deficits dominate the symptom complex of RHD. Affective and communicative deficits accompany them, but pure linguistic deficits (of the kind seen in agrammatic aphasia) are not typical of RHD (Blake, 2018; Blake et al., 2013).

Attentional and Perceptual Deficits

- **Left neglect**—reduced awareness of the left side of the body and generally reduced awareness of stimuli in the left visual field is called left neglect; may pay attention only to the right side of stimuli (e.g., copying only the right side of the face of a clock); failure to allow for a left margin in writing, reading only the right side of a printed page, bumping into things or people on the left side, and using pockets on only the right side.
- **Denial of illness** (**anosognosia**, lack of awareness of deficits)—may not acknowledge the existence of the paralyzed arm or leg and may be indifferent to admitted deficits or problems.
- **Confabulation regarding disability**—exaggerated claims regarding a disabled body part (e.g., a man with a paralyzed hand may claim to be painting with that hand).
- **Facial recognition deficits** (**prosopagnosia**)—failure to recognize a familiar face until the person begins to speak, difficulty remembering faces shown through pictures, and problems distinguishing faces of older and younger or male and female persons; not due to peripheral visual problems, due to impaired function of the visual association cortex in the occipital lobe
- **Constructional impairment**—difficulty reproducing block designs, drawing or copying geometric shapes, and reproducing two-dimensional stick figures.
- **Attentional deficits**—reduced awareness and arousal, difficulty sustaining attention, and difficulty in paying selective attention.
- **Disorientation**—topographic disorientation (confusion about space), geographic disorientation (not knowing where one is), and reduplicative paramnesia (e.g., a patient's belief that he has two left legs or two wives).
- **Visuoperceptual deficits**—difficulty recognizing line drawings; drawings that are distorted in size, dimension, or orientation; and drawings that are superimposed on another.

Affective Deficits

- Understanding emotions expressed by other people
- Describing emotions expressed on printed faces in storybooks
- Recognizing emotions expressed in isolated verbal productions
- Understanding emotional tone of voice
- Expressing emotions (not necessarily *experiencing* emotions)

Communicative Deficits

- **Impaired communicative effectiveness**—deficits associated with RHD are not so much related to syntactic and morphologic aspects of language as to an overall communicative effectiveness and comprehension of abstract meanings.
- **Prosodic deficits**—difficulty understanding prosodic meanings of other people's speech; lack of prosodic variations in one's own speech, resulting in monotone, impaired stress patterns, reduced speech rate, and lack of affect.

- **Impaired (disorganized) discourse and narrative skills**—confusion between significant and irrelevant or trivial pieces of information in a picture description or conversational speech, resulting in premature inferences during discourse, and unelaborated narratives.
- **Confabulation and excessive speech**—excessive inference; too much attention to minor details; and saying too much, which borders on confabulation.
- **Difficulty understanding implied, alternate, or abstract meanings**—failure to grasp the overall meaning of situations or stories; difficulty understanding the central message of conversation; difficulty in describing the underlying theme of a picture or a story; literal interpretation of proverbs and sayings; inferencing deficits; and problems in appreciating humor, sarcasm, and irony.
- **Pragmatic deficits**—problems in conversational turn taking, topic maintenance, and maintaining eye contact, as well as rambling, excessive speech with little communicative value, and impulsive speech.
- **Other communicative deficits**—naming problems, especially of collective nouns (e.g., problem saying "flowers," but no problem naming a particular type of flower); difficulty comprehending complex verbal material; and impaired oral reading of sentences.

Assessment of Right Hemisphere Disorder

Assessment of RHD can be client specific, standardized, or both.

- A quick bedside screen may involve holding a brief conversation with the client to assess the current behavioral status. A few questions about time, day, and date; repeating a few common words; describing a picture or two will help establish the need for standardized testing. Screening tests include the *Mini Inventory of Right Brain Injury–Second Edition* (MIRBI-2; Pimental & Knight, 2000) for visual scanning, integrity of gnosis (finger identification, tactile perception, two-point discrimination), integrity of body image, reading and writing, drawing, and affective and abstract language; *Burns Brief Inventory* (Burns, 1997) for visuospatial skills, prosody, abstract language, orientation, attention, and memory; and *Mini-Mental State Examination–Second Edition* (Folstein & Folstein, 2001) for naming, attention, and calculation.
- Right hemisphere disorder diagnostic tests include:
  - The *RIC Evaluation of Communication Problems in Right Hemisphere Dysfunction–Third Edition* (RICE-3; Halper, Cherney, & Burns, 2010) includes five subtests to evaluate cognitive and communicative deficits associated with right-hemisphere brain damage as well as nonverbal communication skills. In addition, the protocol includes an interview schedule and observation of a patient's interaction with others.
  - The *Right Hemisphere Language Battery–Second Edition* (RHLB-2; Bryan, 1995) helps assess comprehension of spoken and printed metaphors, inferred meanings, appreciation of humor, and discourse.
  - The *Test of Visual Neglect* (Albert, 1973) helps assess neglect by asking the patient to cross out short lines randomly printed on a page.

- The *Behavioral Inattention Test* (BIT; Wilson, Cockburn, & Halligan, 1987) contains both paper-and-pencil tests and techniques to assess neglect in such functional tasks as reading maps, menus, and newspapers and using a telephone.

- Client-specific measures include language samples, narratives, and discourse. The clinician may assess visual–perceptual deficits by asking the client to draw simple pictures (e.g., the face of a clock, a human face). Attentional and perceptual deficits, described previously, may be noted, as well.

Treatment of Right Hemisphere Disorder

There is evidence to support communication treatment and sentence- and discourse-level treatment (Blake, 2018; Blake et al., 2013; Davis, 2014; Hegde, 2018a, 2018d; Tompkins, 2012). The following treatment targets and strategies are appropriate to most clients, although treatment must always be tailored to individual needs:

- **Denial and indifference**. The clinician provides immediate feedback on errors to increase awareness of problems. Video-recorded sessions to give visual feedback on errors are helpful.
- **Impaired attention**. This involves drawing attention to treatment stimuli, giving specific directions, repeating such directions throughout treatment, reinforcing attention during discourse training, and stopping the patient whenever he or she wanders away from the topic of discourse.
- **Impulsive behavior**. Treatment includes nonverbal signals to wait a few seconds before giving an impulsive response (e.g., using a hand gesture or a tone that signals the patient to wait). Also helpful are such verbal stimuli as "Wait for a few seconds and then tell me."
- **Discourse problems**. Useful techniques include story retelling and story generation with hierarchical cues.
- **Pragmatic impairments**. Helpful techniques include video-recorded conversations that show appropriate and inappropriate pragmatic behaviors to draw the patient's attention to such behaviors. The clinician may also give frequent reminders to maintain eye contact, continue talking on the same topic, and so forth.
- **Impaired reasoning**. The clinician can use activities that require reasoning (e.g., planning a vacation) and prompt and reinforce correct and logically sequenced descriptions.
- **Impaired inference**. Helpful treatment techniques include use of pictures that depict situations that require inference and reinforcement for correct inferences.
- **Impaired comprehension of metaphors and idioms**. Treatment involves practice in the correct interpretation of metaphors and idioms by asking the client to select printed statements or make comments that give literal, metaphoric, and implied meanings.
- **Visual neglect**. Visual scanning techniques, known to be effective, include repeated practice on cancellation tasks, finding and picking up specific objects, and reading printed text. The clinician may draw thick and colorful line on the left margins of printed pages to force attention to the text on the left side; teach the patient to keep a finger on the left side of the page; point to the beginning of each line; give frequent verbal prompts to pay attention to the neglected side of the body; fade

the physical stimuli and prompts; and, generally, provide plenty of positive reinforcement for attending to objects on the left side and to the left side of the body. Isolated computer-based training is not effective.

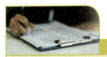

SUMMARY

- The right hemisphere specializes in processing holistic gestalt stimuli, visual and spatial information, facial recognition, drawing, and copying.
- Patients with injury to the right hemisphere manifest attentional, perceptual, affective, and communicative deficits with reasonably intact grammar.
- Client-specific and standardized methods may be used to assess patients with RHD.
- Treatment is targeted at impaired attention and behavior, pragmatic communication problems, impaired reasoning and inference, and visual neglect.

TRAUMATIC BRAIN INJURY

Traumatic brain injury (TBI), also known as **craniocerebral trauma**, is injury to the brain sustained by physical trauma or external force. TBI is a frequently encountered medical emergency. Brain injuries can be open-head (penetrating), closed-head (nonpenetrating), or mild traumatic brain injury (mTBI), also known as **concussion**. Assessment includes client-specific and standardized measures and is dependent upon the patient's level of post-accident consciousness. The two most common approaches to treatment of patients with TBI include the cognitive rehabilitation approach and the behavioral communication treatment approach (Adamovich, 1997; Coelho, 2011; Cooper & Golfinos, 2000; Davis, 2014; Hallowell, 2017; Hegde, 2018a, 2018b, 2018c, 2018d; Hegde & Freed, 2017; Kimbarow, 2016; Payne, 2014).

Definition and Incidence of TBI

Traumatic brain injury is injury to the brain sustained by physical trauma or external force. It does not include brain damage due to strokes, tumors, or progressive or transient neuropathologies. Clinicians should search online to get the latest demographic data on brain injury, as the numbers change annually. Websites of the National Institute of Neurological Diseases and Strokes, Brain Injury Association of America, and Centers for Disease Control and Prevention may be visited for recent statistics.

- Estimates of the incidence of TBI vary within a range of about 150–250 cases per 100,000 persons in the United States; annually, about 1.6 million individuals sustain TBI.

- The prevalence rates are highest for two age groups: 0–4 years and 15–19 years. For the age group 75 and older, the prevalence is higher than it is for the general population (about 300 per 100,000 persons).
- More males than females are affected. For every female with a TBI, there are three to five males with TBI.
- TBI is a significant problem for people living in high-density urban areas, many of whom are from linguistically and culturally diverse backgrounds. There is limited but suggestive evidence that TBI is more common among African Americans and Hispanic Americans than the rest of the national population (Wallace, 1998).
- More than 1.1 million emergency department visits and about 265,000 hospitalizations occur per year due to TBI. Annually, 52,000 deaths are due to TBI. Moderate to severe TBI may leave 75,000 with some degree of disability (Cooper & Golfinos, 2000).

Common Causes of TBI

- Falls, the most common cause, account for 35% of TBIs. Children and the elderly are especially vulnerable.
- Automobile accidents, including pedestrian injuries, account for 20% of TBI; 15% of pedestrians sustain TBI due to automobile accidents. Motorcycle riders have a higher risk of TBI than car drivers. A full 17% of injuries sustained in automobile accidents are TBIs.
- Head striking stationary objects or being struck by moving objects cause about 16% of TBIs.
- Assaults and interpersonal violence (including child and spousal abuse) account for about 10% of TBIs.
- Sports-related concussion is a leading cause of TBI in student and professional athletes.
- Battlefield blasts cause polytrauma (multisystem injuries), because blasts cause injuries to other organs and systems in addition to the brain (Coelho, 2011). About 22% of wounded service personnel may have TBI; closed-head injuries are the most common form, accompanied by communication disorders (Norman et al., 2014).
- Other causes include alcohol and drug abuse, serious preexisting learning disorders, psychiatric disturbances, and prior history of TBI.

Types and Consequences of TBI

Open-head (penetrating) and **closed-head (nonpenetrating)** injuries are two traditional classifications of TBI; **blast (multisystem) injuries** and **concussion (mild traumatic brain injury)** are the more recent third and fourth varieties. Each variety produces unique neuroanatomic and behavioral consequences.

- **Open-head brain injuries** involve a fractured or perforated skull, torn or lacerated meninges, and an injury that extends to brain tissue. High-velocity missiles (e.g., bullets) and low-velocity impacts (e.g., blows to the head) are the most frequent causes of such penetrating brain injuries.
- **Closed-head brain injuries** involve no open wound in the head, no penetration of a foreign substance into the brain, and a damaged brain within the skull. Even when the skull is fractured, the

injury is classified as closed-head (nonpenetrating) if the meninges are intact. Such nonpenetrating injuries may be of the acceleration–deceleration type or the nonacceleration type.

- **Acceleration–deceleration injuries** are more serious than non-acceleration injuries. In acceleration–deceleration, a head is set into motion by physical forces. When the head begins to move, the brain inside is still static. Soon the brain begins to move. When the head stops moving, the brain keeps moving inside the skull and, thus, strikes the skull on the opposite side of the initial impact. The brain injury at the point of impact (e.g., a blow to the head) is called the **coup injury**; the injury at the opposite side of the impact caused by the moving brain striking the skull is called the **contrecoup injury**. The moving brain is lacerated, or torn, because of the bony projections on the base of the skull. The acceleration–deceleration movement of the head in an automobile accident is an example.
- **Non-acceleration injuries** occur when a restrained head is hit by a moving object. A collapsing car crushing the head of a mechanic working under it is an example. A great deal of force may crush the head and kill a person; in most cases, however, nonacceleration injuries produce much less serious consequences for the brain and the behavior of the person, even though they may fracture the skull.
- **Blast injuries** cause both closed-head and open-head injuries; however, closed-head injuries are much more common (up to 88%) than open-head injuries (12%). Explosions raise atmospheric pressure waves that spread and affect such air-filled organs as the ear and lungs, and organs surrounded by fluid-filled cavities, such as the brain and spinal cord.
- **Concussion** or **mild traumatic brain injury** (mTBI) is a form of closed-head injury in which consciousness is lost for less than 20 minutes; often related to sports activities and battlefield blasts.
- Consequences of TBI include both immediate (primary) and delayed (secondary) effects:

  - Immediate or subsequent death, loss of consciousness, coma, destruction of brain tissue, diffuse axonal injury, diffuse vascular injury, brainstem injury, focal lesions, infection, reduced cerebral blood flow, increased blood pressure, swelling of the brain tissue, hydrocephalus, and various types of hematomas (accumulation of blood in an area of the brain)
  - Increased intracranial pressure; ischemic brain damage (damage due to lack of blood); seizures; and long-term physical, language, and cognitive deficits
  - Confusion and disorientation; posttraumatic amnesia and posttraumatic stress syndrome; dysphagia; behavior changes, including hallucinations, delusions, and confabulations; poor emotional control; social withdrawal; irritability; childishness; and unreasonable behaviors

- Communication disorders associated with TBI include

  - an initial mutism that may last varying periods of time;
  - confused language, naming difficulties, perseveration of verbal responses, reduced word fluency, difficulty initiating conversation, lack of turn taking in conversation, problems in topic initiation and maintenance, lack of narrative cohesion, impaired prosody, imprecise language, difficulty with abstract language, auditory comprehension deficits;

- generally impaired social interaction;
- reading and writing problems; and
- motor speech disorders, typically dysarthria.

General Assessment of Persons With TBI

In the assessment of persons with TBI, it is critical to gather a comprehensive case history, observe the client, interview family members and health care workers, and review medical records to understand the nature and extent of the TBI.

- **Initial bedside assessment**. The client regaining consciousness may be inconsistent, disorganized, disoriented, restless, distracted, and irritated. The initial assessment may be done at the bedside. Typically, a few questions about the time, place and person orientation and about the events surrounding the brain injury may be asked to screen the current condition of the client. Clinicians may select one of the TBI scales evaluated and recommended by the American Congress of Rehabilitation Medicine (2010). Some examples of screening tests are *Brief Test of Head Injury* (BTHI; Helm-Estabrooks & Hotz, 1991), which assesses orientation and follows commands and other relevant behaviors, and *Montreal Cognitive Assessment* (MoCA; Nasreddine et al., 2005), a 10-minute screening tool that assesses visuospatial skills, attention, concentration, working memory, language, and orientation to time and place.
- Traumatic brain injury diagnostic tests include:

  - The *Coma Recovery Scale–Revised* (CRS-R; Giacino, Kalmar, & Whyte, 2004) assesses auditory, visual, motor, and oral communication and arousal parameters.
  - The *Scales of Cognitive Ability for Traumatic Brain Injury* (SCATBI; Adamovich & Henderson, 1992) assesses perception, orientation, organization, recall, and reasoning.
  - The *Glasgow Coma Scale* (Teasdale & Jennett, 1974) helps make an initial assessment of eye opening, motor responses (e.g., flexing the body in response to pain), and verbal responses.
  - The *Galveston Orientation and Amnesia Test* (GOAT; Levin, O'Donnell, & Grossman, 1979) assesses amnesia, orientation, and memory.
  - The *Disability Rating Scale* (DRS; Rappoport, Hall, Hopkins, Belleza, & Cope, 1982) assesses changes in patients with head injury; it helps assess eye opening, verbal responses, motor responses, feeding, toileting, and so forth.
  - The *Rancho Los Amigos Levels of Cognitive Function* (Hagen & Malkamus, 1979) assesses cognition and behavior at the levels of no response, generalized response, localized response, confused–agitated, confused–inappropriate, confused–appropriate, automatic–appropriate, and purposeful–appropriate.
  - The *Cognitive Linguistic Quick Test* (CLQT; Helm-Estabrooks, 2001) is a 15–30-minute assessment of attention, memory, executive function, language, and visuospatial skills.

- **Assessment of memory impairments**. Posttraumatic amnesia (loss of memory for events following the trauma) and pretraumatic amnesia (loss of memory for events preceding the trauma) may be assessed by an interview in which client-specific questions surrounding the trauma may be asked.

- **Assessment of executive functions.** Planning, organizing, initiating and completing various activities are subsumed under executive functions. These may be assessed by asking the client to describe how he or she might plan a vacation, organize a picnic, prepare a special meal, and so forth.

Assessment of Communicative Deficits Associated With TBI

Pure linguistic problems may not be severe or significant in patients with TBI. Articulatory or phonological disorders may be noted only if the patient sustained injury to the cerebellum, brainstem, or peripheral nerves. The patient's verbal expressions may be grammatically correct.

Assessment procedures may include selected tests of aphasia and client-specific procedures that the clinician develops (Coelho, 2011; Davis, 2014; Hallowell, 2017; Hegde, 2018a, 2018c; Kimbarow, 2016). The *Scales of Cognitive and Communicative Ability for Neurorehabilitation* (SCCAN; Milman & Holland, 2012) assesses cognitive–communicative deficits and functional ability and measures oral expression, orientation, memory, speech comprehension, reading comprehension, writing, attention and problem solving.

- Initial and persistent communicative problems that must be assessed include the following:

  - **Dysarthria.** Spastic dysarthria or mixed dysarthria in some patients with TBI has been noted; these disorders may be assessed with standard dysarthria assessment tools (described in the next chapter).
  - **Confused language.** If evident initially, this may be assessed with standard interviews and bedside examinations.
  - **Auditory comprehension problems.** Possibly more pronounced for complex or abstract material; both clinical examinations and selected standardized assessment tools may be helpful in assessing auditory comprehension deficits.
  - **Confrontation naming problems.** Standard naming tests, described in the section on aphasia and client-specific procedures the clinician devises, (e.g., showing objects from the client's environment and asking him or her to name them) will be helpful in assessing these problems.
  - **Perseveration of verbal responses.** Repetitive verbal responses may be observed and recorded during interview and conversations with the patient.
  - **Pragmatic language problems.** Difficulty in initiating conversation, turn taking, selecting appropriate topics for conversation, and maintaining topic and cohesion; rambling; and difficulty understanding the meaning of facial expressions and gestures; best assessed during interview and conversation with the patient.
  - **Reading and writing difficulties.** Reading and writing tests; such client-specific tasks as having the client read familiar print, write to dictation, and copy printed material will help assess these difficulties.
  - **Daily living skills.** Functional math skills (e.g., balancing a checkbook, paying bills, calculating a tip), eating and bathing, and managing medications (e.g., remembering medication dosage and how often to take each dose) may be assessed by interviewing the client and a family member.

- **Client-specific assessment**. Language samples, narrative skill (storytelling and retelling) and discourse sampling (talking on a topic of interest) help assess off-target, disorganized, and tangential responses.

Treatment of Persons With TBI

Of the variety of treatment approaches advocated for patients with TBI, cognitive rehabilitation and direct communication training are the two most important (Hallowell, 2017; Hegde, 2018a, 2018d; Kimbarow, 2016). There is evidence to support the behavioral methods of training communication skills (Togher et al., 2014) and retraining memory skills (Elliott & Parente, 2014).

- **Cognitive rehabilitation** is preferred by some clinicians. In cognitive rehabilitation:

  - Clinicians train such components as attention, visual processing, and memory, which may not result in improved communication.
  - Attempts to improve memory, reasoning skills, and other cognitive functions may be better integrated with communication treatment.
  - Patients with TBI recover their memory skills as their condition improves; nonetheless, memory training (of the kind used with patients with dementia) is known to produce beneficial results (Elliott & Parente, 2014).

- **Communication treatment** for patients with TBI often involves direct behavioral procedures. The goals should be functional, and the initial emphasis should be effectiveness of communication, not grammatical correctness. Family members should be involved in treatment.

  - Training communication partners as well as the patient is more effective than training only the patient (Togher, McDonald, Tate, Power, & Rietdijk, 2013).
  - Systematic reinforcement of attending behaviors, relevant speech, appropriate discourse, topic maintenance, self-correction, and so forth will result in their increase and a concomitant decrease in many inappropriate behaviors.
  - Patient's orientation and attention to place, person, and time may be increased by asking questions about the patient's whereabouts and systematically reinforcing correct responses.
  - Posting written signs to help the patient remember the day of the week, the name caregivers in the hospital, and the times of different daily activities will be useful.
  - The patient's memory for the names of significant people may be increased by asking the patient to name pictures of family members.
  - Variability in activities and schedules may be decreased by initially creating a simple, structured routine with few activities for the patient.
  - The patient's attention to communication partners and topics may be increased to promote better comprehension by giving such signals as "Listen carefully, now," "I want to say something to you," and "Are you listening?"
  - Attention during conversation may be increased by introducing new topics by first giving a warning about topic changes in conversation.

- The client may be taught to ask questions when something said is not clear to him or her by modeling such questions and statements as "What do you mean?" "I don't understand that," "Tell me more about that," and so forth.
- Irrelevant, inappropriate, or tangential responses may be reduced by withholding attention.
- Narrative skills may be taught in graded steps by initially telling a brief and simple story, asking the patient to retell it, and eventually having the client retell more complex stories.
- Discourse skills may be improved by asking the client to give a brief lecture on a topic and prompting details and arguments for and against the stands taken, and by prompt reinforcement of appropriate responses.
- Executive functions may be improved by having the client describe how a certain activity is done (e.g., planning a vacation in another state); prompts and reinforcements will help improve the descriptions.
- Such pragmatic skills as topic maintenance and topic initiation may be integrated into narrative skills teaching by such prompts as "Say more" and "Give details."
- Work- or school-related words, phrases, and narratives may be integrated into communication.
- Tangible reinforcers may be necessary, because some patients with TBI may not respond to verbal reinforcers in the early stages of recovery.
- Self-monitoring skills may be taught by including them at all levels of training.
- Compensatory strategies may have to be taught to handle residual deficits (e.g., writing down instructions and important information, requesting information, requesting some people to speak slowly or repeat, requesting others to write down messages, establishing simple and invariable routines, reducing environmental distractions, and self-cueing).
- Family members and communication partners in professional settings may be taught to recognize, prompt, model, and reinforce appropriate communication and general behavior.
- Community reentry may be promoted by preparing the patient for reentry to school or work.
- Family members, teachers, and supervisors may be educated about the patient's strengths and weaknesses; taught to change their style of communication if needed; and asked, especially teachers or supervisors, to modify demands if necessary.

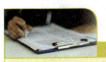

SUMMARY

- Patients with TBI should undergo general assessment as well as assessment of communicative deficits, such as possible dysarthria, pragmatic language and auditory comprehension problems, and written-language deficits.
- The two primary treatment approaches for patients with TBI include the cognitive rehabilitation and communication treatment. These two approaches may be integrated to help the patient reenter the community to the greatest extent possible.

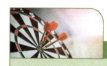

CHAPTER HIGHLIGHTS

- Aphasia is a neurogenic language disorder caused by a stroke and is classified into nonfluent, fluent, and subcortical varieties.
- Varieties of nonfluent aphasia include Broca's aphasia, transcortical motor aphasia, mixed transcortical aphasia, and global aphasia. Varieties of fluent aphasia include Wernicke's aphasia, transcortical sensory aphasia, conduction aphasia, and anomic aphasia. Nonfluent aphasias are generally caused by lesions in the anterior brain structures, and fluent aphasias are caused by lesions in the posterior structures; subcortical aphasia is caused by lesions in the basal ganglia and surrounding structures and the thalamus.
- Relatively intact auditory comprehension and agrammatic, anomic, telegraphic, dysfluent, effortful, and sparse speech characterize nonfluent aphasia. Impaired auditory comprehension and relatively fluent, jargon-filled, and grammatically correct but semantically impaired speech characterize fluent aphasia. Treatment of aphasia targets both auditory comprehension and verbal expression; functional communication is a realistic goal for many severely involved clients.
- Alexia is a reading disorder due to cortical damage. Agraphia is a writing disorder due to cortical damage. Agnosia is a sensory disorder in the absence of peripheral sensory problems.
- Dementia is associated with persistent or progressive deterioration in intellectual functions (cognition, visuospatial skills), language, memory, emotion, and personality. It is often seen in the elderly, is typically progressive, and is reversible in some cases.
- Right hemisphere disorder is a symptom complex including perceptual, attentional, affective, and communicative deficits associated with injury to the right cerebral hemisphere.
- Traumatic brain injury (TBI) is injury to the brain sustained by physical trauma or external force. Open-head (penetrating) brain injuries involve a fractured or perforated skull, torn or lacerated meninges, and an injury that extends to brain tissue. Closed-head (nonpenetrating) brain injuries involve no open wound in the head, no penetration of a foreign substance into the brain, and a damaged brain within the skull. Blast injuries cause both closed-head and open-head injuries. Mild traumatic brain injury (mTBI) also known as concussion, is a form of closed-head injury in which consciousness is lost for less than 20 minutes.

STUDY AND REVIEW QUESTIONS

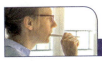

1. A clinician in a hospital setting is asked to evaluate a 64-year-old patient who appears to have dementia. In gathering the case history from the patient's adult daughter, the clinician finds out that the patient began drinking alcohol as a 15-year-old and has been a heavy drinker since that time. A detailed evaluation shows that the patient presents with memory problems, difficulty processing abstract information, and visual–spatial deficits. This patient most likely has

   A. dementia of the Alzheimer's type.
   B. Parkinson's disease.
   C. Wernicke-Korsakoff syndrome.
   D. aphasia.

2. Conduction aphasia is caused by lesions

   A. in the areas supplied by the middle cerebral arteries and the anterior and posterior arteries.
   B. in the region between Broca's area and Wernicke's area, especially in the supramarginal gyrus and the arcuate fasciculus.
   C. in Brodmann's areas 44 and 45 in the posterior-inferior gyrus of the left hemisphere.
   D. in the angular gyrus, the second temporal gyrus, and the juncture of the temporoparietal lobe.

3. Dementia associated with Pick's disease is a part of

   A. Alzheimer's dementia.
   B. frontotemporal dementia.
   C. semantic variant of primary progressive aphasia.
   D. the nonfluent variant of the primary progressive aphasia.

Questions 4–6 refer to the following scenario:

A hospital-based clinician receives a referral of a woman, Fran, who is 76 years old and enjoys walking, swimming, and giving her grandchildren rides. During the initial interview, Fran tells the clinician that she would have to stop her daily walks with her dog, because she believes she is slow when she begins walking and then she would take short, rapid, shuffling steps. She also shares that her writing has become smaller and that her friends and family say that she has been found "expressionless" in the recent days. The clinician also notices decreased intelligibility.

4. Fran probably has

   A. right-hemisphere syndrome.
   B. unilateral upper motor neuron dysarthria.
   C. Alzheimer's dementia.
   D. Parkinson's disease.

5. Based on your diagnosis, you would expect Fran's speech and language to be characterized by

   A. fluency problems, including silent pauses as well as repetitions because of false starts and attempts at self-correction.

   B. quality and rate that are "drunken" and slow, with excessive and even stress.

   C. incoherent, slurred, and rapid speech accompanied by metathetic errors.

   D. monopitch, a harsh and breathy voice, short rushes of speech, imprecise consonants, and respiratory problems.

6. Other symptoms the clinician might expect Fran to manifest would include

   A. chorea, emotional outbursts, schizophrenic-like behaviors, and dysarthria.

   B. hallucinations, mask-like face, and confabulation.

   C. mask-like face, slow voluntary movements, tremors in resting muscles, and disturbed posture.

   D. circumlocutions, repetitive verbal responses, and festinating speech.

7. Functional communication assessment targets

   A. communication in natural or everyday situations.

   B. grammatically correct and complex communication.

   C. comprehension of both daily and academic vocabulary necessary for effective functioning in the "real world."

   D. phonemically correct communication.

8. A hospital-based clinician receives a referral of Mary, a 71-year-old woman. Mary's 35-year-old son says, "Mom just isn't herself anymore; we don't know what's wrong or what to do. We don't know if she had a stroke or what's going on." After talking with Mary in the initial interview, the clinician realizes that he will have to assess Mary in depth to evaluate whether she has aphasia or DAT (dementia of the Alzheimer's type). If Mary has DAT, which of the following symptoms will she show?

   A. Normal syntax except for word-finding problems; good auditory comprehension of spoken language; slurred and rapid speech; disorientation to time and place; visuospatial problems; difficulty with self-care and daily routines; intact repetition skills

   B. Severe problems in recalling remote and recent events; relatively intact syntactic skills; appropriate humor and laughter; disorientation to time and place; intact ability to initiate interactions

C. Severely impaired fluency; severe echolalia; agrammatic and telegraphic speech; intact auditory comprehension skills; no difficulty with self-care or managing daily routines

D. Poor judgment; impaired reasoning; disorientation in new places; widespread intellectual deterioration; empty speech; jargon; incoherent, slurred, and rapid speech; problems in comprehending abstract messages

9. A 54-year-old pastor, Rev. Johnson, has a stroke and takes a leave of absence from his job while he recovers. After a 3–4-month period, he goes back to work, which include preaching sermons on Sunday mornings and visiting church members who are sick. He says that he is "100% back"; however, his parishioners and family notice that he tends to bump into people who walk on his left; when he writes, he does not use the left side of the page. He does not recognize parishioners whom he has known for 30 or more years until they begin to speak. When people tell jokes, he does not laugh or appear to understand the jokes as he used to. He does not detect sarcasm in other people's speech. Rev. Johnson probably has

A. dementia.
B. Wernicke-Korsakoff syndrome.
C. right-hemisphere syndrome.
D. apraxia of speech.

10. A 90-year-old woman in a skilled nursing facility is in the end stages of Alzheimer's dementia. The top treatment priority would be

A. improving her sentence structure.
B. facilitating communication with the staff during daily routines.
C. working on her word retrieval skills.
D. increasing orientation to date and time.

11. You are working with Mr. Thomas, who has been diagnosed with Parkinson's disease. Primary symptoms you can expect to see include

A. difficulty with sequencing motor movements of speech.
B. word retrieval problems and agrammatism.
C. confusion, disorientation, and emotional outbursts.
D. bradykinesia, festination, and cogwheel rigidity.

12. Dementia of the Alzheimer's type is caused by

A. thiamine deficiency.
B. pathological changes of the corpus callosum.
C. neurofibrillary tangles and neuritic plaques.
D. deterioration of neurons in the brainstem.

13. The most significant communication problem associated with right hemisphere disorder is

   A. agrammatic speech.
   B. impaired morphologic production.
   C. severe voice disorders.
   D. overall communicative effectiveness.

14. Primary progressive aphasia is a form of

   A. fluent aphasia.
   B. dementia.
   C. nonfluent aphasia.
   D. subcortical aphasia.

15. You are assessing a 20-year-old man who was involved in an auto accident with severe head injury. The medical report says that the patient has nonpenetrating head injury. In this case, you expect to observe

   A. intact meninges.
   B. torn meninges.
   C. no skull fracture.
   D. an open wound.

References and Recommended Readings at www.advancedreviewpractice.com

STUDY AND REVIEW ANSWERS

1. C. A patient with a history of heavy drinking who presents with memory problems, difficulty processing abstract information, and visual–spatial deficits probably has Wernicke-Korsakoff syndrome.
2. B. Conduction aphasia is caused by lesions in the region between Broca's area and Wernicke's area, especially in the supramarginal gyrus and the arcuate fasciculus.
3. B. Dementia associated with Pick's disease is now a part of the frontotemporal dementia.
4. D. Fran probably has Parkinson's disease.
5. D. Because Fran has Parkinson's disease, you would expect her speech to be characterized by monopitch, a harsh and breathy voice, short rushes of speech, imprecise consonants, and respiratory problems.
6. C. Patients with Parkinson's disease usually present with a mask-like face, slow voluntary movements, tremors in resting muscles, and disturbed posture.
7. A. Functional communication tests seek to assess communication in natural or everyday situations.
8. D. Characteristics of DAT include poor judgment; impaired reasoning; disorientation in new places; widespread intellectual deterioration; empty speech; jargon; incoherent, slurred, and rapid speech; and problems in comprehending abstract messages.
9. C. Rev. Johnson probably has right-hemisphere syndrome, which is characterized by left-side neglect, difficulty recognizing people until they begin to speak, and difficulty detecting sarcasm and humor in other people's speech.

10. B. If a patient is in the end stages of Alzheimer's disease, the number one priority is facilitating communication with staff.
11. D. Patients with Parkinson's disease typically manifest bradykinesia, festination, and cogwheel rigidity.
12. C. Dementia of the Alzheimer's type is caused by neurofibrillary tangles and neuritic plaques.
13. D. The most significant communication problem associated with right hemisphere disorder is overall communicative effectiveness.
14. B. Primary progressive aphasia is a form of dementia, although it starts as aphasia.
15. A. If the patient has nonpenetrating head injury, you expect to observe intact meninges; skull may or may not be fractured and there is no open wound.

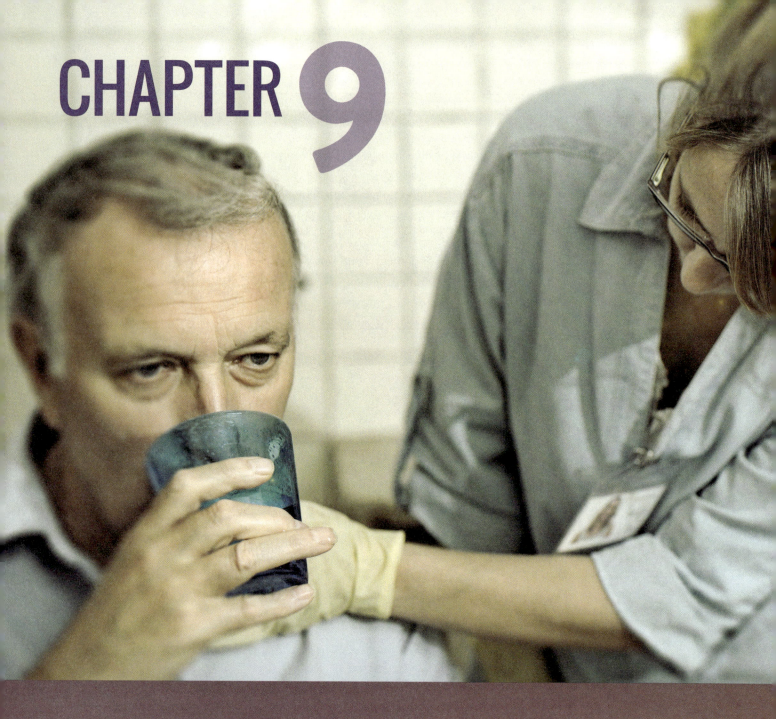

CHAPTER 9

MOTOR SPEECH DISORDERS AND DYSPHAGIA

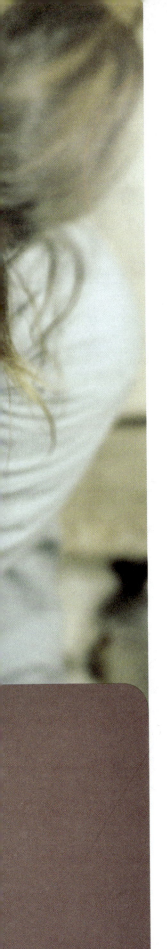

Neuropathologies or brain trauma cause several disorders of communication as well as disorders of swallowing (dysphagia). This chapter provides an overview of the nature, assessment, and treatment of such communicative disorders, which include apraxia of speech and dysarthrias. An overview of swallowing disorders, their common causes, and their assessment and treatment is also provided.

APRAXIA OF SPEECH

Apraxia of speech (AOS) is a neurogenic speech disorder characterized by speech sound production errors combined with prosodic deficiencies. It is hypothesized that patients with AOS have sensorimotor problems in positioning and sequentially moving muscles for volitional speech production. AOS is caused by damage or injury to speech–motor programming areas (e.g., Broca's area) in the dominant hemisphere, often as a result of stroke or other nondegenerative factors. Recent evidence suggests, however, that neurodegenerative diseases also may cause a type of AOS (Duffy & Josephs, 2012). Assessment and treatment for patients with AOS involve detailed procedures related to evaluating and improving articulatory accuracy, speech rate, and self-monitoring (Duffy, 2013; Hegde, 2018a; Hegde & Freed, 2017; Yorkston, Beukelman, Strand, & Hakel, 2010).

Definition and Distinctions

Apraxia of speech is a neurogenic speech sound disorder presumably due to sensorimotor problems in creating motor plans and positioning and sequentially moving muscles for the volitional production of speech. It is clinically characterized predominantly by slower rate of speech, distorted speech sound substitutions and additions, syllable segmentation, articulatory groping, false starts and restarts, prosodic impairments, and longer utterances causing more errors than shorter utterances.

- AOS is primarily an articulatory–phonologic disorder, although its etiology and characteristics are different from those of similar disorders in children. Adult patients with AOS will have acquired articulation normally. Their current articulatory problems are due to recent neuropathology.
- Adults with AOS have unimpaired reflex and automatic acts. The difficulty they have is mostly in executing the voluntary movements involved in speech. AOS is typically associated with prosodic problems (Duffy, 2013).
- AOS is not caused by muscle weakness or neuromuscular slowness. Rather, the brain is unable to generate or send plans to the speech muscles for

appropriate timing, range, and force of contraction. AOS only impacts the motor plans for producing speech.

- Individuals with AOS and no other coexisting disorders will be able to use their articulators for nonspeech movements and will exhibit no difficulty in completing nonverbal aspects of an oral-motor evaluation; breakdowns will be apparent when clients are prompted with speech tasks (Manasco, 2014).

■ It is thought that a disorder of motor programming for speech causes AOS. It more frequently coexists with aphasia, especially Broca's, and less frequently with dysarthria of the unilateral upper motor neuron type. Technically, and in its pure form, AOS should not affect language skills, as it is a speech–motor programming problem. Language skills are affected only when there is a coexisting aphasia.

■ Pure apraxia of speech is rare, but in recent years, it has been observed as the only symptom or as a dominant symptom in patients with either primary progressive aphasia or dysarthria. AOS that is the only, or the dominant, symptom is now called **primary progressive apraxia of speech** (PPAOS), with insidious onset and slow progress, contrasted with stroke-induced AOS, which has a sudden onset, some improvement, and stabilization if the recovery is incomplete.

■ PPAOS is often confused with or subsumed under nonfluent primary progressive aphasia, because patients with that typically exhibit AOS. PPAOS can occur without aphasia, however (Duffy & Josephs, 2012).

■ Apraxia is a basic disorder of volitional movement in the absence of muscle weakness, paralysis, or fatigue; AOS is a special case of apraxia.

■ Nonverbal oral apraxia is a disorder of nonverbal movement involving the oral muscles. AOS is frequently associated with nonverbal oral apraxia.

Neuropathology of AOS

AOS is caused by injury or damage to speech–motor programming areas in the dominant hemisphere; such areas as Broca's and supplementary motor areas often are involved.

■ Certain types of pathology include vascular lesions that cause strokes; specifically affected are the speech programming structures and pathways. In the majority of cases, the cause is a single left-hemisphere stroke; in a few, the cause is multiple strokes.

■ Frontal lesions may be associated with parietal lesions as well. Temporal lobe lesions are observed occasionally but only in combination with lesions elsewhere.

■ PPAOS may be caused by such degenerative neural diseases as Alzheimer's disease, multiple sclerosis (MS), and pathologies that cause primary progressive aphasia.

- Major sites of neuropathology in PPAOS are the premotor and supplementary motor areas and do not follow the cerebral vascular distribution typically found in stroke-induced AOS; lesions may extend to such other areas as the left posterior inferior frontal gyrus (Duffy & Josephs, 2012).

■ AOS can also be caused by left-hemisphere trauma, surgical trauma, tumors in the left hemisphere, and seizure disorders.

General Symptoms of AOS

General symptoms of AOS include impaired oral sensation in some patients. Although not a part of AOS, language disorders typical of damage to the dominant hemisphere may be observed; patients with Broca's aphasia may have a coexisting AOS (Duffy, 2013). When dysarthria is a coexisting condition, facial and lingual weakness may also be present. Some patients may have limb apraxia as well.

- An independent nonverbal oral apraxia (NVOA) is present in many patients. In some cases, there also may be right hemiparesis and sensory deficits.

Communication Deficits in AOS

AOS can range in severity from mild to profound; thus, the following symptoms and characteristics can be present depending on the severity of the disorder:

- Patients with AOS may have an independent problem of auditory processing deficits.
- Most patients have a general awareness of their speech problems, which is commonly manifested by struggle and frustration.
- Patients' initiation of speech may be slow or delayed and appears effortful.
- Patients may use a compensatory strategy of reduced rate of speech to avoid producing errors.
- Presumed speech programming problems and observable speech production errors, such as the ones listed below, are the dominant symptoms of apraxia (Hegde & Freed, 2017):

  - Problems in volitional or spontaneous sequencing of movements required for speech, with relatively unaffected automatic speech
  - High variability of speech errors with changing patterns of errors on repeated attempts; normal production of difficult words on occasion
  - Speech sound substitutions, more common than distortions and omissions of speech sounds; voicing errors possibly frequent, particularly the substitution of a voiceless phoneme for a voiced (e.g., "pet" for "bet"); substitution errors possibly perseverative; phoneme prolongations are also possible
  - More pronounced difficulty with consonants than vowels; more severe problems with affricates and fricatives and consonant clusters; more frequent errors on infrequently occurring sounds
  - Anticipatory substitutions (replacing a phoneme that occurs earlier in the word with one that occurs later; e.g., "lelo" for "yellow")
  - Postpositioning errors (replacing a phoneme that occurs later with one that occurs earlier; e.g., "dred" for "dress")
  - Metathetic errors (switched position of phonemes in words; e.g., "tefalone" for "telephone")
  - Insertion of schwa into consonant clusters or between syllables
  - Increased frequency of errors on longer words (these errors can be highly inconsistent)
  - Trial-and-error groping of the articulators and struggling associated with speech attempts
  - Greater difficulty with word-initial sounds in some cases
  - Easier automatic productions than volitional or purposive productions
  - Attempts at self-correction (**self-repairs**; often unsuccessful)

- Patients with AOS frequently have prosodic problems, which include the following:
  - A slower rate of speech, with difficulty in increasing or changing the rate when requested
  - Silent pauses between words
  - Impaired intonation because of increased duration of consonants and vowels; even stress on syllables; even loudness or restricted range of loudness; limited pitch range
  - Fluency problems including silent pauses, especially at the beginning of speech initiation, and repetitions because of false starts and attempts at self-correction

PPAOS and AOS share most of their speech characteristics; more research is needed to identify the unique features of the former; clinical observations suggest that the patients with PPAOS may produce fewer words per breath group in conversation than those with stroke-induced AOS (Botha et al., 2014).

Assessment of AOS

A detailed case history, careful examination of the medical records, interview of the client and his or her family members, and detailed observation of speech production are necessary to make a diagnosis of AOS in adults (Duffy, 2013; Lowit & Kent, 2011).

- Procedures designed to diagnose aphasia (problems with language production and comprehension, reading, and writing) should be used when the patient shows signs of a coexisting aphasia, often Broca's aphasia (Duffy, 2013; Hegde, 2018a; Hegde & Freed, 2017).
- Assessment of AOS involves the following procedures:
  - Tape-recording the patient's speech samples and transcribing the responses phonetically; taking note of struggle and groping, self-correction, repetition and other forms of dysfluencies, errors of articulation, delayed reaction, facial grimacing, and other behaviors that suggest apraxia
  - Evoking imitative production of a speech sound
  - Evoking repetitive production of syllables (e.g., asking the patient to say "pʌ-pʌ-pʌ," "tʌ-tʌ-tʌ," and "kʌ-kʌ-kʌ" as long and as evenly as possible)
  - Evoking the repetitive production of multiple syllables (e.g., asking the patient to say "pʌ-tʌ-kʌ" as long and as evenly as possible)
  - Evoking the imitative production of progressively longer words when modeling is provided (e.g., asking the patient to imitate such words as *several, tornado, artillery, linoleum, snowman, television, catastrophe, unequivocally, parliamentarian, statistical analysis,* and *Encyclopedia Britannica*)
  - Evoking repeated, imitative production of words and phrases (e.g., asking the patient to say words, such as *artillery, impossibility,* and *disenfranchised,* five times)
  - Evoking the imitative production of sentences
  - Evoking counting responses (e.g., asking the patient to count from 1 to 20)
  - Evoking picture descriptions
  - Assessing oral reading
  - Administering a complete **diadochokinetic test** to assess oral, nonverbal movement (e.g., various tongue, lip, and jaw movements), oral apraxia, or a coexisting dysarthria in case of significant muscle weakness or paralysis

- Assessing limb movements to evaluate limb apraxia by asking the patient to perform certain actions (e.g., demonstrating how an accordion works or how one salutes or waves goodbye)
- Administering a standardized test, such as the *Apraxia Battery for Adults–Second Edition* (ABA-2) (Dabul, 2000)

Treatment of AOS

Behavioral treatment is the most effective in treating AOS (Duffy, 2013).

- Easily produced words (e.g., words of high frequency or those with fewer syllables) need not be initial targets; more difficult words (longer words and low-frequency words), when taught successfully, may promote better generalization.
- Treatment should be primarily concerned with speech movements as opposed to nonspeech movements.
- Treatment should include practice with a variety of sounds and sound combinations. Repeated trials on the same target response ("drill") is essential for initial learning; soon varied targets should be built into successive trials.
- Positive reinforcement for correct responses and corrective feedback for incorrect ones are crucial for learning.
- Treatment targets include articulatory accuracy, slower rate, systematic practice, gradual increase in the rate, and normal prosody.
- Treatment procedures should include instructions, demonstration, modeling, shaping, phonetic placement, frequent cueing, use of rhythm, and immediate positive or corrective feedback.
- Cueing techniques may include tactile cues for placement of articulators, simultaneous production by the clinician and the client, clinician's modeling (immediately followed by client's imitation), delayed imitation (waiting for a few seconds before imitating the clinician's model), and so forth.
- Any special cues and modeling should be faded to promote more spontaneous productions. Contrastive stress tasks, phonetic contrasts, carrier phrases, and singing may all be useful.
- Pushing on the abdomen to achieve vocal fold closure and phonation or use of an artificial larynx may be helpful for a speechless client.
- Such prosthetic devices as a pacing board or a metronome to slow speech rate and improve articulatory proficiency, may be useful during treatment, but their generalized effect has not been established.
- Emphasis on total communication (combined use of verbal expressions, gestures, writing, augmentative devices) may be desirable.
- Teaching accurate (or improved) sound productions in conversational speech should be an important goal. Increasing the speech rate to near normal also should be an important goal.
- Teaching self-monitoring skills and self-correction of errors is important for maintenance.
- Techniques of treating articulation and phonological disorders are generally useful.
- In the case of severe AOS, family members and health care workers should be asked to speak slowly, use shorter sentences, reduce background noise, talk only when the client is focused, and use total

communication. In the case of most severe AOS, augmentative communication techniques may be necessary.

- A coexisting aphasia must be treated as one would ordinary aphasia; however, a more severe disorder (whether it is AOS or aphasia) would require multiple treatment techniques.
- Patients with progressive forms of AOS also are candidates for therapy aimed at improving their daily communication, even if for a temporary duration (Duffy, 2013).
- A specific treatment approach, called sound production treatment (SPT), which has an emphasis on teaching articulation of words with minimal contrast (e.g., *shock–sock*; *conical–comical*), has been found to be effective (Wambaugh, Duffy, McNeil, Robin, & Rogers, 2006).

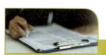

SUMMARY

AOS is a neurogenic speech disorder characterized by sensorimotor problems in positioning and sequentially moving muscles for production of speech. It is caused by damage to speech–motor programming areas in the dominant hemisphere.

- Communication deficits to be assessed and treated in patients with AOS include highly variable speech errors, significant articulatory problems, increased frequency of errors on long words, prosodic problems, and groping and struggling behaviors.
- Assessment of patients with AOS may include detailed, individualized procedures as well as the administration of standardized tests. Treatment should be carefully sequenced to move from automatic, simple productions to less automatic, more spontaneous productions.

THE DYSARTHRIAS

The dysarthrias are a group of neurologically based motor–speech disorders attributable to peripheral or central nervous system pathology, resulting in paralysis, weakness, or incoordination of the muscles involved in speech production. These neuromuscular impairments affect all aspects of speech production. There are seven types of dysarthria: ataxic, flaccid, hyperkinetic, hypokinetic, spastic, mixed, and unilateral upper motor neuron dysarthria. These are shown in Table 9.1. Assessment and treatment of patients with dysarthria involve addressing those problems (Duffy, 2013; Hegde, 2018c; Hegde & Freed, 2017; Sapir, 2014; Yorkston et al., 2010).

Definition of the Dysarthrias

Dysarthrias are neurologically based speech disorders characterized by abnormal strength, speed, range, steadiness, tone, and accuracy of movement involved in speech production. These abnormalities may be evident in respiration, phonation, articulation, prosody, and resonance (Duffy, 2013). The effects of the neural damage that causes dysarthrias, unlike aphasia and apraxia of speech, are pervasive; any and all aspects of speech production may be affected.

(text continues on page 403)

Table 9.1
Summary of Dysarthria Types

Dysarthria type	Lesion site	Neuromotor basis	Common etiologies	Speech characteristics
Ataxic	Cerebellum	Incoordination	Any bilateral or generalized damage to the cerebellum, including: • Degenerative ataxia • Cerebellar strokes • Tumors • Traumatic brain injury (TBI) • Toxic conditions • Inflammatory conditions • Demyelinating disease	**Articulation** • Imprecise consonants • Irregular articulatory breakdowns • Distortion of vowels **Prosody** • Excessive and even stress • Prolonged phonemes and intervals between words or syllables • Slow rate of speech **Phonation** • Monopitch • Monoloud • Harshness **Resonance** • Intermittent hyponasality (not prominent characteristic) **Respiration** • Exaggerated and paradoxical movement during speech production
Flaccid	Lower motor neuron	Weakness and hypotonia	Any damage to LMN connections to muscles and/or the cranial nerves involved in speech production (V, VII, IX, X, XI, XII), including: • Degenerative disease • Motor neuron disease • Progressive bulbar disease • Multiple systems atrophy • Myasthenia gravis • Botulism • Vascular diseases and brainstem strokes • Infections (polio, AIDS) • Guillain Barre syndrome • Surgical trauma	**Articulation** • Imprecise consonants • Weak pressure consonants (more so for lesions of cranial nerve V, VII, XII) **Phonation/Phonatory–Prosodic** • Breathy • Audible inspiration • Harshness • Monopitch • Monoloud or reduced loudness • Short phrases **Resonance** • Hypernasality • Nasal emission • Short phrases **Respiration** • Reduced subglottal air pressure • Weak inhalation

(continues)

Table 9.1 (continued)

Dysarthria type	Lesion site	Neuromotor basis	Common etiologies	Speech characteristics
Hyperkinetic	Basal ganglia and/or basal ganglia connections within central nervous system (CNS)	Abnormal, extra movements	• Huntington's disease • Syndenham's chorea • Brainstem stroke • TBI • Toxic conditions • Metabolic conditions (i.e., tardive dyskinesia) • Tourette's syndrome • Seizure disorders • Spasmodic dysphonia	**Articulation** • Imprecise consonants • Distorted vowels **Prosody** • Slower rate of speech • Prolonged interword intervals • Inappropriate silent periods • Phoneme prolongations • Excess and equal stress • Reduced stress • Short phrases **Phonation** • Monopitch • Monoloud **Resonance** • Hypernasality (mild, in some cases) **Respiration** • Audible inspiration and forced/sudden inspiration or expiration
Hypokinetic	Basal ganglia and/or basal ganglia connections within CNS	Reduced range of motion, rigidity, and reduced movement	• Parkinson's disease (most common cause) • Stroke/vascular disease • Toxic and metabolic conditions (antipsychotic/neuroleptic drug toxicity) • Repeated TBI • Infections (HIV, Creutzfeldt-Jakob disease)	**Articulation** • Imprecise/distorted consonants • Stops sounding more like fricatives • Mushy fricatives **Prosody** • Reduced stress • Inappropriate silent intervals • Short rushes of speech • Variable and increased rate in segments • Short phrases **Phonation** • Monopitch • Monoloud • Low pitch • Harsh and continuously breathy **Resonance** • Mild hypernasality (~25% of cases)

Table 9.1 (continued)

Dysarthria type	Lesion site	Neuromotor basis	Common etiologies	Speech characteristics
Hypokinetic (continued)				**Respiration** • Reduced vital capacity • Irregular breathing • Faster rate of respiration **Fluency** • Repeated phonemes; palilalia less likely
Spastic	Upper motor neuron (Bilateral)	Weakness and spasticity	• Multiple strokes that damage pyramidal and extrapyramidal tracts • Brainstem stroke • Primary lateral sclerosis (PLS) • Multiple sclerosis (MS) • TBI • Brainstem tumor • Viral or bacterial infection of cerebral tissue • Cerebral palsy (children)	**Articulation** • Imprecise consonants • Distorted vowels **Prosody** • Excess and equal stress • Reduced stress • Slow rate • Short phrases **Phonation** • Hyperadduction of vocal folds • Continuous breathy voice • Harshness • Low pitch • Pitch breaks • Strained/strangled voice quality • Monopitch • Monoloud **Resonance** • Hypernasality
Mixed	Damage to various parts of the nervous system	flaccid–spastic ataxic–spastic	• Multiple Sclerosis (MS) • Amyotrophic lateral sclerosis (ALS) • Friedreich's ataxia • Wilson's disease	**Articulation** • Imprecise consonants • Distorted vowels **Prosody** • Excess and equal stress • Reduced stress • Slow rate • Short phrases

(continues)

Table 9.1 (continued)

Dysarthria type	Lesion site	Neuromotor basis	Common etiologies	Speech characteristics
Mixed (continued)				**Phonation** • Hyperadduction of vocal folds • Continuous breathy voice • Harshness • Low pitch • Pitch breaks • Strained/strangled voice quality • Monopitch • Monoloud **Resonance** • Hypernasality • Nasal emission
Unilateral Upper Motor Neuron	Upper motor neuron (Unilateral)	Weakness and spasticity	• Stroke • Neurosurgical trauma • Multiple sclerosis	**Articulation** • Imprecise consonants • Irregular articulatory breakdowns • Some vowel distortions • Sound/syllable repetitions **Prosody** • Slow rate • Increased rate in segments • Excess and equal stress • Short phrases **Phonation** • Harshness/strained harshness • Reduced loudness • Wet hoarseness • Breathiness • Monopitch • Monoloud • Low pitch **Resonance** • Hypernasality • Nasal emission • Combination of hypernasality and nasal emission

Note. Adapted from Manasco (2014).

- Dysarthrias are thus distinct from neurologically based language disorders, such as **aphasia**, and from apraxia of speech, a neurogenic disorder of motor planning (programming) of speech movements, with no muscular weakness or paralysis (Hegde & Freed, 2017).
- The different types of dysarthria share certain characteristics. Impaired muscular control of the speech mechanism and peripheral or central nervous system pathology are common to all forms of dysarthria. Differences in the nature and loci of pathology create different forms of the disorder.
- Dysarthria may be progressive when associated with such degenerative diseases as amyotrophic lateral sclerosis (ALS), typically resulting in flaccid and spastic dysarthrias, and Parkinson's disease, typically causing hypokinetic dysarthria.

Neuropathology of the Dysarthrias

The causes of dysarthrias include the following:

- Nonprogressive neurological conditions that cause dysarthria include strokes, infections, traumatic brain injury, and surgical trauma, as well as such congenital conditions as cerebral palsy, Moebius syndrome, encephalitis, toxic effects from alcohol or drugs, and so forth.
- Degenerative neurological diseases that cause dysarthria include—in addition to previously mentioned Parkinson's disease and ALS—Wilson's disease, progressive supranuclear palsy, dystonia, Huntington's disease, multiple sclerosis, myasthenia gravis, primary progressive aphasia, Pick's disease, Alzheimer's disease, progressive pseudobulbar palsy, and many others (Duffy, 2013).
- Neurotraumatic causes of dysarthria include penetrating head injuries, neck trauma, skull fracture, and surgical trauma.
- Infectious diseases that cause dysarthria include AIDS, Creutzfeldt-Jakob disease, and central nervous system (CNS) tuberculosis.
- Toxic–metabolic causes include botulism, drug toxicity or abuse, carbon monoxide poisoning, dialysis encephalopathy, and many others.

Common sites of lesion include the lower motor neuron, unilateral or bilateral upper motor neuron, cerebellum, and basal ganglia (extrapyramidal system) (Davis & Strand, 2004). See the section "Types of Dysarthria" for more specific information on sites of lesions.

- Pathophysiology and neuromuscular problems include muscle weakness, spasticity, incoordination, and rigidity. There usually is a variety of movement disorders, including reduced or variable range and speed of movement, involuntary movements, reduced strength of movement, unsteady or inaccurate movement, and abnormal tone (increased, decreased, or variable).

Communicative Disorders Associated With Dysarthria

- **Respiratory problems** associated with dysarthria include forced inspirations or expirations that interrupt speech, audible or breathy inspiration, and grunting at the end of expiration.
- **Phonatory disorders** include the following:
  - Pitch disorders characterized by abnormal pitch, pitch breaks, abrupt variations in pitch, monopitch, diplophonia, and shaky or tremulous voice

- Loudness disorders characterized by too-soft or too-loud speech, monoloudness, sudden and excessive variation in loudness, progressive decrease in loudness throughout an utterance, or alternating changes in loudness
- Vocal-quality problems characterized by a harsh, rough, gravelly voice; a hoarse voice (especially the "wet" variety); a continuously or intermittently breathy voice; a strained or strangled voice; effortful phonation; or a sudden and uncontrolled cessation of voice

- **Articulation disorders** include imprecise production of consonants, prolongation and repetition of phonemes, irregular breakdowns in articulation, distortion of vowels, and weak production of pressure consonants.
- **Prosodic disorders** include a slower, excessively faster, or variable rate of speech; shorter phrase lengths; and such linguistic stress problems as reduced, even, or excessive stress. There may also be prolongation of intervals between words or syllables, inappropriate pauses in speech, and short rushes of speech.
- **Resonance disorders** include hypernasality, hyponasality, and nasal emission.

- Other characteristics include slow, fast, or irregular diadochokinetic rate and palilalia (compulsive repetition of one's own utterances with increasing rate and decreasing loudness), as well as decreased intelligibility of speech.

Types of Dysarthria

Ataxic Dysarthria

Ataxic dysarthria results from damage to the cerebellar system. It is characterized predominantly by articulatory and prosodic problems, reflecting predominantly impaired timing and coordination of muscle movements. **Ataxia** (defined as muscular incoordination and irregular movements) is a main factor contributing to this type of dysarthria; hence, the name. Ataxic dysarthria will only appear during movement of the articulators. At rest, these structures will seem normal.

- Motor symptoms created by cerebellar damage are not confined to speech production; thus, ataxia will be manifested in other motor movements. Individuals with ataxic dysarthria will most likely walk with an **ataxic gait**—the feet are broadly spread apart and step irregularly. **Nystagmus**, back and forth rapid eye movement, may also be present. Individuals may also overshoot or undershoot intended movements, known as **dysmetria** (Manasco, 2014).
- Neuropathology that results in ataxic dysarthria includes bilateral or generalized cerebellar lesions, degenerative ataxia (e.g., Friedreich's ataxia and olivopontocerebellar atrophy and late onset autosomal dominant and idiopathic sporadic forms of cerebellar ataxia), cerebellar vascular lesions (due to stroke), tumors, traumatic brain injury, toxic conditions (e.g., alcohol abuse and drug toxicity), and inflammatory conditions (e.g., meningitis and encephalitis), and demyelinating diseases.
- The major characteristics of ataxic dysarthria include the following:

  - **Gait disturbances**—instability of the trunk and head, tremors and rocking motions, rotated or tilted head posture, and hypotonia

- **Movement disorders**—overshooting or undershooting of targets; uncoordinated, jerky, inaccurate, slow, imprecise, and halting movements
- **Respiratory disorders**—exaggerated and paradoxical (simultaneous antagonistic) movement during speech production
- **Articulation disorders**—imprecise production of consonants, irregular articulatory breakdowns, and distortion of vowels
- **Prosodic disorders**—excessive and even stress, prolonged phonemes and intervals between words or syllables, and slow rate of speech
- **Phonatory disorders**—monopitch, monoloudness, and harshness
- **Speech quality**—impression of drunken speech
- **Resonance disorders**—intermittent hyponasality in some individuals (not a prominent feature)

Flaccid Dysarthria

Flaccid dysarthria results from damage to the motor units of cranial or spinal nerves that supply speech muscles (lower motor neuron involvement; damage to the peripheral nervous system).

- A lower motor neuron (LMN) is an efferent portion of a cranial or spinal nerve. All motor plans from the CNS must pass through the LMNs to be executed by muscles. When there is damage to an LMN, motor plans sent from the brain to the muscle cannot reach the muscle or are poorly conducted along the damaged nerve; therefore, the muscles cannot be properly activated for movement. Flaccidity is present for volitional and nonvolitional movement (e.g., stretch reflex) and is characterized by **hypotonia** (low muscle tone) and muscle weakness (Manasco, 2014).
- Only one major muscle group (e.g., the tongue), several muscle groups (affecting either the phonatory or articulatory systems), or all of the muscle groups involved in speech production may be affected, suggesting possible subtypes of flaccid dysarthria (Duffy, 2013).
- Neurological conditions causing flaccid dysarthria include such degenerative diseases as amyotrophic lateral sclerosis (ALS), motor neuron disease, progressive bulbar disease, and multiple systems atrophy (MSA); myasthenia gravis and botulism; vascular diseases and brainstem strokes; infections (e.g., polio, infections secondary to AIDS); demyelinating diseases (e.g., Guillain-Barré syndrome); and trauma due to brain, laryngeal, facial, or chest surgery.
- Specific cranial nerves that may be involved in flaccid dysarthria include the trigeminal (V), facial (VII), glossopharyngeal (IX), vagus (X), accessory (XI), and hypoglossal (XII) nerves. Specific spinal nerve involvement may indirectly affect speech production because of an involved respiratory system. Table 9.2 provides details of flaccid dysarthria resulting from cranial nerve damage.
- The major characteristics of flaccid dysarthria include the following:

  - **Muscular disorders**—weakness, hypotonia, atrophy, diminished reflexes, isolated twitches of resting muscles (fasciculations), contractions of individual muscles (fibrillations), and rapid and progressive weakness with the use of a muscle and recovery with rest
  - **Respiratory weakness**—reduced subglottic air pressure (with spinal nerve involvement), weak inhalation (with damaged phrenic nerve and paralyzed diaphragm)

(text continues on page 408)

Table 9.2

Flaccid Dysarthria Caused by Cranial Nerve Damage

Cranial nerve	Motor innervation	Unilateral damage	Bilateral damage
Trigeminal (V)	**Mandibular branch**—mandibular muscles	Side contralateral to the damaged nerve remains intact Mandible deviates **toward damaged side** when lowered Mild articulatory deficits or slow rate of speech	Weakness/paralysis of both right and left sides Mandible will likely hang open Difficulty closing mouth Articulation is highly affected/is unintelligible Particular phonemes affected: **lingua-alveolar, linguadental, labio-alveolar,** and **bilabial**
Facial (VII)	**Temporal branch**—muscles around the eyes and of the forehead **Zygomatic, buccal,** and **mandibular branches**—muscles of the lower face for lip movement and cheek compression	Lesions often occur prior to division into branches, creating ipsilateral *palsy* (weakness/paralysis), characterized by unilateral: • Lip drooping • Poor labial closure • Ptosis (droopy eyelid) • Difficulty blinking • Decreased eyebrow movement • Smooth forehead • Facial asymmetry • Minor articulation difficulties producing **bilabials** and **labiodentals** but are still able to compensate with unaffected side	Bilateral facial weakness; Possibly unable to bring lips together Inability to produce **bilabials** and **labiodentals** **Vowels** may be distorted if lips are unable to spread and/or be rounded More difficult to visually recognize because face will be symmetrical
Glossopharyngeal (IX)	Innervates stylopharyngeus muscle; possibly supplies motor fibers to pharyngeal plexus	Difficulty raising and dilating pharynx on affected side, impacting swallowing function	Greater impact on swallowing function due to bilateral pharyngeal weakness

Cranial nerve	Motor innervation	Unilateral damage	Bilateral damage
Vagus (X)	**Pharyngeal plexus**—muscles of the pharynx and velum (minus stylopharyngeus and palatoglossus) for elevation of velum and constriction of pharynx **Superior laryngeal branch**—cricothyroid muscle for vocal fold tensing **Recurrent laryngeal branch**—all other intrinsic laryngeal muscles for vocal fold adduction & abduction	**Pharyngeal plexus:** • Ipsilateral weakness • Velum deviates **toward intact side**; velum does not rest at midline • Resonance will be hypernasal but not to extreme extent **Superior laryngeal branch:** • Ipsilateral weakness creating mildly monotonous voice; contralateral side can compensate **Recurrent laryngeal branch:** • Paresis/paralysis of ipsilateral vocal fold creates voice that is breathy and/or hoarse • If vocal fold is paralyzed closer to midline, unaffected vocal fold may still be able to approximate it for phonation	**Pharyngeal plexus:** • Bilateral weakness of velum and uvula • Extreme hypernasality • Velum is centered at midline but hangs low **Superior laryngeal branch:** • Bilateral weakness/paralysis of cricothyroid muscle, creating more significant monotone voice **Recurrent laryngeal branch:** • Bilateral weakness/paralysis of all intrinsic laryngeal muscles (except cricothyroid) • Vocal folds will usually be paralyzed at midline and can potentially compromise respiration • Phonation will be compromised
Accessory (XI)	Assists vagus nerve in innervation of uvula, levator veli palatini, and intrinsic laryngeal muscles **Spinal portion**—sternocleidomastoid and trapezius muscles	Unilateral damage does not have significant effect on speech Shoulder elevation is weakened on affected side Head will have difficulty turning to the side contralateral to the lesion	Bilateral weakness of sternocleidomastoid and trapezius can result in head-and-shoulder weakness and drooping, which may potentially impact respiration, phonation, and resonance, but only mildly
Hypoglossal (XII)	All intrinsic and extrinsic muscles of the tongue (minus palatoglossus) for fine and gross motor movement	Ipsilateral lingual weakness; Tongue deviates **toward weakened side** upon protrusion; Mild to moderate effect on articulation of **lingual stops, lingual fricatives,** and **lingual affricates**	Bilateral weakness of tongue muscles Difficulty/inability to protrude tongue or move tongue in other directions Reduced range of motion of tongue Severe effect on articulation involving any phoneme that relies on lingual movement Atrophy of tongue muscle *Fasciculations* (small, quick muscle contractions) can be observed in the atrophying muscle

Note. Table only lists motor functions of cranial nerves; sensory functions are not in the scope of this content.

Note. Information summarized from Manasco (2014, p. 155–159) and Duffy (2013, p. 108)

- **Phonatory disorders**—breathy voice and audible inspiration
- **Resonance disorders**—hypernasality, nasal emission, and short phrases
- **Phonatory–prosodic disorders**—short phrases, harsh voice, monopitch, and monoloudness or reduced loudness
- **Articulation disorders**—imprecise consonants and weak pressure consonants (more pronounced with lesions of cranial nerves V, VII, and XII)
- **Three disorder clusters**—(1) phonatory incompetence, (2) resonatory incompetence, and (3) phonatory–prosodic insufficiency (Duffy, 2013)

Hyperkinetic Dysarthria

Hyperkinetic dysarthria results from damage to the basal ganglia (extrapyramidal system). It is associated with variable muscle tone and involuntary movements that interfere with speech production. Any or all of the speech systems may be affected, but prosodic disturbances are dominant (Duffy, 2013; Hegde & Freed, 2017).

- Common causes of hyperkinetic dysarthria include degenerative diseases (e.g., Huntington's disease), vascular diseases (brainstem stroke), trauma (head injury), toxic or metabolic conditions (e.g., lithium toxicity, tardive dyskinesia), and many others (Tourette's syndrome, seizure disorders). Spasmodic dysphonia, a voice disorder reviewed in Chapter 7, is caused by extra movement of the vocal folds and is therefore considered a hyperkinetic dysarthria. The cause of hyperkinetic dysarthria may be unknown in the majority of cases. The muscles of the face, jaw, tongue, palate, larynx, and respiration may be involved.
- The major characteristics of hyperkinesias and the resulting hyperkinetic dysarthria include the following:
  - **Orofacial dyskinesia**—abnormal, involuntary, rhythmic or nonrhythmic movements of the orofacial muscles
  - **Myoclonus**—involuntary, rapidly occurring jerks of body parts; may be of single or multiple muscles; hiccups due to diaphragmatic spasms; palatal tremor
  - **Tics**—commonly of the face and shoulders; typically patterned, rapid, and stereotyped
  - **Chorea**—purposeless, random, involuntary movements of body parts
  - **Athetosis**—slow, writhing, purposeless movements; may be a combination of chorea and dystonia
  - **Ballism**—bilateral, involuntary, and irregular movement of the extremities; can be violent
  - **Hemiballism**—unilateral, involuntary, and irregular movement of the extremities; can be violent
  - **Dystonia**—contractions of antagonistic muscles that cause abnormal postures; spasmodic torticollis (intermittent dystonia and spasms of the neck muscles); blepharospasm (forceful and involuntary closure of the eyes due to spasm of the orbicularis oculi muscle)
  - **Spasm**—a muscle contraction that is sudden and involuntary
  - **Tic**—a stereotyped movement that is quick and repetitive and is involuntary

- **Tremor**—rhythmic movements, a common form of involuntary movement
- **Communicative disorders**—specific symptoms depending on the dominant neurological condition (e.g., chorea, dystonia, athetosis, spasmodic torticollis)
- **Respiratory problems**—audible inspiration and forced and sudden inspiration or expiration not typical of other types of dysarthria
- **Phonatory disorders**—voice tremor, intermittently strained voice, voice stoppage, vocal noise, harsh voice, and loudness variations
- **Resonance disorders**—hypernasality in some cases, but typically mild
- **Articulation problems**—imprecise consonant productions, often associated with distorted vowels and hypernasality; slower rate of speech
- **Prosodic disorders**—prolonged interword intervals, inappropriate silent periods, phoneme prolongations, and excess and equal stress; also, monopitch and monoloudness, reduced stress, and short phrases

Hypokinetic Dysarthria

Hypokinetic dysarthria results from damage to the basal ganglia (extrapyramidal system). It may affect all aspects of speech, but voice, articulation, and prosody are typically the most affected. Muscular rigidity and reduced force and range of movement cause the speech problems.

- Hypokinetic dysarthria has a number of causes, but the most common cause is degenerative Parkinson's disease. Other causes include stroke (vascular diseases), toxic and metabolic conditions including antipsychotic or neuroleptic drug toxicity, repeated head trauma, and infections (e.g., HIV, Creutzfeldt-Jakob disease).
- Hypokinetic dysarthria is characterized by the following:
  - **Tremors**—facial, mouth, and limb muscle tremors at rest, diminishing when moved voluntarily
  - **Mask-like face**—infrequent blinking and no smiling
  - **Micrographic writing**—excessively small print
  - **Walking disorders**—slow to begin, then short, rapid, shuffling steps
  - **Postural disturbances**—involuntary flexion of the head, trunk, and arm with difficulty changing positions
  - **Decreased swallowing**—accumulation of saliva in the mouth and drooling
  - **Respiratory problems**—reduced vital capacity, irregular breathing, and faster rate of respiration
  - **Phonatory disorders**—monopitch, low pitch, monoloudness, and harsh and continuously breathy voice
  - **Prosodic disorders**—reduced stress, inappropriate silent intervals, short rushes of speech, variable and increased rate in segments, and short phrases
  - **Articulation disorders**—imprecise or distorted consonants; stops sounding more like fricatives; mushy fricatives

- **Dysfluencies**—more frequently repeated phonemes and less frequently palilalia (e.g., "Yes, yes, yes, yes, yes" that fades into a mumble) (Hegde & Freed, 2017)
- **Resonance disorders**—atypical but mild hypernasality in about 25% of individuals

- Hypokinetic dysarthria is the only dysarthria that creates an increased rate of speech. Because the range of motion of the articulators is reduced, the structures do not move as far for speech production; therefore, the speech of an individual with hypokinetic dysarthria will often speed up until there is a breakdown. This is commonly referred to as **rapid-fire articulation** (Manasco, 2014).
- In addition to these motor speech symptoms, individuals with hypokinetic dysarthria (Parkinson's disease in particular) will also demonstrate several non-speech-motor symptoms as a result of basal ganglia damage, including

  - absence of arm swinging while walking;
  - **akinesia**—absence of movement; immobile posture;
  - **bradykinesia**—a difficulty with the initiation of movement;
  - **festination**—a type of gait characterized by short, shuffling footsteps that progressively quicken; often seem as an attempt to maintain balance;
  - **hypomimia**—diminished facial movement causing a lack of facial expression;
  - **hypokinesia**—a reduced amount and range of motion;
  - **micrographia**—evolution from typical handwriting to abnormally small handwriting; and
  - stooped or hunched posture.

If these hypokinetic symptoms are present due to basal ganglia damage but are **not** the result of Parkinson's disease, these symptoms are referred to as Parkinsonian. Any of the other etiologies described previously (stroke, HIV, etc.) can produce Parkinsonian signs, including hypokinetic dysarthria.

Spastic Dysarthria

Spastic dysarthria results from bilateral damage to the upper motor neurons (direct and indirect motor pathways), creating a predominant spasticity. Lesions in multiple areas, including the cortical areas, basal ganglia, internal capsule, pons, and medulla, are common.

- Spastic dysarthria is caused most commonly by multiple strokes that damage both the pyramidal (direct activation pathway, or DAP) and extrapyramidal (indirect activation pathway, or IAP) tracts, single stroke (if it occurs only in the brainstem and not in the cerebral hemispheres), primary lateral sclerosis (PLS), multiple sclerosis, traumatic brain injury, brainstem tumor, and viral or bacterial infection of the cerebral tissue. In children, cerebral palsy is a common etiology of spastic dysarthria.
- Spastic dysarthria is characterized by the following:

  - **Spasticity and weakness**—bilateral facial weakness, less severe lower face weakness, normal or near normal jaw strength
  - **Movement disorders**—reduced range, force, and speed of movement, loss of fine and skilled movement, and increased muscle tone

- **Articulation disorders**—imprecise production of consonants, distorted vowels
- **Prosodic disorders**: excess and equal stress, slow rate, reduced stress, and short phrases
- **Phonatory disorders**—hyperadduction of vocal folds, continuous breathy voice, harshness, low pitch, pitch breaks, strained and strangled voice quality, monopitch, and monoloudness
- **Resonance disorders**—a predominant hypernasality due to inadequate closure of the velopharyngeal port

Mixed Dysarthrias

Mixed dysarthrias are a combination of two or more pure dysarthrias. All combinations of pure dysarthrias are possible, although a combination of two types is more common than a combination of three or more. The symptom complex may include the major problems of the types that are mixed, but, in some cases, the symptoms of one type may be dominant. The two most common mixed forms are flaccid–spastic dysarthria and ataxic–spastic dysarthria.

- Neurological diseases that produce more widespread or diffuse effects may cause mixed dysarthria; more frequently noted causes include such motor neuron diseases as amyotrophic lateral sclerosis (progressive degeneration of motor neurons), demyelinating multiple sclerosis, Friedreich's ataxia, and the somewhat rare Wilson's disease.
- The mixed flaccid–spastic dysarthria, associated with amyotrophic lateral sclerosis (ALS), is characterized by imprecise production of consonants, hypernasality, harsh voice, slow rate, monopitch, short phrases, distorted vowels, low pitch, monoloudness, excess and equal stress or reduced stress, prolonged intervals, prolonged phonemes, a strained and strangled quality, breathiness, audible inspiration, inappropriate silences, and nasal emission.
- The mixed ataxic–spastic dysarthria, more often associated with multiple sclerosis (MS), is characterized by impaired loudness control, harsh voice quality, imprecise articulation, impaired emphasis, hypernasality, inappropriate pitch levels, decreased vital capacity, breathiness, and sudden articulatory breakdowns.
- The speech symptoms of Wilson's disease are a combination of ataxic and spastic types of dysarthria; reduced stress, monopitch, and monoloudness may be the three most prominent symptoms.
- The speech symptoms of Friedreich's ataxia are a combination of those found in ataxic and spastic types of dysarthria.

Unilateral Upper Motor Neuron Dysarthria

Unilateral upper motor neuron (UUMN) dysarthria results from damage to the upper motor neurons that supply cranial and spinal nerves involved in speech production; while all the previous types of dysarthria are defined physiologically, this one is defined purely in anatomic terms.

- The most common cause of UUMN dysarthria is stroke; nonhemorrhagic or hemorrhagic strokes account for 92% of individuals with this type of dysarthria; neurosurgical trauma and multiple sclerosis are two other infrequent causes; dysarthria due to vascular disorders that produce left-hemisphere lesions may coexist with aphasia or apraxia; dysarthria due to right-hemisphere lesions may coexist with right-hemisphere syndrome.

- UUMN dysarthria is characterized by the following:
  - **Neurological impairments**—unilateral lower face weakness, unilateral tongue weakness, unilateral palatal weakness, and hemiplegia/hemiparesis
  - **Articulation disorders**—imprecise production of consonants, irregular articulatory breakdowns, and some vowel distortions and sound or syllable repetitions
  - **Phonatory disorders**—harsh voice, reduced loudness, strained harshness, wet hoarseness, breathiness, monopitch, monoloudness, and low pitch
  - **Prosodic disorders**—slow rate, increased rate in segments, excess and equal stress, and short phrases
  - **Resonance disorders**—hypernasality or nasal emission, or a combination of the two
  - **Associated disorders**—dysphagia, aphasia, apraxia, and right-hemisphere syndrome

Differentiating Apraxia of Speech From Dysarthria

Table 9.3 summarizes key differences between apraxia and dysarthria.

Assessment of the Dysarthrias

Assessment of the dysarthrias involves multiple procedures because of the wide range of symptoms that must be evaluated (Duffy, 2013; Hegde, 2018a; Hegde & Freed, 2017; Lowit & Kent, 2011; Sapir, 2014; Yorkston et al., 2010). As for any disorder of communication, assessment of dysarthria begins with taking a complete case history, examining the medical records of the patient, and interviewing the patient and the family to understand the patient's past communicative behaviors and current status.

Table 9.3

Differentiating Apraxia of Speech From Dysarthria

Apraxia of speech	Dysarthria
Difficulty/inability to generate and/or send motor plans to muscles for the production of speech	Motor plans are intact, but **neuromuscular weakness or slowness** inhibits the muscles' execution of the motor plan
Unimpaired/error-free automatic, involuntary utterances	**Affects both voluntary and involuntary** utterances
Greater amount of errors for words that are longer and more phonetically complex	**Errors are consistent** regardless of length or complexity of word
Errors are inconsistent and varied	Errors are **predictable and consistent**
Buccofacial–oral apraxia more likely to co-occur	Buccofacial–oral apraxia less likely to co-occur
Normal strength, tone, and range of movement of oral and pharyngeal muscles	**Abnormal** strength, tone, and range of movement of oral and pharyngeal muscles
Can complete non-speech motor tasks during oral–mech exam without difficulty; breakdown will occur on speech tasks	Will have **difficulty performing both non-speech and speech motor tasks**

- Specific to assessing the variety of dysarthric symptoms, most clinicians do the following:
  - Record an extended conversational speech sample and a reading sample.
  - Use a variety of speech tasks, including imitation of syllables, words, phrases, and sentences; production of modeled syllables, words, phrases, and sentences; and sustained phonation (vowel prolongation).
  - Assess the diadochokinetic rate or alternating motion rates (AMRs) and sequential motion rates (SMRs).
  - Assess the speech production mechanism during non-speech activities through the following activities:
    - Observing facial symmetry, tone, tension, droopiness, expressiveness, and so forth
    - Observing the movements of the facial structures as the patient puffs the cheeks, retracts and rounds the lips, bites the lower lip, and so forth
    - Observing the patient's emotional expressions
    - Taking note of the patient's jaw movements and deviation during movement and observing the tongue movements
    - Observing the velopharyngeal mechanism and its movements
    - Assessing nasal airflow by holding a mirror at the nares as the patient prolongs the vowel /i/
    - Assessing laryngeal function by asking the patient to cough, a weak cough being associated with weak adduction of the cords, inadequate breath support, or both
  - Assess respiratory problems by observing the patient's posture and breathing habits during quiet and during speech, taking note of rapid, shallow, or effortful breathing, signs of shortness of breath and irregularity of inhalation and exhalation, and so forth.
  - Assess phonatory disorders through the following activities:
    - Having the patient say "ah" after taking a deep breath and sustain it as steadily and for as long as the air supply lasts
    - Taking note of the patient's pitch, pitch breaks, diplophonia, abrupt variations in pitch, and lack of normal pitch variations
    - Taking note of voice tremors; assessing the presence of diplophonia; and judging vocal loudness, its appropriateness, variations, decay, and alternating changes
    - Judging the quality of voice, including hoarseness, harshness, and breathiness, taking note of strained or effortful voice production or sudden cessation of voice
  - Assess **articulation disorders** by evaluating consonant productions, duration of speech sounds, phoneme repetitions, irregular breakdowns in articulation, precision of vowel productions, phoneme distortions, and the adequacy of pressure consonantal productions.
  - Assess **prosodic disorders** by evaluating the rate of speech, phrase lengths in selected portions of speech, stress patterns in speech, pauses in speech, and the presence of short rushes of speech.
  - Assess **resonance disorders** by making clinical judgments about hyponasality and hypernasality and nasal emission.

- Assess **speech intelligibility** by making clinical judgments as to the percentage of words or phrases understood and by using a rating scale if warranted.
- Assess **muscle strength**, **speed**, **range**, **accuracy**, **tone**, *and* **steadiness of movement involved in speech production** by systematic observations throughout the assessment session. To assess muscle integrity and function, clinicians may use a systematic protocol, such as the one provided by Hegde and Freed (2017).
- Use such standardized tests as the *Assessment of Intelligibility of Dysarthric Speech* (Yorkston, Beukelman, & Traynor, 1984), the *Quick Assessment for Dysarthria* (Tanner & Culbertson, 1999), and *Frenchay Dysarthria Assessment–Second Edition* (FDA-2; Enderby & Palmer, 2008). The *Speech Intelligibility Test for Windows* is also available for making a computerized assessment (Yorkston, Beukelman, & Hakel, 1996). Alternatively, the clinician may use a comprehensive assessment protocol provided by Hegde and Freed (2017).
- Make a differential diagnosis based on a careful analysis of clusters of neurologic and speech symptoms that are predominant in specific types of dysarthria.

Treatment of the Dysarthrias

Goals and Procedures

Treatment of dysarthria includes a wide range of techniques, partly because the communication disorders themselves have a wide range. All aspects of speech production must be addressed in treatment. Treatment goals should be individualized to suit the clusters of problems a patient exhibits. The underlying medical condition (stable, progressive) will influence the degree of improvement (Duffy, 2013; Hegde, 2018c; Hegde & Freed, 2017; Sapir, 2014; Yorkston et al., 2010).

Treatment goals include modifying respiratory, phonatory, articulatory, resonatory, and prosodic problems and increasing the efficiency, effectiveness, and naturalness of communication.

- Treatment goals also include increasing physiological support for speech and teaching self-correction, self-evaluation, and self-monitoring skills. Teaching compensatory behaviors for lost or reduced functions is important, and teaching the use of alternative or augmentative communication systems may be necessary.
- Augmentative and alternative communication (AAC) devices may be recommended for those whose intelligibility is severely affected and for those diagnosed with degenerative disease, such as ALS or Huntington's disease. For these individuals, teaching the device early in the disease progression is key so that they and their caregivers can be accustomed to how the AAC device works and choose the device that might best meet their needs as the disease progresses.
- **Treatment procedures** include intensive, systematic, and extensive trials (drill), instruction, demonstration, modeling (followed by imitation), shaping, prompting, fading, differential reinforcement, and other proven behavioral management procedures. It is generally recognized that treatment of dysarthria (and other neurogenic communication disorders) is essentially behavioral (Duffy, 2013). When necessary, phonetic placement and its variations can be taught. Instrumental feedback or biofeedback may be used when needed.

- Some treatment strategies that are helpful for one dysarthria type may be counterproductive for another. For example, relaxation techniques that are appropriate for treating spasticity should not be used for treating flaccid dysarthria, because the muscles are already too loose and relaxed. The clinician, therefore, should be familiar with the characteristics of each dysarthria and critically appraise whether a treatment strategy is beneficial for the dysarthria being presented.

Specific Treatment Targets

In treating patients with dysarthria, the clinician needs to target specific skills:

- **Modification of respiration** by training consistent production of subglottal air pressure with the help of a manometer or air pressure transducer; training maximum vowel prolongation; shaping production of longer phrases and sentences; teaching controlled exhalation; teaching the client to push, pull, or bear down during speech or nonspeech tasks; using resistive breathing devices to increase breath support for speech by strengthening inspiratory muscles; using a manual push on the client's abdomen; modifying postures that promote respiratory support, including using neck and trunk braces if helpful; and teaching the client to inhale more deeply and exhale slowly and with greater force during speech
- **Modification of phonation** by using biofeedback to shape desirable vocal intensity and training the client in the use of portable amplification systems if the voice is too soft; possibly also training aphonic clients in the use of an artificial larynx and teaching the client to initiate phonation at the beginning of an exhalation
- **Modification of resonance** disorders by providing feedback on nasal airflow and hypernasality by using a mirror, nasal flow transducer, or nasendoscope; training the client to open the mouth wider to increase oral resonance and vocal intensity; and using a nasal obturator or nose clip. For clients with hypernasality, a continuous positive airway pressure (CPAP) machine can be used to strengthen the velum through resistance. This device, commonly used for sleep apnea, pushes air through the nose to keep the velum open. When speaking while using this device, the velum is actively resisting this pressure (Manasco, 2014).
- **Modification of articulation** by training the client to assume the best posture for good articulation; using a bite block to improve jaw control and strength; using such methods as simplifying the target, instruction, demonstration, modeling, shaping, and immediate feedback in teaching correct articulation; using phonetic placement, slower rate, and minimal contrast pairs; providing instructions and demonstrations and teaching self-monitoring skills; using relaxation techniques, such as the jaw-shaking exercise to loosen up muscles of the mandible; and teaching compensatory articulatory movements (e.g., use of tongue blade to make sounds normally made with tongue tip)
- **Modification of speech rate** by using delayed auditory feedback (DAF), a pacing board, an alphabet board, a metronome, or hand or finger tapping, and by reducing excessive pause durations in speech
- **Modification of prosody** by reducing the speech rate and teaching appropriate intonation

- **Modification of pitch** with the help of instruction, modeling, differential feedback, or such instruments as Visi-Pitch
- **Modification of vocal intensity** through behavioral methods of modeling, shaping, and differentially reinforcing greater inhalation, increased laryngeal adduction, and wider mouth opening. The Lee Silverman Voice Treatment (LSVT) (Ramig, Fox, & Sapir, 2004) is a specific therapy protocol for increasing vocal intensity and is commonly used for the hypokinetic dysarthria accompanying Parkinson's disease.

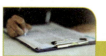

SUMMARY

The dysarthrias are a group of motor–speech disorders resulting from impaired muscular control of the speech mechanism, involving peripheral or central nervous system pathology.

- Dysarthrias are classified into ataxic, flaccid, hyperkinetic, hypokinetic, spastic, mixed, and unilateral upper motor neuron types.
- The oral communication problems that accompany dysarthria include respiratory, articulatory, phonatory, resonatory, and prosodic disturbances that are caused by weakness, incoordination, or paralysis of speech musculature.
- All aspects of speech production need to be assessed to develop a treatment plan that seeks to modify the various speech production problems. Treatment may involve the use of augmentative devices for patients with severe dysarthria.

SWALLOWING DISORDERS

Normal swallowing is a life-sustaining skill. Therefore, impaired swallowing is life threatening. Swallowing disorders (also called dysphagia or deglution disorders) involve impaired execution of the oral preparatory, oral, pharyngeal, and esophageal phases of a normal swallow. Dysphagia may be caused by strokes, traumatic brain injury (TBI), neurodegenerative diseases, and other factors. Assessment of dysphagia involves evaluating the patient's swallowing skills and screening communication skills. Treatment of dysphagia may be direct, indirect, medical, or a combination of these (Hegde, 2018a, 2018b, 2018c; Leonard & Kendall, 2014; Logemann, 1998; Perlman & Schluze-Delrieu, 1997). Although swallowing disorders are not communication disorders, speech–language pathologists are the recognized experts in the assessment and management of swallowing disorders, except for esophageal swallowing disorders, which are handled medically.

The Nature and Etiology of Swallowing Disorders

Dysphagia is impaired swallowing. The impairment may be evident in the oral, pharyngeal, and esophageal stages of swallowing. The patient may have problems chewing food, preparing it for swallow, initiating the swallow, propelling the bolus through the pharynx, or passing the food through the esophagus. There are many causes of swallowing disorders:

- Strokes, especially brainstem and anterior cortical strokes, resulting in poor motor control of structures involved in swallowing; it is the most common cause
- Oral and pharyngeal tumors and various neurologic diseases, including Parkinson's disease, Huntington's disease, amyotrophic lateral sclerosis, multiple sclerosis, progressive supranuclear palsy, myasthenia gravis, muscular dystrophy, dystonia, and dementia
- Surgical or radiation treatment of oral, pharyngeal, or laryngeal cancer; any form of brain, head, neck, or gastrointestinal surgery
- Traumatic brain injury; cervical spine disease
- Poliomyelitis (polio), chronic and obstructive pulmonary disease, and cerebral palsy
- Genetic factors (e.g., dysautonomia, an inherited disorder associated with autonomic imbalance, sensory deficits, and motor incoordination)
- Side effects of certain prescription drugs (e.g., antispasticity, antipsychotic, antibiotic, antiparkinsonian, lipid lowering, antihistamine, corticosteroid, neuroleptic, and many others)

Normal and Disordered Swallow

It is essential for speech–language pathologists who assess and treat swallowing disorders to fully understand the anatomy and physiology of normal swallowing (Corbin-Lewis, Liss, & Sciortino, 2005; Hixon, Weismer, & Holt, 2013; Leonard & Kendall, 2014; Seikel, King, & Drumright, 2010), as well as swallowing disorders (Logemann, 1998).

- Feeding and swallowing are related but separate activities. Feeding is transportation of food from the plate to the mouth; it may be accomplished by self-feeding or feeding by others. Feeding disorders may be evident in individuals with motor impairment (e.g., paralyzed hands) or severe cognitive impairments. Swallowing, on the other hand, is the transportation of food from the mouth to the stomach.
- For the sake of studying it, the normal swallow is divided into oral preparatory (including mastication), oral, pharyngeal, and esophageal phases. These phases are not discrete events, because mastication to eventual transportation of food from the mouth to the stomach is a continuous process with overlapping phases.
- Forms of swallowing disorders may be associated with each of those phases. The following paragraphs contain descriptions of the normal phases of swallow and the disorders found in them.
  - **Oral preparatory phase and its disorders.** In this phase, the food placed in the mouth is first masticated. Mastication is chewing solid or semisolid food and mixing it with saliva. Well-masticated food is prepared for swallow in the oral preparatory phase by making a **bolus** (a rounded mass of food that is ready to be swallowed). Disorders of oral preparatory phase include the following:
    - Problems in chewing food because of reduced range of lateral and vertical tongue movement, reduced range of lateral mandibular movement, reduced buccal tension, and poor alignment of the mandible and maxilla
    - Difficulty in forming and holding the bolus, abnormal holding of the bolus, slippage of food into anterior and lateral sulcus, aspiration (entry of food into the lungs, with serious respiratory complications including aspiration pneumonia) before swallow, due mostly to weak lip closure, reduced tongue movement, and inadequate tongue and buccal tension

- **Oral phase and its disorders.** This phase begins with the anterior-to-posterior tongue action that moves the bolus posteriorly (toward the back of the mouth); the phase ends as the bolus passes through the anterior faucial arches when the swallowing reflex is initiated. Disorders of the oral phase include the following:

    - Anterior, instead of posterior, tongue movement and generally weak tongue movement; reduced range of tongue movement and elevation; tongue thrust (a forward, instead of the normal backward, movement of the tongue); reduced labial, buccal, and tongue tension and strength
    - Decreased tongue sensation may cause premature loss of the bolus over the base of the tongue
    - Food residue in various places (e.g., anterior and lateral sulcus and the floor of the mouth), suggesting incomplete swallow due to tongue and buccinator weakness
    - Premature swallow of solid and liquid food and aspiration before swallow, caused by apraxia of swallow
    - Piecemeal swallow (attempts at swallowing abnormally small amounts of the bolus)

- **Pharyngeal phase and its disorders.** This phase consists of reflex actions of the swallow. Reflexes are triggered by the contact the food makes with the anterior faucial pillars. The pharyngeal phase involves velopharyngeal closure, laryngeal closure by an elevated larynx to seal the airway, reflexive relaxation of the cricopharyngeal muscle for the bolus to enter, and reflexive contractions of the pharyngeal contractors to move the bolus down and eventually into the esophagus. Disorders of the pharyngeal phase include the following:

    - Difficulties in propelling the bolus through the pharynx and into the pharyngoesophageal (PE) sphincter segment; delayed or absent swallowing reflex; nasal and airway penetration of food
    - Food coating on the pharyngeal walls; food residue in valleculae (space between the base of the tongue and the epiglottis) due to reduced base of tongue strength and retraction, on top of airway, in pyriform sinuses, and throughout the pharynx; delayed pharyngeal transit; reduced pharyngeal peristalsis, or the constricting and relaxing movements of the pharynx; pharyngeal paralysis
    - Inadequate closure of the airway; aspiration before and after swallow
    - Reduced movement of the base of the tongue; reduced hyolaryngeal movement; cricopharyngeal dysfunctions

- **Esophageal phase and its disorders.** This swallowing phase is not under voluntary control. It begins when the food arrives at the orifice of the esophagus; food is propelled through the esophagus by peristaltic action and gravity and into the stomach. Bolus entry into the esophagus results in restored breathing and a depressed larynx and soft palate. Disorders of this phase include the following problems, which are generally caused by a weak cricopharyngeus:

    - Difficulty passing the bolus through the cricopharyngeus muscle and past the seventh cervical vertebra

- Backflow of food from esophagus to pharynx; reduced esophageal contractions (due to surgery, neurologic damage, or radiation therapy)
  - Formation of diverticulum (a pouch that collects food); development of tracheoesophageal fistula (a hole); esophageal obstruction (e.g., by a tumor)

- **Achalasia** is a special form of esophageal swallowing disorder due to esophageal motility impairment or a failure of the lower esophageal sphincter to relax; consequently, the food is not passed into the stomach but retained in the esophagus. Achalasia may be confused with eating disorders (EDs) commonly reported in young females (mean age of 18 years) because of food avoidance, vomiting, and other symptoms associated with EDs (Reas, Zipfel, & Rø, 2014).

Assessment of Swallowing Disorders

Such standard procedures as taking a detailed case history; reviewing medical records; and interviewing the patient, family, and health care workers are a part of the total assessment. SLPs assessing swallowing functions through such procedures as videofluoroscopy and endoscopy, should get adequate training before attempting any of those procedures. In addition, the clinician should follow the procedures listed below (Hegde, 2018a; Leonard & Kendall, 2014; Logemann, 1998):

- Before beginning a formal assessment of swallowing, assess the client's ethnocultural background, food habits (e.g., meat eating or vegetarian), preferred and avoided foods and liquids, and any dietary restrictions due to health problems or cultural background.
- Screen speech, voice, language, and writing skills using the clinical interview. Note errors of articulation, voice quality, pitch and loudness characteristics, and the presence of hyponasality and hypernasality.
- Screen concrete and abstract language comprehension by giving a few simple verbal commands and by asking the patient to give the meaning of common proverbs and phrases. Differences or deviations in the use of language, if any, may be noted to better assist the treatment process.
- Conduct a basic oral-mechanism examination to determine lingual, labial, and buccal strength and range of motion.
- Conduct a laryngeal examination with indirect laryngoscopy or endoscopy to inspect the base of the tongue, vallecula, epiglottis, pyriform sinuses, vocal folds, and ventricular folds and their functioning.
- Administer test swallows, taking into consideration the patient's medical condition and the type of swallowing disorder. Collect the necessary materials (laryngeal mirror, tongue blade, cup, spoon, straw, syringe, and foods of various consistencies).
- Correctly position the patient for test swallows. For example, in the case of tongue weakness and bolus manipulation problems, the patient should tilt his head downward as food is placed in the mouth and tilt the head backward when the swallow is initiated. In the case of hemilaryngectomy, delayed triggering of swallowing reflex, and inadequate laryngeal closure, the patient should tilt his head downward to hold the food in the valleculae until the reflex is triggered.
- Appropriately place the food in the mouth. For example, place food in the more normal side of the mouth or use a straw or syringe to place liquids posteriorly.

- Use different kinds of foods in evaluating test swallows. For example, use liquid foods or foods of thin consistency when the patient has limited oral control and foods of thicker consistency when the patient's swallowing reflex is delayed.
- Give appropriate instructions for head position and swallowing.
- Manually examine the swallowing movements by placing the index finger just below the chin, the middle finger on the hyoid, and the third and fourth fingers at the top and bottom of the thyroid to take note of the submandibular, hyoid, and laryngeal movements during swallowing or aspiration.
- Conduct a videofluorographic assessment (modified barium swallow, also known as dynamic swallow study) with varied food consistency and quantity to evaluate oropharyngeal swallow involving lateral and anterior–posterior (AP) plane examinations (Leonard & Kendall, 2014).
- Conduct a flexible endoscopic evaluation of swallowing (FEES) using food and liquid of different consistencies and quantities to evaluate laryngeal penetration of food, aspiration, food residue, and completeness of swallow.
- Conduct a manometric assessment with the help of an esophageal manometer, which measures pressure in the upper and lower esophagus.
- Conduct an electromyographic assessment by attaching electrodes on structures of interest (e.g., oral, laryngeal, or pharyngeal muscles). Conduct an endoscopic assessment to examine the movement of the bolus until it triggers the pharyngeal swallow and any food residue after swallow.
- Conduct an ultrasound examination to measure tongue movement and hyoid movement.

Treatment of Swallowing Disorders

Clinicians who treat patients with swallowing disorders should always take into account the patient's cultural background. Patients may have food preferences or religious beliefs that affect the type of food and the timing of feeding that occur as part of treatment.

Direct, indirect, neurorehabilitation, and medical procedures help treat swallowing disorders. Speech–language pathologists are involved in both direct and indirect treatment, and their methods are entirely behavioral (Doeltgen & Huckabee, 2012; Hegde, 2018c; Leonard & Kendall, 2014; Logemann, 1998; Poorjavad, Moghadam, Ansari, & Daemi, 2014).

Direct Treatment of Swallowing Disorders

In direct treatment, food or liquid is placed in the patient's mouth to shape appropriate swallowing. Direct treatment is designed to reduce problems that are evident in the different stages of swallow. The following paragraphs describe direct treatment goals and procedures of the various swallow disorders:

- **Treatment of disorders of the oral preparatory phase of the swallow** involves teaching the patient to better masticate food and generally better handle food in the mouth. The clinician may teach the patient to do the following:

  - Press the tongue against the hard palate.
  - Keep the food on the more mobile side of the tongue or on the stronger side of the mouth.
  - Apply a gentle pressure with one hand on the damaged cheek to increase cheek tension.
  - Keep the head tilted to the stronger side to maintain food on that side.

- Tilt the head forward to keep the food in the front of the mouth until ready to swallow.
- Tilt the head back to promote the swallow.
- Hold the bolus in the anterior or middle portion of the mouth.

■ **Treatment of disorders of the oral phase of the swallow** involves teaching the patient to do the following:

- Place the tongue on the alveolar ridge and initiate a swallow with an upward and backward motion to prevent tongue thrust swallow.
- Compensate by placing food at the back of the tongue and then initiating a swallow.
- Compensate for tongue elevation problems by placing food posteriorly in the patient's oral cavity, placing a straw almost at the level of the faucial arches to help the patient swallow liquid, and then tilting the patient's head back and letting gravity push the food from the oral cavity into the pharynx.
- Compensate for reduced buccal tension by instructing the patient to use his or her tongue to clear the lateral sulci (known as a **lingual sweep**).
- Compensate for disorganized anterior-to-posterior tongue movement by holding the bolus against the palate with the tongue and beginning the swallow with a strong, single, posterior movement of the tongue.

■ **Treatment of disorders of the pharyngeal phase of the swallow** can be carried out by teaching the patient to do the following:

- Tilt the head forward (chin tuck) while swallowing to compensate for delayed or absent swallowing reflex. Tilting the head down widens the valleculae, so the bolus collects there, giving more time for the swallow to be triggered.
- Switch between liquid and semisolid swallows so that the liquid swallows help clear the pharynx to compensate for reduced peristalsis.
- Swallowing multiple times for a single bolus to help clear pharyngeal residue to compensate for reduced peristalsis and base-of-tongue strength.
- Tilt the head toward the stronger side if the patient has a unilateral paralysis in lingual function, unilateral laryngeal paralysis, decreased laryngeal elevation, poor epiglottic inversion, and/or decreased PES opening.
- Turn the head to the weak side if there is weak pharyngeal contraction on one side of the pharynx. This forces the bolus to travel down the intact side.
- Tilt the head forward while swallowing or placing pressure on the thyroid cartilage on the damaged side to improve laryngeal closure.

■ **Treatment of disorders of the esophageal phase of the swallow** is medically handled; however, speech–language pathologists may counsel the patient to

- avoid certain foods (e.g., coffee, alcohol, citrus juices, fatty foods);
- eat small portions of food and eat 2–3 hours before bedtime; elevate the head of the bed;
- lose weight if overweight;
- stop smoking; and
- stay in an upright position for 30 minutes after eating.

Indirect Treatment of Swallowing Disorders

Indirect treatment of swallowing disorders does not involve food. Instead, various exercises and swallowing-related skill training, designed to improve muscle strength, are prescribed and practiced (Argolo, Sampaio, Pinho, Melo, & Nobrega, 2013; Athukorala, Jones, Sella, & Huckabee, 2014).

Oral–motor control exercises are numerous, and each is designed to reduce a particular problem. For example, various exercises are designed to do the following:

- Increase the range of tongue movements (e.g., raising the tongue, holding the tongue as high as possible, alternating raising and lowering the tongue).
- Increase buccal tension (e.g., stretching the lips as tightly as possible and saying "ee," rounding the lips tightly and saying "oh," and rapidly alternating between "ee" and "oh").
- Increase the range of lateral movements of the jaw (e.g., wide opening and sideways movement of the jaw) and of tongue resistance (e.g., pushing the tongue against a tongue depressor); strengthen lip closure (e.g., stretching the lips to stimulate the production of /i/; puckering the lips tightly; tightly closing the lips).

Some exercises are designed to **stimulate the swallow reflex** by doing the following:

- Touch the base of the anterior faucial arch with a laryngeal mirror dipped in ice water for about 10 seconds (thermal stimulation).
- Ask the patient to swallow after the stimulation without food.
- Practice liquid swallow after stimulation.
- Progressively increase the consistency of food introduced after stimulation.

Other exercises are designed to improve adduction of tissue at the top of the airway by using lifting and pushing motions to improve laryngeal adduction, which protects the airway during swallowing (e.g., holding his or her breath, the patient pushes down on the chair or pulls up on it; subsequently, the patient may lift or push with simultaneous voicing).

To increase base of tongue strength, the Masako maneuver can be used, in which the patient holds the anterior portion of the tongue between his or her upper and lower teeth by gently biting down. The patient then swallows (only saliva) while keeping the tongue between the teeth. The Masako maneuver (tongue hold) is technically an exercise and not a maneuver. The primary intent of this technique is to improve the strength and movement of the posterior pharyngeal wall when swallowing. Base-of-tongue strength can also be improved using resistive sucking exercises. For example, the patient can suck a thicker consistency, like pudding, through a straw. This requires the back of the tongue to work harder against the resistance. It can be made even more difficult by attaching paperclips along the middle of the straw—the more paperclips, the more resistance.

Specific Swallow Maneuvers

Swallow maneuvers are techniques designed to compensate for specific problems associated with dysphagia; they help the patient gain some degree of control over certain involuntary aspects of swallowing.

These maneuvers are supported only by weak data, and better studies are needed (Ashford et al., 2009). A few common maneuvers include the following:

- The **supraglottic swallow** helps close the airway at the level of the vocal folds to prevent aspiration. The patient is asked to hold the food in the mouth, take a deep breath and hold it soon after initiating a slight exhalation, swallow while holding the breath, and cough soon after the swallow.
- The **super-supraglottic swallow** helps close the airway before and during swallow; the procedure also promotes false vocal fold closure. The patient is asked to inhale and hold the breath tightly by bearing down (an action that tilts the arytenoids and helps close the false folds) and swallow while holding the breath and bearing down. The patient coughs soon after the swallow using this technique as well.
- The **effortful swallow** helps increase the posterior motion of the tongue and increase pharyngeal pressure. The patient is asked to squeeze as hard as possible while swallowing; this may be more effective when combined with infrahyoid motor electrical stimulation (Park, Kim, Oh, & Lee, 2012).
- The **Mendelsohn maneuver** helps elevate the larynx and, thus, widens the cricopharyngeal opening. The patient is first educated about the laryngeal elevation, then asked to palpate the laryngeal elevation when swallowing saliva, and, finally, taught to hold the laryngeal elevation during swallowing for progressively longer durations.

Neuromuscular Rehabilitation for Swallowing Disorders

Neuromuscular rehabilitation consists of three main procedures: (1) neuromuscular electrical stimulation (NMES) of the neck muscles to improve swallowing, (2) transcranial magnetic stimulation, and (3) transcranial direct current stimulation. Case study and clinical results seem to suggest positive effects of these procedures, but better controlled experimental research is needed before they can be recommended for routine practice (Clark, Lazarus, Arvedson, Schooling, & Frymark, 2009; Doeltgen & Huckabee, 2012).

Computer Applications in Treatment

Several applications are available for use on computers, iPads, iPods, and iPhones (e.g., a program called iSwallow). It illustrates various swallow maneuvers and exercises (Leonard, Kendall, McKenzie, & Goodrich, 2014).

Medical Treatment of Swallowing Disorders

Surgeons are mostly involved in the medical treatment of swallowing disorders, as most of the medical procedures are surgical. These procedures include the following:

- **Cricopharyngeal myotomy.** In this procedure, the cricopharyngeal muscle is split from top to bottom to create a permanently open sphincter for swallowing. Fibers of the inferior constrictor above and the esophageal musculature below also may be slit. Eating may be resumed within a week. This procedure is recommended for patients with Parkinson's disease, amyotrophic lateral sclerosis, and oculopharyngeal dystrophy whose main problem is cricopharyngeal dysfunction.

- **Esophagostomy.** Designed for patients who cannot tolerate oral feeding, the procedure involves inserting a feeding tube into the esophagus and stomach through a hole (stoma) that has been surgically created through the cervical esophagus.
- **Gastrostomy.** Also designed for patients who cannot tolerate oral feeding, this procedure involves insertion of a feeding tube into the stomach through an opening in the abdomen; blended table food is directly transported to the stomach.
- **Nasogastric feeding.** Yet another surgical method for patients who cannot tolerate oral feeding. A tube, inserted through the nose, pharynx, and esophagus into the stomach, feeds the patient.
- **Pharyngostomy.** In this variation of non-oral, surgical feeding methods, a tube is inserted into the esophagus and stomach through a hole that has been surgically created through the pharynx.
- **Teflon injection into the vocal folds.** This is a surgical implant method designed to improve airway closure during swallowing. Teflon is injected into a normal or reconstructed vocal cord or any remaining tissue on top of the airway to increase the muscle mass that helps close the airway.

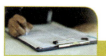

SUMMARY

Dysphagia, which involves impaired execution of the oral, pharyngeal, and esophageal phases of a swallow, can be caused by many factors, including stroke and TBI.

- Phases of swallowing include the oral preparatory phase, oral phase, pharyngeal phase, and esophageal phase. A thorough assessment involves evaluation of all these phases.
- Treatment for dysphagia should take cultural factors into account. It can be direct, indirect, medical, or a combination of these. In direct treatment, food and liquid are placed in the patient's mouth to shape appropriate swallowing. In indirect treatment, food is not involved; exercises to improve muscle strength are practiced. Medical treatment may involve various surgical procedures.

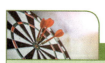

CHAPTER HIGHLIGHTS

- Apraxia is a motor planning disorder due to cerebral damage. Apraxia of speech is a speech–motor planning disorder due to cerebral damage; it is characterized by articulation errors and difficulty in executing volitional movements needed for speech, with relatively intact automatic movements.

- Dysarthria is a speech–motor disorder due to impaired muscular control of the speech mechanism, involving peripheral or central nervous system pathology and affecting respiratory, articulatory, phonatory, resonatory, and prosodic aspects of speech.
- Dysphagia is a swallowing disorder involving impaired execution of the oral preparatory, oral, pharyngeal, and esophageal phases of swallow; a type of dysphagia found in young females that is often confused with EDs is called achalasia. Patients with dysphagia may receive direct treatment, indirect treatment, medical treatment, or a combination; specific swallow maneuvers and manipulation of body positions (especially the head and neck) also are parts of treatment. Disorders of the esophageal phase are handled only medically.

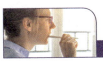

STUDY AND REVIEW QUESTIONS

1. A clinician in a hospital setting is asked to evaluate a 64-year-old patient who appears to have dysarthria as a result of a TBI from falling and hitting the back lower portion of his head. A detailed motor speech evaluation shows that the patient presents with slurred speech, imprecise consonants, distorted vowels, slow rate of speech, and excess and even stress. The patient's motor movements are described by the nursing staff as "clumsy" and "uncoordinated." Based on the given information, the clinician would most likely classify the patient's dysarthria as

- **A.** Hyperkinetic dysarthria.
- **B.** Hypokinetic dysarthria.
- **C.** Ataxic dysarthria.
- **D.** Flaccid dysarthria.

2. Which of the following dysarthria is associated with Parkinson's disease?

- **A.** Spastic dysarthria
- **B.** Flaccid dysarthria
- **C.** Hypokinetic dysarthria
- **D.** Hyperkinetic dysarthria

3. Amyotrophic lateral sclerosis results in which kind of mixed dysarthria?

- **A.** Spastic–ataxic dysarthria
- **B.** Flaccid–spastic dysarthria
- **C.** Hypokinetic–spastic dysarthria
- **D.** Flaccid–ataxic dysarthria

4. Which of the following is characteristic of apraxia of speech but not dysarthria?

- **A.** Consistent errors regardless of length and complexity of utterance
- **B.** Difficulty performing both non-speech and speech motor tasks
- **C.** Predictable errors
- **D.** Normal strength, tone, and range of movement of oral and pharyngeal muscles

5. Purposeless, random, involuntary movements of body parts associated with hyperkinetic dysarthria is known as

    A. myoclonus.
    B. chorea.
    C. tics.
    D. tremors.

6. Which of the following is *not* a disorder of the pharyngeal phase of the swallow?

    A. Decreased laryngeal elevation
    B. Reduced tongue base retraction
    C. Decreased upper esophageal sphincter (UES) opening
    D. Premature spillage over the base of the tongue

7. For which of the following disorders of swallowing would it be *inappropriate* to recommend tilting the head to the strong side?

    A. Unilateral weak pharyngeal constriction
    B. Decreased laryngeal elevation
    C. Decreased upper esophageal sphincter (UES) opening
    D. Incomplete epiglottic inversion

8. Apraxia of speech is often associated with

    A. lesions in Broca's area.
    B. lesions in Wernicke's area.
    C. lesions in subcortical structures.
    D. lesions in the occipital area.

9. Dysarthria is

    A. a speech disorder in the absence of muscle weakness or paralysis.
    B. a speech disorder never associated with aphasia.
    C. a single disorder with a unitary etiology.
    D. a speech disorder associated with muscle weakness or paralysis.

10. Of the following symptoms, the one associated with dysarthria is

    A. even and consistent breakdowns in articulation.
    B. impaired syntactic structures.
    C. forced inspirations and expirations that interrupt speech.
    D. an invariably slower rate of speech.

11. A clinician in a skilled nursing facility (SNF) receives a note that Dick, a new 80-year-old patient, has been transferred to her facility. The note states that Dick was assessed by the clinician in the previous SNF, but there is no diagnosis in the papers that have been sent from the previous clinician. However, the previous clinician reported that Dick manifested the following symptoms: general awareness of his speech problems, significant articulation problems, problems with volitional speech with relatively intact automatic speech, more difficulty with consonants than vowels, intonation and fluency problems, and trial-and-error groping and struggling associated with speech attempts. Therapy was recommended. Dick most likely has

- **A.** hyperkinetic dysarthria.
- **B.** unilateral upper motor neuron dysarthria.
- **C.** right-hemisphere syndrome.
- **D.** apraxia of speech.

12. Lucien, a 22-year-old male, is hospitalized after sustaining traumatic brain injury from a motor vehicle accident. There is no injury to the cerebellum, brainstem, or peripheral nerves. When assessing Lucien, the clinician might expect to find

- **A.** dysarthria, confused language (e.g., confabulation), auditory comprehension problems, confrontation naming problems, perseveration of verbal responses, pragmatic language problems, and reading and writing difficulties.
- **B.** dysarthria, confused language (e.g., confabulation), auditory comprehension problems, no confrontation naming problems, and agrammatic or telegraphic speech.
- **C.** confrontation naming problems, perseveration of verbal responses, pragmatic language problems, intact reading and writing skills, and echolalia.
- **D.** severely impaired fluency, severe echolalia, agrammatic and telegraphic speech, and intact auditory comprehension skills.

13. Which of the following is considered an *exercise* for patients with dysphagia and should not be performed with food?

- **A.** Masako maneuver
- **B.** Supraglottic swallow
- **C.** Mendelsohn maneuver
- **D.** Effortful swallow

14. Which of the following would be *inappropriate* to recommend for a patient with dysphagia due to poor base-of-tongue retraction?

- **A.** Use of the chin tuck strategy
- **B.** Swallowing multiple times for one bolus
- **C.** Lingual sweep of lateral sulci
- **D.** Effortful swallow

15. A clinician is asked to give a workshop to graduate students about evaluation of patients with swallowing disorders. She discusses evaluation in depth. Which one of the following facts in the clinician's workshop would be *inaccurate*?

   A. An ultrasound examination can measure oral tongue movement and hyoid movement.
   B. A manometric assessment can assess the preparatory phase of the swallow using posterior and lateral plane examinations.
   C. An electromyographic assessment can be conducted by attaching electrodes on structures of interest (e.g., oral, laryngeal, or pharyngeal muscles).
   D. A laryngeal examination can be conducted with indirect laryngoscopy or endoscopic examination to inspect the base of the tongue, vallecula, epiglottis, pyriform sinuses, vocal folds, and ventricular folds.

References and Recommended Readings at www.advancedreviewpractice.com

STUDY AND REVIEW ANSWERS

1. C. Based on the evaluation results and given information, the patient most likely has ataxic dysarthria.
2. C. Hypokinetic dysarthria is associated with Parkinson's disease
3. B. Amyotrophic lateral sclerosis is the degeneration of both upper and lower motor neurons, resulting in mixed flaccid–spastic dysarthria.
4. D. Normal strength, tone, and range of movement of oral and pharyngeal muscles are characteristic of apraxia of speech. Individuals with dysarthria will have abnormal strength, tone, and range of movement of oral and pharyngeal muscles.
5. B. Purposeless, random, involuntary movements of body parts associated with hyperkinetic dysarthria is known as chorea.
6. D. Premature spillage over the base of the tongue is a disorder of the oral phase of swallowing, not pharyngeal phase.
7. A. If a patient has unilateral weak pharyngeal constriction, it would be more appropriate to recommend that they turn their head to the weak side, rather than tilting it to the strong side.
8. A. Apraxia of speech is often associated with lesions in Broca's area.
9. D. Dysarthria is a speech disorder associated with muscle weakness or paralysis.
10. C. Of the stated disorders, the one associated with dysarthria is forced inspirations and expirations that interrupt speech.
11. D. Dick probably has apraxia of speech, which is characterized by general awareness of his speech problems; significant articulation problems; problems with volitional speech with relatively intact automatic speech; more difficulty with consonants than vowels; intonation and fluency problems; and trial-and-error groping and struggling associated with speech attempts.

12. A. Dysarthria, confused language (e.g., confabulation), auditory comprehension problems, confrontation naming problems, perseveration of verbal responses, pragmatic language problems, and reading and writing difficulties are typical in patients with traumatic brain injury.
13. A. The Masako maneuver is considered an exercise. The patient should only swallow their saliva.
14. C. Instructing the patient to sweep their tongue in their lateral sulci would be appropriate if the patient had oral residue in the sulci due to reduced buccal tension, not if the patient has poor base-of-tongue retraction.
15. B. It would be inaccurate to state that manometric assessment can assess the preparatory phase of the swallow using posterior and lateral plane examinations.

CHAPTER 10

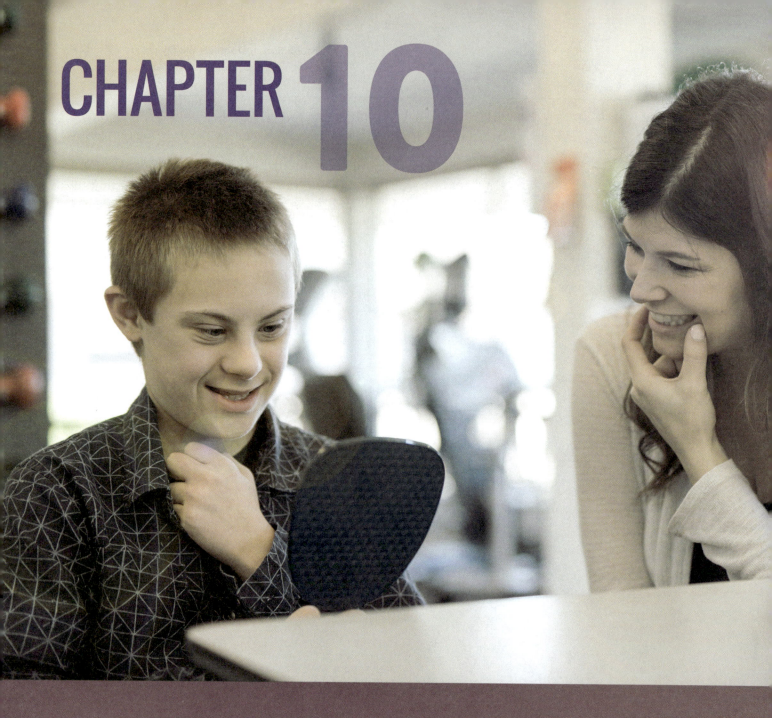

CLEFT PALATE, CRANIOFACIAL ANOMALIES, AND GENETIC SYNDROMES

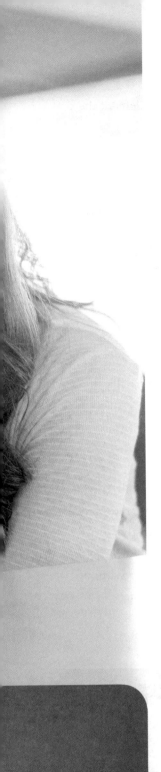

In the 21st century, the profession of speech–language pathology has expanded to include service delivery to a greater number and variety of clients with communication disorders and their families. This includes clients with cleft palate and craniofacial anomalies. According to the Centers for Disease Control and Prevention (2017), in the U.S. each year, about 4,440 babies are born with a cleft lip with or without a cleft palate. Clefts that occur with no other major birth defects are one of the most common types of birth defects in the U.S. Because of this, speech–language pathologists (SLPs) are more than ever in need of information regarding issues related to craniofacial anomalies and genetic syndromes. This chapter discusses these areas and their implications for SLPs as they attempt to provide high-quality, appropriate service delivery to an ever-growing and changing population.

CRANIOFACIAL ANOMALIES AND CLEFT PALATE

Craniofacial anomalies, mostly due to genetic factors, create many clinical conditions and syndromes, some of which are associated with communication disorders. In this section, major craniofacial anomalies, including clefts of the lip and palate, and some major genetic syndromes that are associated with communication disorders are reviewed (Allori et al., 2017; Kummer, 2014; Perry, Kuehn, Sutton, & Fang, 2017; Peterson-Falzone, Hardin-Jones, & Karnell, 2009).

Craniofacial Anomalies

- **Craniofacial anomalies** are abnormalities of the structures of the head and face. These abnormalities are congenital and, in many cases, due to genetic factors.
- A variety of factors have been demonstrated or hypothesized to cause craniofacial anomalies. Clefts of the lip and the soft palate are better known to SLPs, but there are hundreds of genetic syndromes with craniofacial anomalies that are associated with communication disorders (Jung, 2010; Paul, Norbury, & Gosse, 2018; Zajac & Vallino, 2016).
- Selected syndromes with significant association with communication disorders are summarized later in this chapter under "Genetic Syndromes."

Cleft Lip

- A **cleft** is an opening in a normally closed structure. Cleft lip, therefore, is an opening in the lip, usually the upper lip. Lower lip clefting is very rare.

Clefts of the lips alone are also rare; they are usually associated with cleft of the palate. Clefts of the palate are often not associated with cleft lips, however.

- Cleft lips are more often unilateral (Figure 10.1) than bilateral (Figure 10.2), and they occur more frequently on the left side than on the right side. Rare bilateral lip clefts have an even greater tendency to coexist with palatal clefts than unilateral left lip clefts do.
- Cleft lips alone rarely result in speech disorders and are less frequently associated with other genetic anomalies than palatal clefts.
- Clefting is a congenital disorder; it is present at the time of birth. A congenital disorder may or may not be inherited.

Cleft Palate

General Facts

- **Palatal clefts** are various congenital malformations resulting in an opening in the hard palate, the soft palate, or both. These malformations are due to disruptions of the embryonic growth processes, resulting in a failure to fuse structures that are normally fused.
- Cleft palates may be a part of a genetic syndrome with other anomalies. It is now believed that clefting of the lip and palate is etiologically different from clefting of the palate only.
- The incidence of palatal clefts in different populations varies. In the U.S. population, about 1 in 600–750 live births may be diagnosed with clefting. The highest to the lowest incidence rates are found among Native Americans, Japanese, Chinese, Whites, and African Americans, in that order.
- Generally, males tend to exhibit a higher frequency and greater severity of cleft lip (with or without cleft palate) than females, who tend to exhibit higher frequency of palatal clefts (without the cleft lip).

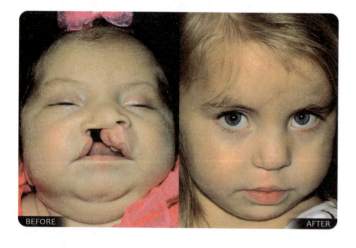

Figure 10.1 Complete unilateral cleft of the lip and palate. Used with permission from Dr. Derek Steinbacher; www.dereksteinbacher.com.

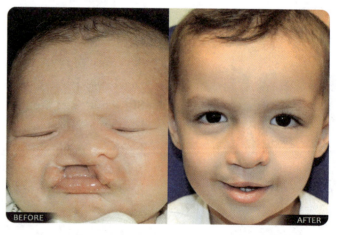

Figure 10.2 Complete bilateral cleft of the lip and palate. Used with permission from Dr. Derek Steinbacher; www.dereksteinbacher.com.

Overview of the Embryonic Growth of the Facial Structures

The most crucial period for genetic malformations is the embryonic period, which consists of the first 7–10 weeks of gestation. Most new organs emerge in the embryonic period. The 4th to the 6th week of pregnancy poses the greatest threat of embryonic disruptions, as it is the most sensitive period of growth. This period is characterized by the following:

- Multiplication of embryonic cells during the first few weeks
- Development of three layers of cells from which different organs emerge
- Development of a marked bend in the top portion of the embryo, creating a bulge that becomes the primitive forebrain by the end of the 3rd week
- Development of a groove known as the **stomodeum**, which is the primitive mouth and nose
- Development of the **frontonasal process**, which develops into the nose, the central part of the upper lip, and the primary palate
- Development of two **maxillary processes**, which form most of the face, mouth, cheeks, and the sides of the upper lip; most of the hard palate; the alveolar ridge; and the soft palate
- Development of the **upper lip** and the **primary palate** (by the end of the 7th week). The upper lip does not develop as a single structure, hence it is prone to clefting. The nose and the midline of the upper lip are formed out of one structure, and the two sides of the lip are formed out of another structure. As a result, the cleft of the lip typically appears at either the right or the left side of the nose.
- Development of the two **mandibular processes**, giving rise to the lower jaw (mandible), lower lip, and chin—all formed and fused by the end of the 4th or 5th week
- Development of the mandible, which moves to a lower and more normal position
- Growth of the tongue, which initially lies higher, at the level of the nose, dropping down to its normal position when the jaw develops
- Growth of the hard and soft palates, identifiable at the 5th week of gestation
- The two shelves of the maxillary bone that form the hard palate remaining in a vertical position, on either side of the high-placed embryonic tongue, until the tongue drops, when the palatal shelves move in an upward and lateral manner and toward each other to form the roof of the mouth
- Fusion of the two shelves of the hard palate at the midline between the 8th and 9th weeks; this is a front-to-back fusion, a fact reflected in the clefting process. Also, fusion of the maxillary shelves with the triangular premaxillary bone (the primary palate) occurs, thus separating the mouth from the nose.
- Growth of the muscles of the soft palate, initially as two separate halves. Palatal bones, as they move toward the midline, also bring the two halves of the soft palate together. By the 12th week, the muscle mass from the two sides fuses to form the soft palate.

Etiology of Clefts

Clefts are related to a variety of genetic, chromosomal, environmental, and mechanical factors. Some of the more common factors are as follows.

Genetic Abnormalities

Clefts of the lip and palate are often associated with the following:

- Autosomal dominant inheritance in some syndromes (e.g., Apert syndrome, Stickler syndrome, Van der Woude syndrome, Waardenburg syndrome, and Treacher Collins syndrome)
- Recessive genetic inheritance in some syndromes (e.g., orofacial–digital syndrome)
- X-linked inheritance in some syndromes (e.g., oto-palatal–digital syndrome)
- Chromosomal abnormalities (e.g., Trisomy 13)

Environmental Teratogenic Factors

The following are external factors that affect the genetic material:

- Fetal alcohol syndrome
- Illegal drug use
- Side effects of some prescription drugs (e.g., anticonvulsant drugs or thalidomide, a sedative)
- Rubella

Mechanical Factors

The following are factors that may also be related to clefting:

- Intrauterine crowding
- Twinning
- Uterine tumor
- Amniotic ruptures

Classification of Clefts

Clefts are classified in different ways. No system of classification captures the variations and combinations found in clefts. Therefore, none is universally accepted, although today there are several preferred classifications. Clefts vary in extent, often measured in thirds ($1/3$, $2/3$, or $3/3$) and widths.

- The major types of clefts include the following:
  - Cleft lip (complete or incomplete, unilateral or bilateral)
  - Cleft of alveolar process (unilateral, bilateral, median, or submucous)
  - Cleft of pre-palate (combination of previous types with or without pre-palate protrusion or rotation)
  - Cleft of the palate (of the soft palate, of the hard palate, or submucous)
  - Cleft of pre-palate and palate (any combination of clefts of the pre-palate and palate)
  - Facial clefts other than pre-palate and palate (e.g., such rare forms as horizontal clefts, lower mandibular clefts, lateral oro-ocular clefts, and naso-ocular clefts)

- Children might also manifest **microforms**, which are minimal expressions of clefts, including a hairline indentation of the lip or just a notch on the lip. Microforms are revealed only through laminographic examination.
- Microforms include **submucous clefts** (also called **occult cleft palate**), in which the surface tissues of the soft or hard palate fuse but the underlying muscle or bone tissues do not.
- In a submucous cleft of the soft palate, there is a midline deficiency or lack of muscular tissue, as well as incorrect positioning of the muscles. A **bifid** (or cleft) **uvula** may be present.
- In a submucous cleft of the hard palate, there is a bony defect in the midline or center of the bony palate. This can be felt as a depression or notch in the bony palate if the palate is palpated with a finger as part of an intraoral examination.
- Usually, a child with a submucous cleft palate presents with hypernasal speech. Ear infections may also be present.
- An **occult submucous cleft** is only detectable by X-ray examination and nasopharyngoscopy (viewing the palate through a small tube that is placed through the nose).
- Treatment may consist of surgery, placement of a prosthetic device to compensate for velopharyngeal incompetence (VPI), therapy to reduce hypernasality, or a combination of these.
- Children with cleft palate frequently have dental problems. There may be supernumerary (extra) teeth. Specifically, children with bilateral cleft lip and palate commonly have **hypodontia**, or missing teeth (Suzuki et al., 2017).

Congenital Palatopharyngeal Incompetence
- Congenital palatopharyngeal incompetence (CPI) is not a form of clefting but, rather, is a related disorder. It refers to impaired velopharyngeal closing-valve functioning.
- CPI is characterized by significant impairment of velopharyngeal functions as revealed by videofluoroscopy or endoscopy, which reveal inadequate velopharyngeal closure, although the laryngeal structures appear normal.
- CPI may be caused by a short palate, an occult submucous cleft palate, reduced muscular mass of the soft palate, a deep or enlarged larynx, incorrect insertion of levator muscles (insertion to hard palate instead of the normal insertion to soft palate), or a combination of such factors.
- People with CPI typically have hypernasal speech, which ranges from mild to severe. They can benefit from speech therapy, surgery, prostheses, or a combination of these.

Communication Disorders Associated With Clefts

Hearing Loss
- Children with clefts are prone to middle ear infections and hearing loss. The most common cause of hearing loss in children with cleft palate is otitis media. Otitis media with effusion compromises movement of the ossicular chain and the tympanic membrane (see Figure 10.3). Thus, conductive hearing loss is the most common type of loss in children with clefts.

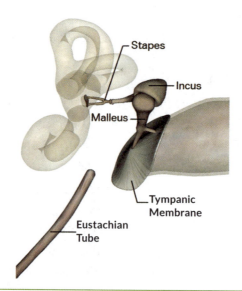

Figure 10.3 The ossicular chain and the tympanic membrane. Used with permission from Anatomage.

- Eustachian tube dysfunction is also prevalent in children with clefts. This creates conditions conducive to conductive hearing loss especially.
- In babies with cleft palate, Eustachian tube dysfunction is probably mostly related to the lack of contraction of the tensor veli palatini muscle and compromised compliance of the lateral tubal wall. (The tensor veli palatini muscle flattens, tenses, and lowers the soft palate while simultaneously opening the Eustachian tube.)
- After palatal reconstructive surgery, tensor veli palatini dysfunction improves but may never normalize. Chronic otitis media with effusion continues to be a problem after palatal surgery. The incidence of hearing loss in the cleft palate population is about 58%. Usually, the hearing loss is bilateral and conductive, but not necessarily symmetrical.

Speech Sound Disorders
Speech sound disorders (SSDs) are more significant if the palatal cleft is not repaired early or the repair is inadequate. SSDs include errors such as those described below:

- Greater difficulty with unvoiced sounds than with voiced sounds, pressure consonants, audible or inaudible nasal air emission, and distortion of vowels
- Specifically, difficulty with sibilants (e.g., /s/, /z/), as well as high pressure stops (e.g., /b/, /p/) and fricatives (e.g., /f/, /v/)
- Compensatory errors, including various types of substitutions that help compensate for the inadequate closure of the velopharyngeal mechanism, such as substitutions of stops, fricatives, and affricates with unusual (often posterior) movements and posture of the tongue to stop the air or to produce friction noise (e.g., substitution of glottal stops for stop consonants, substitution of laryngeal fricatives for fricatives, and substitution of pharyngeal affricates for affricates)
- Specific difficulty with affricates, fricatives, and plosives if velopharyngeal closure is inadequate

Language Disorders

Language disorders may not be as significant as articulation disorders unless other conditions are associated; language is normal in many cases. Common problems include the following:

- Initially delayed language development, with significant improvement as the child grows older; normal language possible by age 4 or so
- Significant language disorders in children whose clefts are a part of genetic syndromes that include hearing loss, developmental disabilities, sensory problems, and so forth
- Relatively normal receptive language skills, with delays in expressive language

Laryngeal and Phonatory Disorders

Children with palatal clefts tend to exhibit a higher prevalence of laryngeal and vocal disorders, which may include the following:

- Vocal nodules
- Hypertrophy and edema of the vocal folds
- Vocal hoarseness, reduced vocal intensity, reduced pitch variations, and strangled voice
- Resonance disorders characterized by hypernasality, hyponasality, denasality, or a combination

Assessment of Children With Clefts

- Assessment of children with cleft palate includes all the standard procedures (e.g., case history, interview of the parents and the child if appropriate).
- The main concern is to assess speech sound production and velopharyngeal adequacy. It is also important to screen hearing and assess language (Vallino, Ruscello, & Zajac, 2017).

Assessment of Velopharyngeal Function

- Most SLPs work as part of an interdisciplinary cleft palate team when they assess children. These teams consist of professionals, such as the oral surgeon, plastic surgeon, geneticist, pediodontist, prosthodontist, and others.
- It is recommended that routine speech and language evaluations be a part of the cleft palate team evaluation for every child, starting before the early postnatal period of treatment. SLPs should also routinely be involved with assessments as children grow older.
- Procedures for assessment of velopharyngeal function include judgments about hypernasality and hyponasality, the presence of which indicates velopharyngeal inadequacy. In many cases, instrumental measures can supplement clinical perceptions related to the adequacy of velopharyngeal functioning (Perry, Kuehn, Sutton, & Fang, 2017).
- Objective assessment of the velopharyngeal mechanism includes an earlier mentioned endoscopic examination of the velopharyngeal mechanism (**nasopharyngoscopy**). In nasopharyngoscopy, a nasopharyngoscope is passed through the middle meatus and back to the area of velopharyngeal closure. The examiner can then observe the posterior and lateral pharyngeal walls, as well as the nasal aspect of the velum and the adenoid pad, as the client produces sentences.

- Objective assessment also includes a videofluoroscopic examination of the velopharyngeal mechanism in order to observe the movements of the soft palate, the lateral pharyngeal wall, the posterior pharyngeal wall, and the tongue as the client produces consonant–vowel combinations, voiced and voiceless fricatives, and selected phrases.
- When assessing velopharyngeal closure, an oral manometer can be helpful. The patient either sucks from or blows into a mouthpiece as forcefully as possible. The inhalation task gives a negative reading, while the exhalation task yields a positive pressure reading from manometer gauges. The clinician obtains a ratio by comparing pressures achieved in the nostrils-occluded and the nostrils-open conditions.
- A normal ratio of 1.00 suggests adequate velopharyngeal closure. Ratios of less than 1.00 may indicate velopharyngeal incompetence (VPI), reduced intelligibility, and hypernasal speech in patients with cleft palate. Ratios of less than 0.89 especially indicate these phenomena.
- KayPENTAX Inc. sells the nasometer, a computer-based system that measures nasalance. **Nasalance** is a ratio formed between oral and nasal sound pressures, which is expressed as a percentage. The patient speaks syllables or words, and the nasometer measures nasalance during this task. Use of the nasometer can be most helpful in objectively assessing velopharyngeal function.
- Some teams use **cephalometric analysis** to evaluate velopharyngeal structures and their functional relationships; this analysis informs decisions about surgery, therapy, and others. Cephalometric analysis depends upon cephalometric radiography, which studies relationships between bony and soft tissue landmarks.
- Cephalometric analysis is especially used to scientifically analyze the size and range of motion of the soft palate and related structures. The Cephalometric Assessment of Velopharyngeal Structures (CAVS) is a computer program designed to analyze the ratio relationship between the depth of the nasopharynx and the length of the soft palate.
- A ratio of 60–80 generally indicates adequate tissue for velopharyngeal closure for speech. If ratios are higher than 80, this usually means that the velum is too short or the nasopharynx is too deep. If this is the case, there may be inadequate soft palate tissue to reach the posterior pharyngeal wall, and speech therapy alone will be insufficient for the patient.
- A ratio of less than 60 is usually found when the nasopharynx is too shallow or the soft palate is too long. This may indicate a tendency for hyponasality, cul-de-sac nasality, or mixed nasality.
- Assessment also includes an orofacial examination to take note of the clefts in the lip, the hard palate, and the soft palate, as well as adequacy of the surgical repair of the cleft, facial abnormalities indicative of a genetic syndrome, and the velopharyngeal mechanism.

Assessment of Speech Sound Disorders
- Assessment of SSDs in children with clefts includes standard procedures used in assessing similar disorders in children without clefts.
- However, special considerations are given to assess the kinds of errors and compensatory error patterns that are typical of children with cleft palates (e.g., pressure consonants) (Allori et al., 2017).

- Many clinicians administer the *Iowa Pressure Articulation Test* (a subtest of the *Templin Darley Test of Articulation*) (Templin & Darley, 1969) as well as other standardized tests of articulation and phonological skills.
- It is important for clinicians to obtain speech samples, because connected speech samples yield information about children's overall intelligibility, as well as the effect of context and natural prosodic patterns.

Assessment of Language Disorders
- Assessing language disorders in children with clefts includes standard procedures used in assessing both language comprehension and production. Assessment of expressive language skills is especially important, as these tend to lag behind receptive language skills.
- It is important to gather a comprehensive language sample to analyze the use of semantic, syntactic, morphologic, and pragmatic use of language.

Assessment of Phonatory Disorders
- Assessing phonatory disorders in children with clefts includes standard procedures used in assessing voice disorders in children with no clefts.
- The clinician makes clinical judgments about voice-quality deviations (e.g., hoarseness, harshness, breathiness).
- He or she also assesses vocally abusive behaviors, evaluates pitch and loudness of voice, and may conduct an instrumental assessment of voice disorders (e.g., with the use of Visi-Pitch or the phonatory function analyzer).

Assessment of Resonance Disorders
- Assessment of resonance disorders includes assessing hypernasality in conversational speech by making clinical judgments.
- Rating of hypernasality in connected speech by two or more clinicians may also take place, and assessing hyponasality may be necessary.
- Instrumentation is increasingly being used to evaluate the presence and severity of resonance disorders, as previously discussed (for a detailed explanation, see Vallino et al., 2017).

Treatment of Children With Clefts
- Treatment of children with clefts is a team effort involving several specialists, including oral surgeons, pediatricians, orthodontists, otolaryngologists, psychologists, and speech–language pathologists. Often, the surgical repair of the palate is the major initial treatment implemented.
- Traditionally, decisions for surgery have involved the Rule of 10s—waiting until the child has reached a weight of 10 pounds and the age of 10 weeks and has a hemoglobin of 10. Exceptions are sometimes made, but following the Rule of 10s helps to minimize the risk of general anesthesia, maximize the child's healing capacity, and facilitate the aspects of surgical repair based on the child's size.

Surgical Management of the Clefts

The following types of surgery are common for patients with clefting:

- **Primary surgery for the clefts** is the initial surgery, in which the clefts are closed.
- **Secondary surgeries for clefts** are done to improve appearance and functioning after the initial closure of the clefts.
- **Lip surgery** is done to close unilateral or bilateral clefts of the lip; this is typically done when the baby is about 3 months old or weighs about 10 pounds.
- **Palatal surgery** is done to close the cleft or clefts of the palate; this is typically done when the baby is 9–24 months.
- **V-Y retroposition** or the **Veau-Wardill-Kilner** method (see Figure 10.4) of surgery is done to repair the cleft of the palate. Single-based flaps of palatal mucoperiosteum are raised on either side of the cleft and brought together and pushed back to close the cleft; this push-back (retropositioning of the flaps) lengthens the palate and improves chances of velopharyngeal approximation.

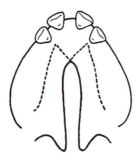

A. Incision on either side of the cleft

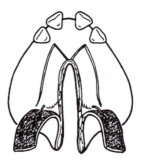

B. Two flaps of tissue freed from the bone

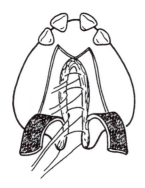

C. Margins of the cleft pared

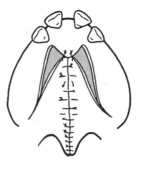

D. Flaps brought together, pushed back, and sutured

Figure 10.4 The Veau-Wardil-Kilner operation. From *Introduction to Communicative Disorders* (5th ed.), by M. N. Hegde, forthcoming, Austin, TX: PRO-ED. Copyright by PRO-ED, Inc. Reprinted with permission.

- The **von Langenbeck surgical method** is performed to repair the cleft of the palate by raising two bipedicled (attached on both ends) flaps of mucoperiosteum, bringing them together and attaching them to close the cleft; this leaves denuded bone on either side and does not lengthen the palate.
- **Delayed hard palate closure** is a surgical procedure in which the cleft of the soft palate is closed first, and the cleft of the hard palate is closed later.
- **Pharyngeal flap** is a secondary palatal surgical procedure in which a muscular flap is cut from the posterior pharyngeal wall, raised, and attached to the velum; the openings on either side of the flap allow for nasal breathing, nasal drainage, and production of nasal speech sounds. The flap helps close the velo-pharyngeal port and thus reduce hypernasality (see Figure 10.5).
- **Pharyngoplasty** is another surgical procedure in which a substance, such as Teflon, silicone, dacron wool/silicone gel bag, or cartilage, may be implanted or injected into the posterior pharyngeal wall to make it bulge and thus help close the velopharyngeal port.

Treatment of Speech Sound Disorders

- For children with cleft palate, it is very important to focus on increasing intelligibility. Research has shown that typically developing children make negative social and personal attribute judgments about children with cleft palate based solely on their speech intelligibility (Lee, Gibbon, & Spivey, 2017).
- Treatment of SSDs resulting from a cleft palate is sequenced from sounds, syllables, words, phrases, and sentences, in that order.
- The following treatment procedures are recommended:
  - More visible sounds are taught before less visible sounds, except for the linguadentals.
  - Stops and fricatives are taught before other classes of sounds.

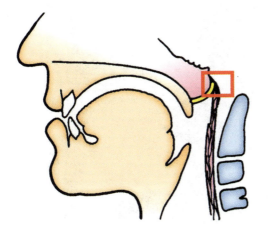
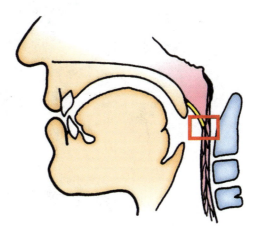

Figure 10.5 Pharyngeal flap surgical procedure.

- Training on /k/ and /g/ may be inappropriate if the child's velopharyngeal functioning is inadequate.
- If stimulable, fricatives, affricates, or both may be trained; in any case, they may be trained after stops are mastered.
- Frequent presentation of auditory and visual cues and modeling may be helpful.
- Compensatory articulatory positioning, where appropriate, may be taught.
- The clinician may teach the child to avoid posterior articulatory placements and to articulate with less effort and facial grimacing.
- Tactile cues and instruction to improve tongue positioning may be useful.
- Some children benefit from a minimal pairs approach, especially if they delete final consonants. For example, the SLP can contrast pairs, such as *bee-beach*, *cow-couch*, *bye-bike*, *lie-line*, and others.

■ Research has not shown that work on non-speech, oral–motor blowing exercises is helpful for children with cleft palates (Ruscello, 2008). Clinical outcome research is needed to assess the efficacy of exercises, such as blowing horns, on the speech production of children with SSDs associated with cleft palate.

■ A promising technique for improving a child's speech sound production is electropalatography (EPG). In EPG, an orthodontist designs an artificial palate that contains 62 embedded electrodes connected to a computer. The palate is fitted in the child's mouth (somewhat like a retainer; see Figure 10.6a), and when the tongue contacts the electrodes during speech production, articulatory patterns can be seen on the computer screen (see Figure 10.6b).

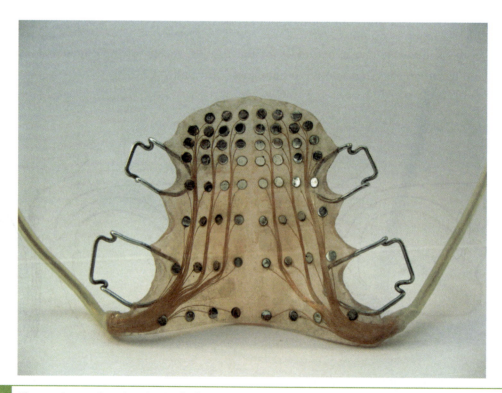

Figure 10.6a Electropalatography palate Copyright © Rose Medical Solutions Ltd. www.rose-medical.com.

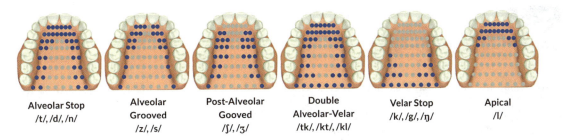

Figure 10.6b Electropalatography articulatory patterns. Copyright © Rose Medical Solutions Ltd. www.rose-medical.com.

- EPG is ideal for children with cleft palate, because they can receive immediate visual feedback about tongue placement for speech sounds. This makes it much easier for the SLP to teach correct articulator placement.

Treatment of Language Disorders

- Most SLPs work with parents to help them learn techniques for language stimulation with their infants and children with cleft palate. When necessary, formal language treatment may be offered if this language stimulation is not sufficient.
- It may be especially important to stimulate expressive language, as it tends to be more delayed than receptive language, as previously stated.

Treatment for Resonance Disorders

- Hypernasality due to VPI should not be treated until (a) there is surgical or prosthetic efficacy to improve the physiological functioning, and (b) the child is capable of velopharyngeal closure but is using previously established inappropriate compensatory articulation patterns that can be modified.
- Children with mild hypernasality may respond positively to therapy techniques alone. However, children with more severe symptoms of velopharyngeal anatomical insufficiency or neuromuscular incompetency usually need surgical or prosthetic intervention, or both, before speech therapy can succeed.
- Speech–language pathologists can use voice therapy techniques to reduce hypernasality. These techniques include increased vocal loudness, discrimination training to distinguish oral from nasal resonance, lowered pitch, and encouragement of increased oral opening.
- Biofeedback instruments to reduce hypernasality (e.g., Tonar II) may also be useful. A previously mentioned adaptation of the Tonar II is the nasometer (KayPENTAX Inc.), a non-invasive computer-based system that measures the relative amount of oral-to-nasal energy in a client's speech. The client receives visual feedback to help him or her reduce the amount of hypernasality in speech.
- In order to successfully assess and treat children with VPI, clinicians need to be well trained and qualified. Clinicians will usually work on teams with other professionals and use appropriate instrumentation to assess and treat persons with VPI adequately.
- In children with VPI, the velopharyngeal port does not close during production of non-nasal sounds.

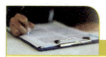

SUMMARY

- Craniofacial anomalies, such as cleft lip and palate, are due mostly to genetic factors, although environmental and mechanical factors may also play a role.
- Persons with clefts of the palate have communication disorders associated with the clefts. These disorders include hearing loss as well as disorders of speech, language, resonance, and voice.
- When assessing children with clefts, a multidisciplinary team approach is needed to assess velopharyngeal incompetence as well as speech, language, phonatory, and resonance disorders.
- Intervention for children with clefts usually consists of surgical management combined with treatment of disorders of speech, language, resonance, and voice.

GENETIC SYNDROMES

A **syndrome** is a constellation of signs and symptoms that are associated with a morbid process; a genetic syndrome is such a constellation with a known genetic basis.

Many genetic syndromes are associated with communication disorders. Syndromes that involve the craniofacial complex and those that affect general intellectual functions tend to produce the most significant effects on communication. Some of the most common syndromes that affect communication include the following (Paul et al., 2018).

Genetic Syndromes Associated With Communication Disorders

Angelman Syndrome

- Angelman syndrome (AS) was first described by Dr. Harry Angelman, an English physician. It usually involves a normal prenatal and birth history, normal head circumference, and no obvious birth defects. It occurs when chromosome 15 is duplicated from the father or deleted from the mother.
- Usually AS is diagnosed between 3–7 years of age, although developmental delay may be apparent by 6–12 months of age. Though the developmental delay is present, these children do not show regression.
- Symptoms include seizures, a stiff and jerky gait, laughter and a happy demeanor, an easily excitable personality, hypermotoric behavior, hand-flapping movements, and a short attention span.
- Most children with AS have few or no words; nonverbal communication and verbal receptive skills are higher than verbal expressive skills.

Apert Syndrome

- Apert syndrome may be caused by spontaneous autosomal dominant mutations. The gene and locus of Apert syndrome is FGR2 at 10q25–26. Its transmission is limited because of the low reproductive capacity of affected people.

- Its physical characteristics include syndactyly (digital fusion) involving the second, third, and fourth digits and craniosynostosis, resulting in smaller anterior–posterior skull diameter, flat frontal and occipital bones and high forehead, increased intracranial pressure, and compensatory growth in cranial structures.
- Other physical characteristics include midfacial hypoplasia (underdevelopment), an arched and grooved hard palate, conductive hearing loss in some individuals, class III malocclusion, irregularly placed teeth, thickened alveolar process, long or thickened soft palate, and cleft of the hard palate in 25–30% of cases.
- Communication problems include a tendency toward hyponasality, forward carriage of the tongue, and articulation disorders involving mostly alveolar consonants (e.g., /s/ and /z/) and labiodental sounds (e.g., /f/ and /v/).
- Some people with Apert syndrome have normal intelligence, while others exhibit mild to moderate intellectual disability.

Cri du Chat Syndrome
- Cri du chat syndrome is caused by an absence of the short arm of the fifth chromosome (known as 5p). Its physical characteristics include a high-pitched cry of long duration; the cry resembles that of a cat (hence the name) in the infant.
- Other physical characteristics include low-set ears, a narrow oral cavity, laryngeal hypoplasia, microcephaly, hypertelorism, micrognathia, and oral clefts.
- Communication problems include articulation and language disorders typically associated with intellectual disability.

Crouzon Syndrome
- Crouzon syndrome is caused by autosomal dominant inheritance, with varied expression in individuals. Its physical characteristics include **craniosynostosis** (fusion of the cranial suture, especially that of the coronal) and hypoplasia of the midface, maxilla, or both.
- Other physical characteristics include a small maxillary structure, sphenoethmoidal synchondroses, ocular **hypertelorism** (eyes that are far apart), protrusion of the eyeballs, strabismus, a parrotlike nose, facial asymmetry and tall forehead, malocclusion class III in some cases, a highly arched palate, shallow oropharynx, a long and thick soft palate, and **brachycephaly** (short head).
- Communication problems include conductive hearing loss in some individuals, articulation disorders associated with hearing loss and abnormalities of palatal oral cavity structures, hyponasality, and language disorders.

Down Syndrome
- Down syndrome is caused by an extra whole number chromosome 21, resulting in 47, rather than the normal 46 chromosomes. Physical characteristics include generalized hypotonia; a flat facial profile; small ears, nose, and chin; and brachycephaly.

- Other physical characteristics include midface dysplasia, shortened oral and pharyngeal structures, a narrow and high arched palate, a relatively large and fissured tongue that tends to protrude, a short neck with excess skin on the back of it, hyperflexible joints, cardiac malformations in about 40% of cases, and short fingers.
- Communication problems include conductive loss in many cases and sensorineural loss in some. There may be language delays and disorders, especially deficient syntactic and morphological features accompanied by relatively better vocabulary skills. Hypernasality and nasal emission, breathier voice, and articulation disorders may also be present.

Fragile X Syndrome
- Fragile X syndrome is the leading inherited cause of intellectual disability in males. This syndrome is caused by an expansion of the nucleic acid cytosine-guanine-guanine (CGG), which repeats too often on the fragile X mental retardation gene (FMR1), located on the bottom end of the X chromosome.
- Physical characteristics include a large, long, and poorly formed pinna, a big jaw, enlarged testes, and a high forehead.
- Persons with Fragile X syndrome may manifest mood instability, anxiety, seizures, aggression, sleep disturbances, and attention deficits (Levin, 2017).
- Most males with Fragile X syndrome have intellectual disability. During childhood, this intellectual disability is mild-moderate, becoming more severe in adulthood.
- Communication problems include jargon, perseveration, echolalia, inappropriate language or talking to oneself (more often in the male), lack of gestures and other nonverbal means of communication that normally accompany speech, voice problems, and articulation disorders.
- Males with Fragile X syndrome may avoid eye contact, withdraw socially, have limited attention spans, be hyperactive, and have autistic-like social deficiencies. Generally, adolescent and adult males with Fragile X syndrome have delays in pragmatic, semantic, phonologic, and syntactic aspects of language. Syntax is especially affected (Estigarribia, Martin, & Roberts, 2013; Oakes, Kover, & Abbeduto, 2013). Speech intelligibility may be compromised. Early intervention is crucial with this population.

Hurler's Syndrome
- Hurler's syndrome is a rare, congenital metabolical disease caused by an autosomal recessive deficiency of X-L iduronidase. It occurs in approximately 1 out of 10,000 births. Most children with Hurler's syndrome die in their early teens or sometimes even before they are 10 years old.
- In the 1800s and early 1900s, Hurler's syndrome was called "gargoylism." The name changed around 1919–1920. The syndrome is characterized by dwarfism, a hunchback, intellectual disability, short and thick bones, coarse facial features with a low nasal bridge, sensorineural deafness, and noisy respiration. There is vocal fatigue and hoarseness because of the deposition of metabolites in the larynx.

- Children with Hurler's syndrome also usually have a protuberant abdomen, angina pectoris, frequent chest infections, decreased joint mobility, and thickening of the coronary arteries. Their hands may be short, wide, and thick.
- Children with Hurler's syndrome also have thick, everted lips; a large tongue; and small, malformed teeth. Thus, they frequently have compromised intelligibility.

Landau-Kleffner Syndrome

- The causes of Landau-Kleffner syndrome (LKS) are unknown. LKS is a rare childhood neurological disorder whereby formerly healthy children ages 3–7 years lose their ability to comprehend language and then to speak it. This loss and resulting aphasia can be gradual or sudden (National Institute of Neurological Disorders and Stroke, 2017).
- Some children are left with severe, permanent language disorders. Others regain many of their language abilities over a span of months or years. For some children, relapses and remissions occur.
- Abnormal brain wave patterns have been detected through EEG in persons with LKS. It is estimated that 80% of affected children develop epilepsy. They usually have infrequent seizures that may or may not be accompanied by convulsions; these seizures usually occur at night.
- Some children develop accompanying behavior disorders, such as hyperactivity, aggressiveness, and depression. Treatment usually involves medications (e.g., anti-convulsants and corticosteroids) and speech–language therapy.

Marfan Syndrome

- Marfan syndrome is an autosomal, dominant inherited disorder caused by mutations in the FBN1 gene. It affects the body's connective tissue and may include bone overgrowth and loose joints. Overgrowth of the ribs can cause the sternum to bend inward or push outward. Intelligence is not affected.
- About 70% of people with Marfan syndrome have restrictive lung disease. Restrictive lung disease prevents the chest from expanding fully. When the lungs cannot expand fully, respiration is affected and breathing becomes more difficult. This can lead to shortness of breath during speech.

Moebius Syndrome

- Moebius syndrome has a heterogeneous causation, including agenesis or aplasia of the motor nuclei of the cranial nerves. There is sporadic, unpredictable occurrence in most cases and autosomal dominant inheritance in some cases.
- Its physical characteristics include involvement of facial and hypoglossal nerves in most cases and of the trigeminal nerve in some cases.
- There is also bilabial paresis and weak tongue control for lateralization, elevation, depression, and protrusion; unilateral or bilateral paralysis of the abductors of the eye; limited strength, range, and speed of movement of articulators; feeding problems in infancy; and a masklike face.
- Communication problems include conductive hearing loss in only a few cases and delayed language in some cases, especially in children with frequent hospitalizations. There may also be articulation

disorders ranging from mild to severe, with bilabial, linguadental, and lingua-alveolar sounds affected more than the others.

Pierre-Robin Syndrome

- Pierre-Robin syndrome is caused by autosomal recessive inheritance in most cases. In some cases, this syndrome may be a part of Stickler syndrome, in which case autosomal dominant inheritance may be the genetic basis.
- Its physical characteristics include mandibular hypoplasia, a cleft of the soft palate (but typically not associated with cleft of the lips), velopharyngeal incompetence, a deformed pinna and low-set ears, and temporal bone and ossicular chain deformities.
- In addition, these children are born with **glossoptosis**, a condition in which the tongue is positioned posteriorly, often causing blockage of the airway and pharynx. Naturally, this affects breathing and feeding.
- Feeding problems are often present, and these exist due to difficulty coordinating breathing, sucking, and swallowing. Many infants require alternative methods of feeding, including the use of a **nasogastric tube** (a tube that runs up the nose and into the stomach) or a **gastrostomy tube** (G-tube), which is placed directly into the stomach for feeding.
- Communication problems include unilateral or bilateral conductive hearing loss associated with otitis media and cleft palate, delayed language and articulation disorders, hypernasality and nasal emission, articulation disorders, and hypercompensatory articulation.
- Language delay may also be present (Alencar, Marques, Bertucci, & Prado-Oliviera, 2017).

Prader-Willi Syndrome

- Prader-Willi syndrome (PWS) is suspected to be caused by autosomal dominant inheritance and deletion in the region of the long arm of chromosome 15 (15q11–15q13) in some cases.
- Its physical characteristics include low muscle tone, early feeding difficulties, failure to thrive initially, obesity after the first year, excessive eating, and underdeveloped genitals.
- Many children with Prader-Willi syndrome have imprecise articulation, oral–motor difficulties that contribute to poor articulation, and hypernasality. Some also exhibit flat intonation patterns, a slow speaking rate, a harsh or hoarse vocal quality, and abnormal vocal pitch due to clinical characteristics given in the list below.
- Children with PWS frequently also have developmental delays and intellectual disability. Many have impaired expressive and receptive language skills, with expressive skills being more impaired than receptive skills. These speech–language characteristics can result from clinical features of Prader-Willi syndrome, which are listed below. However, a continuum of abilities ranges from nonverbal individuals to those who develop normal speech and language skills by adulthood.
- Clinical characteristics of individuals with Prader-Willi syndrome that can contribute to speech and language problems include the following:

- **Hypotonia**—slow movement of articulators, stretching of laryngeal muscles, and poor velopharyngeal movement, which can contribute to slow rate of speech, imprecise articulation, hyper- or hyponasality, and variations in vocal pitch and quality
- **Altered growth of the larynx** as a result of endocrine dysfunction, which leads to pitch variations
- In the mouth, **narrow overjet**, **micrognathia, and narrow palatal arch**, which contribute to reduced intelligibility and articulation skills
- **Tooth decay** due to reduced output of saliva and hypoplasia of the enamel, which contribute to reduced intelligibility and articulation skills
- **Cognitive sequencing problems and intellectual disability**, which contribute to delayed receptive and expressive language skills, as well as poor narrative skills
- **Behavioral disturbances**—stubbornness, temper tantrums, emotional lability, compulsive behavior, argumentativeness, poor social relationships, and difficulty detecting social cues, which contribute to poor pragmatic skills

- At this time, new medical treatments are being used with individuals who have Prader-Willi syndrome. These include use of growth hormones, as well as surgical procedures to reduce hypernasality.

Russell-Silver Syndrome
- Russell-Silver syndrome is suspected to be caused by genetic factors, although information about etiology is very scarce. Babies with Russell-Silver syndrome have low birthweight, are small for their gestational age, and are considered to have dwarfism.
- Physical characteristics include asymmetry of the arms or legs; a disproportionately large head; craniofacial disproportion; mandibular hypoplasia; a high, narrow palate, and **microdontia** (abnormal smallness of the teeth).
- Communication problems often include hypernasality, feeding problems in infancy, articulation disorders, expressive and receptive language disorders, and an abnormally high-pitched voice.

Tourette Syndrome
- Tourette syndrome is an inherited neurological disorder which becomes evident in early childhood or adolescence. It is characterized by uncontrollable vocal sounds (tics) and repeated involuntary movements. Sometimes the tics include involuntary, inappropriate words and phrases, such as swear words and other obscene language (coprolalia).
- It is currently estimated that in the U.S., 1 out of every 160 children between ages 5 to 17 years has Tourette syndrome (Tourette Association of America, 2017).
- Tourette syndrome affects males three or four times more often than females and affects persons from all ethnic backgrounds.
- No one knows what causes Tourette syndrome; however, some researchers speculate that it is due to an abnormality in the genes affecting the brain's metabolism of neurotransmitters, such as serotonin, norepinephrine, and dopamine.

- Usually, the first symptoms are facial tics, such as eye blinking; however, tics can include grimaces or nose twitching. In time, other motor tics may appear, including neck stretching, head jerking, body twisting and bending, and floor stamping. Tics "go up and down," increasing and decreasing in frequency, location, and type; that is, symptoms may subside for weeks or months and then recur.
- As stated, people with Tourette syndrome may utter unacceptable sounds, words, or phrases. Commonly, they clear their throats, grunt, sniff, cough, shout, yelp, or bark. Some may demonstrate echolalia and may repeat actions unnecessarily and obsessively.

Treacher Collins Syndrome
- Treacher Collins syndrome is caused by autosomal dominant inheritance in most cases and spontaneous mutation in some. Its physical characteristics include underdeveloped facial bones, including mandibular hypoplasia (small chin) and malar (cheek) hypoplasia, dental malocclusion and hypoplasia, and downwardly slanted palpebral fissures.
- Other characteristics include **coloboma** (lesion or defect, usually a cleft) of the lower eyelid, stenosis or atresia of the external auditory canal, malformations of the pinna, and middle and inner ear malformations.
- There is usually a high hard palate, a cleft palate in about 30% of cases, a submucous cleft in some cases, a short or immobile soft palate, and sucking and swallowing problems in infancy.
- Communication problems include congenital, bilateral, conductive hearing loss in many cases and sensorineural loss in some cases, as well as language disorders typically associated with hearing impairment.
- Other communication problems include hypernasality and nasal emission in cases with clefts and VPI, as well as articulation disorders consistent with hearing loss and oral structural deviations.

Trisomy 13
- In Trisomy 13, the baby has an extra copy of chromosome 13 and is thus born with 47 instead of 46 chromosomes. The incidence of Trisomy 13 is approximately 1 in 5,000 live births.
- Trisomy 13 is associated with many life-endangering, severe birth defects. These include congenital heart defects, severe brain anomalies, spina bifida, severe eye defects, cleft lip and palate, and polydactyly (extra fingers, toes, or both).
- Many babies with Trisomy 13 have midline facial deformities and a midline cleft lip. This usually indicates the presence of **holoprosencephaly**, or the failure of the brain to divide into two hemispheres.
- A number of babies with Trisomy 13 die before their first birthdays, usually from a cardiac or central nervous system event. If babies live, they have profound intellectual disability, as well as feeding difficulties, which require nasogastric feeding.

Turner Syndrome

- Turner syndrome occurs only in females and is caused by a missing or deformed X chromosome in most cases. A similar syndrome that occurs in both males and females is called **Noonan syndrome**.
- The physical characteristics of Turner syndrome include ovarian abnormality, resulting in absence of menstruation and infertility; congenital swelling of the feet, neck, and hands; cardiac defects; webbing of the neck (excess skin over the neck); and a low posterior hairline.
- Other physical characteristics include a broad chest with widely spaced nipples, **cubitus valgus** (elbows bent outward or away from the midline), pigmented skin lesions, a narrow maxilla and palate, and **micrognathia** (abnormally small lower jaw).
- Further physical characteristics include anomalies of the auricle, including low-set, elongated, and cup-shaped ears; thick earlobes; a high arched palate; a cleft palate in some cases; and evidence of right hemisphere dysfunction.
- Communication problems include sensorineural hearing loss in many cases (usually noticed after the 10th year); middle ear infections during infancy and early childhood; conductive loss in some cases; language and articulation disorders consistent with hearing impairment; and visual, spatial, and attentional problems.

Usher Syndrome

- Usher syndrome is caused by autosomal recessive inheritance in most cases and is X-linked in rare cases. This syndrome may affect 50% of individuals who are deaf and blind.
- Its physical characteristics include night blindness in early childhood, limited peripheral vision as visual problems worsen, eventual blindness, and cochlear abnormalities.
- Communication problems include sensorineural loss, language and articulation disorders consistent with hearing impairment, and hypernasality and nasal emission.

Velocardiofacial Syndrome

- Velocardiofacial syndrome (VCFS) is the syndrome most commonly associated with a cleft palate, usually a cleft of the soft palate. VCFS is also called **Shprintzen syndrome** after Dr. Robert Shprintzen, who first described this condition in 1978.
- Though the exact cause of VCFS is not known, it is known to be a genetic disorder. A small part of chromosome 22, known as 22q11.2, is missing in most people with VCFS. VCFS is an autosomal disorder; only one parent needs to have the gene in order to pass it on to the children. VCFS has also been called **DiGeorge sequence**.
- In addition to cleft palate, over 180 other anomalies are associated with VCFS. Not every child has all anomalies, nor is any one anomaly present in all children with VCFS.
- Major anomalies include middle ear infections, learning problems, speech and feeding problems, and unique facial characteristics. Usually, cleft palate and/or velopharyngeal insufficiency is present.
- Craniofacial characteristics include a wide nose, small ears, almond-shaped eyes, micrognathia, microcephaly, and an elongated face.

- Children with VCFS may have significant language difficulties as well as articulation disorders and intellectual disability. Intelligence is generally in the low–normal range.
- The neonatal period of babies with VCFS is especially challenging. Feeding problems and failure to thrive are common, and often doctors refer these infants to SLPs for feeding therapy.
- Feeding problems are frequently complicated by generalized and pharyngeal hypotonia, oral apraxia, laryngeal and vascular anomalies, and nasal regurgitation and nasal vomiting. Special feeding strategies carefully implemented can help to make gastrostomies and nasogastric tubes unnecessary.

Williams Syndrome

- Williams syndrome (WS) is a rare genetic disorder that affects an estimated 1 out of every 20,000 babies. Sometimes WS is called **elfin-face syndrome**, because people with WS have a physical resemblance to elves. They are often small boned and short, with a long upper lip, wide mouth, full lips, small chin, upturned nose, and puffiness around the eyes.
- WS is caused by an abnormality on chromosome 7, including a gene that makes the protein elastin. Elastin provides elasticity and strength to blood vessel walls. Specifically, it is thought that the developmental and medical problems of people with WS are caused by the deletion of approximately 25 genes on one copy of chromosome 7q11.23.
- Most people with WS have IQs between 50 and 70; however, they can show high intelligence in certain areas, such as music, language, and interpersonal skills. Children with WS often have charming personalities; they are courteous, gregarious, and loving and are unafraid of strangers (which worries their parents).
- WS causes a varied profile of medical and developmental problems; each child's profile is unique. Some children have an elevated blood calcium level, or hypercalcemia, which can cause extreme irritability. Sometimes it is necessary for these children to undergo medical or dietary intervention.
- Most children with WS have narrowed pulmonary arteries and a narrowed aorta. These problems can range from mild to severe and may necessitate surgical intervention.
- Children with WS may also have abnormalities of dental occlusion or bite, as well as small, widely spaced teeth. Usually these problems can be corrected with orthodontia.

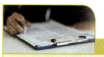

SUMMARY

- Many genetic syndromes are associated with communication disorders. Those syndromes often cause disorders of speech, language, voice, and resonance.
- Some individuals are born with genetic syndromes. One of the most common is Down syndrome.
- Many but not all syndromes are accompanied by language disorders, intellectual disability, and speech sound disorders. There may also be hearing and feeding problems.
- Persons with syndromes frequently benefit from a multidisciplinary team approach that addresses a wide variety of medical, speech, language, hearing, and other needs.

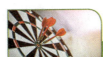

CHAPTER HIGHLIGHTS

- Speech–language pathologists treat persons with clefts of the lip, palate, or both. A multidisciplinary team approach is usually necessary.
- Craniofacial anomalies, such as cleft lip and, palate are due mostly to genetic factors, although environmental and mechanical factors may also play a role.
- Persons with clefts of the palate have communication disorders associated with the clefts. These disorders include hearing loss as well as disorders of speech, language, resonance, and voice.
- When assessing children with clefts, it is necessary to evaluate velopharyngeal competence as well as speech, language, phonatory, and resonance disorders. Use of appropriate instrumentation is very helpful.
- Intervention for children with clefts usually consists of surgical management combined with treatment of disorders of speech, language, resonance, and voice.
- Many genetic syndromes are associated with communication disorders. Syndromes that involve the craniofacial complex and those that affect general intellectual functions tend to produce the most significant effects on communication.
- One of the most common syndromes is Down syndrome. Tourette Syndrome has become increasingly common.
- Many but not all syndromes are accompanied by language disorders, intellectual disability, and speech sound disorders. There may also be hearing and feeding problems.
- Persons with syndromes frequently benefit from a multidisciplinary team approach that addresses a wide variety of medical, speech, language, hearing, and other needs.

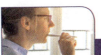

STUDY AND REVIEW QUESTIONS

1. You have been asked to give an in-service to a group of students who wish to eventually specialize in service delivery to children with cleft palates and their families. The students want to know detailed information about in utero development of the hard and soft palate (among other things). You can accurately tell them that in utero, the hard palate fuses between the developmental ages of

    A. 1 and 2 weeks.
    B. 5 and 6 weeks.
    C. 8 and 9 weeks.
    D. 10 and 12 weeks.

Questions 2–4 refer to the following scenario:

A clinician in a private practice is approached by the parents of Tommy D., a 5-year-old boy. The parents want to place Tommy in kindergarten in the fall but say, "We know there's something wrong with him—we're just not sure what." According to Tommy's parents, he is a "sweet, lovable boy who will go to anybody. He likes to sing a lot, too." Because the parents live in a rural area, health care access has been limited. After seeing Tommy for the first time, the clinician refers his parents to a neurologist because she suspects that Tommy has a syndrome. He is small for his age and has an elfin-like appearance characterized by a small chin, turned-up nose, puffiness around the eyes, a long upper lip, and a wide mouth. His teeth are small and widely spaced.

2. The clinician suspects that Tommy has

  A. Williams syndrome.
  B. Apert syndrome.
  C. Moebius syndrome.
  D. Turner syndrome.

3. This syndrome is caused by a rare genetic disorder that affects an estimated 1 out of every 20,000 babies. It is caused by

  A. a missing part of chromosome 22, known as 22q11.
  B. an expanded number of cytosine-guanine-guanine (CGG) nucleic acid repeats on a specific gene on one of the distal ends of the X chromosome.
  C. a spontaneous autosomal dominant mutation, whose gene and locus is FGR2 at 10q25–26.
  D. the deletion of approximately 25 genes on one copy of chromosome 7q11.23.

4. The clinician knows that she will probably end up seeing Tommy for intervention if his parents are able to bring him on a weekly basis. She will probably be working on which of the following goals?

  A. Pragmatics, to increase Tommy's ability to interact with others
  B. Oral–motor coordination, because children with this syndrome usually have oral–motor coordination problems, which contribute to decreased intelligibility
  C. Overall expressive and receptive language, because children with this syndrome generally have IQs of 50–70 (although some have good language skills)
  D. Morphological skills, because although children with this syndrome usually have above average IQs, they frequently delete bound morphemes from the beginnings and ends of words

5. A condition in which the surface tissues of the soft or hard palate fuse but the underlying muscle or bone tissues do not is called

  A. fusion disorder.
  B. submucous or occult cleft palate.
  C. class III palatal cleft.
  D. submucosal cleft class IV.

6. Though cleft palate is often caused by genetic factors, it can also be related to mechanical factors. Which one of these is NOT a mechanical factor related to cleft palate?

  A. Intrauterine crowding
  B. Twinning
  C. Uterine tumor
  D. Illegal drug use by the birth mother

7. Children with bilateral cleft lip or palate may have problems with their teeth. A common problem for these children is

    A. supernumerary teeth.

    B. teeth erupting out of the hard palate.

    C. hypodontia or missing teeth.

    D. teeth that are too small.

8. The surgical method of cleft palate repair that involves raising two bipedicled flaps of mucoperiosteum, bringing them together, and attaching them to close the cleft is called the

    A. von Langenbeck surgical method.

    B. V-Y retroposition.

    C. Veau-Wardill-Kilner method.

    D. pharyngeal flap procedure.

9. A child comes to a clinic with her mother for articulation therapy. The mother tells the clinician that her daughter has Hurler's syndrome. Hurler's syndrome is caused by

    A. autosomal recessive deficiency of X-L iduronidase.

    B. a spontaneous autosomal dominant mutation of FGR 2 at 10q25–26.

    C. autosomal dominant inheritance and deletion in the region of the long arm of chromosome 15 (15q11–15q13).

    D. an expanded number of cytosine-guanine-guanine (CGG) nucleic acid repeats on a specific gene on one of the distal ends of the Y chromosome.

10. A school-based clinician is assessing the velopharyngeal adequacy of Janie K., a 17-year-old immigrant high school student from the Philippines. Janie was born with a cleft of the palate and lip; there was no repair until her family came to the United States when Janie was 16 years old. In the Philippines, Janie and her family lived on Tablas, a small and rural island, where surgery was unavailable. Though the repair surgery in the United States a year ago was successful and Janie now has a more aesthetically pleasing appearance and better speech, there is still audible nasal emission and hypernasality when she speaks. The clinician plans to refer her to a local craniofacial team, but he also wants to conduct as thorough an examination as he can despite the lack of instrumentation available at his school site. He does have access to an oral manometer. He uses this to provide a beginning point from which to refer Janie to the craniofacial team. After obtaining a ratio by comparing pressures achieved in the nostrils-occluded and the nostrils-open conditions, the clinician concludes that Janie especially needs to be referred to the craniofacial team for possible further surgery or a pharyngeal flap. When he used oral manometry, the clinician probably found that Janie

    A. had a ratio of 1.0.

    B. had a ratio of 1.2.

    C. had a ratio of .96.

    D. had a ratio of .87.

11. In infants and children with cleft palates, Eustachian tube dysfunction is probably mostly related to the lack of contraction of the

    A. levator veli palatini muscle.

    B. veli palatini muscle.

    C. tensor veli palatini muscle.

    D. palatopharyngeus muscle.

12. You are serving a child with a repaired cleft palate. Marissa is 11 and still somewhat unintelligible, manifesting difficulty with some speech sounds. To help her, you employ a specialized procedure. In this procedure, an orthodontist will design an artificial palate containing 62 embedded electrodes connected to a computer. This will be fitted into Marissa's mouth, and when her tongue contacts the electrodes during speech production, articulatory patterns can be seen on the computer screen. This procedure is called

    A. electropalatography.
    B. electroglottography.
    C. palatomyography.
    D. myomanometry.

13. A child from Apple City transfers to Middleton City, and his file indicates that he has been receiving speech–language services in Apple City. To the chagrin of the Middleton City clinician, some pages of the report from the SLP in Apple City are missing. However, on the first page, it is indicated that this child has Moebius syndrome. He also has a history of frequent hospitalizations. The Middleton City clinician can probably expect to find that this child

    A. has low muscle tone, a history of early feeding difficulties, initial failure to thrive, obesity after the first year, and underdeveloped genitals.
    B. has underdeveloped facial bones, including mandibular hypoplasia, malar hypoplasia, dental malocclusion, and downwardly slanted palpebral fissures.
    C. has a small maxillary structure, sphenoethmoidal synchondroses, ocular hypertelorism, facial asymmetry including a tall forehead, and brachycephaly.
    D. may have delayed language and an articulation disorder, as well as bilabial paresis and weak tongue control for lateralization, elevation, depression, and protrusion; a masklike face; a history of feeding problems in infancy; and unilateral or bilateral paralysis of the abductors of the eye.

14. A clinician is a member of a cleft palate team that asks her to conduct an objective assessment of an 8-year-old child's velopharyngeal mechanism. The clinician decides to do nasopharyngoscopy, in which a nasopharyngoscope is passed through the middle meatus and back to the area of velopharyngeal closure. This will enable the clinician to observe the child's

    A. adenoid pads and anterior pharyngeal walls as the child prolongs /s/.
    B. posterior and lateral pharyngeal walls, as well as the adenoid pad, as the child sustains /ɑ/.
    C. nasal aspect of the velum and the adenoid pad as the child produces CVC words.
    D. posterior and lateral pharyngeal walls, as well as the nasal aspect of the velum and the adenoid pad, as the child produces sentences.

15. You have received a referral of Akhtar, a 4-year-old refugee child from a Dari-speaking family from Afghanistan. Akhtar has never been evaluated or received speech–language services. Before you meet Akhtar, you speak with the doctor, who explains that Akhtar has midface dysplasia, a high and narrow arched palate, a relatively large and fissured tongue that protrudes, hearing loss, and speech sound disorder. Akhtar also has generalized hypotonia and brachycephaly (small head). You can confidently conclude that Akhtar has

   A. Crouzon syndrome.
   B. Cri du chat syndrome.
   C. Down syndrome.
   D. Hurler syndrome.

16. You are on a cleft palate and craniofacial anomalies team that evaluates children with cleft palates. When a child has a resonance problem, the team decides whether the child will benefit from speech therapy alone or more intensive medical intervention (e.g., surgery) is needed. As part of the assessment process, cephalometric analysis is used. In cephalometric analysis, the Cephalometric Assessment of Velopharyngeal Structures computer program analyzes the ratio relationship between the length of the soft palate and the depth of the nasopharynx. Which one of the following statements best summarizes a key principle that guides treatment decisions?

   A. A ratio of less than 60 is usually found when the soft palate is too short and the nasopharynx is too shallow.
   B. A ratio of less than 60 is usually found when the nasopharynx is too deep or the soft palate is too long.
   C. A ratio of 60–80 generally indicates adequate tissue for velopharyngeal closure for speech.
   D. If a ratio is higher than 80, this means the nasopharynx is too shallow or the velum is too long.

17. You are providing support for a man with Marfan syndrome; he has difficulties with respiration, and you are working on breathing techniques. He shares with you that he and his wife want to have a child, and they are concerned about their child possibly having Marfan syndrome. You refer him to a genetic counselor, who will share with him that Marfan syndrome is

   A. an autosomal, dominant inherited disorder caused by mutations in the FBN1 gene.
   B. an autosomal recessive disorder caused by mutations in the FBN1 gene.
   C. a partial deletion syndrome caused by mutations in the FBN2 gene.
   D. not genetically transferred to offspring, so the parents do not need to be concerned.

18. As part of your job in a public-school district, you serve several preschools. You get an urgent call from a parent at one of the schools. She states that her daughter Michelle (age 4), who previously had typical language skills, has suddenly "lost her words," and is having seizures. She shares that Michelle "is so much more hyper now, and we don't know what's wrong." The mom shares that they have an appointment with Michelle's pediatrician to find out more about what is happening. You support this decision, especially because you suspect that Michelle has

   A. Williams syndrome.
   B. Landau-Kleffner syndrome.
   C. Treacher Collins syndrome.
   D. Pierre-Robin syndrome.

19. In your private practice, a father brings his 5-year-old son, Jordan, to see you. The kindergarten teacher has noticed that Jordan "talks kind of funny," and sometimes other children make fun of him. Justin was born with a cleft palate and has had repair surgery, and he has a history of conductive hearing loss secondary to otitis media with effusion. During your evaluation of Jordan's speech, you note that he is especially having difficulty producing affricates, fricatives, and plosives. This is probably because he is having continued difficulty with

   A. vocal nodules.
   B. hypertrophied adenoids.
   C. velopharyngeal closure.
   D. maxillary deficiency.

20. You are serving in a juvenile detention facility and receive a referral of Max, a 16-year-old with documented Fragile X syndrome. Which of the following will you expect to find when you evaluate Max?

   A. Attention deficits, a large tongue, sleep disturbances, and a high, protruding forehead
   B. Speech sound disorders, normal intelligence, expressive language delays, and micrognathia
   C. Gargoylism, tracheal stenosis, brachycephaly, and hypertonia
   D. Intellectual disability and delays in pragmatic, semantic, phonologic, and syntactic aspects of language, with syntax being especially affected

References and Recommended Readings at www.advancedreviewpractice.com

STUDY AND REVIEW ANSWERS

1. C. In utero, the hard palate fuses between the developmental ages of 8 and 9 weeks' gestation.
2. A. Because Tommy is small for his age and has an elfin-like appearance characterized by a small chin, turned-up nose, puffiness around the eyes, a long upper lip, and a wide mouth with small and widely spaced teeth, he probably has Williams syndrome.
3. D. Williams syndrome is caused by the deletion of approximately 25 genes on one copy of chromosome 7q11.23.
4. C. The clinician will probably work on increasing overall expressive and receptive language, because children with Williams syndrome generally have IQs between 50 and 70 (although some of these children have good language skills).
5. B. A condition in which the surface tissues of the soft or hard palate fuse but the underlying muscle or bone tissues do not is called submucous or occult cleft palate.
6. D. Illegal drug use by the birth mother is not a mechanical factor related to clefting.
7. C. Children with bilateral clefts of the palate and lip commonly have hypodontia, or missing teeth.
8. A. The surgical method of cleft palate repair that involves raising two bipedicled flaps of mucoperiosteum, bringing them together, and attaching them to close the cleft is called the von Langenbeck surgical method.

9. A. Hurler's syndrome is caused by autosomal recessive deficiency of X-L iduronidase.
10. D. When the clinician did oral manometric testing, he probably found that Janie had a ratio of .87. Anything below .89 is especially indicative of problems.
11. C. In infants and children with cleft palates, Eustachian tube dysfunction is mostly related to the lack of contraction of the tensor veli palatini muscle.
12. A. This procedure is called electropalatography.
13. D. A child with Moebius syndrome can be expected to have possible delayed language and an articulation disorder, as well as bilabial paresis and weak tongue control for lateralization, elevation, depression, and protrusion; a masklike face; a history of feeding problems in infancy; and unilateral or bilateral paralysis of the abductors of the eye.
14. D. Nasopharyngoscopy enables the clinician to observe the posterior and lateral pharyngeal walls, as well as the nasal aspect of the velum and the adenoid pad, as the child produces sentences.
15. C. Akhtar has Down Syndrome, which is characterized by generalized hypotonia, brachycephaly, midface dysplasia, a high and narrow arched palate, and a relatively large and fissured tongue that tends to protrude. Persons with Down syndrome may also have hearing loss and speech sound disorder.
16. C. A ratio of 60–80 generally indicates adequate tissue for velopharyngeal closure for speech.
17. A. Marfan syndrome is an autosomal, dominant inherited disorder caused by mutations in the *FBN1* gene
18. B. In Landau-Kleffner syndrome, children may experience sudden loss of language, seizures, and hyperactivity.
19. C. If a child with a repaired cleft palate specifically has continued difficulty with fricatives, affricates, and plosives, this generally indicates continued inadequate velopharyngeal closure.
20. D. Teen boys with Fragile X syndrome commonly show intellectual disability and delays in pragmatic, semantic, phonologic, and syntactic aspects of language, with syntax being especially affected.

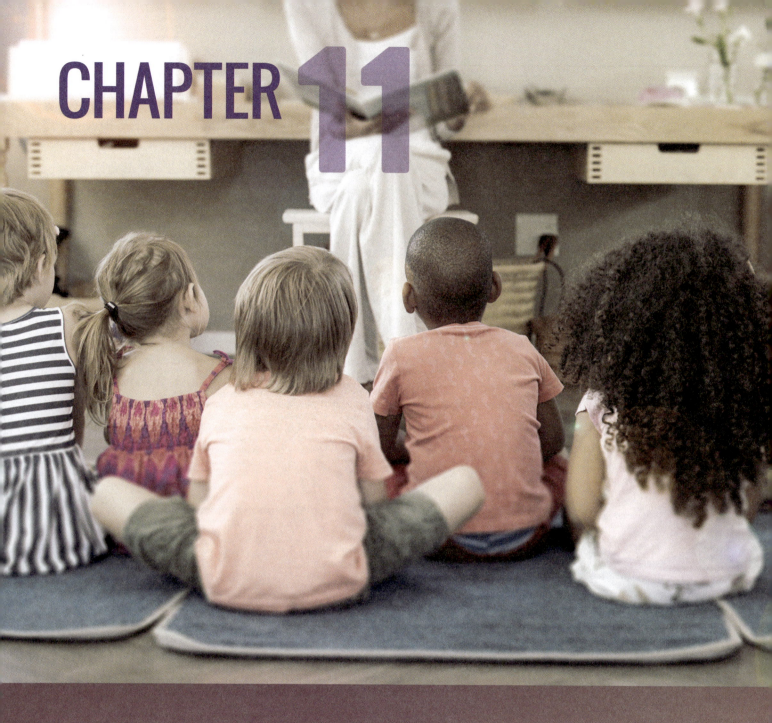

CHAPTER 11

COMMUNICATION DISORDERS IN MULTICULTURAL POPULATIONS

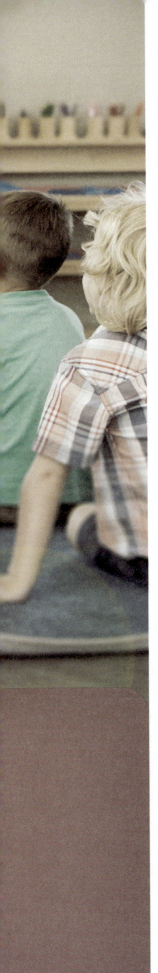

The United States population has been likened to a kaleidoscope that is constantly changing colors and becoming more and more diverse. By the year 2055, the U.S. will not have a single racial or ethnic majority. The number of foreign-born persons in the U.S. has more than quadrupled since 1965 and is expected to reach 78 million by 2065 (Pew Hispanic Research Center, 2018).

With increasing numbers of culturally and linguistically diverse (CLD) adults and children in the United States, the number of people who have disorders of communication is also growing. Clinicians frequently find themselves attempting to effectively serve an increasingly diverse client group, and it is imperative that they be as culturally competent and knowledgeable as possible (Roseberry-McKibbin, 2018).

This chapter presents foundational issues concerning serving CLD clients. The speech–language characteristics of African American, Hispanic, and Asian clients and the ramifications for assessment and treatment are described. The chapter discusses the differentiation of language differences from language impairments in CLD children who are English learners (ELs) and describes how issues of second-language acquisition and bilingualism can affect service delivery. Knowledge of second-language acquisition and bilingualism is critical to a fair and unbiased assessment of the language skills of EL children. Considerations in the use of standardized tests, alternatives to standardized tests, and important concepts in working with interpreters in the assessment process are reviewed. The section on treatment considerations discusses issues related to treatment of EL children with language impairments, as well as considerations for CLD adults with neurologically based disorders of communication.

FOUNDATIONAL ISSUES

Because of the increasing number of CLD people living in the United States, speech–language pathologists (SLPs) need to understand basic cultural characteristics that can affect service delivery to this population. The American Speech-Language-Hearing Association (ASHA, 2017) has developed policies and position statements that provide guidance for clinicians who work with CLD clients.

General Cultural Considerations

Basic Principles

- When working with CLD clients of all ages, it is important to have a basic understanding of what culture is. Culture is a dynamic, multifaceted phenomenon that is influenced by many variables.
- **Culture** can be viewed as a framework through which actions are filtered, as individuals go about the business of daily living. It includes the beliefs, behaviors, and values of a group of people (Battle, 2012a).
- Speech–language pathologists must develop cultural competence (Fogle, 2019). This can be done in many ways. The culturally competent SLP is one who (a) is actively in the process of becoming aware of his or her own assumptions; (b) actively attempts to understand the worldview of his or her culturally diverse clients and families; and (c) is actively developing and practicing culturally relevant, sensitive, and appropriate service delivery skills and practices.
- For example, the culturally competent SLP, when faced with a child or adult client who speaks a different language than the SLP, would engage the services of a trained interpreter to be present for assessment and intervention procedures.
- It is important for SLPs to develop as much cultural sensitivity as possible. This can be done through a variety of activities that focus on continually learning more about the cultures of the clients served.
- Reading literature, conducting home visits, and talking to families and community members about the culture in question will help clinicians become sensitive to and aware of cultural variables that can affect service delivery.
- A danger of attempting to understand any cultural group is that stereotyping and overgeneralizing may occur. **Stereotypes** can be viewed as a means of categorizing others based upon perceptions that are incomplete.
- Ideally, SLPs should understand **tendencies** of various cultural groups, so that clients and families can be viewed as individuals within the general framework of their community and culture.
- Professionals must keep in mind the great heterogeneity within cultural groups. It is optimal to take a situational approach, wherein each individual is viewed as unique, with shifting needs, characteristics, and strengths.
- One way to view each individual as unique is to learn the name of the geographic or cultural group given by its members and use this name. For example, if a client is from Mexico, this client may be described as Mexican or Mexican American, not Hispanic. A client from the Philippines may be described as Filipino American, not Asian. This shows respect for individuals and acknowledgment of their unique heritage.

Variables Influencing Individual Behavior Within a Culture

- A number of variables influence the behavior of individuals within a culture. The combination of general cultural practices and individual characteristics of people within cultures influences service delivery to those clients and their families.

- Potential variables of influence upon individuals include the following (Moore & Montgomery, 2018; Roseberry-McKibbin, 2018; Spector, 2017):

  - **Educational level**, which may be quite basic (e.g., a few years of schooling) or sophisticated and extensive
  - **Language(s) spoken**, including the prestige of the language(s) in the area of residence and the level of skill in each language
  - Length of residence in an area
  - **Country of birth** (foreign born or native born), which relates to immigrant or refugee status versus being born in the United States
  - Urban versus rural background
  - Gender
  - Religion
  - Age
  - Generational membership
  - Socioeconomic status and upward class mobility
  - Neighborhood and peer group
  - Degree of acculturation into mainstream American life
  - **Outmarriage** (marriage to someone from a different ethnic background) status
  - **Individual choice** within the intrapersonal realm (for example, choosing what church to attend)

- Immigrants who come to the United States are incorporated into society by the processes of acculturation and assimilation. **Acculturation** refers to the process by which immigrants assume American cultural attributes (e.g., cultural norms and values).
- **Assimilation** is the process of their incorporation into the cultural and social networks of the host society (e.g., place of residence, family, leisure activities, work). It refers to the degree to which immigrants give up their culture of origin and take on the characteristics of the new culture.
- There are various levels of acculturation. Immigrants who are **bicultural** are fully involved in both their own and the host cultures. They maintain their native language and become fluent in the new language, too. They maintain many of their own cultural practices and adopt the host culture's practices, as well. They are comfortable going back and forth between the two cultures.

ASHA Guidelines Regarding Multicultural Issues

- Due to the increasing cultural and linguistic diversity in the United States, ASHA has developed policies, position statements, and guidelines regarding service delivery to CLD clients (ASHA, 2017).
- ASHA's Office of Multicultural Affairs and its Multicultural Issues Board are active in the creation and implementation of these guidelines. Copies of guidelines and policies are available; interested readers can contact the national office in Rockville, Maryland. ASHA has also created Special

Interest Division 14 (SID #14), Communication Disorders and Sciences in Culturally and Linguistically Diverse Populations.
- It is important to have a basic knowledge of the various position statements in order to provide effective service delivery consistent with ASHA's policies.
- ASHA has continually attempted to address the issue of effective service delivery to members of various cultural and linguistic groups. For example, ASHA developed a focused initiative relevant to improving services to members of CLD populations. ASHA has developed a practice portal to help SLPs build their cultural competence.

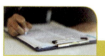

SUMMARY

- The increasing number of culturally and linguistically diverse people living in the United States makes it imperative for clinicians to be sensitive to cultural issues that affect service delivery. Clinicians must become culturally competent.
- A number of variables, such as age and generational membership, affect the behavior of individual clients from various cultures.
- ASHA has published guidelines regarding effective service delivery to clients from linguistically and culturally diverse backgrounds.

SPEECH–LANGUAGE CHARACTERISTICS OF CLD CLIENTS

When attempting to ascertain whether clients are manifesting speech–language differences or impairments, it is important to have a basic understanding of how various dialects and languages influence the production of Mainstream American English (MAE). It is also critical to remember that within each language group, there is great diversity. For example, the Philippines, a country the size of Arizona, has more than 87 mutually intelligible languages.

Unfortunately, it is common in the United States for adults and especially children to be labeled as having an impairment or "disorder" when, in fact, they are merely manifesting speech–language differences attributable to their primary language or dialect. For example, clients whose first language is Spanish, or an Asian language, manifest characteristics of articulation, morphology, and syntax that differ from patterns of MAE. Clients who speak a dialect of American English may also manifest such characteristics. In this section, we discuss dialects of American English, African American English (AAE), Spanish-influenced English, and English influenced by Asian languages.

Dialects of American English

- In the United States, MAE is used in government communications, printing, national television newscasts, and many businesses. Many consider MAE to be the official language of the United States.

- Every language is spoken somewhat differently by different subgroups of a linguistic community. MAE has several dialects; each one has characteristic sound patterns, including typical expressions and unique accents.
- Dialectal differences are due to several interrelated factors, including geographic region, socioeconomic level, speaking situation, and subgroup membership.
- People living in different parts of the United States develop variations of language use and production. Based on geographic regions, specialists have identified 10 major dialects of MAE: New York City, Eastern New England, Western Pennsylvania, Appalachian, Southern, Middle Atlantic, Central Midland, Southwest, Northwest, and North Central (see Figure 11.1).

African American English

General Background

- African American English (AAE) has undergone many changes in nomenclature over the years. It has been called Black Dialect, Black English, Black English Vernacular, African American Language, and Ebonics. The changes in nomenclature have been due in part to increasingly sophisticated understanding of AAE and to changes in sociolinguistic theory. Today, AAE is viewed as a systematic, rule-governed dialect of general American English (Goldstein & Iglesias, 2017).
- Use of AAE is influenced by a number of factors, including retention of some African language patterns, geographic region, socioeconomic status, education, gender, age of the speaker, and bonding between members of the African American community.
- A number of West African languages have impacted modern-day AAE: Bambara, Ewe, Fanta, Fon, Fula, Ga, Ibibio, Ibo, Imbundu, Kimbundu, Longo, Mandinka, Mende, Twi, Wolof, and Yoruba.

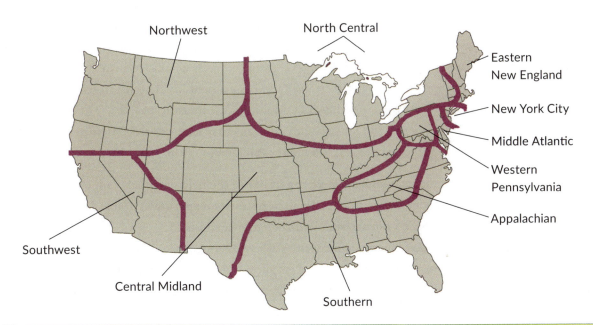

Figure 11.1 The major dialects of American English. From *Introduction to Communicative Disorders* (5th ed.), by M. N. Hegde, forthcoming, Austin, TX: PRO-ED. Copyright by PRO-ED, Inc. Reprinted with permission.

Misconceptions About AAE

There are some widespread assumptions and misconceptions about AAE and its speakers, and these are listed below. So that AAE speakers are not mistakenly identified as having disorders, it is important to be aware of these misconceptions (Battle, 2012b; Pearson, Conner, & Jackson, 2013; Roseberry-McKibbin, 2018):

- **All African Americans speak AAE**. Some African Americans speak AAE; some do not. Some code-switch back and forth between MAE and AAE depending on variables such as topic, listener, and communicative intent. Most African Americans who are socialized primarily with Anglos generally speak MAE.
- **AAE is spoken only by African Americans**. AAE may be spoken by people of any ethnic or linguistic background. Non-African Americans may speak AAE if their primary peer group is composed of African Americans. For example, some Puerto Rican students in New York City speak AAE, and some Anglo students in Oakland, California, speak AAE.
- **AAE is a substandard form of Mainstream American English**. Some people historically took a "deficit perspective"; a major premise of this view was that African Americans were cognitively unable to learn MAE. The **ethnolinguistic theory** of today states that AAE is a dialect in its own right; its roots can be traced to many languages of West Africa, as previously suggested.
- **AAE does not have a regular, predictable system**. In previous decades, it was believed that AAE was unpredictable and not rule governed. Today, it is widely known that AAE is a rule-governed system in which patterns can be predicted based on rules.
- **If children speak AAE, their use of AAE must be discontinued**. Some experts believe that speakers of AAE should become "bilingual" or "bidialectal" so that they can fluently speak both AAE and MAE. In this optimal situation, individuals preserve their culture, heritage, and community dialect, as well as learn a style of speaking that is required in some daily situations, school learning experiences, and future places of employment.
- **Use of standardized language tests with AAE speakers is a nonbiased indicator of actual language knowledge and skill**. Many currently used assessment instruments in schools are normed and standardized on Anglo, middle-class, monolingual English speakers. These tests have been criticized as being inappropriate for use with African American children (Battle, 2012b; Oetting, McDonald, Seibel, & Hegarty, 2016; Roseberry-McKibbin, 2018).

Many standardized tests of morphosyntactic skill, especially in the field of speech–language pathology, are biased against AAE speakers (and those from other non-English backgrounds). Table 11.1 shows examples of bias against speakers of AAE on formal, standardized language tests.

It is recommended that when clients who speak AAE are assessed, alternative forms of assessment be used. These alternative forms of assessment include language sample analysis, contrastive analysis, and description of children's functional communication skills. It is also recommended that standardized tests of aphasia be appropriately modified for adults who speak AAE (Payne, 2014).

Characteristics of AAE Morphology, Syntax, and Articulation

- Before testing AAE speakers, it is critical to know which aspects of their speech and language are reflective of AAE rules and which are indicative of an underlying speech or language impairment. Many

Table 11.1

Examples of Bias Against Speakers of AAE on Formal Language and Intelligence Tests

1. Grammatical judgment items.

Examiner: Tell me whether the following sentences are correct or incorrect:

Them girls is having a good time.
The boys is going to the party.
We don't have no time to talk to you.

2. Sentence repetition tasks.

Examiner: Repeat these sentences after me. Remember to say them EXACTLY as I say them!

Neither of the children are using the swings.
They had been hungry.
She looks at the big, brown dog.

3. Grammatical closure tasks.

Examiner: I am going to say some sentences. I want you to fill in the word that is missing. For example, "A rose is a flower, and a daisy is a flower. Daisies and roses are both _____." Now you do some:

Today I play the marimba; yesterday I _____ the marimba.
I have a cat, and you have a cat; we have two _____.
Today Sue is going to the store; yesterday she _____ going to the store.

4. Receptive grammatical tasks.

Examiner: We are going to look at some pictures. Each page has three pictures. When I say a sentence, you point to the picture that goes with the sentence I say. Here's the first picture.

Show me "The cats are playing in the garden."
Now show me "He played baseball."
Point to "They have been painting the fence."

5. Articulation and phonological tasks. Most tests of articulation and phonology are normed on Anglo children. The speech–language pathologist must remember to take into account the unique characteristics of AAE when assessing articulation and phonology.

Note. From *Multicultural Students With Special Language Needs: Practical Strategies for Assessment and Intervention* (4th ed., p. 244), by C. Roseberry-McKibbin, 2014, Oceanside, CA: Academic Communication Associates. Copyright 2014 by Academic Communication Associates. Reprinted with permission.

SLPs take children who speak AAE in the public schools onto their caseloads for "remediation" of AAE. Not only is this illegal but it is often unsuccessful, as well.

- Some adult speakers of AAE, however, may elect to become bidialectal, choosing to become proficient in MAE as well as AAE. Being bidialectal enables these speakers to maintain their use of AAE while also being able to use MAE for purposes such as conducting business with non-AAE speakers.

- Parents may also choose elective intervention for their children so that their children can become bidialectal. This elective intervention cannot be provided in the public school setting; however, parents may seek these services through universities and private practices.

- When SLPs are aware of the typical characteristics of AAE, they can distinguish between a speech–language difference and a speech–language impairment in children who speak AAE. Table 11.2 shows the characteristics of AAE morphology and syntax, while Table 11.3 shows the characteristics of AAE articulation and phonology. Table 11.4 shows some examples of acceptable utterances by speakers of AAE.

Spanish-Influenced English

General Background

- The term **Hispanic** is a label of convenience used to refer to people who reside in the United States but were born in or trace the background of their families to one of the Spanish-speaking Latin American nations or to Spain or Portugal. The term may also be used to refer to people from Caribbean countries, such as Cuba. The term **Latino** is also frequently used.
- **Hispanic** is used as an ethnic label by the U.S. Bureau of the Census; it does not denote a race. Most Hispanics are racially mixed, including combinations of American Indian, African Black, and European White. The majority are **mestizo**, having both a European and an Indian heritage. Most Hispanics prefer to be referred to according to their country of origin (e.g., Cuban American, Mexican American).
- Hispanics constitute one of the fastest-growing segments of the U.S. population. Today, 55 million people or 17% of the American population are of Hispanic origin (National Hispanic Heritage Month, 2017).

Spanish-Language Characteristics and Considerations

- The diversity among Spanish speakers is great. Although Spanish is spoken in Spain and most of Latin America, there are variations, which are reflected mostly in pronunciation and some vocabulary.
- Spanish speakers in the United States may speak different dialects or varieties of Spanish (Goldstein & Iglesias, 2017). The two major Spanish dialects in the United States are southwestern (e.g., Mexican) and Caribbean (e.g., Puerto Rican). Thus, clinicians must consider the individual client's background and origins, which are reflected in the variety of Spanish used, and not assume that each Spanish-speaking client can be viewed in the same way (Brice, 2015).
- Spanish-speaking individuals who learn English as a second language may manifest differences with MAE in articulation of sounds and in morphosyntactic structures. There are many structural differences between English and Spanish, especially with respect to morphology.
- These differences are not indicative of an underlying language impairment requiring intervention but are differences that are typical and to be expected. It is important for professionals who work with Spanish-speaking clients to understand foundational information regarding Spanish-influenced English. Table 11.5 describes the articulation characteristics of Spanish and the possible influences on pronunciation of English. Table 11.6 describes the morphosyntactic characteristics of Spanish and possible influences on English production.

Table 11.2

Characteristics of African American English Morphology and Syntax

AAE characteristic	Mainstream American English	Sample AAE utterance
Omission of noun possessive	That's the woman's car. It's John's pencil.	That the *woman* car. It *John* pencil.
Omission of noun plural	He has two boxes of apples. She gives me 5 cents.	He got two box of *apple*. She give me 5 *cent*.
Omission of third-person singular present-tense marker	She walks to school. The man works in his yard.	She *walk* to school. The man *work* in his yard.
Omission of *to be* forms, such as *is* and *are*	She is a nice lady. They are going to a movie.	She a nice lady. They going to a movie.
Present tense used regardless of person and number	They are having fun. You are a smart man.	*They is* having fun. *You is* a smart man!
Lack of person–number agreement with past and present forms of *to be*	You are playing ball. They are having a picnic.	You *is* playing ball. They *is* having a picnic.
Present-tense forms of auxiliary *have* omitted	I have been here for 2 hours. He has done it again.	I *been* here for 2 hours. He *done* it again.
Past-tense endings omitted	He lived in California. She cracked the nut.	He *live* in California. She *crack* the nut.
Past *was* used regardless of number and person	They were shopping. You were helping me.	They *was* shopping. You *was* helping me.
Multiple negatives; each additional negative form, adding emphasis to the negative meaning	We don't have any more. I don't want any cake. I don't like broccoli.	We don't have *no* more. I don't never want *no* cake. I don't *never* like broccoli.
None substituted for *any*	She doesn't want any.	She don't want *none*.
Perfective construction; *been* used to indicate that an action took place in the distant past	I had the mumps when I was 5. I have known her for years.	I *been had* the mumps when I was 5. I *been* known her.
Done combined with a past-tense form to indicate that an action was started and completed	He fixed the stove. She tried to paint it.	He *done fixed* the stove. She *done tried* to paint it.
The form *be* used as the main verb	Today she is working. We are singing.	Today *she be* working. *We be* singing.
Distributive *be* used to indicate actions and events over time	He is often cheerful. She's kind sometimes.	*He be* cheerful. *She be* kind.
Pronoun used to restate the subject	My brother surprised me. My dog has fleas.	My brother, *he* surprise me. My dog, *he* got fleas.
Them substituted for *those*	Those cars are antiques. Where'd you get those books?	*Them* cars, they be antique. Where you get *them* books?
Future tense *is* and *are* replaced by *gonna*	She is going to help us. They are going to be there.	She *gonna* help us. They *gonna* be there.
At used at the end of *where* questions	Where is the house? Where is the store?	Where is the house *at*? Where is the store *at*?
Additional auxiliaries often used	I might have done it.	I *might could* have done it.
Does replaced by *do*	She does funny things. It does make sense.	She *do* funny things. It *do* make sense.

Note. From *Multicultural Students With Special Language Needs: Practical Strategies for Assessment and Intervention* (5th ed., pp. 70–71), by C. Roseberry-McKibbin, 2018, Oceanside, CA: Academic Communication Associates. Copyright 2018 by Academic Communication Associates. Reprinted with permission.

Table 11.3

Characteristics of African American English Articulation and Phonology

AAE characteristic	Mainstream American English	African American English
/l/ phoneme lessened or omitted	tool always	too' a'ways
/r/ phoneme lessened or omitted	door mother protect	doah muddah p'otek
f/voiceless th substitution at end or middle of word	teeth both nothing	teef bof nufin'
t/voiceless th substitution at beginning of word	think thin	tink tin
d/voiced th substitution at beginning, middle of word	this brother	dis broder
v/voiced th substitution at end of word	breathe smooth	breave smoov
Consonant-cluster reduction	desk rest left wasp	des' res' lef' was'
Differing syllable stress patterns	guitar police July	**gui**tar **po**lice **Ju**ly
Verbs ending in /k/ changed	liked walked	li-tid wah-tid
Metathesis	ask	aks ("axe")
Devoicing of final voiced consonant	bed rug cab	bet ruk cap
Possible deletion of final consonant	bad good	ba' goo'
i/e substitution	pen ten	pin tin
b/v substitution	valentine vest	balentine bes'
Diphthong reduction	find oil pound	fahnd ol pond
n/ng substitution	walking thing	walkin' thin'

Note. Characteristics may vary depending on variables, such as geographic region. From *Multicultural Students With Special Language Needs: Practical Strategies for Assessment and Intervention* (5th ed., pp. 72–75), by C. Roseberry-McKibbin, 2018, Oceanside, CA: Academic Communication Associates. Copyright 2018 by Academic Communication Associates. Reprinted with permission.

Multicultural Populations **471**

Table 11.4

Examples of Acceptable Utterances by Speakers of African American English

Mainstream American English	African American English
That boy looks like me.	That boy, he look like me.
If he kicks it, he'll be in trouble.	If he kick it, he be in trouble.
When the lights are off, it's dark.	When the lights be off, it dark.
It could be somebody's pet.	It could be somebody pet.
Her feet are too big.	Her feet is too big.
I'll get something to eat.	I will get me something to eat.
She is dancing, and the music's on.	She be dancin' an' the music on.
What kind of cheese do you want?	What kind of cheese you want?
My brother's name is Joe.	My brother name is Joe.
I raked the leaves outside.	I rakted the leaves outside.
After the recital, they shook my hand.	After the recital, they shaketed my hand.
They are just standing around.	They is just standing around.
He is a basketball star.	He a basketball star.
They are in cages.	They be in cages.
It's not like a tree or anything.	It not like a tree or nothin'.
He does like to fish.	He do like to fish.
They are going to swim.	They gonna swim.
Mom already repaired the car.	Mom done repair the car.

Note. From *Multicultural Students With Special Language Needs: Practical Strategies for Assessment and Intervention* (5th ed., p. 74), by C. Roseberry-McKibbin, 2018, Oceanside, CA: Academic Communication Associates. Copyright 2018 by Academic Communication Associates. Reprinted with permission.

English Influenced by Asian Languages

General Background

- Asians originate primarily from three geographic regions:

  - **Southeast Asia**: the Philippines, Laos, Cambodia, Thailand, Indonesia, Singapore, Burma, Vietnam, and Malaysia
  - **South Asia**: Sri Lanka, Pakistan, and India
  - **East Asia**: Japan, Korea, and China

- Many Asians originate from countries in the Pacific Rim, which includes all nations and regions that touch the Pacific Ocean.
- Asian Americans are the fastest-growing racial group in the U.S. The estimated number of Asians in the U.S. is currently 21–22 million; 74% of Asian adults are foreign-born (U.S. Census Bureau, 2017).

Table 11.5

Articulation Differences Commonly Observed Among Spanish Speakers

Articulation characteristics	Sample English patterns
/t/, /d/, /n/ may be dentalized (tip of tongue placed against the back of the upper central incisors)	
Final consonants often devoiced	*dose/doze*
b/v substitution	*berry/very*
Deaspirated stops (sounds like speaker is omitting the sound because it is said with little air release)	
ch/sh substitution	*Chirley/Shirley*
d/voiced *th*, or z/voiced *th* (voiced *th* does not exist in Spanish)	*dis/this, zat/that*
t/voiceless *th* (voiceless *th* does not exist in Spanish)	*tink/think*
Schwa sound inserted before word-initial consonant clusters	*eskate/skate* *espend/spend*
Words end in 10 different sounds: a, e, i, o, u, l, r, n, s, d	May omit sound at end of word
/h/ silent in words beginning with /h/	*'old/hold, 'it/hit*
/r/ tapped or trilled (tap /r/ might sound like the tap in the English word *butter*)	
No /ʤ/ (e.g., *judge*) sound in Spanish; possible substitution of y	*Yulie/Julie* *yoke/joke*
Frontal /s/ (Spanish /s/ produced more frontally than English /s/)	Some speakers may sound like they have frontal lisps
ñ pronounced like y (e.g., *baño* pronounced bahnyo)	
5 vowels—a, e, i, o, u (ah, ɛ, ee, o, u)—and few diphthongs in Spanish; possible vowel substitutions include: i/ɪ substitution ɛ/æ, ɑ/æ substitutions	*peeg/pig, leetle/little* *pet/pat, Stahn/Stan*

Note. From *Multicultural Students With Special Language Needs: Practical Strategies for Assessment and Intervention* (5th ed., p. 101), by C. Roseberry-McKibbin, 2018, Oceanside, CA: Academic Communication Associates. Copyright 2018 by Academic Communication Associates. Reprinted with permission.

Speech–Language Characteristics and Considerations

- Some of the most widely spoken Asian languages in the United States are Chinese, Filipino, Vietnamese, Japanese, Khmer, and Korean.
- Many Asian languages have numerous dialects that may or may not be mutually intelligible. For example, as previously stated, there are over 87 mutually unintelligible dialects in the Philippines.
- Some groups have no written language and rely on oral traditions.
- Vietnamese, Chinese, and Laotian are tonal languages; each tone change (toneme) is phonemic in nature and represents a meaning change. For example, in Mandarin, "ma" can mean *mother, horse, scold, flax,* or *curse* depending on the tone used in pronouncing it.

Table 11.6

Language Differences Commonly Observed Among Spanish Speakers

Language characteristics	Sample English utterances
Adjective comes after noun.	The house green is big.
s is often omitted in plurals, possessives, and regular third-person present tense.	We have five *plate* here. The *girl* book is brown. The *baby* cry.
Past-tense *–ed* is often omitted.	We *walk* yesterday.
Double negatives are used.	I *don't* have *no* more.
Negative imperatives may be used.	*No* touch the hot stove (*no* used instead of *don't*).
"No" may be used before a verb to signify negation.	The kid *no* cross the street.
Superiority is demonstrated by using "more" before an adjective, similar to the use of *más* in Spanish.	This cake is *more* big.
The adverb often follows the verb.	He drives very fast his motorcycle.
Pronoun modifiers are used.	This is the book *of my sister.*
Articles may be used with body parts.	I bruised *the* knee.
Have may be used in place of the copula.	I *have* 12 years (instead of I *am* when talking about age)
Articles are often omitted.	Papa is going to store.
When the subject has been identified in the previous sentence, it may be omitted in the next sentence.	Mama is sad. Lost her purse.

Note. From *Multicultural Students With Special Language Needs: Practical Strategies for Assessment and Intervention* (5th ed., p. 100), by C. Roseberry-McKibbin, 2018, Oceanside, CA: Academic Communication Associates. Copyright 2018 by Academic Communication Associates. Reprinted with permission.

- Some characteristics of Asian languages follow:
  - Mandarin has four tonemes, Cantonese has seven, Northern Vietnamese has six, and Central and Southern Vietnamese both have five.
  - Japanese, Khmer, and Korean are not tonal languages.
  - Chinese, Vietnamese, and Laotian are basically monosyllabic.
  - Chinese and Vietnamese have no consonant blends.
  - Many Asian languages, such as Chinese, do not have inflectional markers.
  - Some Asian languages (e.g., Indonesian, Japanese, and Tagalog) do not have specific gender pronouns (do not differentiate between *he, she, it*).
  - Asian speakers' prosody or intonation in English may sound very "choppy" and monotonous to native English speakers.
  - Some Asian speakers may sound hypernasal in English.

- It is difficult to provide generalities about Asian speakers' English patterns due to the vast variety in Asian languages and dialects. Thus, the examples in Tables 11.7 and 11.8 may or may not be representative of various clients; each must be assessed on an individual basis.

Table 11.7

Language Differences Commonly Observed Among Asian Speakers

Language characteristics	Sample English utterances
Omission of plurals	Here are two *piece* of toast. I got five *finger* on each hand.
Omission of copula	He *going* home now. They *eating*.
Omission of possessive	I have *Phuong* pencil. *Mom* food is cold.
Omission of past-tense morpheme	We *cook* dinner yesterday. Last night she *walk* home.
Past-tense double marking	He *didn't went* by himself.
Double negative	They *don't* have *no* books.
Subject–verb–object relationship	I messed *up it*.
Differences/omissions	He *like*.
Singular present-tense omission or addition	*You goes* inside. *He go* to the store.
Misordering of interrogatives	You are going now?
Misuse or omission of prepositions	She is *in* home. He goes to school 8:00.
Misuse of pronouns	*She* husband is coming. She said *her wife* is here.
Omission or overgeneralization of articles	*Boy* is sick. He went *the home*.
Incorrect use of comparatives	This book is *gooder* than that book.
Omission of conjunctions	You I going to the beach.
Omission, lack of inflection on auxiliary *do*	She not take it.
Omission, lack of inflection on forms of *have*	He *do not* have enough. She *have* no money. We been the store.

Note. From *Multicultural Students With Special Language Needs: Practical Strategies for Assessment and Intervention* (5th ed., p. 129), by C. Roseberry-McKibbin, 2018, Oceanside, CA: Academic Communication Associates. Copyright 2018 by Academic Communication Associates. Reprinted with permission.

Table 11.8

Articulation Differences Commonly Observed Among Asian Speakers

Articulation characteristics	Sample utterances
Possible deletion of final consonants in English	*ste/step* *li/lid* *ro/robe* *do/dog*
Possible truncation of polysyllabic words or emphasis on wrong syllable	*efunt/elephant* *diversity/DIversity*
Possible devoicing of voiced cognates	*beece/bees* *pick/pig* *luff/love* *crip/crib*
r/l confusion	*lize/rise* *clown/crown*
/r/ omitted entirely	*gull/girl* *tone/torn*
Reduction of vowel length in words	Words sound choppy to Americans
No voiced or voiceless *th*	*dose/those* *tin/thin*
Epenthesis (addition of *uh* sound in blends, at end of words)	*bulack/black* *wooduh/wood*
Confusion of *ch* and *sh*	*sheep/cheap* *beesh/beach*
/æ/ nonexistent in many Asian languages	*block/black* *shock/shack*
b/v substitutions	*base/vase* *Beberly/Beverly*
v/w substitutions	*vork/work* *vall/wall*
p/f substitutions	*pall/fall* *plower/flower*

Note. From *Multicultural Students With Special Language Needs: Practical Strategies for Assessment and Intervention* (5th ed., p. 130), by C. Roseberry-McKibbin, 2018, Oceanside, CA: Academic Communication Associates. Copyright 2018 by Academic Communication Associates. Reprinted with permission.

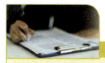

SUMMARY

- Knowledge of the influence of a primary language or dialect on English production is critical for differentiating speech and language differences from impairments in CLD speakers.
- Speakers of African American English, Spanish, and Asian languages have unique and predictable characteristics, based on primary-language influence, that are signs of differences and not impairments.
- These differences do not need to be remediated; however, some speakers may seek elective intervention so that their productions may more closely approximate those of Mainstream American English speakers.

LANGUAGE DIFFERENCES AND LANGUAGE IMPAIRMENT

Clinicians are continually confronted with the need to distinguish language differences from language impairment (LI). This challenge is influenced by the unique processes of second-language acquisition and by the nature of bilingualism and language proficiency. Knowledge of basic facts about acquiring a second language can help clinicians make accurate decisions in distinguishing language differences from LIs in EL children (Brice, 2015; Paul, Norbury, & Gosse, 2018; Roseberry-McKibbin, 2018).

Differentiating Language Differences From Language Impairments

- When clinicians are confronted with EL students who appear to be struggling in school, the first question they usually ask is, "Does this student have a language difference or an LI?" In other words, can the problems be traced to cultural differences or the student's lack of facility with English, or is there an underlying LI that requires special education intervention?
- Bloom and Lahey (1978) defined **language** as a system of symbols used to represent concepts that are formed through exposure and experience. Clinicians must ask about students' environmental and linguistic exposure and experience.
- Some EL students do not have the environmental and linguistic exposure and experience that teachers assume they do. They may come from nonliterate backgrounds, for example, or from backgrounds where the language is oral only and has not been put in written form.
- Unfortunately, statistics indicate that EL students are disproportionately affected by poverty, and this is another factor relevant to environmental and linguistic exposure (Gusewski & Rojas, 2017). Some clinicians do not stop to ask themselves whether students have had any of the usual mainstream experiences that are inherently assumed, like exposure to literacy or experience with preschool.
- This is often where deficits in students are created: When students' exposure and experiences are different from those expected in the mainstream school environment, clinicians and other professionals may assume that there are deficits inherent in the students themselves.
- If students' background experiences and exposure to life situations and linguistic models are different from those expected by schools, it follows that their language, which represents their unique backgrounds, will not be consistent with that expected by the school.

- This difference in students' backgrounds and schools' expectations can lead to misdiagnosis of students and consequent inappropriate placement into special education. Historically in U.S. schools, disproportionate numbers of EL children have been placed in special education unnecessarily.
- Children who speak more than one language can be properly diagnosed as having an LI only if they manifest language-learning difficulties both in the primary language and in English. Legally, it must be proven that the student in question has an LI that underlies both languages.
- If a student has typical abilities in the primary language and is having difficulty with English, this student does not need special education remediation services such as speech–language therapy. Rather, the student needs other services, such as bilingual education, to facilitate English-language learning (see Figure 11.2).

Acquiring a Second Language

- In assessing any child to differentiate a language difference from an LI, it is necessary to know what "typical" behavior is. A major challenge confronting clinicians is that typical behavior varies widely even among monolingual children. When one is attempting to work with EL students, the picture becomes far more complex.

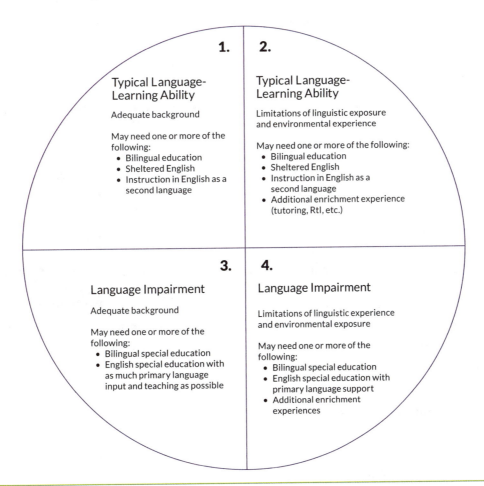

Figure 11.2 The diagnostic "pie." From *Multicultural Students With Special Language Needs: Practical Strategies for Assessment and Intervention* (5th ed., p. 240), by C. Roseberry-McKibbin, 2018, Oceanside, CA: Academic Communication Associates. Copyright 2018 by Academic Communication Associates. Reprinted with permission.

- Sometimes ELs who demonstrate typical second-language acquisition processes can spuriously appear to have underlying LIs. To avoid making inaccurate diagnoses of such learners, it is important to be familiar with typical processes of second-language acquisition (Cummins, 2017; Roseberry-McKibbin, 2018).

Typical Processes of Second-Language Acquisition

- **Interference** or **transfer** refers to an error in a student's second language (L2) that is directly produced by the influence of the first language. Interference can occur in all areas: syntax, morphology, phonology, pragmatics, and semantics. For example, a child from an Asian-language background might say, "The mom have two book." This would be an example of interference (also called transfer) from the first language, not an LI.
- Some students, when learning an L2, go through a **silent period**, in which there is much listening and comprehension and little output. It is believed that children are using this time to comprehend the new language before producing it. The silent period can last anywhere from 3 to 6 months, although estimates vary.
- **Code-switching** can be defined as the alternating or switching between two languages at the word, phrase, or sentence level; this behavior is part of natural bilingual development and is used by normal bilingual speakers worldwide.
- If use of the first language is discontinued or diminished, it is common for the second-language learner to experience **language loss**—that is, to lose skills in that first language. Because English is the dominant language of society in the United States, children often experience language loss of the first language; it is replaced by English, or L2.
- If an EL has experienced first language loss and is still acquiring English, he or she may appear to be low functioning in both languages. Many clinicians might conclude that low functioning in the first language as well as L2 is indicative of an LI, when it actually is a result of the loss of first-language skills.

Considerations for Second-Language Acquisition in Internationally Adopted Children

- In the United States in the 21st century, some parents have adopted children from Russia, Taiwan, China, and other countries; the number of these children in the United States has declined substantially in the past several years. Between the years 2004 and 2016, the number of internationally adopted children dropped by almost 80% (U.S. Department of State, 2017). Many of these children lived in orphanages in their home country until they were adopted by their American parents.
- Some of these children may show delays in their primary language as well as English because of the environmental conditions in their home country. Many children who live in orphanages in other countries experience very limited cognitive–linguistic stimulation in their primary languages. Of course, conditions vary from country to country.
- Recent research has highlighted several facts regarding the linguistic and cognitive development of internationally adopted children (Ellesef, 2013; Glennen, 2015; Hwa-Froelich, 2012; Hwa-Froelich, Matsuo, & Jacobs, 2017):

- Age of adoption is a critical factor in language development. The younger the children are when they are adopted, the greater their progress in language development after living in the United States for a period of time.
- Adopted children's language skills should be assessed immediately after they arrive in the United States and at regular intervals thereafter to evaluate progress in receptive and expressive English language skills.
- Language attrition of first language (L1) tends to happen very rapidly, because many adopted children have underdeveloped L1 foundations to begin with, due to limited linguistic stimulation in the orphanage in which they lived in their home country.
- For many children, receptive English language skills increase more rapidly than expressive skills.
- While many adopted children benefit from therapy for overall language skills, the area of social–pragmatic skills may need special focus. This area can present challenges, even after students are performing in a typical fashion in classroom academic tasks.
- Working with the parents of adopted children is imperative, especially since some children present challenges in multiple areas (e.g., fine and gross motor skills, cognitive skills, behavior). Parents benefit from support and specific instruction (Roseberry-McKibbin, 2018).

Basic Interpersonal Communication Skills and Cognitive–Academic Language Proficiency

- Before EL students are evaluated for the possible presence of an LI, it is important to understand what type of English fluency they possess. Basic Interpersonal Communication Skills (BICS) is oral language fluency that facilitates social interaction in daily life. There is surrounding context, and

Table 11.9

Conversational and Academic Language Fluency

Basic Interpersonal Communication Skills (BICS)	Cognitive–Academic Language Proficiency (CALP)
Involves oral language only	Involves oral and written language
Developed for social interaction in daily life	Gained primarily through schooling
Learned naturally in daily environments	Mostly taught explicitly in academic settings
Context embedded	Context reduced
Involves shared reality between speakers	Assumes listener knowledge; usually minimal shared reality
Supported by paralinguistic cues (e.g., gestures, facial expression, intonation)	Not usually supported by paralinguistic cues
Used in casual, informal communication	Usually used in reading, writing, formal oral communication
Formulaic language sometimes used	Formulaic language rarely used; characterized by specialized vocabulary, grammar, and discourse patterns

Note. From *Multicultural Students With Special Language Needs: Practical Strategies for Assessment and Intervention* (5th ed., p. 221), by C. Roseberry-McKibbin, 2018, Oceanside, CA: Academic Communication Associates. Copyright 2018 by Academic Communication Associates. Reprinted with permission.

communication between speakers is informal and casual (Cummins, 2017; Roseberry-McKibbin, 2018).

- Cognitive–Academic Language Proficiency (CALP; Cummins, 2017; Roseberry-McKibbin, 2018) refers to oral and written language skills that are gained primarily through schooling. CALP is mostly taught in academic settings and is used in reading and writing (see Table 11.9).

- Generally, CALP takes longer to develop than BICS. By some estimates, BICS to a native-like level in 2–3 years, while CALP can take 5–10 years to become commensurate with that of native speakers (Cummins, 2017). Speech–language pathologists (SLPs) and other special education professionals must realize that EL students with solid BICS still may be in the process of developing CALP (Paradis, 2016).

- Formal tests of language skills in English often rely upon well-developed CALP; the EL student who can hold a casual conversation in English may still have difficulty with the context-reduced, formal language tasks that are so common on standardized tests of language skills.

- This difficulty is due to typical processes of second-language acquisition, not to LI. The gap between BICS and CALP must not lead to erroneous labels of "language impairment" if the student is indeed a typically developing child who merely shows a normal, to-be-expected BICS–CALP gap.

- It is ideal for EL students to participate in bilingual education programs that nurture the first language while teaching English. This prevents loss of the first language and helps students experience the great benefits of fluent bilingualism.

- Many European countries value multilingualism so much that they promote a policy of trilingualism in schools. In Switzerland, for example, students cannot graduate from high school unless they speak three languages fluently.

- Unfortunately, some United States citizens have a negative attitude toward bilingualism and believe that it has negative cognitive and social effects on children. Thus, the availability of strong, theoretically sound bilingual programs in the United States is limited.

Simultaneous and Sequential Bilingualism

- Researchers have broadly delineated two types of bilingualism: simultaneous and sequential. **Simultaneous bilingual acquisition** occurs when two languages are acquired simultaneously from infancy.

- This phenomenon, in which two languages are spoken to a child beginning in early infancy, can also be called **infant bilinguality**. Such children acquire two languages simultaneously in natural communication situations, and this bilingual development closely parallels monolingual development. Children who acquire two languages simultaneously in naturalistic situations seem to do so with minimal interference.

- **Sequential bilingual acquisition** involves a situation where the child is exposed to the second language after he is exposed to the first language. If a child is exposed to a second language after 3 years of age, he is usually viewed as a sequential bilingual. Some students may acquire the second language with minimal interference; others may experience difficulties.

- If a student is introduced to an L2 before the L1 competency threshold has been reached, the development of L1 may be arrested or may regress while the child is focusing on L2 development.
- Since L2 proficiency is partially a function of L1 competence, a condition of "limited bilingualism" may occur, in which the student does not fully develop either language. For a period of time, these students may obtain low test scores in both L1 and L2 and consequently appear to have a language impairment.
- Thus, when clinicians are working with EL students in the schools, it is necessary, when a student appears to be "low functioning," to ask how the student developed both languages—simultaneously or sequentially?
- If the languages were developed sequentially, was L1 stable and developed enough so that acquisition of L2 was beneficial? If not, the student's seemingly limited academic performance and limited skills in both languages could result from acquisition of L2 when the underlying system was not yet stable.

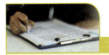

SUMMARY

- When clinicians attempt to distinguish a language difference from a language impairment in EL students, they must take into account factors of second-language acquisition and bilingual development.
- Typical processes of second-language acquisition include transfer, silent period, code-switching, and language loss. BICS and CALP are two types of language proficiency that clinicians should be aware of in assessing students. For many students, BICS takes 2–3 years to develop to a native-like level, while CALP can take 5–10 years.
- If internationally adopted children are being evaluated, the contribution of their unique background circumstances to language development must be taken into account.
- In distinguishing language differences from impairments, it is critical to ask whether a child has developed her two languages simultaneously or sequentially.
- In many cases, errors in judgment and consequent inappropriate placement of EL students can be avoided if clinicians are aware of second-language–learning factors. The greater the understanding clinicians have of these factors, the more unbiased and appropriate will be the services provided to EL students in the schools.

ASSESSMENT OF EL STUDENTS

Culturally fair and nonbiased assessment of EL students is an issue affecting schools across the United States (Arias & Friberg, 2017; Kraemer & Fabiano-Smith, 2017; Moore & Montgomery, 2018; Roseberry-McKibbin, 2018). A major consideration for all schools is state and federal mandates governing assessment of and intervention for EL children. Clinicians must also look carefully at the typical practice of using standardized tests for assessment of language impairment; most of these tests are biased against EL students. Clinicians are increasingly using alternatives to standardized tests and working with interpreters from the students' cultures who can help ensure that assessment is fair and unbiased.

Legal Considerations

- A number of laws affect service delivery to EL students. A key law currently in practice, the Individuals With Disabilities Education Improvement Act of 2004, specifically mandates the following:

  - All children, regardless of disability, are entitled to an appropriate and free education.
  - Testing and evaluation materials and procedures must be selected and administered so that they are not racially or culturally discriminatory.
  - Testing and evaluation materials must be provided and administered in the language or other mode of communication in which the child is most proficient unless it is clearly not feasible to do so.
  - Tests must be administered to a child with a motor, speech, hearing, visual, or other communication disability, or to a bilingual child, so as to reflect accurately the child's ability in the area tested, rather than the child's limited English-language skill.
  - Multicultural education is to be considered in guaranteeing equal educational opportunities for minorities with handicaps.

- The Every Student Succeeds Act (ESSA; signed by President Obama in December 2015) indicates that English-language proficiency is considered an academic indicator of accountability for American schools. Students who are ELs need to take math and reading tests along with their monolingual English-speaking peers (U.S. Department of Education, 2017).

Considerations in the Use of Standardized Tests

Foundational Concepts

- Many clinicians rely entirely on the use of standardized tests to evaluate EL students' language abilities and to plan intervention, even though standardized tests are generally heavily biased against members of EL populations.
- If clinicians continue to use these formal tests with EL students, they should at least be aware of the tests' potential legal, psychometric, cultural, and linguistic limitations in terms of validity and reliability.
- It is important to be familiar with the assumptions underlying formal, standardized tests. When clinicians are familiar with these assumptions, they can modify standardized tests so the tests are less biased.

Formal Test Assumptions

- The development of formal tests has grown out of a framework that is Western, literate, and middle class. For these and many other reasons, formal tests are often very biased against EL students.
- Formal tests are based on many inherent assumptions that clinicians may be only partially aware of. These assumptions are extremely important to consider when working with EL students. They hold that test takers (students) will (Roseberry-McKibbin, 2018)

  - follow the cooperative principle, performing to the best of their ability and trying to provide relevant answers;

- attempt to respond even when test tasks don't make sense;
- understand test tasks (e.g., fill in the blank, point to the picture);
- have been exposed to the information and experiences inherent in a test; and
- feel comfortable enough with the examiner in the testing setting to perform optimally.

■ These assumptions cannot be made with regard to many EL students. For example, some students come from cultural backgrounds where it is considered respectful to be silent in the presence of an unfamiliar adult. Cultural differences may cause students not to optimally display their competence and abilities when taking standardized tests.

■ Many formal, standardized tests that involve storytelling assume that children come from a literate narrative tradition. In such a tradition, narratives are highly structured, are decontextualized, and follow specific patterns. It is assumed that the speaker will provide explicit information for and *inform* the listener.

■ However, some children (e.g., African American and Native American children) come from *oral* narrative traditions in which listener knowledge is assumed. The speaker's job is to *entertain* the listener; storytelling is not as structured. Clinicians must not mislabel these children as having language problems if they do not produce narratives according to mainstream expectations.

■ A test's **ecological validity** refers to the extent to which it reflects the child's actual, daily environment and life experience. Most standardized tests that are normed on monolingual English-speaking children do not possess ecological validity when administered to ELs.

Translating Standardized Tests

■ Translated versions of English tests are often used with EL students. There are many difficulties with using translated English tests, so it is best to avoid this practice.

■ Differences in structure and content between English and the primary language raise questions of comparability of scores. Many words cannot be translated directly from one language to another. For example, some Asian languages do not have pronouns; translating *she* or *he* versus *it* into those languages is impossible.

■ Psychometric properties of tests, such as validity, reliability, sample sizes, and norming populations, do not carry over to translated versions.

■ Translation assumes that EL students have the same life experiences and background as the norming population, when they often do not.

Tests Developed in Primary Languages

■ Many clinicians believe that they can obtain valid assessments of EL students' language skills if they use tests specifically developed in the students' primary languages. For example, Spanish-speaking students can be given Spanish tests. However, there are some problems with this, as well.

■ One major problem is the great heterogeneity of various minority populations. For example, many dialects of Spanish exist, and Spanish-speaking children come from such different countries as Cuba, Mexico, the Dominican Republic, and Spain. Also, Spanish-speaking students raised in different parts of the United States use different vocabulary words for some items.

- A second difficulty is that there is little developmental data on languages other than English. Some Spanish norms for articulation have been developed, but few easily accessible, established language or articulation development norms exist for languages other than English.

Selecting, Administering, and Interpreting Standardized Tests

- When professionals are considering which tests to use with EL students, they must keep in mind the following:

  - **Purpose of the test**. Is it for screening or in-depth evaluation?
  - **Construct validity**. What theory was used in the test's creation? Is any theory mentioned? Is it appropriate for this particular student?
  - **Appropriateness of test content**. Professionals can have native speakers review the test; they also can get help in field-testing the assessment instrument so that they can change or delete items that most of the children miss.
  - **Adequacy of norms**. How was the standardization sample selected? Are the students who are being tested represented in the norming and standardization processes?

- There are ways in which professionals can alter the administration of standardized tests so that EL students will perform optimally and reflect their true abilities (Roseberry-McKibbin, 2018).

  - Omit biased items that the student will probably miss.
  - Test beyond the ceiling.
  - Complete the assessment over several sessions.
  - Have a parent or another adult who is trusted by the child administer test items under the clinician's supervision.
  - Give instructions in both English and L1.
  - Rephrase confusing instructions.
  - Give extra examples, demonstrations, and practice items.
  - Give the student extra time to respond.
  - Repeat items when necessary.
  - If students give "wrong" answers, ask them to explain and write down their explanations. Score items as correct if they are correct in students' cultures. Record all responses.

- There are also ways that professionals can interpret standardized tests to effectively reduce bias.

  - Review test results with family members and other people from the student's culture to gain additional insight into the student's performance.
  - Interpret overall test results in a team setting. If professionals review and interpret results alone, errors are more likely.
  - Don't identify a student as needing special education solely on the basis of test scores. Use informal measures to supplement standardized test scores.
  - Ascertain if students' errors are typical of other students with similar backgrounds.

- When writing assessment reports, be sure to include cautions and disclaimers about any departures from standard testing procedures. In addition, discuss how the student's background may have influenced testing results.

Alternatives to Standardized Tests

Basic Principles

- Because the use of standardized tests poses many difficulties when professionals are evaluating EL students, the use of nonstandardized, informal procedures and instruments for the assessment of EL students has become increasingly frequent.
- One major advantage of informal testing is that it can be matched to students' curriculum. Another major advantage is that it takes into account the fact that EL students are often very capable in their own milieus and very functional in their own worlds. Formal testing seldom taps these students' individualized, functional skills in their own environments.
- The assessment wheel of a team approach to comprehensive assessment (see Figure 11.3) illustrates the necessity of combining informal assessment strategies with more formal testing for EL students. It is important to carry out thorough assessments that include a case history, language proficiency testing, environmental observations, and dynamic assessment.

Specific Alternatives to Standardized Assessment

- Instead of relying exclusively on standardized tests for assessing EL students, clinicians can do the following (Arias & Friberg, 2017; Ebert & Pham, 2017; Paradis, 2016; Paul et al., 2018; Roseberry-McKibbin, 2018):

  - **Obtain a thorough case history** of the student's development in all domains: linguistic, cognitive, physical, academic, and others. It is very important to ascertain the student's history of exposure to the first language and English.
  - **Use observations in a variety of naturalistic contexts**, evaluating the student's ability to interact in various everyday situations. Professionals can observe students in the classroom, at recess, at lunch, in the library, in the home, and in a variety of other settings.
  - **Use questionnaires** administered to teachers, parents, and others who interact with the student on a regular basis. Use of questionnaires gives a much broader picture of the student's communication functioning in daily contexts. It also helps the professionals doing the assessment to work as part of a team and not carry the entire responsibility for assessing the EL student.
  - **Use narratives** appropriate to the student's background to assess the student's ability to construct narratives as well as retell stories she or he has heard.
  - **Use the portfolio method of assessment**, in which samples of the student's work are gathered over time. These work samples can be analyzed to see how much learning is taking place.
  - **Use language samples** to evaluate the student's communication skills in everyday contexts with various interlocutors.

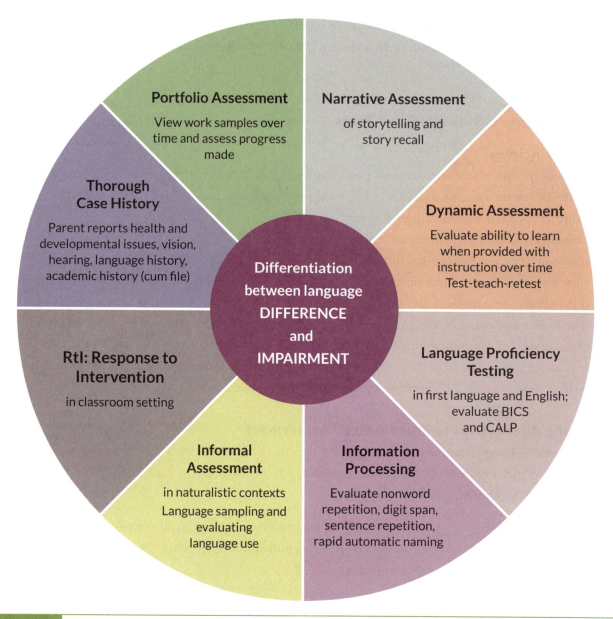

Figure 11.3 Team approach to comprehensive assessment: assessment wheel for ELs. From *Multicultural Students With Special Language Needs: Practical Strategies for Assessment and Intervention* (5th ed., p. 267), by C. Roseberry-McKibbin, 2018, Oceanside, CA: Academic Communication Associates. Copyright 2018 by Academic Communication Associates. Reprinted with permission.

- **Use school records** of the student's achievement and performance. Cumulative files (permanent records kept for each student) often contain helpful information that allows the clinician to track a student's performance over time.
- **Use conceptual scoring,** where students' answers in both the first language and English are counted in the overall total language score. This helps clinicians more accurately estimate students' bilingual skills.
- **Use a dynamic approach to assessment** in which a student is evaluated over time in a test-teach-retest format. Many students come from backgrounds of reduced exposure to

mainstream school concepts and vocabulary and may do poorly in formal testing situations that rely on their current knowledge rather than on their ability to learn.

- A dynamic approach is highly preferable to a static approach in which the student is tested in one or two assessment sessions, because dynamic assessment evaluates a student's ability to learn when provided with instruction. If a child responds poorly to dynamic assessment, this may be a sign that she has a genuine language impairment.
- One increasingly popular form of dynamic assessment is **response to intervention** (RtI). The use of RtI encompasses a number of components. A primary one is having teachers and other support personnel use specialized, scientifically based instruction in the regular education classroom with students who are struggling academically.
- This instruction is given above and beyond the regular teaching that occurs on a daily basis. For example, a resource specialist might come into the classroom and work with a small group of students using a specialized computer program to help them learn to decode polysyllabic words more efficiently. If such specialized, above-and-beyond instruction is insufficient to produce desired changes in students' performance, then special education referrals are made (Moore & Montgomery, 2018).
- Today, assessment of working memory (also called information processing) skills is a popular way to distinguish language differences from LIs in EL students. These working memory or information processing tasks circumvent the problem of limited English skills and possible lack of assumed background knowledge. For example, a student may be asked to repeat increasingly longer strings of nonsense words (e.g., "Say *kah, mih, fuh, kay*"). This task does not tap previous linguistic knowledge or background exposure.
- In a number of current studies, nonword repetition tasks have successfully differentiated between typically developing and LI students from such language backgrounds as Spanish, Czech, Italian, French, Vietnamese, Portuguese, and others (Brandeker & Thordardottir, 2015; le Clerq et al., 2017; Kapantzoglou, Restrepo, Gray, & Thompson, 2015; Paradis, 2016).
- The *Comprehensive Test of Phonological Processing Skills–Second Edition* (CTOPP-2; Wagner, Torgeson, Rashotte, & Pearson, 2013) has a nonword repetition task that can be used with EL students who are suspected of having an LI. Of course, scoring would need to be linguistically and culturally sensitive; the EL student's performance would need to be compared with that of similar peers, not that of the standardization sample.

Working With Interpreters in the Assessment Process

- Due to the national shortage of trained professionals who speak a language other than English, schools are increasingly turning to interpreters for assistance in the assessment and treatment of EL students. The clinician who is utilizing the services of an interpreter for assessment of EL students has ethical responsibilities to carry out. The clinician needs to make sure that he or she does the following (Langdon & Saenz, 2016; Roseberry-McKibbin, 2018):
  - Makes sure that the permission for assessment form indicates that the services of an interpreter will be used during the assessment

- Makes clear in the assessment report that the services of an interpreter were used
- Recognizes the limitations of interpreted tests
- Allows interpreters to carry out only those activities for which they have been trained
- Allows the interpreter time before the student arrives to organize test materials, read instructions, and clarify any areas of question
- Gives the interpreter background information about the student who is to be tested
- Prepares the interpreter for each testing session and debriefs the interpreter afterwards
- Shows the interpreter how to use tests and makes sure the interpreter feels comfortable with the testing
- Ensures that the interpreter does not protect the student by hiding the extent of the student's limitations or disabilities
- Supervises the interpreter during the testing session and watches for possible inappropriate behaviors, such as recording the assessment data incorrectly, prompting the student or giving clues, or using too many words
- Reminds the interpreter to write down all the student's behaviors seen during testing, even if the behaviors seem extraneous to the immediate task
- Considers the interpreter's observations but does not place responsibility for the placement decision on the interpreter

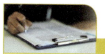

SUMMARY

- Federal law mandates nondiscriminatory, culture-fair testing for EL students. However, many clinicians use standardized, formal tests that are biased against EL students.
- If clinicians use those tests, they must be aware of potential forms of bias and try to control for them as much as possible.
- Many clinicians are increasingly turning to nonstandardized, informal assessment, which is much more valid in assessing the true language-learning abilities and skills of EL children. Interpreters can be a valuable part of this process.
- If the clinician does not speak the child's language, he or she is responsible for engaging the services of a trained interpreter to assess the child's first language.
- Response to intervention, or RtI, uses scientifically based instruction in the regular education classroom in addition to regular instruction. If students do not respond in a satisfactory manner to RtI, at that point they are referred for special education evaluation.

TREATMENT CONSIDERATIONS IN SERVICE DELIVERY TO CLD CLIENTS

EL children with language impairments that underlie both the primary language and English can be served through different delivery models. Treatment should always be individualized and should be linguistically and culturally appropriate for the particular student involved. CLD adults who have neurologically based disorders of communication have unique needs that must be taken into consideration when providing services.

Children With Language Impairments

Basic Principles

- As previously stated, students should not be diagnosed as having a language impairment (LI) if "problems" are observed only in English. If the student truly has an LI, problems in communication should be evident in both English and the primary language.
- An LI affects a child's ability to learn any language. Exposure to two or more languages is not the cause of a disability. Bilingual children with underlying LI will have difficulty learning any language.
- State and federal laws provide some specific guidelines for considering service options for EL students. Often EL children do need assistance but do not qualify for special education.
- It is illegal for clinicians in the public schools to place EL students into special education to work on improving their English. Only a small number of EL students are truly eligible for special education services, including speech–language therapy.
- If EL students do not qualify for speech–language services but need support in learning English, clinicians can help teachers find other options, such as bilingual education, English as a Second Language (ESL) programs, and others.

Service Delivery Models

- If EL students do qualify for special education services, including speech–language therapy, the following service delivery models can be considered (Roseberry-McKibbin, 2018):

  - A bilingual special education classroom
  - A monolingual, English, special education classroom with primary-language support through a bilingual teacher, tutor, or others
  - Pull-out services (speech–language therapy, resource support, or both) in the primary language
  - Pull-out services in English with primary-language support
  - Consultative, collaborative service provision in which the EL child remains in the regular classroom and the teacher receives assistance from special education personnel or ESL or bilingual staff
  - Placement in a regular bilingual education or ESL classroom with support from special education treatment professionals

- If a student is more proficient in the primary language than in English, carrying out treatment in the primary language is usually much more efficient and effective.
- If an EL child is exposed to English in school, some professionals worry that conducting therapy in the child's stronger, primary language will have negative effects.
- However, research shows that EL children with LI can and do learn two languages effectively; research also shows that EL students with intellectual disability and autism spectrum disorder can

become successfully bilingual (Duran, Hartzheim, Lund, Simonsmeier, & Kohlmeier, 2016; Ijalba, 2016; Kay-Raining Bird, Genesee, & Verhoeven, 2016; Hampton, Rabagliati, Sorace, & Fletcher-Watson, 2017).

- If children are cut off from their primary language, this can have many negative effects.
- Ideally, intervention activities should accomplish the following goals:
  - Acknowledge students' cultural and linguistic backgrounds and experiences and promote self-esteem
  - Support the development of both the first language and English
  - Focus on development of vocabulary skills
  - Promote effective communication and interaction among students
  - Include reading, writing, listening, and talking; literacy should always be incorporated
  - Be related to the classroom curriculum, including the Common Core State Standards
  - Build relevant cognitive processing skills such as increasing processing speed
- It is critical for intervention to involve not just therapy in a pull-out model but also intervention in the child's classroom setting. Clinicians must, as much as possible, see that they collaborate with classroom teachers to help children succeed in the academic and social settings of the classroom. In the classroom-based intervention model, the clinician will go into the classroom and serve the child there, supporting the child's access to the curriculum.
- Clinicians should work closely with children's families and include caregivers as collaborators in the development of treatment goals. It is also very helpful to work with people from the families' cultures in order to promote treatment success.

Serving CLD Adults: Prevalence and Incidence Rates of Medical Conditions and Communication Disorders

- Clinicians must be aware that some CLD groups have higher prevalence and incidence rates of communication disorders or related medical conditions than others. (**Prevalence** refers to the current number of individuals; it is a head count. **Incidence** refers to the future occurrence of such an event in a population.)
- The presence of communication disorders and related medical conditions is related to several variables. These variables include, but are not limited to, language barriers, poverty, lack of health insurance, poor diet, and lack of access to medical services (Battle, 2012a; Payne, 2014; Qualls, 2012; Spector, 2017).
- Hispanics tend, as a group, to have the following:
  - Low prevalence of esophageal cancer
  - High prevalence of cardiovascular disease
  - Higher prevalence of strokes and diabetes (especially adult-onset diabetes) than Whites
  - Higher prevalence of heart disease
  - High incidence of malignant neoplasms
  - Overall low smoking rate

- African Americans tend, as a group, to have the following:
  - High prevalence of traumatic brain injury, especially due to gunshot wounds in youth
  - High prevalence of strokes and hypertension
  - High prevalence of multi-infarct dementia
  - High prevalence of laryngeal, esophageal, and lung cancers
  - High prevalence of heart disease
  - Low incidence of cleft palate, especially cleft lip
  - Overall low smoking rate

- Asian Americans tend, as a group, to have the following:
  - High prevalence of cleft palate, especially in Japanese and Chinese Americans
  - High prevalence of nasopharyngeal cancer, especially in Chinese Americans
  - High prevalence of malignant neoplasms
  - High prevalence of heart disease
  - High prevalence of strokes
  - Low prevalence of Alzheimer's disease, especially in Chinese Americans
  - Overall low rates of alcoholism and smoking

- Native Americans tend, as a group, to have the following:
  - Generally low prevalence of lung cancer
  - High prevalence of cleft palate
  - High prevalence of otitis media
  - Generally high rate of smoking
  - High prevalence of alcoholism and fetal alcohol syndrome

- Awareness of the above-listed tendencies can help clinicians be sensitive to the needs of clients from various ethnocultural groups, thus increasing the efficacy and thoroughness of the assessment and treatment processes.

Potential Sociocultural and Linguistic Barriers to Service Delivery

In the United States and across the world, people with disabilities do not receive the health care they need and have poorer health than their nondisabled peers (World Health Organization [WHO], 2018). People with disabilities are more than twice as likely to find health care providers' skills and facilities inadequate; they are nearly three times more likely to be denied health care and four times more likely to receive inferior treatment (WHO, 2018). The WHO Global Disability Action Plan 2014–2021 seeks to address these disparities.

- When working with CLD clients and their families, it is important to recognize any barriers to full utilization of clinical services. Such barriers might include the following:
  - Overclassification of EL children as needing special education services
  - Client health care access problems (e.g., lack of health insurance), leading to underdiagnosis of problems such as middle ear infections

- Client presenting with more advanced states of communication disorders and related medical problems, caused by lack of health care and, thus, opportunities to prevent problems or treat them at an early stage
- Client's and family's lack of English proficiency, and a lack of interpreters to serve as liaisons with the health care system
- Client's and family's distrust of traditional, Western medicine and rehabilitation
- Lack of transportation to and from health care facilities

Adults With Neurologically Based Disorders of Communication

Basic Issues

- The aging population is the most rapidly growing group in our country. Due to recent advances in health care, people are living longer. The U.S. Census Bureau (2017) predicted that by the year 2060, there will be 100 million persons in the U.S. who are older than 65. The number of foreign-born persons over 65 will have increased by 294.8% to approximately 28 million.
- As stated earlier, increasing numbers of CLD people are living longer. Members of CLD groups tend to have a higher prevalence of neurological impairments (typically found in older people) than is found in the general population. This is due to many factors, including poverty and lack of health insurance and preventive care (Payne, 2014; Spector, 2017).
- The leading cause of neurological impairments is strokes. Strokes are associated with the following:

  - **Hypertension**, which may result in hemorrhagic strokes. Hypertension is prevalent among many CLD adults, especially African Americans.
  - **Arteriosclerosis**, a major etiological factor in strokes. In many CLD communities, arteriosclerosis is associated with high cholesterol levels. Also, foods that are high in salt and fat content (e.g., pork) are major causes of arteriosclerosis; these foods are popular in African American and Hispanic communities.
  - **Sickle cell anemia**, which primarily affects people of African and Mediterranean descent. Areas of the brain supplied by small blood vessels don't get enough oxygen, which may cause a stroke.
  - **Diabetes**, which affects Hispanics, in particular. Mexicans and Puerto Ricans have a rate of (adult-onset) diabetes two to three times higher than the rate in the White population. Diabetes is associated with an increased risk of stroke.
  - **AIDS**, which is often associated with IV drug use, a pervasive problem in large urban areas.
  - **Alcohol abuse**, which is a serious problem in many CLD groups because so often it begins in the early to middle teen years. This places abusers at high risk for neurological impairments, such as strokes, involving linguistic and cognitive deficits. Heavy, life-long alcohol abuse can also lead to **Wernicke-Korsakoff Syndrome**, a neurological disorder caused by thiamine deficiency. Memory, vision, coordination, and balance may be affected.
  - **Drug abuse**, which is very high in urban areas. Many inner-city residents have difficulties with drug abuse, and drugs such as crack (a vasoconstrictor) can cause strokes.

Theories Regarding Stroke Recovery in Bilinguals

- It is important to be aware of whether a stroke patient speaks more than one language. In one actual case, a bilingual English-Russian patient had a stroke and spoke only Russian afterward. The hospital staff, not having checked the patient's records, thought she was using jargon.
- During the acute recovery phase (approximately 4 weeks after the onset of aphasia), a patient might experience substantial change across either or both languages, dramatic differences between the languages, or both.
- There are several recovery theories that have been described for bilingual stroke patients (Paradis, 2004). The most common type of recovery is **synergistic and differential recovery**; 95–98% of stroke patients experience this.
- In this type of recovery, both languages are impaired but not necessarily to the same degree. One language may be more affected than the other. Both languages may eventually recover but not necessarily at the same rate.

Sociocultural Considerations in Rehabilitation: Implications for Assessment and Treatment

- It is important to consider individual patients' premorbid status, as well as their functional needs within their personal life contexts. For example, many older African Americans have strong church connections; therapy activities could address daily communication skills that are centered around church activities.
- Clinicians must evaluate the family's culture in terms of the appropriateness of the rehabilitation goal of independence for the patient. Encouragement of independence may be offensive in some cultures.
- For example, some Hispanic families believe it is their duty to take care of the patient with the neurological impairment. Requiring the patient to attend rehabilitation and become independent could be looked on as disrespectful and cause shame to the family.
- Socioeconomic status has a great impact on CLD patients' potential for utilizing rehabilitation services. Unfortunately, many elderly CLD adults tend to have little money or insurance.
- Family relationships are an important consideration. For example, African Americans tend to be more involved than Whites in providing help across the generations, and the extended family network is often much greater for African Americans than for Whites. Asian families tend to be highly involved in caring for ill or infirm family members. Clinicians can utilize family members for support.
- It is important to assess premorbid educational levels and vocational attainments of patients, because they affect assessment and treatment. Patients who have less formal education pre-stroke may not recover language skills as well as those with more formal education.
- Socioeconomic status and educational attainment affect patients' acceptance of and belief in conventional rehabilitation, especially when the rehabilitation involves technology. For example, if an elderly person from a low-income Hmong refugee family needs to have an MRI or CT scan to determine if he has had a stroke, the family may resist the procedure because they have not been exposed to "high-tech" neurodiagnostic procedures.

- Religion also may play a role in patients' and families' acceptance of rehabilitation. Some families believe in folk healers, not traditional medicine. Other families believe that a disability caused by a stroke, for example, is the will of a supreme being, and thus rehabilitation would go counter to religious beliefs (Roseberry-McKibbin, 2018; Spector, 2017).
- When assessing bilingual patients, it is imperative that the clinician assess skills in both the primary language and English. Assessment should be carried out as soon as possible and should focus on the most dominant language.
- The clinician, if he or she does not speak the patient's language, should utilize the services of a certified interpreter to evaluate the patient in his or her first language.
- Clinicians should ascertain which is the most appropriate language to use in rehabilitation of CLD clients. Factors to consider in making this decision include the following:
  - The patient's premorbid language history
  - The availability of an interpreter
  - The patient's abilities (both oral and written) in each language
  - Whether the patient will return to a home or work setting
- For clients with swallowing disorders, clinicians must ascertain their food preferences and possible religious restrictions pertaining to consumption of food and beverages. For example, during the month of Ramadan, many Muslims do not take food or liquid between sunrise and sunset.

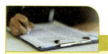

SUMMARY

- An EL child is considered to have an LI only if he or she has language-learning difficulties that underlie both the primary language and English.
- EL children in the schools who manifest LIs can be served through a variety of service delivery models. Treatment activities for these children should be culturally appropriate and should assist the children in becoming effective communicators in their environments. Family involvement is critical.
- Adults with neurologically based communication disorders, such as those resulting from strokes, may recover their languages in various ways after the stroke. Clinicians should be sensitive to these clients' bilingual status and the way it affects recovery.
- Assessment and treatment should occur in the patient's strongest language if possible. Treatment must be functional for the individual patient's environment and appropriate for his or her cultural background.

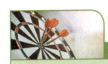

CHAPTER HIGHLIGHTS

- The increasing numbers of culturally and linguistically diverse (CLD) persons in the United States have created a great need for SLPs to develop cultural sensitivity and knowledge about how to best provide appropriate service delivery. ASHA has developed guidelines and policies regarding optimal service delivery to people from multicultural backgrounds.
- Speakers of African American English, Spanish, and the Asian languages manifest unique phonological, morphological, semantic, and syntactic characteristics and patterns that differ from those of Mainstream American English. These characteristics and patterns are indicative not of a disorder but of a difference. Errors caused by interference, or transfer from the first language, indicate a communication difference.
- It is important to take into account the influence of the primary language or dialect so that CLD clients are not misdiagnosed as having a language disorder. Some CLD individuals may choose to participate in elective speech–language therapy so that they can improve their Mainstream American English skills for vocational and other purposes.
- A great challenge for SLPs is to differentiate between language differences and language impairments (LIs) in children who speak more than one language. Frequently, there is a mismatch between the skills and abilities these children bring to the schools and the schools' expectations of these children. This mismatch often creates deficits in EL students who have typical underlying language-learning ability.
- Part of accurately differentiating between a language difference and a language impairment is knowledge of typical second-language acquisition processes. The processes of interference (transfer), silent period, code-switching, and language loss can appear to be symptoms of a language impairment; however, these processes are normal and common. Whether children are developing a second language simultaneously with or sequentially to the first language also has an impact on development.
- EL children learning a second language manifest different types of language fluency. Basic Interpersonal Communication Skills (BICS) often develops faster than Cognitive–Academic Language Proficiency (CALP). For many students, BICS develop to a native-like level in 2–3 years, where CALP can take 5–10 years. Thus, there may be a BICS–CALP gap in which BICS is better developed than CALP. Clinicians must not erroneously interpret this gap as evidence of a language impairment.
- Federal law mandates that assessment of EL children be fair, nondiscriminatory, and conducted in the children's most proficient language. Because most clinicians use standardized tests normed on English-speaking children, fair and nonbiased assessment of EL children is a great challenge.

- Clinicians can make alterations in standardized testing to make testing less biased. Optimally, however, they should use nonstandardized, informal assessment measures such as dynamic assessment, working memory measures, questionnaires administered to adults who are familiar with the child's daily communicative functioning, and language samples. Use of response to intervention or RtI techniques is becoming increasingly popular. Using the services of well-trained interpreters can also be very helpful.
- Some EL students have underlying language impairments; they are not able to learn any language adequately. A number of service delivery options are available for these children. Treatment methods and activities should focus on improving functional communication, literacy, and knowledge of school curriculum and language; they should also be culturally appropriate. It is imperative to include families in the treatment process.
- CLD adults tend, as a group, to be more predisposed to strokes than the general population. This is due to such related factors as diabetes, hypertension, and arteriosclerosis. Assessment and treatment of CLD adults with neurologically based communication disorders must consider many variables, such as family support, religious beliefs, educational and vocational background, socioeconomic status, and other sociocultural variables.

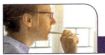

STUDY AND REVIEW QUESTIONS

1. Xu Fang is a 7-year-old girl in an all-English-speaking second-grade classroom. Xu's parents emigrated from mainland China 8 years ago; Xu was born in the United States. She came to an all-English kindergarten speaking only Mandarin; kindergarten was her first exposure to English on a regular basis. She had no prior preschool experience in either Mandarin or English. The second-grade teacher has referred Xu for a speech–language evaluation because he says that, although she interacts well with her English-speaking classmates on the playground, she is "behind" her classmates in written language skills (e.g., spelling, reading). Xu definitely demonstrates a gap. Based on her background, you can state that

   A. because BICS develops faster than CALP, Xu is probably developing in an appropriate manner, and at this time, evaluation for a possible language impairment is not necessary.

   B. because Xu has been in an all-English-speaking classroom setting for at least 2 years, her CALP should be as well developed as her BICS. Her difficulties are a red flag, and a speech–language assessment should be conducted.

   C. Xu's CALP should actually develop faster than her BICS, because Chinese parents are known to focus on academic skills at home; thus, her BICS–CALP gap is a red flag that she may have an underlying language impairment.

   D. Xu's BICS–CALP gap may indicate a possible intellectual disability, and she should be evaluated by the school psychologist.

2. A teacher has referred Isaiah Brown to you for an evaluation. Isaiah is an African American kindergartener who is reportedly doing well in class academically. When you observe him on the playground with his peers, you see that he has many friends and does not appear to have problems interacting appropriately with other children. Isaiah's friends do not appear to have any difficulty understanding what he says. However, the teacher is concerned because, she says, "I think Isaiah pronounces some of his sounds wrong. I think he needs speech therapy." When you conduct a speech screening with Isaiah, you will remember: Which of the following is a typical variation of African American English and not a sign of a disorder?

   A. v/f substitution in word-final position
   B. Production of [æks] instead of [æsk]
   C. w/r substitution in all word positions
   D. initial consonant deletion

3. A classroom teacher refers a 9-year-old African American male student to you because she is concerned about his intelligibility. This teacher is anxious to avoid the mistake of mislabeling this student as having a "speech disorder" if he is merely manifesting characteristics of African American English (AAE). When you screen the boy, you find that he makes the following substitutions: d/m, f/n, and m/n. You would

   A. let the classroom teacher work with the student because this is such a mild problem.
   B. do nothing, knowing that boys mature more slowly than girls.
   C. do nothing, realizing that this is normal for speakers of African American English.
   D. treat the student, because this is a sign of a speech sound disorder involving substitutions of other sounds for nasals.

4. In an adolescent speaker of African American English, which of the following utterances would be an example of the use of the perfective construction, with *been* used to indicate an action that took place in the distant past?

    A. "I been had a marble collection when I was 7."
    B. "Our family been gonna do it."
    C. "I might been coulda done it."
    D. "He been done it again."

5. Consuelo is a Mexican American, Spanish-speaking, 6-year-old first grader, who is in the process of learning English. Her parents emigrated from Mexico 3 years ago; thus, she was exposed first to Spanish at home and to English in kindergarten at the age of 5 years 3 months. Consuelo's mother tells you that during the summer before kindergarten, Consuelo attended an English-speaking preschool. The first-grade classroom teacher shares that she thinks Consuelo may have a speech sound disorder but is not sure. The teacher provides you with some examples of things Consuelo has said in the past few weeks. Some of these examples are due to interference or transfer from Spanish. As you look at the examples, which one of the following would *not* be based on interference from Spanish and thus atypical for her in terms of predictable productions based on Spanish influence?

    A. t/th substitutions in word-initial positions (e.g., *tin/thin*)
    B. Devoicing of final consonants (e.g., *beece/bees*)
    C. v/f substitutions in word-initial and word-final positions (e.g., *vine/fine, roove/roof*)
    D. j/ʤ substitutions (e.g., *yava/java*)

6. Which one of the following is a predictable production for speakers of Asian languages as a result of language interference (transfer)?

    A. "He be to bed going now."
    B. "I see cat the little."
    C. "Yesterday she cook a pot of soup."
    D. "We no not be drivin' over there."

7. A 74-year-old bilingual Asian gentleman has had a stroke, and you are seeing him for therapy. He is recovering both his primary language and his English skills, but you are working only in English. There are no interpreters available, unfortunately, and the family has indicated that they would prefer treatment to be conducted in English anyway, since many of the patient's grandchildren speak English fluently. Which one of the following productions would be an example, on the patient's part, of English influenced by his primary language and not the stroke?

    A. "They coming over here now."
    B. "I done got to eat breakfast now."
    C. "She not have no dollar in her purse."
    D. "We be havin' many fun."

8. A high school teacher refers a Japanese-speaking 10th grader, Kosuke, to you for an evaluation. Kosuke and his family have been in the United States for 2 years; the father was brought to the United States for a 3-year computer project in a major American city. The family will be returning to Japan next year. Kosuke's teacher says that, although he is doing well academically, he is "hard to understand sometimes." She says that the other students don't make fun of Kosuke, but they don't always seem to follow what he is saying. The teacher wonders if he could benefit from intervention for an "articulation disorder." You conduct a screening. Which one of the following articulatory–phonological characteristics would NOT be predictable based on Kosuke's first language of Japanese?

   A. Substitution of a/æ (e.g., *sock/sack, fong/fang*)
   B. Final-consonant deletion (e.g., *be–/bed, po–/pot*)
   C. r/l confusion (e.g., *laise/raise, clown/crown*)
   D. d/t substitution (e.g., *din/tin*)

9. Which one of the following is *not true*, according to the Individuals With Disabilities Education Improvement Act of 2004?

   A. Testing must be administered in a way that is not racially or culturally discriminatory.
   B. Testing and evaluation materials must be provided and administered in the language or other mode of communication in which the child is most proficient unless it is clearly not feasible to do so.
   C. Testing must be administered to a bilingual child so as to reflect accurately the child's ability in the area tested, rather than reflecting limited English-language skill.
   D. Mandatory consent in the primary language is always required.

10. A teacher has referred a third-grade boy to you for a speech–language assessment. She is concerned because she feels that he is academically "behind his peers." He and his family are Cambodian refugees, and they have been in the United States for 8 months. Because the boy has been in refugee camps most of his life, his schooling in Cambodia was quite limited. His parents tell you that they estimate that he has had approximately 1½ years of schooling in Cambodia. The teacher is concerned that the boy may have an underlying language impairment, and she wonders if he is eligible for speech–language services. What would be the best combination of assessment techniques to use with him?

   A. Dynamic assessment, language samples in Cambodian, and observations of his interaction with family members and other Cambodian children
   B. Use of the *Peabody Picture Vocabulary Test–Fourth Edition* and the *Test of Language Development–Primary: Fourth Edition*, translated into Cambodian; dynamic assessment; and language samples in Cambodian
   C. Use of a district-developed test for Cambodian students in your geographic area and administration of questionnaires to the boy's teachers and family
   D. Use of formal, standardized tests in English combined with observations of the boy's interactions, in Cambodian, with peers and family members

11. You are working in a school district where there is an influx of immigrants from Russia. These immigrants have come to your area because there are Russian churches that have sponsored them. In the last few years, over 50,000 Russian families have moved in. Teachers are beginning to refer some Russian students to you for assessment for language impairment, saying that the students are "not learning English fast enough." You consult with the pastor of a local Russian church, Pastor Soldantenkov, who is highly regarded in his community, and share with him the stories of some of the students who have been referred to you. As he listens, Pastor Soldantenkov tells you that many families in his church had difficulty leaving Russia and, though they now live in the United States, want to limit their interactions with Americans as much as possible. Many parents wish to "preserve the Russian language and culture" and want to limit their children's exposure to English and American culture in general. Which of the following can you *not* conclude about the Russian students referred to you based on your conversation with Pastor Soldantenkov?

   A. It is possible that instead of having language impairments, these students are typical language learners who have had limited assimilation into American mainstream society.

   B. The families of these students who have been referred to you are bicultural, and this is part of the problem that the students are having in school.

   C. The families of these students have limited acculturation into American life, and this factor may be influencing the students' performance in school.

   D. The reluctance of the families to assimilate into American culture might be a factor that is influencing the students' interaction with other students who are native speakers of English, and this may be related to the Russian students' learning English more slowly.

12. A monolingual, English-speaking speech–language pathologist is working in a Head Start in a city with many EL children. In the last year, EL children from over 15 different cultural and linguistic groups have come to the Head Start speaking only their primary languages. The ideal plan for dealing with the needs of these children is to

   A. encourage them not to speak their primary languages and to speak English as much and as quickly as possible.

   B. tolerate the children's use of their primary languages and speak to them solely in English, hoping that they will eventually "pick up" English and discontinue using their primary languages.

   C. hire bilingual aides from the neighboring communities and use their services to help the children maintain their primary languages and learn English, also.

   D. assume that these children probably have language impairments in their primary languages and hire bilingual speech–language pathologists to assist in remediation.

13. A teacher refers José E. to you for a speech–language evaluation. José, a Puerto Rican American second grader who speaks Spanish and English with equal fluency, transferred to your school district 3 months ago from another district in your state. In his previous district, he was in a bilingual classroom where his primary language of Spanish was maintained and he was exposed to English, also. According to his report card from the previous district, "José does well speaking both Spanish and English. I [the teacher] think he is beginning to show a preference for English. José is performing adequately in all academic areas." The second-grade teacher at your school, who teaches only in English, feels that after 3 months in her classroom, "José is catching on slowly. I wonder if he needs special education." Your best course of action would be to

A. ask José's parents to sign a permission form so that he may be assessed immediately in English using only English tests, since English is apparently beginning to be his preferred language.
   B. use a variety of English screening instruments to screen José's English ability because these instruments are ecologically valid for him.
   C. do nothing at the present time and tell the teacher that you will wait for 6 months to see how José progresses in his classroom.
   D. use a dynamic assessment model to evaluate José's language-learning ability and combine this with classroom observations over the next 2–3 months to evaluate his progress.

14. Mr. Nehru is a gentleman from India who has had a stroke and now has aphasia. His family reports that before the stroke, he spoke both Hindi and English fluently. In planning for therapy, you, as a monolingual English-speaking speech–language pathologist, think about the possibility of incorporating work on English idioms. Which one of the following is NOT a consideration in terms of whether to make comprehension and expression of English idioms a treatment goal?

   A. Mr. Nehru's oral and written abilities in both English and Hindi
   B. Your own interest in English idioms and whether you consider them important in therapy for a stroke patient
   C. Whether Mr. Nehru will return to his work setting, where his colleagues speak English, or now spend all of his time at home, where his family speaks primarily Hindi
   D. Mr. Nehru's educational and vocational history

15. A fifth-grade teacher refers Mia to you. Mia speaks Tongalese. She and her family have been living in the United States for 3 years, and Mia has been enrolled in U.S. schools for that whole time. However, she has been sick a great deal and missed many days of school. The family is most helpful, and Mia's parents do their best to do assignments with her at home. However, their conversational English is limited, and they do not read or write in English at all. When you talk to the teacher, he states that Mia has friends and gets along well in the classroom, but she especially struggles in the area of reading. The school team meets and decides to utilize an RtI (response to intervention) approach to discern whether Mia has a language and experiential difference or a language impairment. In the RtI model

   A. Mia's teacher will implement the use of scientifically based instruction in the regular education setting to provide her with additional reading support; if this is insufficient to improve her performance, the special education team will evaluate her for possible special education services.
   B. Mia will automatically undergo an extensive special education evaluation that will determine her possible need for pull-out speech–language therapy and academic support from the resource specialist.
   C. Mia will automatically undergo an extensive special education evaluation that will determine her possible need for placement in a self-contained special education classroom.
   D. the classroom teacher will continue "business as usual," providing no extra or additional instruction and assessing whether Mia makes progress.

16. Mrs. Elizaga, a 70-year-old Filipino woman, has had a stroke. Her first and dominant language is Tagalog. She speaks some English. You do not speak Tagalog but know that you need to evaluate her Tagalog skills. As a culturally competent clinician, you will

    A. evaluate her in English only; after all, she is in the U.S. and needs to be evaluated in our mainstream language.

    B. ask a family member to come and gather a language sample in Tagalog and help you analyze it and figure out goals based upon this sample.

    C. ask the medical facility to provide you a certified, highly trained Tagalog interpreter to gather a case history and evaluate Mrs. Elizaga's Tagalog skills, following up with some English assessment as well.

    D. have Mrs. Elizaga's family fill out a form indicating whether or not Tagalog or English is her dominant language and asking for their input on best assessment practices.

17. You observe a Spanish-speaking child on the school playground. The teacher is concerned about Manuela's language skills, and you are starting by general observations in regular school settings. You hear Manuela speaking with her friends and saying things like "Yulie (Julie) has a shirt red," and "I want to estart playing with duh tederball (tetherball)." You are observing evidence of

    A. a clinically significant speech sound disorder.

    B. a clinically significant language disorder.

    C. clinically significant speech and language disorders.

    D. transfer from Spanish.

18. Rohini is a 6-year-old speaker of Telegu from India. Her family moved to the U.S. 6 months ago because her mother is a doctor and wanted expanded opportunities in the U.S. Rohini speaks primarily Telegu and almost no English. Rohini is one of three children. Her mother confides that Rohini stands out from her two other siblings in that she "just didn't catch on to English" as fast as they did. She also shares that Rohini was slow to develop her language milestones in Telegu, not speaking her first word in Telegu until she was 2 years old. You are a monolingual English-speaking SLP and know that given the "red flags" from the mother's description, you need to do a thorough evaluation to ascertain whether or not Rohini has a language disorder or just a language difference that will resolve with time. However, you do not speak Telegu. What is the best choice in this situation?

    A. Not test Rohini at all—wait and see if time will make a difference

    B. Obtain the services of a trained interpreter and have him or her evaluate Rohini in Telegu

    C. Administer standardized tests in English because, after all, Rohini needs to succeed in American schools

    D. Have Rohini's mother fill out a detailed case history form and use the results to guide your decision

19. A test's **ecological validity** refers to the extent to which it reflects

   A. the child's actual, daily environment and life experience.
   B. culture-fair assessment practices.
   C. grade-level appropriate content.
   D. procedures which have been proven nondiscriminatory for ELs.

20. You are a new clinician, considering using a new test with an EL student. You are asking questions like "What theory was used in the test's creation?" "Is any theory mentioned?" or "Is it appropriate for this particular student?" You are questioning the test's

   A. concurrent validity.
   B. reliability.
   C. construct validity.
   D. theoretical reliability.

References and Recommended Readings at www.advancedreviewpractice.com

STUDY AND REVIEW ANSWERS

1. A. Because BICS develops faster than CALP, Xu is probably developing in an appropriate manner, and at this time, no evaluation for a possible language impairment is necessary.
2. B. Many typically developing speakers of African American English show metathesis in productions like [æks] instead of [æsk]. However, a w/r substitution is not common and probably indicates an articulation problem that is not related to the use of African American English. Typically developing African American students also do not make v/f substitutions or delete consonants in word-initial position.
3. D. The listed substitutions are not commonly found in speakers of African American English, so this student has a disorder involving substitutions of other sounds for nasals.
4. A. In an adolescent speaker of African American English, the utterance "I been had a marble collection when I was 7" would be an example of the use of the perfective construction with *been*, indicating an action that took place in the distant past.
5. C. v/f substitutions in word-initial and word-final positions (e.g., *vine/fine, roove/roof*) would *not* be typical for a Spanish-speaking 6-year-old girl who is in the process of learning English, in terms of predictable productions based on Spanish influence.
6. C. "Yesterday she cook a pot of soup" would be a predictable utterance for a speaker of most Asian languages. The other utterances would not be predictable based on the influence of any Asian language.
7. A. A 74-year-old Asian gentleman who has had a stroke and is receiving therapy in English could say, "They coming over here now" as an English utterance influenced by his primary language and not the stroke.

8. D. Predictable utterances for a Japanese-speaking 10th grader, based on his primary language of Japanese, would be substitutions of a/ae (e.g., *sock/sack, fong/fang*), final consonant deletion (e.g., *be–/bed, po–/pot*), and r/l confusion (e.g., *laise/raise, clown/crown*). However, a d/t substitution would not be typical for a Japanese speaker.

9. D. This statement, "mandatory consent in the primary language is always required" is not true; it is not part of the IDEA 2004.

10. A. Practices that are discouraged in evaluating ELL children include translated English tests and the use of formal, standardized tests administered in English. It would be ideal to use dynamic assessment, language samples in Cambodian, and observations of interactions with family members and other Cambodian children.

11. B. You cannot assume this because immigrants who are *bicultural* are fully involved in both their own and the host culture. They maintain their native language and become fluent in the new language, too. They maintain many of their own cultural practices and adopt the host culture's practices, as well. They are comfortable going back and forth between their own and the host culture.

12. C. It would be ideal to hire bilingual aides from the neighboring communities and use them to help the children maintain their primary languages and learn English also. Research shows that with children, it is best to maintain and nurture their primary languages and also introduce English so that they (ideally) eventually become proficient bilingual speakers.

13. D. Use a dynamic assessment model to evaluate José's language-learning ability and combine this with classroom observations over the next 2–3 months to evaluate his progress. Assessing José in English only is not valid, and English screening instruments are not ecologically valid for him. It would be best to assess his ability to learn language and to observe him in the classroom for the next few months to see whether he progresses appropriately. If he does not, then the bilingual speech–language pathologist can undertake a formal evaluation of his Spanish and English skills.

14. B. You need to consider Mr. Nehru's Hindi and English oral and written abilities, as well as whether he will return to his work setting, where his colleagues speak English, or will now spend all of his time at home, where his family speaks primarily Hindi. Your own preferences as a monolingual English-speaking speech–language pathologist are irrelevant to Mr. Nehru's needs and individual situation.

15. A. In the RtI model, Mia's teacher will implement the use of scientifically based instruction in the regular education setting to provide her with additional reading support; if this is insufficient to improve her performance, the special education team will evaluate her for possible special education services.

16. C. Because Tagalog is Mrs. Elizaga's dominant language, you should ask the medical facility to provide you a certified, highly trained Tagalog interpreter to gather a case history and evaluate her Tagalog skills. Because she speaks some English, you can follow up with some English assessment.

17. D. If a Spanish-speaking child says things like "Yulie (Julie) has a shirt red," and "I want to estart playing with duh tederball (tetherball)," these are signs of transfer from Spanish, not a clinically significant speech or language disorder.

18. B. Obtain the services of a trained interpreter and have him or her evaluate Rohini in Telegu. It is not ethical to do nothing at all, because there are some definite "red flags." But it is illegal to only administer standardized tests in English. It is best to utilize the services of a trained Telegu-speaking interpreter to evaluate Rohini in her first language.
19. A. A test's *ecological validity* refers to the extent to which it reflects the child's actual, daily environment and life experience.
20. C. When you are asking questions like "What theory was used in the test's creation?" "Is any theory mentioned?" or "Is it appropriate for this particular student?" you are questioning the test's construct validity.

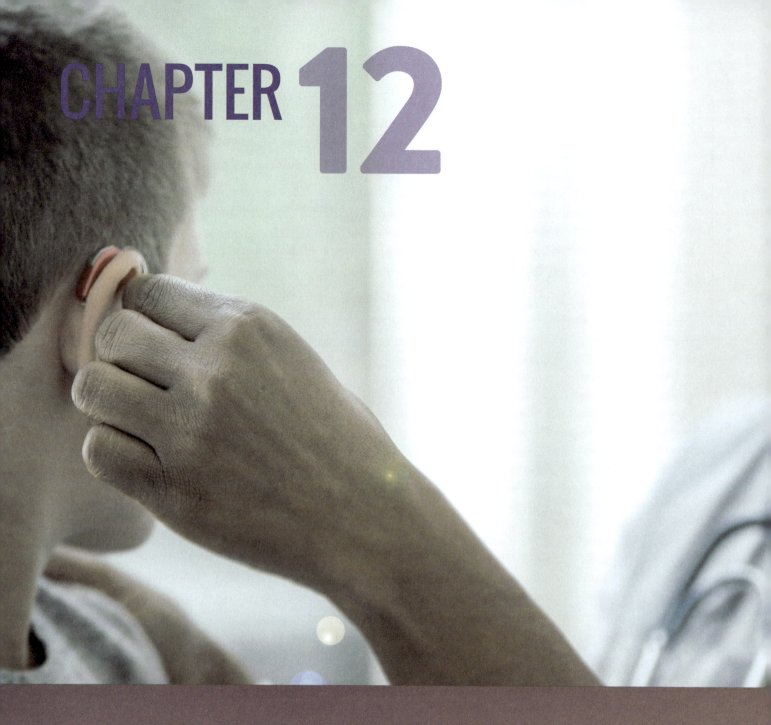

CHAPTER 12

AUDIOLOGY AND HEARING DISORDERS

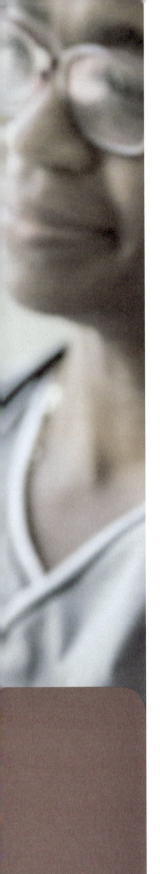

It is estimated that in the United States, approximately 50 million persons experience hearing impairment, depending on the definition of hearing impairment that is used. In the United States, 3 out of every 1,000 children are born deaf or hard of hearing. One in five teens has a hearing loss, and 60% of veterans returning from Afghanistan and Iraq have a hearing loss accompanied by tinnitus (Hearing Health Foundation, 2014).

Audiology is the study of hearing, its disorders, and the measurement and management of those disorders. The birth of the audiology profession occurred during World War II. Many returning servicemen had impaired hearing and needed rehabilitation; this need gave rise to the profession of audiology.

Audiologists are health care professionals who provide a comprehensive array of services to diagnose, treat, and prevent hearing impairment and its associated communication disorders. They work in a variety of settings, such as hospitals or medical center facilities and school settings. Some audiologists work in residential health care facilities, industries, universities, and other related agencies. Others work in nonresidential health care facilities, such as physicians' practices, private clinics, and community speech and hearing centers. The largest number of audiologists are currently employed in a medical environment.

Audiology as a profession has expanded into new areas of service. These areas include ear canal inspection and cerumen management, neonatal hearing screening, auditory electrophysiology, and multisensory modality monitoring in operating rooms where patients are undergoing tumor removal (especially nerve VIII tumors).

In the 21st century, many universities are offering a professional doctorate in audiology (AuD). In this model, students enroll in a 3- to 4-year program (similar to that required for dentistry and optometry). The early years are primarily devoted to academic training and the later years to clinical training. At the end of the program, students receive the AuD and may practice independently.

In 2007, the AuD became the entry-level degree for audiologists nationwide. Until that time, a master's degree was required. For those audiologists who received their audiology degree prior to 2007, they are not required to obtain the AuD degree to continue practicing audiology. However, they are not being "grandfathered" in terms of automatically receiving the AuD degree just because they are practicing audiologists.

ANATOMY AND PHYSIOLOGY OF HEARING

The ear is divided into three sections: the outer ear, the middle ear, and the inner ear. Efficient functioning of these sections of the ear is necessary for normal hearing. However, the auditory nervous system must also be intact in order for sound to be carried to its ultimate destination, the cortex, where it is interpreted. Figure 12.1 shows two views of the ear.

The Outer Ear

The outer ear is composed of two parts:

- The **auricle** or **pinna** (the most visible part of the ear, composed primarily of cartilage), which funnels the sound to the ear canal and helps localize sound
- The external auditory canal (also called the external auditory meatus), which goes from the pinna to the tympanic membrane or eardrum

The external auditory canal is a muscular tube, made up mostly of cartilage. The tube is not straight but curves slightly like an S. Thus, a specialist who examines the ear canal must first pull the pinna up and back to insert the **otoscope** (an instrument for examining the ear) into the canal.

- The external auditory canal is, on the average, approximately 2.5 cm (1 inch) long and resonates sounds that enter it. The resonant frequency of the ear canal is about 2500 Hz. The canal ends at the tympanic membrane, or eardrum.
- The external auditory canal has special cells that secrete wax, or **cerumen**. The functions of cerumen include lubricating and cleansing the canal and protecting the ear from fungi, bacteria, and small insects.
- Cerumen should be removed only by an audiologist or another trained medical professional. Use of Q-tips to remove cerumen actually impacts the cerumen, making it press against the tympanic membrane; this makes hearing more difficult.

The Middle Ear

The middle ear is an air-filled cavity separated from the outer ear by the **tympanic membrane**. The three small bones in the middle ear form the **ossicular chain**. The **Eustachian tube** connects the middle ear to the nasopharynx.

Tympanic Membrane

The **tympanic membrane** is elastic, thin, and cone-shaped. It is flexible and tough and vibrates in response to sound pressure. The entire tympanic membrane responds to low-frequency sounds, but only certain portions respond to high-frequency sounds.

- It is easy to damage the tympanic membrane. It can be ruptured by a Q-tip, a hairpin, or other objects inserted into the ear. Explosions and sudden pressure changes can also rupture the tympanic membrane.
- A damaged or punctured tympanic membrane may heal spontaneously. However, repeated ruptures could cause scar tissue, which reduces the membrane's mobility.

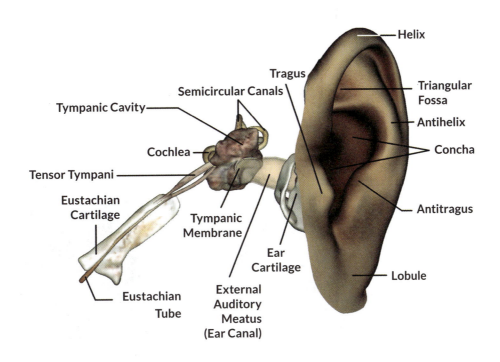
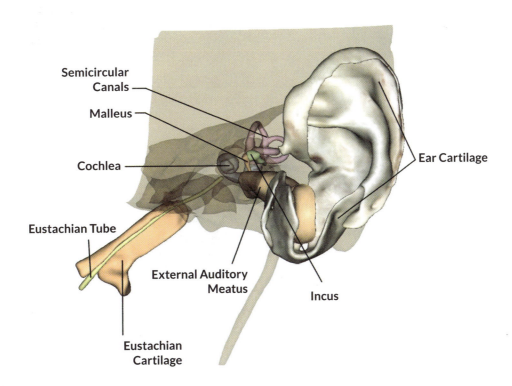

Figure 12.1 Two views of the ear. Used with permission from Anatomage.

510　Chapter 12

Ossicular Chain

The **ossicular chain**, suspended in the middle ear by ligaments, is composed of three tiny bones: the malleus, incus, and stapes.

- The first and largest of the three bones is called the **malleus** (Latin for *hammer*) because it resembles a hammer. One end of the malleus is embedded in the tympanic membrane. Because of this attachment, the vibrations of the tympanic membrane are transmitted to the malleus.

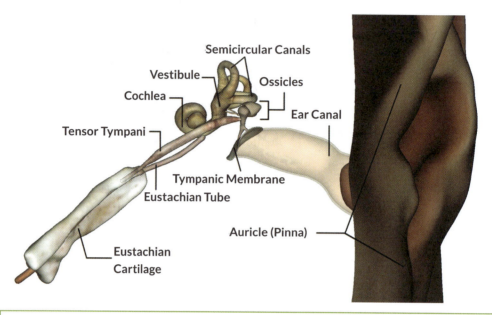

Figure 12.2　Ossicular chain. Used with permission from Anatomage.

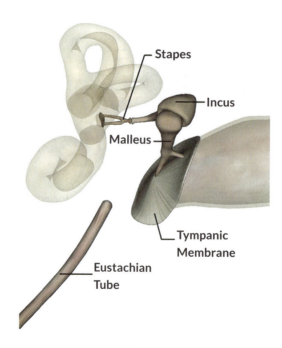

Figure 12.3　Middle ear. Used with permission from Anatomage.

- The malleus is attached to the second bone, which is called the **incus** (Latin for *anvil*). The malleus and incus are connected in a tight joint that permits very little movement.
- The incus is attached to the third bone, called the **stapes** (Latin for *stirrup*). The footplate, or other end of the stapes, is inserted into the oval window, a small opening that leads to the inner ear.
- The ossicular chain transmits sound efficiently and with no distortion. It also amplifies incoming sound by approximately 30 dB before transmitting it into the fluids of the inner ear.

Muscles and Reflexes

Two small muscles in the middle ear dampen the vibrations of the tympanic membrane and the ossicular chain: the tensor tympani and the stapedius muscles.

- The **tensor tympani** is innervated by cranial nerve V (the trigeminal nerve). The **stapedius** muscle, the smallest muscle in the body, is innervated by cranial nerve VII (the facial nerve).
- The stapedius muscle stiffens the ossicular chain so that its vibrations are reduced. The tensor tympani muscle tenses the tympanic membrane so that its vibrations are reduced. Figure 12.2 and Figure 12.3 depict the ossicular chain and the middle ear.
- When a person hears very loud noises that could damage the ears, the middle ear muscles contract in a reflexive action called the **acoustic reflex**. The acoustic reflex stiffens the middle ear system, especially the tympanic membrane.

Eustachian Tube

Also known as the auditory tube, the **Eustachian tube** connects the middle ear with the nasopharynx. The Eustachian tube goes from the anterior middle ear wall to the posterior wall of the nasopharynx.

- The Eustachian tube helps maintain equal air pressure within and outside the middle ear. The nasopharyngeal end of the tube can be opened by yawning or swallowing. This ventilates the middle ear by letting in fresh air.
- The opening of the Eustachian tube is assisted by the contraction of the **tensor veli palatini**. The tensor veli palatini helps with opening the Eustacian tube during yawning and swallowing.
- The Eustachian tube can also allow germs and infections to spread into the middle ear, causing hearing problems. This is especially common in infants, whose Eustachian tubes are more horizontal than those of adults.
- Infants with a cleft of the palate frequently have Eustachian tube dysfunction, making them vulnerable to conductive hearing loss (described in its own section later in this chapter).

The Inner Ear

The **inner ear** is the most complex of the three divisions of the ear. It begins with the **oval window**, which is a small opening in the **temporal bone** that houses the inner ear. Through the movement of the footplate of the stapes in the oval window, the inner ear receives the mechanical vibrations of sound. Figure 12.4 shows the round and oval window.

- The inner ear is a system of interconnecting tunnels called **labyrinths** within the temporal bone. The tunnels are filled with a fluid called **perilymph**.

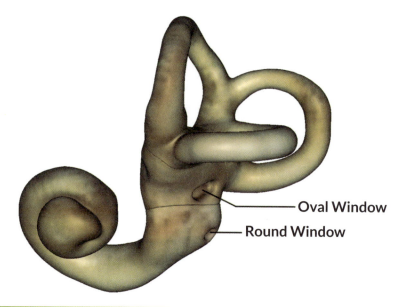

Figure 12.4 Round window and oval window. Used with permission from Anatomage.

- There are two major structures in the inner ear, each with separate functions. The first is the **vestibular system**, which contains three **semicircular canals**. The semicircular canals are responsible for equilibrium. Thus, the vestibular system is related to movement, balance, and body posture. The vestibular system is shown in Figure 12.5.
- The second major structure in the inner ear is the **cochlea**. The cochlea is snail shaped and resembles a coiled tunnel. When stretched, the human cochlea measures about 3.8 cm (1.5 inches). It is filled with **endolymph**, a type of fluid.

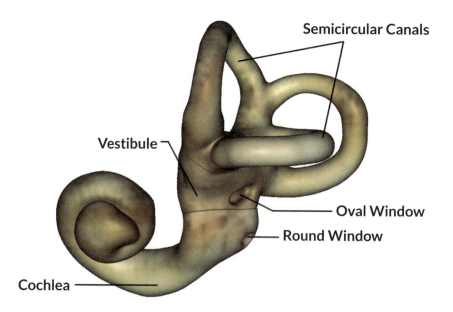

Figure 12.5 Vestibular system. Used with permission from Anatomage.

- The floor of the cochlear duct is called the **basilar membrane**, which contains the **organ of Corti**. The organ of Corti is bathed in endolymph and contains several thousand hair cells, or **cilia**, which respond to sound vibrations. Each ear contains approximately 15,500 hair cells.
- The vibrations created by the footplate of the stapes into the oval window create wavelike movements in the perilymph. Through **Reissner's membrane**, those movements are transmitted to the endolymph. The endolymph then transmits the movements to the **basilar membrane**.
- Different portions of the basilar membrane respond best to sounds of different frequencies. The tip, or apex, of the membrane is thicker, wider, and more lax than the base. At the base, the membrane is thinner, narrower, and stiffer than at the tip.
- Low-frequency sounds stimulate the apex, and high-frequency sounds stimulate the base. The stimulating sound signals set off waves in the fluid, which in turn create movements of the membrane.
- The hair cells in the organ of Corti respond to the vibrations of the basilar membrane. The vibrations create a shearing force on those cells. At that point, the mechanical forces of vibrations are transformed into electrical energy, which can stimulate nerve endings.
- This energy transformation within the organ of Corti is critical, because the nerve fibers that carry the sound to the brain do not respond to mechanical vibrations—only to electrical impulses.

The Auditory Nervous System

Cranial nerve VIII (the acoustic nerve) picks up the neural impulses created by the movement of the hair cells in the cochlea. This nerve, also called the vestibulocochlear nerve, is a bundle of neurons with two branches. Figure 12.6 shows the vestibulocochlear nerve.

- The **vestibular branch** is concerned with body equilibrium or balance. The **auditory**, or **acoustic**, **branch** supplies many hair cells of the cochlea and conducts electrical sound impulses from the cochlea to the brain.

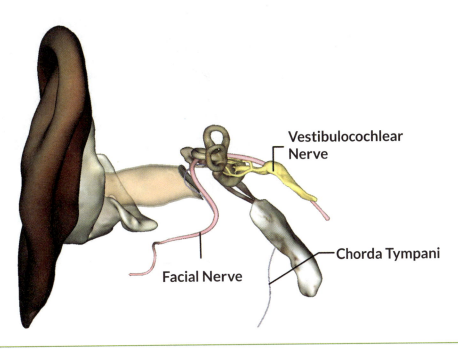

Figure 12.6 Cranial nerve VIII (the acoustic nerve). Used with permission from Anatomage.

- The auditory division of the acoustic nerve has many endings in the cochlea. These nerve endings are in contact with the hair cells to pick up the sound vibrations that are transformed into neural impulses.
- Approximately 30,000 nerve fibers of the auditory nerve exist in the cochlea. The auditory nerve exits the inner ear through the **internal auditory meatus**.
- The nerve impulses carried by the right and left auditory pathways enter the brainstem. The auditory pathways up to this point (the brainstem) are considered **peripheral** (related to structures outside the brain). Beyond the brainstem, the pathways are considered **central** (within the brain).
- At the **cerebellopontine angle**, the auditory nerve exits the temporal bone through the internal auditory meatus and enters the brainstem. At the brainstem level, most of the auditory nerve fibers from one ear **decussate** (cross over) to the opposite side, forming **contralateral pathways**.
- Some, however, continue on the same side, forming **ipsilateral pathways**. This crossover of signals allows the brain to compare the sounds received from each of the two ears. It helps the brain localize and interpret sounds.
- From the brainstem, the acoustic nerve fibers project sound to the temporal lobe of the brain. The temporal lobe contains the primary auditory area, which is responsible for receiving and interpreting sound stimuli. The temporal lobe, with its primary auditory area, is shown in Figure 12.7.

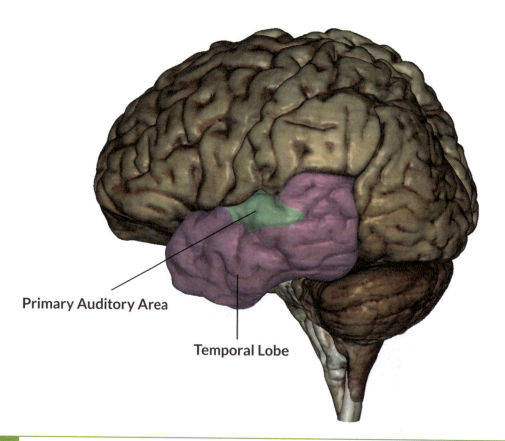

Figure 12.7 Temporal lobe and primary auditory area. Used with permission from Anatomage.

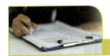

SUMMARY

The outer ear, composed of the auricle and the pinna, funnels sound to the middle ear. The tympanic membrane, which separates the outer ear from the middle ear, vibrates in response to sound.

- Sound is then responded to by the ossicles, which conduct the sound to the inner ear. The vestibular system and cochlea are the major structures of the inner ear. Here energy is converted to electrical impulses, which stimulate the acoustic nerve.
- The auditory branch of the acoustic nerve carries electrical sound impulses from the cochlea to the brain, where the sound is interpreted in the primary auditory area of the temporal lobe.

ACOUSTICS: SOUND AND ITS PERCEPTION

Acoustics, a branch of physics, is the study of sound as a physical event. Psychoacoustics is the study of sound as the psychological experience of hearing. Speech is the most important acoustic signal for humans to perceive. (For a more in-depth discussion of acoustics, see Chapter 2) Humans perceive sound in terms of frequency (pitch) and intensity (loudness). Hearing can be measured in terms of sound pressure (SPL) or hearing level (HL).

The Source of Sound

The source of sound is mechanical vibrations of an elastic object. The vibrations create waves of disturbance. The waves then travel through a gas, a liquid, or a solid—these are called **mediums**. The mediums must be elastic to carry sound. To be called a sound, the disturbance of the molecules must be audible.

- There are many sources of sound: the vocal folds, the strings of an instrument, a tuning fork, and others. The vibrations of a tuning fork illustrate a source of sound. A tuning fork, when struck, vibrates at a single frequency.
- Vibrations occur in **cycles**, or repeated patterns of movement that are measured per second. **Frequency** refers to the number of times a cycle of vibration repeats itself within a second. A tone of single frequency is called a **pure tone**. A tone of single frequency that repeats itself is called a **simple harmonic motion** or **sinusoidal motion**. Two or more sounds of differing frequencies create a **complex tone**.
- The vibrations that make up a complex tone may be periodic or aperiodic. As illustrated in Figure 12.8, **periodic** vibrations have a pattern that repeats itself at regular intervals until it is stopped by external action. **Aperiodic** vibrations do not have such a pattern; they occur at irregular intervals.

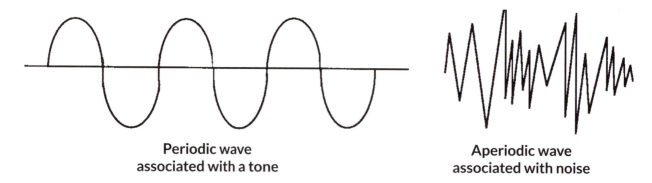

Figure 12.8 Periodic and aperiodic sound waves. From *Introduction to Communicative Disorders* (5th ed.), by M. N. Hegde, forthcoming, Austin, TX: PRO-ED. Copyright by PRO-ED, Inc. Reprinted with permission.

Sound Waves

When an object such as a guitar string moves back and forth, it displaces nearby air molecules, causing them to move, too. This in turn causes movement in molecules lying farther and farther away from the vibrating object. These movements are called **sound waves**.

- The molecules near the vibrating object swing back and forth while remaining where they are (they do not move from one point to another). These swings disturb adjacent molecules, which then swing back and forth, thus disturbing the molecules next to them, and the process continues.
- The back-and-forth movements of the molecules change the air pressure because the movements consist of an instance in which the molecules are compressed together (**compression**) and an instance in which they are farther apart (**rarefaction**). Rarefaction can also be thought of as expansion. As Figure 12.9 illustrates, a single cycle consists of one instance of compression and one instance of rarefaction within a second.

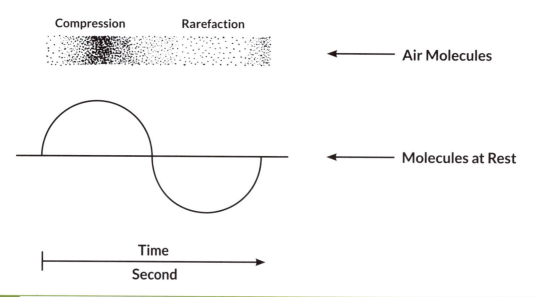

Figure 12.9 A tone of a single Hz (1cps) containing one instance of rarefaction and one instance of compression of air molecules in 1 second. From *Introduction to Communicative Disorders* (5th ed.), by M. N. Hegde, forthcoming, Austin, TX: PRO-ED. Copyright by PRO-ED, Inc. Reprinted with permission.

- The term **hertz** (Hz) refers to cycles per second. For example, 200 Hz means that there are 200 cycles of compression and rarefaction in 1 second. It means the same thing as 200 cps, or cycles per second.

Frequency and Intensity

The human ear is capable of responding to frequencies in the range of 20 Hz to 20000 Hz. Some animals, such as dogs and dolphins, can hear sounds of much higher frequency.

- Variations in the frequency of vibratory cycles cause the sensation of different pitches. **Pitch** changes are basically changes in frequency. Pitch is the perceptual correlate of changes in frequency. Pitch is perceptual; frequency is physical.
- As well as varying in frequency, sounds vary in **intensity**. Changes in intensity are changes in the **loudness** of sounds. Loudness is a perceptual phenomenon; intensity is a physical phenomenon.
- Intensity is related to **amplitude**, which is the extent of displacement of the molecules in their to-and-fro motion. The greater the range of displacement, the greater the amplitude of the sound. And the greater the amplitude of sound, the greater the intensity of that sound. Tones of different amplitude in the context of different frequencies are illustrated in Figure 12.10.
- The human ear is sensitive to a wide range of intensity—perhaps 10 trillion units, as measured on a linear scale that has an absolute zero point and equal numerical increments.
- Because measuring these large numbers is cumbersome, scientists use a **logarithmic scale**. On such a scale, one number is multiplied by itself a specified number of times.
- On a logarithmic scale, the ear is sensitive to 130 units called decibels (dB). A **decibel** is ¹/₁₀ of a bel, the basic unit of sound pressure measurement named after Alexander Graham Bell.

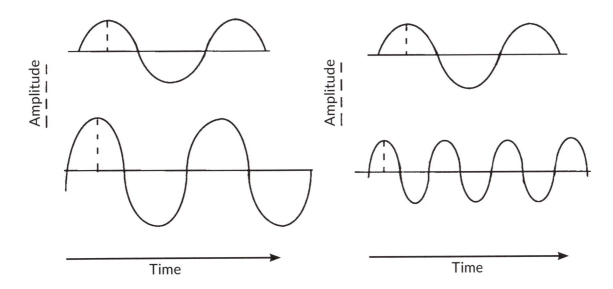

These two sound waves have the same frequency but different amplitude.

These two sound waves have the same amplitude but different frequency.

Figure 12.10 Amplitude in the context of frequency. From *Introduction to Communicative Disorders* (5th ed.), by M. N. Hegde, forthcoming, Austin, TX: PRO-ED. Copyright by PRO-ED, Inc. Reprinted with permission.

Sound Pressure Level and Hearing Level

The decibel is a measure of sound pressure; it also measures the intensity of one sound against another.

- The value of **sound pressure** is the square root of **power**, which is measured in **watts**. The pressure is measured in terms of **pascal** (Pa). The intensity of a sound is expressed in terms of decibels at a certain **sound pressure level** (SPL).
- For example, normal speech usually varies between 50 and 70 dB SPL. Very loud sounds, such as those of an airplane, may be as high as 100 dB SPL. People feel pain when sound level reaches 140 dB SPL.
- SPL is different from **hearing level** (HL), which is the lowest intensity of a sound necessary to stimulate the auditory system. Hearing level is the decibel level used on audiometers; it is the decibel level of sound referenced to audiometric zero.
- The auditory system is not equally sensitive to all frequencies at the same intensity. The human ear is most sensitive to sounds ranging between 1000 and 4000 Hz. Thus, to stimulate the auditory system, tones of 1000–4000 Hz can be less intense than tones of other frequencies. This differential sensitivity of the human ear to different frequencies creates complications in the measurement of hearing and hearing loss.
- To deal with this problem, scientists first determined the SPLs necessary to stimulate the auditory system at different frequencies in a large number of people with normal hearing. Then those SPLs were considered the 0 dB HL. For example, to stimulate the healthy normal ear of a young adult, a tone of 250 Hz must have a sound pressure level of 25.5 dB SPL. For the same purpose, a sound of 1000 Hz needs only 7 dB SPL.
- In measuring hearing with an audiometer, the actual SPL values needed to stimulate the auditory system of a typical person at those two frequencies were set at 0, although in the case of the 250 Hz tone, the SPL value is higher than in the other tone (1000 Hz). Similarly, for all the frequencies that are tested on an audiometer, the amount of energy needed to stimulate the auditory system has been set at 0.

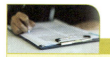

SUMMARY

Sound must travel through a medium and create an audible disturbance of molecules to be heard. Sound occurs in cycles, each of which consists of one instance of compression and one instance of rarefaction.

- Humans hear sounds in various frequencies at various intensity levels and respond differentially to different frequencies. Human responses to sound can be measured by several means, including sound pressure level and hearing level.

THE NATURE AND ETIOLOGY OF HEARING LOSS

The development of hearing begins in utero; fetuses can respond to sound in the first trimester of development. Babies localize and discriminate sound with increasing skill as they grow older. Sound is conducted to the inner ear through either air or bone conduction. In people with hearing impairment, this process is disrupted through hearing loss of a conductive, sensorineural, or mixed nature. Some people also experience hearing loss due to auditory nervous system impairments.

Normal Hearing

Auditory Development

Normal hearing is made possible by the complex working of the outer, middle, and inner ear, as well as the auditory nerve and auditory areas of the brain. Normal hearing also involves a set of skills that develop over time.

- During the fetal development period, babies can hear in utero—in fact, a 20-week-old fetus responds to sound. Newborns can respond differentially to sounds of different intensity and frequency.
- By 3–4 months of age, babies turn their heads toward sources of sound. Three-month-old babies respond to the mother's voice more consistently than to anyone else's voice.
- As babies grow older, they respond more precisely to auditory stimuli. Sounds are better discriminated and localized. By 6 months of age, an infant can localize speech that is very soft. Young babies with normal hearing can hear better than adults.

Air and Bone Conduction of Sound

In people with normal hearing, sound is conducted to the inner ear by two means: air conduction and bone conduction.

- In the process of **air conduction**, sound waves strike the tympanic membrane. The movement of the tympanic membrane causes the ossicles to move, creating movement of the fluids of the inner ear. These movements cause vibrations in the basilar membrane of the cochlea.
- The hair cells supplied by the acoustic nerve respond to these vibrations, and the sound is carried to the brain by the acoustic nerve. In this process, sound travels through the medium of air. Thus, the process is described as air conduction.
- The process of **bone conduction** is different. The fluids of the inner ear are housed in the skull. The larger bones of the skull conduct sound, as does the ossicular chain of the middle ear. The skull bones vibrate in response to airborne sound waves, causing movements in the inner ear fluids. Thus, bones have conducted the sound to the inner ear.
- Air and bone conduction result in the same kind of cochlear activity, in which the hair cells are displaced. Normally, air- and bone-conducted movements are integrated. It is only in certain kinds of hearing loss that the two can be distinguished.

The Nature of Hearing Impairment

Hearing impairment is an increasing health and educational problem. Many more people are living longer, manifesting hearing problems associated with the aging process.

- One phenomenon observed in the 21st century is the increasing number of younger adults who present with hearing losses. Today, more than half of all hearing-impaired persons are younger than 65 years of age. Most people with hearing loss are Baby Boomers, between the ages of 54 and 74 years. Baby Boomers are defined as being born between the years 1944 and 1964. One out of six Baby Boomers is hearing impaired (Martin & Clark, 2014). The increased use of personal music players and earbuds has been a major contributor to this phenomenon.
- Recent research has found that many young African Americans who listen to rap music on their portable listening devices exceed recommended volume levels for listening (Fligor, Levey, & Levey, 2014). A contributor to this phenomenon may be that to fully appreciate the bass notes in rap, music must be played at a higher volume.
- In addition, more newborn babies are at risk for hearing impairment. Advanced medical technology has enabled more fragile, high-risk, preterm infants to be saved; these infants are more vulnerable to hearing problems than healthy, full-term infants (Driscoll & McPherson, 2010).
- Factors that place a child at risk for hearing loss include anatomic malformations of the head and neck, maternal history of drug or alcohol abuse, certain maternal diseases such as rubella, or syphilis during pregnancy. Parents can also carry a gene or genes for hearing loss. If the genetic component is a recessive gene, it is possible for neither parent to have a hearing loss.
- Hearing impairment can be very mild, but may still create academic difficulties and problems in communication. It can also be severe to profound, causing major difficulties in articulation, resonance, and comprehension and reception of speech. The range of hearing loss in dB HL and the corresponding categories are shown in Table 12.1.
- The term *hearing impaired* refers to the condition of being hard of hearing or deaf.
- Degrees of hearing loss range from slight to profound. Slight hearing loss is between 16 to 25 dB HL; mild is between 26 to 40 dB HL; moderate is between 41 to 55 dB HL; moderately severe is between 56 to 70 dB HL; severe is between 71 to 90 dB HL; and profound is 91+.
- Children and adults who are **deaf** are those who cannot hear or understand conversational speech under normal circumstances.
- The term *Deaf* with an uppercase *D* refers to deafness as a cultural identity.
- People who have a hearing impairment may have one of several kinds of hearing losses: conductive, sensorineural, or mixed. Some people also manifest central auditory or retrocochlear disorders, which are special categories.

Conductive Hearing Loss

In conductive hearing loss, the efficiency with which the sound is conducted to the middle or inner ear is diminished. In pure conductive hearing loss, the inner ear, acoustic nerve, and auditory centers of the brain are all working normally. The person's bone conduction is also fairly normal (normal bone conduction refers to the skull bones, not the ossicular chain).

Table 12.1

Range and Categories of Hearing Loss With the Corresponding dB HL

Hearing loss	Characteristics
Up to 15 dB	Normal hearing in children. In adults the upper limit of normal hearing may extend to 25 dB.
16 to 40 dB	Mild hearing loss in children: difficulty hearing faint or distant speech—may cause language delay in children. In adults the range is between 25 and 40 dB.
41 to 55 dB	Moderate hearing loss: delayed speech and language acquisition; difficulty in producing certain speech sounds correctly; difficulty following conversation.
56 to 70 dB	Moderately severe hearing loss: can understand only amplified or shouted speech.
71 to 90 dB	Severe hearing loss: difficulty understanding even loud and amplified speech; significant difficulty in learning and producing intelligible oral language.
91+ dB	Profound hearing loss: typically described as deaf; hearing does not play a major role in learning, producing, and understanding spoken speech and language.

Note. From *Introduction to Communicative Disorders* (5th ed.), by M. N. Hegde, forthcoming, Austin, TX: PRO-ED. Copyright by PRO-ED, Inc. Reprinted with permission.

- Even when the bones of the ossicular chain are not conducting sound, the bones of the skull do. Thus, conductive hearing loss is never profound; there is always some hearing left because of bone conduction created by the skull bones.
- Consequently, people with conductive hearing loss can hear their own speech well. Thus, they tend to speak too softly, especially when there is background noise, which they cannot hear as well as their listeners can.
- There are many causes of conductive hearing loss. These include abnormalities of the external auditory canal, the tympanic membrane, or the ossicular chain of the middle ear.
- Birth defects, diseases, and foreign bodies can also block the external ear canal. Some children born with cleft palate or other craniofacial anomalies may have **aural atresia**, in which the external ear canal is completely closed. Atresia is often associated with **microtia**, in which the pinna is very small and deformed.
- Another birth defect, **stenosis**, results in an extremely narrow external auditory canal. In these cases, most sound waves will not strike the tympanic membrane.
- **External otitis**, caused by bacteria or viruses, is a fairly common infection of the skin of the external auditory canal; this is a cause of conductive loss. This infection, commonly found in swimmers, results in the swelling of the tissue of the external auditory canal. Consequently, sound transmission is reduced.
- Foreign objects in the ear canal, such as beans, paper clips, and seeds, can block the ear canal and impede hearing. **Bony growths** and tumors may appear in the external ear canal, blocking the transmission of sound to the middle and inner ears.

- **Otitis media**, also known as **middle ear effusion**, is an infection of the middle ear that is often associated with upper-respiratory infections and Eustachian tube dysfunction. Figure 12.11 shows an audiogram representing the typical hearing loss seen in people with otitis media accompanied by effusion.

  - Otitis media occurs frequently in infants and children but rarely in adults. Differences in the incidence rate of otitis media have also been found among racial groups. African Americans have the lowest rate; the highest rates exist among Aborigines, Alaskan Eskimos, and Native Americans. These differences in incidence rates may be related to differences in the structure and function of the Eustachian tube among racial groups.

- Otitis media usually creates a conductive hearing loss of 20–35 dB HL, which often goes undetected by regular pure-tone screenings, which are carried out at 25 dB HL. There are three types of otitis media: serous, acute, and chronic.

- In **serous otitis media**, the middle ear is inflamed and filled with watery or thick fluid. The Eustachian tube is blocked and thus does not allow fresh air to ventilate the middle ear. The middle ear thus becomes airtight; soon the air inside is thinned out and the pressure is reduced.

  - The increased air pressure outside the ear begins to push the tympanic membrane inward, reducing its mobility. The retracted membrane vibrates inefficiently, resulting in conductive hearing loss.

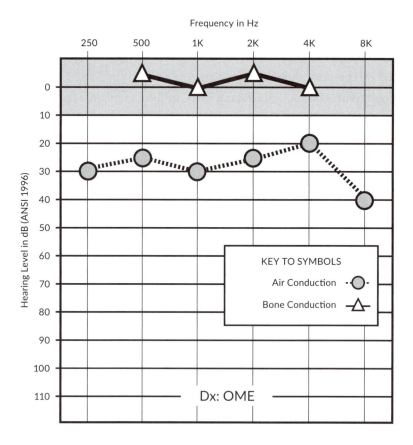

Figure 12.11 An audiogram representing the effects of otitis media with effusion (OME).

Serous otitis media is frequently treated with antibiotics and **pressure equalizing (PE) tubes**. These tiny tubes are inserted through the tympanic membrane, ventilating the middle ear and restoring hearing.

- In **acute otitis media**, there is sudden onset due to infection. A quick buildup of fluid and pus causes moderate to severe pain. The child has a fever and may experience vertigo. The buildup of pressure in the middle ear may rupture the tympanic membrane, giving instant relief as pus is discharged from the ruptured membrane. Hearing loss can occur when the tympanic membrane has ruptured.

  - Acute otitis media is treated with medical and surgical procedures. In a surgical procedure known as **myringotomy**, small incisions are made in the tympanic membrane to relieve the pressure.

- In **chronic otitis media**, there is permanent damage to middle ear structures. This is frequently due to erosion of ossicles, cholosteotoma, or atrophy or perforation of the tympanic membrane.

  - When the tympanic membrane is involved, it is permanently ruptured with or without associated middle ear diseases. Many patients may have a painless, foul-smelling discharge from the ear. Antibiotics may be prescribed if an infection is present. In a surgical procedure known as **myringoplasty**, the perforated tympanic membrane is surgically repaired.

- Mild and nonrecurrent otitis media generally does not cause permanent hearing loss. Permanent loss is more likely to result from chronic disease. However, even mild and fluctuating conductive hearing loss associated with prolonged middle ear infections in young children can adversely affect their speech and language development.

- **Otosclerosis** is another common cause of conductive hearing loss. It may be inherited and is more common in women than in men. It is found primarily among Whites worldwide.

  - In otosclerosis, a new, spongy growth starts on the footplate of the stapes. Consequently, the stapes becomes rigid, and the footplate does not move enough into the oval window to create pressure waves in the inner ear fluid. Figure 12.12 shows an audiogram representing the typical hearing loss seen in people with otosclerosis.

- **Carhart's notch**, frequently found in those patients with otosclerosis, is a pattern of bone-conduction thresholds characterized by reduced bone-conduction sensitivity predominantly at 2000 Hz.

- A disease called **otospongiosis** causes the stapes to become too soft to vibrate. The diseased or fixated stapes is surgically removed in a procedure called a **stapedectomy**. A synthetic prosthesis of wire or Teflon replaces the removed stapes, often dramatically improving hearing postsurgically.

- Other causes of conductive hearing loss include collapsed ear canals, impacted cerumen, ossicular fixation, and disarticulation of the ossicular chain. Figure 12.13 shows an audiogram representing the typical hearing loss seen in people with disarticulation of the ossicular chain, also called **ossicular discontinuity**.

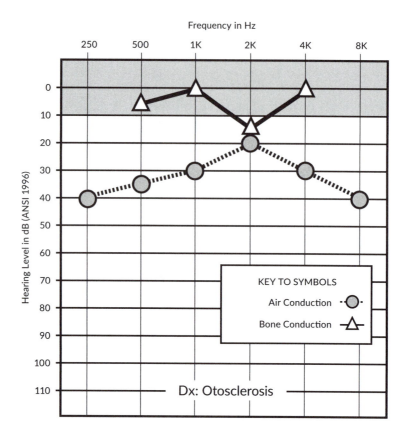

Figure 12.12 An audiogram representing the effects of otosclerosis.

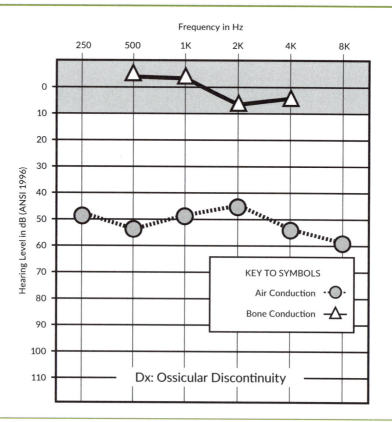

Figure 12.13 An audiogram representing the effects of ossicular discontinuity.

Sensorineural Hearing Loss

In **sensorineural hearing loss**, the middle ear may conduct sound efficiently to the inner ear, but damage to the hair cells of the cochlea (**sensori**) or to the acoustic nerve (**neural**) prevents the brain from receiving the neural impulses of the sound.

- Sensorineural loss is permanent, because neither the damaged hair cells or the acoustic nerve is repairable. The person with sensorineural loss may experience very mild to profound deafness along the continuum of frequencies.
- Because bone as well as air conduction is impaired, people with sensorineural loss have difficulty hearing themselves, as well as others. This may cause them to speak more loudly than is typical of others.
- Sensorineural loss is not necessarily the same across all frequencies; some frequencies may be more adversely affected than others. The higher frequencies tend to be more profoundly affected by sensorineural loss than the lower frequencies.
- A potential symptom of sensorineural hearing loss is recruitment. **Recruitment** refers to a disproportionate increase in the perceived loudness of sound when it is presented with linear increases in intensity. Recruitment makes a person hypersensitive to intense sounds and must be considered during hearing aid fitting.
- People with sensorineural hearing loss may experience severe effects on their speech and language. Articulation, resonance, and even voice may be affected. There are many causes of sensorineural hearing loss.

  - **Prenatal causes** of hearing loss include events that occur during pregnancy to damage the fetus's hearing. Certain drugs taken by the mother, especially during the 6th and 7th week of pregnancy, can cause cochlear damage in the fetus. In addition, children born to alcohol- and drug-addicted mothers may have sensorineural hearing loss.
  - **Ototoxic** drugs reach the inner ear through the bloodstream and damage the cochlear hair cells or the acoustic nerve fibers in children and adults. Antibiotic drugs of the "mycin" family (kanamycin, meomycin, streptomycin) are especially ototoxic. These powerful antibiotics should only ever be used in cases of severe, life-threatening infections, such as those related to kidney malfunctioning. In such cases, profound hearing loss may be an undesirable but unavoidable side effect.
  - **Genetic factors**, including a dominant or recessive gene(s) for hearing loss
  - **Noise** is another factor that can induce sensorineural hearing loss. Prolonged exposure to intense noises (e.g., loud music, electric drills, airplanes, explosives) usually damages the cochlear hair cells. The resulting sensorineural hearing loss is usually the most profound between 3000 Hz and 6000 Hz (see Figure 12.14).

A healthy, average person should hear normally up until about age 60 years if his or her unprotected ears have not been exposed to loud levels of noise. Unfortunately, it is estimated that between 5 million and 30 million Americans are occupationally exposed to noise levels greater than 85 dB. It is estimated that one fourth of these workers will develop a permanent hearing loss that will probably be accompanied by

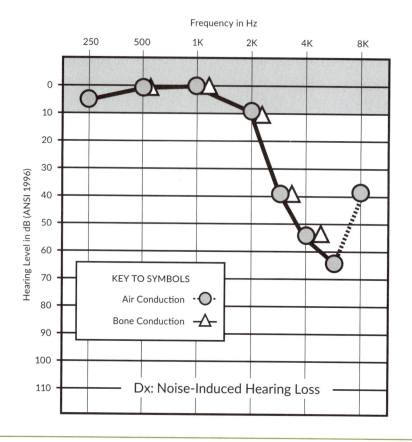

Figure 12.14 An audiogram representing the effects of excessive noise exposure.

tinnitus (a ringing or buzzing sound in the ears). It is very important for workplaces to help their employees protect their hearing when loud levels of noise are present.

- Today, noise is one of the leading causes of sensorineural hearing loss in young and middle-aged American adults. The vast majority of high school and college students own a personal music device, and most are not informed about listening levels that are safe (DeBonis, 2015).
- **Birth defects** in some children may be responsible for sensorineural hearing loss. For example, the auditory nerve or cochlea may not have developed normally by the time the baby is born, or portions of the inner ear may be missing.
- Viral and bacterial diseases can also result in sensorineural hearing loss in children. Bacterial meningitis and mumps are two such causes.
- The acronym STORCH refers to major causes of hearing loss in fetuses and newborns and stands for the following:
  - **Syphilis**, which some children contract from the mother at the time of birth, can cause inner ear damage.
  - **Toxoplasmosis**, a disease transmitted through the placenta, is often contracted when the pregnant mother handles cat feces or contaminated raw eggs or meat.
  - **Rubella**, or German measles, can be transferred to the fetus through the placenta.

- **Cytomegalovirus**, the most common cause of viral hearing loss, is a herpes-type virus transmitted by close contact with infected children and also through sexual contact.
- **Herpes simplex**, transmitted from the mother to the fetus, also can cause hearing loss.

■ A tumor called an **acoustic neuroma** can develop on the acoustic nerve and cause sensorineural loss by slowing nerve conduction of sound impulses to the brain.

■ **Presbycusis**, a hearing impairment in older people, is due to the effect of aging and is associated with sensorineural hearing loss. It affects the high frequencies especially, resulting in a sloping high-frequency loss (see Figure 12.15). Patients often have difficulty understanding speech, especially under challenging listening conditions, such as noisy parties.

■ **Meniere's disease** is a condition that causes fluctuating sensorineural hearing loss, usually in adults. It is attributed to excessive endolymphatic fluid pressure in the membranous labyrinth, which causes Reissner's membrane to become distended.

- Symptoms of Meniere's disease include hearing loss, spells of dizziness or vertigo, a sense of fullness in the ear, and **tinnitus**, a ringing or buzzing sound in the ears. Currently, no cure for this disease is available.

■ Most sensorineural hearing loss can be helped importantly by medical and surgical intervention, especially when the intervention is utilized soon after the hearing loss occurs. People who have

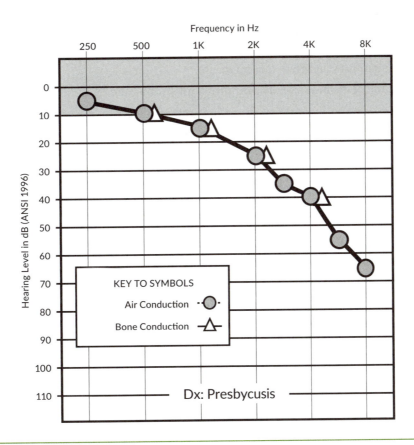

Figure 12.15 An audiogram representing the effects of presbycusis.

sensorineural hearing loss may rely on a combination of approaches including early education (for children), amplification or restoration (via cochlear implants) of sound, and speech–language therapy. These and other habilitative services are described later in this chapter.

Mixed Hearing Loss

Mixed hearing loss occurs when neither the middle ear nor the inner ear is functioning properly. Any of the several conditions that cause conductive and sensorineural hearing loss can, in some combination, cause a mixed loss.

- Mixed losses may be caused by the presence of two separate disorders in the same ear. For example, a child could have a sensorineural loss *and* a temporary conductive loss in the same ear caused by **otitis media**.
- Another cause of mixed losses could be a single pathology, such as advanced otosclerosis or a head injury, that affected both sensorineural and conductive systems. A mixed loss affects both air and bone conduction, but air conduction is affected more than bone conduction.

Auditory Nervous System Impairments

Central Auditory Disorders

The central auditory system includes the brainstem, where the auditory nerve terminates; the fibers that project sound to the auditory centers of the brain; and those auditory centers themselves.

- The term **central auditory processing** refers to the effectiveness and efficiency with which the central nervous system uses auditory information.
- **Peripheral hearing problems** result from problems in the outer, middle, or inner ear (excluding the auditory nerve). **Central auditory disorders** refer to hearing losses due to disrupted sound transmission between the brainstem and the cerebrum as a result of damage or malformation. The temporal cortex of the brain may receive incorrect information, or the person may process information incorrectly.
- Put differently, central auditory processing disorder can be viewed as a disorder in a person's ability to take in a spoken message, interpret it, and make it meaningful.
- Central auditory disorders can be caused by tumors, traumatic brain injury, HIV, asphyxia during birth, various genetic disorders, infections such as meningitis and encephalitis, metabolic disturbances, cerebrovascular diseases, drug- or chemical-induced problems, central degenerative diseases such as Alzheimer's disease, and demyelinating diseases such as multiple sclerosis.
- There is controversy in the literature about the existence, nature, and treatment of central auditory disorders (DeBonis, 2015; Nelson, 2010). Empirical evidence is limited, and many researchers do not support "central auditory disorder" as a valid diagnostic label, although others do.
- People with central auditory disorders may have no significant peripheral hearing loss. Routine speech recognition tests in quiet environments and typical pure-tone threshold tests are not sensitive to central auditory disorders.

- Difficulty understanding distorted speech is a major symptom of central auditory disorders. In some of the central auditory tests, speech may be presented at low intensity, compressed in time, masked with noise, periodically interrupted, or filtered by eliminating certain frequencies of speech. **Dichotic listening** tasks, in which the listener must process different messages presented simultaneously to both ears, are also used.
- Although everyone has some difficulty understanding distorted speech, those with central auditory disorders have great difficulty.
- For example, when there is a lesion in the temporal lobe of the brain, filtered-speech test scores may be worse in the ear opposite the damaged side (contralateral) than in the ear on the side of the damage. People with central auditory disorders usually also have abnormal auditory discrimination because speech sounds are distorted at the cortical level.
- Patients with central auditory disorders typically manifest the following characteristics (DeBonis, 2015; Geffner & Ross-Swain, 2012; Pakulski, 2014b):
  - Poor auditory discrimination (as stated)
  - Poor auditory integration
  - Poor auditory sequencing skills
  - Poor auditory closure (e.g., recognizing that "_anta _aus" is "Santa Claus")
  - Difficulty listening when background noise exists
  - Poor auditory attention
  - Poor auditory memory
  - Poor auditory localization, or ability to locate a sound source in the environment
  - Difficulty understanding rapid speech and other forms of auditory input that are characterized by reduced redundancy
  - Difficulty following melodic and rhythmic elements of music
  - Overall academic problems, including challenges with reading, writing, and spelling
  - Difficulty with vocabulary and pragmatics skills

Behavioral intervention programs for children with central auditory processing disorders can be described as a tripod with three components: (a) using direct intervention or remediation techniques aimed at improving auditory skill, (b) helping the child use compensatory strategies to manage the deficit, and (c) modifying the environment to minimize adverse learning conditions. Sometimes, FM systems (described later in this chapter under "Communication Learning") are successful in helping children with central auditory processing disorders.

Retrocochlear Disorders

People with **retrocochlear** pathology have damage to the nerve fibers along the ascending auditory pathways from the internal auditory meatus to the cortex. Thus, these disorders usually consist of pathology involving the cerebellopontine angle (mentioned earlier, in the "Auditory Nervous System Impairments" section) or cranial nerve VIII.

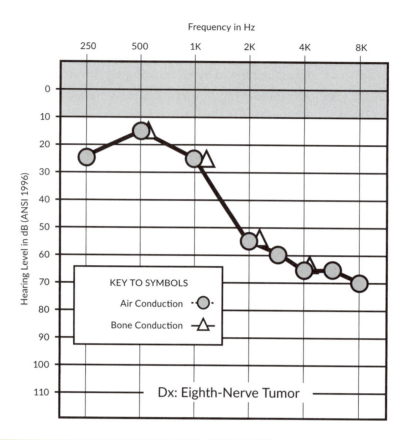

Figure 12.16 An audiogram representing the effects of an eight-nerve acoustic tumor.

- Retrocochlear pathology is usually caused by unilateral tumors or **acoustic neuromas**. The patient often experiences a unilateral high-frequency hearing loss that may be accompanied by tinnitus and dizziness, as well as a general feeling of disequilibrium (see Figure 12.16). When the affected ear is stimulated, acoustic reflexes are usually absent or present at elevated levels.
- Patients with acoustic neuromas may also experience alterations of facial sensation and movement because the facial and trigeminal nerves are compromised. There may be pain and headache in the ear and mastoid region and a feeling of "fullness" in the affected ear. Due to compression of the brainstem and cerebellum, the patient may experience problems with balance.
- Symptoms of retrocochlear disorders are often subtle, because patients have normal ability to detect pure tones, as well as normal speech recognition in quiet. To help determine the presence of retrocochlear pathology, many audiologists use degraded speech signals, which involve speech that is interrupted, accompanied by noise, or filtered.
- It is challenging to make an audiological diagnosis of acoustic neuroma. Because acoustic neuromas grow very slowly, the patient may not notice the ever-so-gradual loss of hearing until the acoustic neuroma is quite large and there is a serious hearing loss.
- If the patient is relatively young and physically active, balance problems may be harder to detect than they would be in older, more sedentary patients. In these older patients, balance problems would be noticed earlier.

- It is not difficult to confuse the symptoms of acoustic neuroma with the symptoms of Meniere's disease. Auditory brainstem responses (described in the "Assessment of Hearing Impairment" section of this chapter) are a frequently used electrophysiologic measure because they are the easiest to obtain and interpret and because they assist in differential diagnosis.
- Retrocochlear disorders may be caused by **von Recklinghausen disease**, an inherited disease characterized by the presence of numerous small tumors that grow slowly along various peripheral nerves. When they grow along cranial nerve VIII, they may initially be mistaken for acoustic neuroma. Patients with this disease may die if the tumors become malignant.
- Brainstem lesions, or tumors that appear in the brainstem at levels above cranial nerve VIII, are so rare that patients often die because the tumors are undiagnosed. Even if they are detected and surgery ensues, the surgery itself may create problems (e.g., facial paralysis). Some lesions are inoperable because they lie so deep in the brainstem.

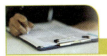

SUMMARY

Hearing is a phenomenon that begins even before babies are born and continues to develop throughout early childhood. Through air and bone conduction, sound reaches the inner ear and is sent to the brain for interpretation.

- However, some people have conductive, sensorineural, or mixed hearing losses, which disrupt the transmission of sound. People with auditory nervous system impairments such as central auditory and retrocochlear disorders also experience difficulties with sound transmission.
- It is important to accurately identify the type of hearing impairment so that appropriate treatment may be provided.

ASSESSMENT OF HEARING IMPAIRMENT

Assessment of hearing impairment has been greatly improved by new technology and sophisticated instrumentation techniques that permit increasingly accurate diagnoses of hearing problems. An initial hearing screening rules out the need for more intensive testing for most people. For those who need such testing, pure-tone and speech audiometry are standard assessment procedures, as is acoustic immittance testing, which evaluates middle-ear function. Electrophysiological audiometry and medical imaging incorporate highly specialized diagnostic methods and instruments to evaluate auditory mechanism functioning. Children and infants may be tested by special methods appropriate for their age group. Once children and adults have been tested, the test results are interpreted and recommendations for treatment can be made.

Audiometry: Basic Principles

An **audiometer** is an electronic instrument that generates and amplifies pure tones, noise, and other stimuli for testing hearing. Advanced audiometers are computerized.

- The audiometer generates tones at the frequencies of 125, 250, 500, 750, 1000, 1500, 2000, 3000, 4000, and 8000 Hz. The audiologist can select the frequency and vary the intensity of the sound stimulus through use of a dial that increases or **attenuates** (decreases) the intensity of the sound.
- The person to be tested sits in a specially constructed soundproof booth. This booth eliminates interference from ambient noise in the environment.
- During air-conduction testing, the client wears earphones held in place by a steel headband fitting across the top of the head. The earphones deliver the sound stimulus directly to the ear. The client can respond by holding up a hand or by pressing a switch that lights up a small lamp on the audiometer.

Pure-Tone Audiometry

The **pure-tone** hearing test is carried out to determine the threshold of hearing for selected frequencies. A **threshold** is an intensity level at which a tone is faintly heard at least 50% of the time it is presented. Each tone is presented several times to reliably establish a threshold.

- Audiologists test hearing at selected frequencies. Usually, a tone of 1000 Hz is presented first, because it is most easily detected. Next, tones of 2000, 4000, and 8000 Hz are tested, in that order. Finally, the tones of 500, 250, and 125 Hz are tested. All these frequencies are tested because they are the most important for human speech, which falls in the range of 100 to 8000 Hz.
- Typically, to begin, 1000 Hz is presented at 30 dB. If the participant does not respond to this tone, it should be increased to 50 dB and up to 60 dB if the subject still fails to respond; then up in 10 dB intervals until the subject responds to the tone. Once the subject responds, decrease by 10 dB until there is no response. Then, increase in 5 dB increments until there is a response. Once there is a response, decrease by 10 dB again. This "down 10 dB, up 5 dB" pattern repeats until the **threshold** is found—this is the lowest dB level that can be identified in 3 out of 6 times. This process is repeated for each of the different frequencies tested in both ears.
- Both ears are tested, one at a time. The person is asked to listen and press the response switch immediately when even a faint sound is heard.
- **Bone-conduction testing** assesses the sensitivity of the sensorineural portion of the auditory mechanism. The method is as follows: A bone vibrator is placed on the forehead or behind the test ear. When the sound strikes the bones of the skull, the bones vibrate and thus stimulate the fluid in both inner ears. Thus, it is difficult to determine which ear heard the sound and which did not.
  - To overcome this problem, the audiologist uses a procedure called **masking**, in which noise is sent through a headphone at a level that is strong enough to mask the tone heard in the opposite ear.
- Even in **air-conduction testing**, masking is used when hearing in one ear is markedly better than hearing in the other ear. That is, the better ear is masked when the poorer ear is tested, so that the client does not respond only because the sound is heard in the better, untested ear.

Speech Audiometry

A person's pure-tone thresholds do not indicate how well he or she understands speech. **Speech audiometry** measures how well a person understands speech and discriminates between speech sounds.

- The audiologist first determines a **speech reception threshold**, defined as the lowest or softest level of hearing at which the person can understand 50% of the words presented. To make this determination, a list of **spondee words** is used; these words are two-syllable words with equal stress on each syllable (e.g., *baseball, hotdog, cowboy, birthday*).
- The spondee words are either played through a recorder or spoken by the audiologist. When the client hears the words through the headphones, he or she writes them down or says them out loud.
- Another assessment made by an audiologist is based on a **word discrimination** or **word recognition** test. This test establishes how well a person discriminates between words by having the client correctly repeat monosyllabic words such as *cap* and *day*.
- Because the purpose of this test is to determine speech comprehension rather than speech threshold, the words are presented at a level of loudness that is comfortable for the person being tested.
- The speech discrimination score is the percentage of presented words that the client correctly repeats. This score helps identify people who can hear but not understand speech. People with sensorineural hearing loss are most likely to show this problem.

Acoustic Immittance

Acoustic immittance refers to a transfer of acoustic energy. An energy transformation takes place when a sound stimulus reaches the external ear canal and strikes the tympanic membrane.

- The tympanic membrane and middle ear structures offer **impedance**, or resistance, to the flow of sound energy. **Admittance**, a counterpart of impedance, is a measure of the amount of energy that flows through the system.
- Both very low and very high impedance suggests pathology within the auditory system. For example, a child with middle ear fluid may demonstrate high impedance. An adult with a broken ossicular chain may show low impedance. Tympanometry and acoustic reflex thresholds are two common acoustic immittance measures.
- **Tympanometry** is a procedure in which acoustic immittance is measured with an electroacoustic instrument called an **impedance bridge** or **impedance meter**.

  - This instrument allows the audiologist to place a sound stimulus in the external ear canal with an airtight closure and measure changes in the acoustic energy as the sound stimulates the auditory system. The instrument also helps create either negative or positive changes within the ear canal. Acoustic immittance is altered by such air pressure changes.

- The impedance meter can also measure **acoustic reflex**, a simple reflex response of the muscles attached to the stapes bone. The acoustic reflex is elicited in both ears by a relatively loud sound presented to either ear. The reflex response involves a stiffening of the ossicular chain, presumably to protect the ear from potential damage.
- Acoustic reflex testing is valuable in detecting middle ear diseases, including those that are not associated with hearing loss.

Other Methods

Electrophysiological Audiometry

Electrophysiological audiometry is an objective measure of auditory mechanism functioning. In response to sound, the cochlea, acoustic nerve, and auditory centers of the brain generate measurable electrical impulses. These impulses are recorded as changes in the background electrical activity of the brain.

- Such electrical changes produced by sound stimuli are called **auditory-evoked potentials**. Usually, abnormal patterns of electrical activity in reaction to a sound stimulus indicate a hearing loss.
- **Electrocochleography** is the procedure for measuring the electrical activity of the cochlea in response to sound. The electrocochleogram (ECoG) generated by this testing is a response consisting primarily of the compound action potential that occurs at the distal portion of cranial nerve VIII. Electrocochleography is most useful in monitoring cochlear function in operating rooms to simplify the placement of electrodes.
- **Auditory brainstem response (ABR)** is a technique used to record the electrical activity in the auditory nerve, the brainstem, and the cortical areas of the brain. It is useful in detecting brainstem diseases. It is also very helpful in testing the hearing of newborn infants.
- If the blood supply to the cochlea is interrupted or the nerve is severed or otherwise damaged when surgeons are operating on tumors or other masses near nerve VIII, either results in hearing loss for the patient.
- It is most helpful for an audiologist to be present during such surgeries. The audiologist uses auditory-evoked potential monitoring to measure the function of nerve VIII and provide feedback to the surgeon during the surgery.

Medical Imaging

- **Computerized axial tomography** is an important tool in otological diagnosis. It can help detect small tumors as well as brain lesions (e.g., infections, strokes) that cause hearing impairment.
- **Magnetic resonance imaging** is best for imaging the internal auditory canals, base of the skull, and pituitary gland regions to evaluate the possible presence of pathology affecting the auditory system. MRI is especially helpful in detecting acoustic neuromas or tumors.

Hearing Screening

It is time-consuming to test patients with a complete battery of hearing tests. However, it is important to identify people who may have a hearing problem. Hearing screening is a quick, preliminary way to determine whether the person being tested has normal hearing or may have a hearing problem and therefore needs further, more in-depth testing.

- The three major groups of individuals who undergo hearing screening include newborns, schoolchildren, and adults in professions in which they are exposed to potentially hazardous levels of noise.
- In hearing screening, pure tones are presented at 20–25 dB. Only the frequencies of 500, 1000, 2000, and 4000 Hz are tested. Testing usually takes place in a quiet room and may be done with individuals or groups.

- Some people undergo acoustic immittance testing as a part of the screening. In public schools, this is rare; usually, schoolchildren undergo pure-tone audiometric screening only.

Assessment of Infants and Children

It is important to detect hearing loss in infants as soon as possible, because early intervention can reduce its effects on speech and language acquisition.

- Various committees and health boards, such as the Joint Committee on Accreditation of Health Organizations and the Department of Health and Human Services, are encouraging all hospitals to include universal newborn hearing screening programs. Universal hearing screening for newborns is becoming increasingly implemented across the United States.
- In many hospital neonatal units, there are two primary types of newborn screening: otoacoustic emissions (OAE) and auditory brainstem response (ABR) audiometry (Welling, 2014).
- Because infants and some young children cannot give voluntary responses, hearing assessment procedures depend mostly on reflexive responses elicited by loud sounds. These sounds may include electronic instruments, toys, or bells. Testing of this type is most effective in eliciting reflexive responses from infants between birth and 6 months of age.
- **Visual reinforcement audiometry**, often used with older infants, involves presenting a sound and seeing whether the infant will turn his or her head toward the sound. This response is measured by presenting sound from different directions and noting the infant's response.
- **Behavioral observation audiometry** is a test that is used to when visual reinforcement audiometry is not possible. It is often used with infants who are less than six months of age or who are not able to turn their heads in the direction of a sound.
- **Play audiometry** uses games and is often used for children between the ages of two and four years. For example, a child will be asked to drop a toy in a box every time a tone is heard.
- In **operant audiometry**, a child's hearing is tested by conditioning voluntary responses to sound stimuli. Operant audiometry is best for children who are challenging to test using traditional audiometric means. Children with intellectual disabilities, attention-deficit disorder, and behavioral disorders often benefit from operant audiometry procedures.

Interpretation of Hearing Test Results

Before audiologists make recommendations about the habilitation of a person with hearing impairment, they consider audiological test results and information gathered from a variety of sources, which include the following:

- A case history and interview
- A comprehensive speech and language assessment
- Otological records from the patient's otologist
- Any general medical reports that include information relative to the patient's hearing and overall health
- For children, reports from regular and special education teachers

Hearing losses can be judged as follows:

- Mild (16–40 dB)
- Moderate (41–55 dB)
- Moderately severe (56–65 dB)
- Severe (66–89 dB)
- Profound (90+ dB)

- **Unilateral losses** are those found only in one ear, whereas **bilateral losses** affect both ears. The degree of loss may be the same in both ears, or there may be a difference between the ears.
- **Audiograms** are graphs that display the results of air- and bone-conduction tests. A typical audiogram shows the HL in dB for both bone- and air-conducted tones for the tested frequencies.
- Figure 12.17 shows an example of conductive hearing loss. The bone-conducted hearing is normal bilaterally, because the sound is delivered directly to the inner ear through bone conduction. However, when sound is delivered to the outer ear, there is a hearing loss. The **air–bone gap** indicates that the loss is conductive.

  - An air–bone gap can be further described as the difference between a bone-conduction hearing threshold and an air-conduction hearing threshold for a given frequency in the same ear. A difference between the air- and bone-conduction frequencies that averages 10 dB or more implies a conductive hearing loss.

- When the hearing is not significantly better in one ear, it is not necessary to use masking noise. Therefore, in Figure 12.18, unmasked bone-conduction thresholds are represented by different symbols. The audiogram shows that the person's hearing is better for some frequencies than others, which is typical of sensorineural hearing loss.
- Figure 12.19 shows an audiogram representing a mixed hearing loss. A sensorineural component is evident, because the thresholds are higher than normal when the sound is delivered directly to the cochlea via bone conduction. However, the air-conduction thresholds are also elevated. The difference between the air- and bone-conduction thresholds indicates a probable conductive hearing loss, as well.
- Figure 12.20 illustrates an audiogram of a noise-induced hearing loss. The difference in air- and bone-conduction thresholds indicates the sensorineural nature of the loss. There is also a notable diagnostic sign of noise-induced loss: a greater loss between 3000 and 6000 Hz.

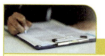

SUMMARY

Primary methods of assessing hearing impairment include pure-tone and speech audiometry, acoustic immittance, and electrophysiological audiometry.

- Whether children or adults are assessed, it is important to accurately interpret the hearing test results, so that appropriate management of the hearing impairment may be undertaken.

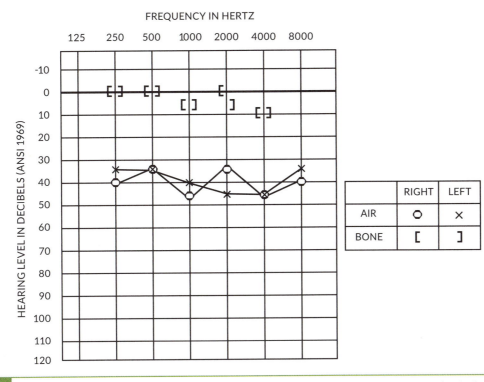

Figure 12.17 An audiogram illustrating conductive hearing loss. From *Introduction to Communicative Disorders* (3rd ed., p. 396), by M. N. Hegde, 2001, Austin, TX: PRO-ED. Copyright 2001 by PRO-ED, Inc. Reprinted with permission.

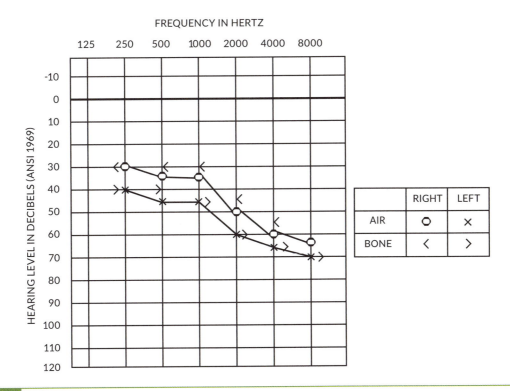

Figure 12.18 An audiogram illustrating sensorineural hearing loss. From *Introduction to Communicative Disorders* (3rd ed., p. 396), by M. N. Hegde, 2001, Austin, TX: PRO-ED. Copyright 2001 by PRO-ED, Inc. Reprinted with permission.

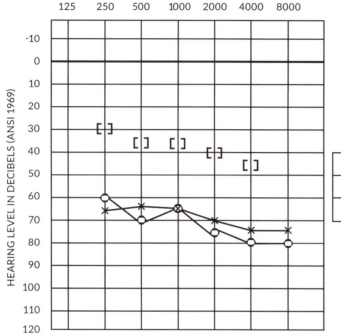

Figure 12.19 An audiogram showing a mixed hearing loss. From *Introduction to Communicative Disorders* (4th ed., p. 522), by M. N. Hegde, 2010, Austin, TX: PRO-ED. Copyright 2010 by PRO-ED, Inc. Reprinted with permission.

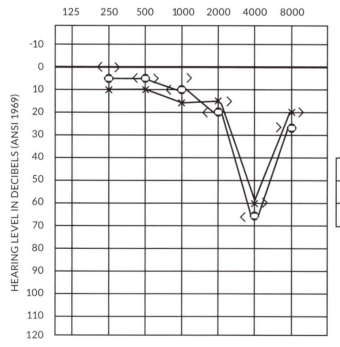

Figure 12.20 An audiogram showing a noise-induced hearing loss. From *Introduction to Communicative Disorders* (4th ed., p. 523), by M. N. Hegde, 2010, Austin, TX: PRO-ED. Copyright 2010 by PRO-ED, Inc. Reprinted with permission.

MANAGEMENT OF HEARING IMPAIRMENT

Hearing impairments can range from mild to profound, and management of hearing impairment reflects this continuum. Depending upon the type and extent of the hearing loss, people with hearing impairment often manifest difficulties in articulation, language, voice, fluency, and resonance. Amplification devices, such as hearing aids, cochlear implants, tactile aids, and assistive devices, are often used in aural rehabilitation. Communication learning may also be part of treatment, which involves methods such as auditory habilitation; speech reading; cued speech; oral language therapy; and speech, rhythm, and voice therapy. There are two broad approaches to communication learning: verbal approaches, which involve speech, and nonverbal approaches, which involve sign language.

Communication Disorders of People With Hearing Impairment

General Principles

Without normal hearing, children may learn signs, gestures, and other modes of manual communication. However, spoken language is affected.

- Hearing supports the acquisition and production of speech and language in several ways. Hearing makes infants aware of environmental and speech sounds. Hearing also makes it possible to understand spoken language. Those who cannot hear and understand speech usually need special assistance.
- Hearing is also necessary in monitoring one's own production of speech and language. Self-monitoring enables people to monitor *how* they speak, as well as what they say. People with hearing impairments have challenges in monitoring their speech, language, and voice productions.
- The extent of adverse effects of hearing impairment on speech, language, and voice depends on many variables—especially the **age of onset** of the hearing loss and the **degree of the loss**.
- **Congenital** hearing loss, or loss present at birth, has a greater impact than hearing loss acquired later in adult life. Children with **prelingual deafness** become deaf before they acquire speech and language, whereas children with **postlingual deafness** have a hearing impairment that occurred after age 5.
- The prognosis for speech and language acquisition in hard-of-hearing and deaf children depends on several factors:
  - How early in life professional help is given
  - The quality and scope of services the child receives
  - The early fitting and full-time use of hearing technologies that provide access to environmental sounds and spoken language
  - The extent to which the parents help their deaf child
  - The presence of other disabling conditions (e.g., blindness, brain damage)

In judging the impact of the hearing impairment on the patient's daily life, audiologists can have adults and older children carry out self-assessments. These typically involve questionnaires in which people evaluate the impact of the hearing loss on many aspects of their daily life and functioning.

Speech Disorders

Children with hearing impairments who are unmeliorated by hearing technologies have difficulty learning speech sounds because they cannot hear these sounds well, if at all. People with untreated profound deafness distort many vowels and almost all consonants. Omissions, substitutions, and distortions of sounds are common. Early, full-time use of appropriate hearing technologies, including hearing aids, cochlear implants, and FM systems, can provide most children access to speech sounds (also called "audibility") across the frequency range.

It is common for people with unmeliorated hearing impairment to manifest the following speech problems:

- Distortion of sounds, especially fricatives and stops
- Omission of initial and final consonants
- Consonant cluster reduction
- Substitution of voiced consonants for voiceless consonants (e.g., g/k)
- Omission of /s/ in almost all positions of words
- Substitution of nasal consonants for oral consonants (e.g., *mat/bat*)
- Increased duration of vowels
- Imprecise production of vowels (e.g., diphthongization of vowels)
- Epenthesis, or adding a schwa sound to consonant blends (e.g., sətap/stap)

Language Disorders

Some individuals who are deaf use language well; for example, there are accomplished writers who are deaf. However, many prelingually deaf people are likely to exhibit problems with language (Koehlinger, Van Horne, & Moeller, 2013).

Language problems of many prelingually deaf who do not have good access to sound via hearing technologies include the following:

- Use of a limited variety of sentence types
- Use of sentences of reduced length and complexity
- Difficulty comprehending and producing compound, complex, and embedded sentences
- Occasional irrelevance of speech, including non sequiturs (utterances that do not relate to the topic at hand)
- Provision of insufficient background information to the listener
- Limited oral communication, including lack of elaborated speech and reluctance to speak
- Difficulty understanding proverbs, metaphors, and other abstract utterances
- Slower acquisition of grammatical morphemes
- Omission or inconsistent use of many morphemes, including past tense and plural inflections, third-person singular *–s*, indefinite pronouns, present progressive *–ing*, articles, prepositions, and conjunctions
- Poor reading comprehension
- Writing that reflects oral language problems (e.g., deviant syntax, limited variety of sentence types, omission of grammatical morphemes)

Voice, Fluency, and Resonance Disorders

Problems in voice, fluency, and resonance depend heavily on the degree of hearing loss and the amount of intervention a person has experienced.

Voice, fluency, and resonance problems in many people who are deaf include the following:

- Hypernasal resonance on non-nasal sounds
- Hyponasal resonance on nasal sounds
- Abnormal phrasing, flow, and rhythm of speech
- Monotone speech with lack of appropriate intonation
- Improper stress patterns, including excessive pitch inflections
- Restricted pitch range
- Inappropriately high pitch
- Rate of speech that is too slow or too fast
- Pauses at inappropriate junctures
- Inefficient breathing, including breathiness
- Deviations in voice quality, including hoarseness and harshness

Aural Rehabilitation: Basic Principles

Aural rehabilitation is an educational and clinical program implemented by a team of professionals. It is designed to help people with hearing losses achieve their full potential.

Aural rehabilitation includes several key components (DeBonis, 2015; Hull, 2013; Pakulski, 2014b; Welling, 2014):

- An evaluation of the hearing loss
- An assessment of the patient's communicative needs (including the patient's self-assessment)
- Determination of the availability of human and financial resources to support hearing habilitation
- Prescription and fitting of a hearing aid
- Auditory therapy especially family centered auditory approaches that involve the parents and all members of a child's family in the language learning process
- Use of amplification systems in communication and educational training sessions
- Focus on communication patterns in the environment
- Addressing the impact of social, vocational, psychological, and educational factors of the hearing loss
- Counseling the person with the hearing impairment and his or her family
- Recommending additional services if needed
- Periodic reevaluation of the client's status

Many specialists are involved in aural rehabilitation. They include the following:

- The **audiologist**, who is primarily responsible for the aural rehabilitation components listed above
- The **otologist**, who monitors the health of the ear (and performs such ear surgeries as stapedectomy and tympanoplasty and prescribes medication for middle ear diseases)

- The **speech–language pathologist**, who supports the development of communicative competence in the domains of articulation, language, pragmatics, conversational skills, literacy, resonance, voice, and fluency
- In schools, the **educator of the deaf**, a special educator who teaches communication methods such as American Sign Language, as well as academic subjects, to children with hearing impairments
- The **vocational counselor**, who helps individuals investigate and make decisions about careers and vocational programs

Professionals carrying out aural rehabilitation have historically focused intensive efforts on speech reading and auditory habilitation. Today, there is a greater focus on hearing aid fitting and/or cochlear implantation and orientation, learning to use the amplified signal modifying the environment and communication patterns within the environment, and early identification and intervention.

It is recommended that those who interact with children with hearing loss communicate with **acoustic highlighting**, which involves emphasis on key words, shorter sentences, increased repetition and redundancy, a slower speaking rate, nearness to the listener, increased pitch and rhythm, and emphasis on the ends of sentences (Pakulski, 2014b).

Amplification

An important part of aural rehabilitation of people with hearing impairment is amplification of sound and speech. Sound and speech can be amplified through several means, including hearing aids, cochlear implants, tactile aids, and assistive devices.

- When children and adults with hearing losses are considered candidates for amplification, there are two major considerations. First, do they truly need the amplification? Second, are they motivated to use the amplification and care for any amplification devices properly? Patient motivation is a major factor in deciding upon appropriate amplification.

Hearing Aids

Most traditional hearing aids are small electronic devices that are worn inside the ear unilaterally or bilaterally, depending upon the needs of the client. Hearing aids amplify sound and deliver it to the ear canal. An ear mold, though not part of the hearing aid itself, is necessary for using the aid.

- The cost of hearing aids can be great; for example, a pair of state-of-the-art hearing aids can cost up to $8,000 or more. This makes access to hearing aids prohibitive for many people, as health insurance companies are increasingly transferring costs to consumers. Many insurance companies will not pay for hearing aids at all.
- To save money, some people may wear only one hearing aid. However, it is a widely accepted fact that wearing hearing aids in both ears is optimal. There are several basic types of hearing aids (DeBonis, 2015; Hall, 2014; Martin & Clark, 2014):
  - The **behind-the-ear model**, which fits behind the ear and has an internal receiver (most children wear this type of aid); the components of the device are all contained in the same case: either behind the ear or in the ear.

- The **in-the-canal model**, which fits in the ear canal and is less visible. The receiver in the canal (RIC) model has a case behind the ear that contains the aid's amplifier and microphone and a small bud that contains the receiver located inside the ear canal. A tube connects the case to the receiver.
- The **completely-in-the-canal model**, which is smaller and even less visible than the in-the-canal model and terminates close to the tympanic membrane
- The **in-the-ear model**, which is a smaller unit that fits within the concha of the external ear.

■ The **analog hearing aid** is not often used. They create patterns of electric voltage that correspond to the sound input. All analog hearing aids consist of the same basic components: a microphone, an amplifier, a receiver, a power source (batteries), and volume control. Analog hearing aids now comprise a very small proportion of the total—approximately 10%.

■ Digital hearing provide superior sound and connectivity to other devices (i.e., Bluetooth) and now comprise 90% of the market.

■ Hearing aid **transducers** include the **microphone**, which picks up sound, and the **receiver**, which delivers the sound to the ear. These transducers convert one form of energy into another.

■ The microphone converts the sound energy into electrical energy. The **amplifier** is where the electrical signals are fed and signals are amplified, which is then delivered to the receiver. The amount of amplification applied to the signal is called **gain**. The receiver, housed in the ear mold, converts the electrical energy back into sound waves. The following figure is a schematic representation of how the parts of a hearing aid work to amplify sound and transmit it to the ear. Figure 12.21 displays a hearing aid schematic.

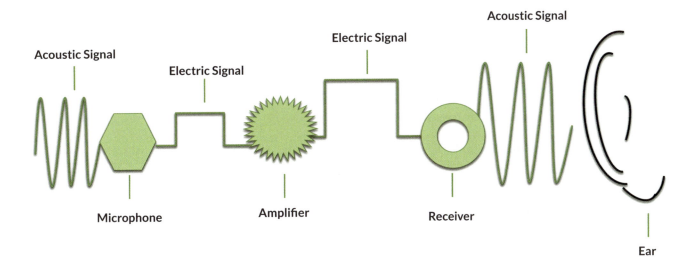

Figure 12.21 Hearing aid schematic.

The more recently developed **digital hearing aid** contains microcomputer technology. Whereas the microphone of a traditional analog hearing aid creates a continuously variable voltage pattern that is analogous to the sound input, a digital aid rapidly samples the input signal and converts each sample into a binary system of zeros and ones. Those numbers are then processed by a computer housed in a unit worn on the body.

- Digital aids have several advantages:
  - They are more flexible than analog aids and can be modified to adapt to each patient's pattern of hearing loss and communicative needs.
  - Digital processing helps amplify selected frequencies for which hearing loss is greater.
  - Digital aids are more effective than analog aids in reducing irritating loud noises, such as dogs barking and vacuums running.
  - Digital aids provide a better **signal-to-noise ratio**; that is, they are more effective than analog aids in clearly separating speech from background noise, which also is more effectively suppressed.

- Advances in technology have greatly improved the quality of hearing aids. Advances include highly sensitive microphones, ear molds that are custom made for each person, and amplifiers that amplify sound with minimal to no distortion.

- State-of-the-art hearing aids are **programmable**, in that they can be programmed to provide different types of amplification depending upon the setting. For example, the wearer could choose among different settings depending upon whether she would be at a party (with background noise) or watching TV alone at home.

- Unfortunately, a recent trend related to hearing aids is that some companies are selling them on the Internet. In some cases, companies send hearing aids directly to the consumer, who is expected to use the accompanying fitting software to program his own hearing aid. It is important for professionals to counsel all patients against participating in these situations (Bramble, 2013).

- Most hearing aid technology is computerized, meaning that hearing aid specifications, testing procedures, and prescriptive fitting methods are programmed by software.

- Most hearing aids (such as those previously described) are air-conduction hearing aids. **Bone-conduction hearing aids** are of several varieties.
  - Bone-anchored hearing aids (BAHA) are also called bone-anchored devices. They are used with people who have conductive hearing losses, single-sided deafness, unilateral hearing losses, or those who cannot wear "in the ear" or "behind the ear" hearing aids. Bone-anchored hearing aids use surgically implanted abutment to transmit sound and bypass the external auditory canal and the middle ear.
  - Ponto hearing implants are osseointegrated hearing implants with a titanium fixture and abutment. They are surgically implanted in the bone behind the external ear. They are used with an external bone conduction sound processor. The Ponto receives sound via the ear canal, eardrum, and ossicles, and through bone conduction. The sound is transmitted directly through the skull and jaw bone. The outer and middle ear is bypassed.

- Selection of a hearing aid is a process involving several steps:
  - An ear examination by an otologist to identify any physical condition of the ear that may contra-indicate the use of amplification
  - Diagnostic tests administered by an audiologist to help determine the extent and type of hearing loss
  - A hearing aid evaluation, conducted by an audiologist, in which various models are tested to determine the best aid for the individual's needs
  - Evaluation of whether the patient needs **monaural** (one ear only) or **binaural** (both ears) amplification

Several decades ago, it was deemed unethical for audiologists to sell hearing aids for profit. ASHA did not permit audiologists to sell hearing aids until the 1970s. Today, a hearing aid can be purchased from several sources, including audiologists and hearing aid dealers.

Cochlear Implants

Hearing aids are an invaluable tool for many people with hearing loss. However, some people with more severe hearing losses cannot benefit from hearing aids. The recent technology of cochlear implants may profit those individuals.

- **Cochlear implants** are electronic devices. They are surgically placed in the cochlea and other parts of the ear and deliver the sound directly to the acoustic nerve endings in the cochlea. Although the patient may be severely hearing impaired, there is often a large residual population of primary cochlear neural elements; a cochlear implant can take advantage of those residual elements.
- Cochlear implants differ from hearing aids primarily in that the hearing aid delivers amplified sound to the ear canal, whereas cochlear implants deliver electrical impulses, converted from sound, directly to the auditory nerve. Basically, cochlear implants replace the nonfunctioning inner hair cell transducer system.
- Cochlear implants can be thought of as "prosthetic cochleas." They consist of four elements, as follows:
  - A **microphone** picks up sound and converts it to electrical impulses.
  - The microphone is connected to a **processor**, which is placed behind the ear or sits entirely over the internal magnet. The battery-operated processor suppresses extraneous noise and selects sounds salient to comprehending speech. In some cochlear implants, the microphone and processor are contained in the same unit, either on the ear mold or on the body.
  - Those sounds are then sent to an **external transmitter coil**, which is magnetically held on the head via the magnet in the internal cochlear implant.
  - Digitized information is sent across the skin to the internal cochlear implant receiver/stimulator via radio waves.
  - The internal receiver/stimulator package picks up the radio signal from the outside transmitter coil and sent via a thin wire to an electrode array which is threaded into the cochlea by the surgeon.

- Unlike early cochlear implants that had only one channel (one active electrode), all cochlear implants now have multiple channels or electrodes. Each electrode channel stimulate different areas of the cochlea to produce various tonal perceptions and a more accurate representation of sound.
- Cochlear implants today are used with people who have moderate to profound sensorineural hearing loss and do not sufficiently benefit from hearing aids. Contemporary cochlear implants provide open set word discrimination (ability to understand speech without seeing the speaker's face) as well as access to environmental sounds and music. Most cochlear implant recipients are able to use a voice telephone without assistance.
- Candidates for cochlear implants are selected after an evaluation by teams of specialists. These specialists include audiologists, speech pathologists, educators of the deaf, psychologists, and otologists. Advances in cochlear implants and surgical refinements have made it possible for those patients with residual hearing to retain some, if not most, of their residual hearing.
- Candidacy for cochlear implantation has changed over the years. In the past, only those with **bilateral** (two ears) profound hearing loss who could no longer benefit from the use of hearing aids were candidates for a cochlear implant. Today, however, cochlear implants can be used with people who have mild to moderate low-frequency hearing loss with profound high-frequency deafness.
- Candidacy should be determined using a multitude of variables. The team of specialists should consider the audiogram, speech understanding scores, medical considerations, lifestyle, and hearing history to determine if their patient is a candidate for cochlear implantation. These variables should also be considered when deciding the most appropriate internal and external device for that patient.
- Hybrid cochlear implants, which combine a hearing aid for low frequencies, with a cochlear implant at higher frequencies, were approved by the Food and Drug Administration (FDA) in 2014.
- Cochlear implant surgery is typically performed as an outpatient procedure. The surgery is performed under general anesthesia and takes approximately 1–3 hours. The procedure is considered a routine surgery with low risk.
- Contemporary cochlear implants provide open set word discrimination (ability to understand speech without seeing the speaker's face) as well as access to environmental sounds and music. Most cochlear implant recipients are able to use a telephone without assistance. Candidates for cochlear implants are selected after an evaluation by a team of specialists. These specialists include audiologists, speech pathologists, educators of the deaf, psychologists, and otologists. Advances in cochlear implants and surgical refinements have made it possible for those patients with residual hearing to retain some, if not most, of their residual hearing. For more information on cochlear implant advances, go to www.acialliance.org.
- Candidates implanted with a hearing preservation cochlear implant and maintaining low-frequency acoustic hearing can wear an external processor, which provides both acoustic and electrical stimulation in the same ear. Cochlear implants, which combine a hearing aid for low frequencies with a cochlear implant at higher frequencies, were approved by the FDA in 2014.
- Prelingually deaf children who receive cochlear implants at an early age and appropriate habilitation follow-up have a substantially higher likelihood of developing listening and spoken language that is at, or near, the level of typically hearing peers (Geers & Hayes, 2011; Niparko et al., 2010). Cochlear implants help maximize these children's potential and may positively affect the auditory

system's ability to mature (Sharma, Nash, & Dorman, 2009). Children today are receiving cochlear implants as young as 6 months of age.

- The number of children who are receiving cochlear implants early in life is on the rise. Recent research has shown that the earlier children receive a cochlear implant, the better their speech and language skills are later (Caselli, Rinaldi, Varuzza, Giuliani, & Burdo, 2012; Pakulski, 2014b; Szagun & Stumper, 2012). It is important, however, to confirm the infants hearing through behavioral audiometry so as to not implant a child with significant residual hearing.

- Some members of the Deaf community have shown resistance to cochlear implants. Some question the ethics of having others make decisions for children who are too young to choose if they would like to reside in the Deaf community or try to interact in the hearing world (DeBonis, 2015). These individuals view deafness as a culture, not as a pathologic medical condition. There is a move to acknowledge the cultural values of the Deaf population and view the differences between deaf and typically hearing people as cultural differences rather than deviations from the norm.

- The **central electroauditory prosthesis** (CEP), typically called a brainstem implant, is a more current development in implant technology. The CEP directly stimulates the cochlear nucleus of the auditory nerve at the brainstem level. When the cochlea and its hair cells are damaged to such an extent that a cochlear implant will not work, implants of electrodes may carry the sound to the auditory nerve fibers at the brainstem. More research is needed to establish the usefulness of the CEP.

Assistive Devices

New technologies have been created to support the communication needs of individuals who are deaf and hard of hearing. Some can be used alone, whereas others must be used in conjunction with interpreters, speech reading (discussed later in this chapter), or other support systems.

- **Safety alerting devices** help people with hearing impairment gain information through flashing lights or vibrators on common devices. These devices help people know, for example, when the doorbell rings or a burglar alarm goes off.
- **Closed-captioning** on television provides subtitles on the screen to help people who are deaf know what is happening in a TV program.
- **Telecommunication devices for the deaf** (TDDs) allow people who are deaf to use the telephone. The TDD is a portable terminal that both sends and receives typed messages via telephone.

Communication Learning

General Guidelines

It is important to consider the impact of hearing loss on all aspects of a patient's life. Hearing loss often creates educational challenges for children and vocational challenges for adults (Ambrose, Fey, & Eisenberg, 2012; Pakulski, 2014a).

- Acceptance of a hearing loss can vary from culture to culture. It is important to be sensitive to culturally determined reactions such as embarrassment or the belief that God has given a family a deaf child as a cross to bear (Roseberry-McKibbin, 2014).

- When working with children who have a hearing loss, it is important to begin speech and language habilitation as early as possible. The family should be involved in speech and language habilitation and stimulation activities and their input and opinions given serious consideration in terms of what techniques and methods are used.
- By agreeing upon the goals of habilitation and the techniques used to achieve those goals, clinicians and parents form a "therapeutic alliance" (Bordin, 1979) that is known to be critical for high outcomes in clinical settings.
- The child must be under appropriate medical and audiological management, including being fitted with a customized hearing aid or a cochlear implant as appropriate. The child and parents should be trained in proper care and use of the hearing technology.
- Clinicians who serve children should work closely with classroom teachers and with educators of the deaf. The development of auditory skills must be integrated into the child's educational and speech–language programs.
- Children must be placed in appropriate educational settings. Those settings exist along a continuum from full inclusion in the general education classroom to enrollment in a residential school for the deaf. Federal law mandates that a child be placed in the Least Restrictive Environment (LRE) that will allow him or her to access curricular content and achieve the goals outlined on the IEP.
- Many adults who begin wearing hearing aids continue to have psychosocial difficulty. Wearing hearing aids does not automatically alleviate challenges like hearing in noise, talking on the telephone, and other situations. Some adults may experience depression and decreased physical activity in addition to psychosocial difficulty.
- Adults with hearing loss are more likely than adults with normal hearing to acquire dementia. In a 6-year study, the cognitive abilities of adults ages 75–84 with hearing loss declined 30–40% faster than those of older adults whose hearing was normal (Hearing Health Foundation, 2014).
- Clinicians who work with adults frequently need to provide personal adjustment counseling for these adults and their families. This counseling should focus on dealing constructively with the impact of the hearing loss, adjusting to hearing aid use, and modification of the environment for optimal hearing.
- Older people with hearing loss may be served through clinics, senior citizen centers, and nursing homes and other long-term health care facilities. The patient's living setting must be carefully considered as aural rehabilitation efforts are carried out.

Auditory Habilitation

Auditory habilitation is designed to teach a person with hearing impairment to listen to amplified or electrically transmitted sounds, recognize their meanings, and discriminate sounds from each other.

- Individuals who use hearing aids generally undergo a **hearing aid orientation**, which is provided by an audiologist or sometimes by a hearing aid dealer. The person is instructed in use and care of the hearing aid. For those who receive cochlear implants, there is also an orientation program in use of the device as well as suggested rehabilitation programs.

- An **FM system** is a wireless assistive listening system that can be used in group or individual treatment sessions. In a classroom, for example, it allows the teacher and the child or children to move about within a certain range. The children and teacher both wear receiving and transmitting units so they can hear and talk with each other. The FM system may connect to the child's personal hearing technology (hearing aid, cochlear implant, osseointegrated implant, etc.) or it can enhance the sound signal to the room.
- Ambient or extraneous noise in school classrooms is approximately 60 dB. The signal-to-noise ratio (S/N ratio or SNR), the difference in dB between the stimulus of interest (usually the teacher's voice) and competing background noise, is often negative; that is, the teacher's voice cannot be adequately heard due to the background noise. When this situation occurs, students often are off task and do not pay attention.
- This negative S/N ratio is very detrimental to children with hearing impairments, and FM or other assistive devices are extremely beneficial in such situations. The Acoustical Society of America is currently working toward recommendations and an action plan to reduce ambient noise and other acoustical barriers in classrooms.
- Auditory habilitation goals for children with hearing impairments range from highly structured analytical tasks, including discrimination of environmental sounds, discrimination of speech sounds and word pairs, and discrimination of phrases and sentences to conversation-based, meaningful tasks such as barrier activities, board games, and show-and-tell.

Speech Reading

Previously known as lipreading, **speech reading** involves deciphering speech by looking at the face of the speaker and using visual cues to understand what the speaker is saying.

- In speech reading, the listener watches the movements of the lips, jaw, and tongue, as well as the shape of the lips and mouth. The speaker's gestures, hand movements, and facial expressions are also observed to understand the total message being conveyed.
- In English, only 30% of sounds are visible on the face. These include the labials /v/, /f/, /m/, /p/, and /b/. The labials are **homophenous**; that is, they look the same and may be confusing. Other sounds are less visible and very difficult to read.
- Ideally, speech reading should be supplemented with other means of communication.

Cued Speech

Cued speech is speech produced with manual cues that represent the sounds of speech. It may be used to supplement speech reading.

- Cued speech differs from sign language, as it is composed of only eight signs or hand configurations for consonants and four signs for vowels.
- The hand gestures that constitute cued speech are often helpful in assisting a person with hearing impairment to distinguish among homophenous sounds.
- Research has demonstrated that people with hearing impairment benefit when the speaker uses cued speech. Nicholls and Ling (1982) showed that correct speech reading of syllables increased

from 30% without cues to 84% with cues. A challenge in using cued speech is that speakers must be able to speak and cue simultaneously.

Speech–Language Communication: General Principles

The aforementioned communication methods help people who are deaf to understand speech that is spoken to them. To be fully successful communicators, however, they must also learn to express themselves to others. Successful expression requires focused habilitative techniques.

- Oral language habilitation should begin as early as possible. Language stimulation programs are best carried out in both clinical and educational settings, as well as the home. These programs should involve cooperative efforts of a team consisting of an audiologist, family members, a speech–language pathologist, and an educator of the deaf.
- Parents of infants who are deaf should speak to their children as much as possible, talking about and labeling things in the environment. Caretakers can integrate visual with auditory stimulation by showing objects and naming them simultaneously, as well as demonstrating actions when they are described.
- Initially, it is best to select and highlight functional words that children need in their daily environments, always modeling by incorporating single words into natural phrases and sentences. Subsequently, the goals for children will be expanded to target their use of phrases and sentences, just as would be expected of children with typical hearing.
- Clinicians should also focus on other structures and concepts that are especially difficult for children with communication challenges, including hearing impairment. These include the following:
  - Grammatical morphemes such as past tense *–ed* and plural *–s*
  - Question forms, including those with Wh-words and interrogative reversals
  - Complex syntactic structures, such as "if . . . then" statements and embedded clauses
  - Higher-level thinking-with-language concepts, such as:
    - Terms with dual meanings (e.g., *rock, pound*)
    - Antonyms (e.g., *up–down, light–dark*) and synonyms (e.g., *happy–joyful*)
    - Proverbs (e.g., "A penny saved is a penny earned")
    - Abstract terms (e.g., *lighthearted, flimsy*)
- Children with hearing impairment are at risk for delays in language pragmatics. Clinicians, therefore, often include therapy goals for conversational skills such as turn taking, topic initiation, topic maintenance, and eye contact.
- It is important to use visual cues in therapy sessions. These visual cues can include hand gestures, facial expressions, toys and other manipulatives, pictures, printed letters, books, and other visuals to supplement auditory input.

Speech, Rhythm, and Voice Training

In teaching speech sound production, it is important to balance the use of auditory and visual cues. Clinicians can use charts, pictures, and other visuals to assist children in correct sound production.

- Clinicians must pay special attention to affricates, fricatives, and stops. These sounds are especially difficult for children with hearing impairment.
- The voice–voiceless distinction is also critical for children with hearing impairment to learn. Clinicians can contrast the cognates /p/ and /b/, for example, through visual and tactile means.
- Clinicians must address any voice abnormalities, such as hoarseness, harshness, high pitch, and monotone. Clients must learn to speak with proper volume, especially avoiding excessive loudness. Work with proper respiration—especially proper breath support—can be helpful.
- Resonance problems such as hypernasality and hyponasality must also be addressed. Clinicians may need to help clients balance oral–nasal resonance and avoid cul-de-sac resonance (defined in Chapter 7).
- Goals in the area of prosody may include teaching normal intonation, smooth flow of speech, and modifying pauses that are placed inappropriately or are of inappropriate length.
- If a child does not have auditory access to speech through hearing technology, it is very helpful to use mechanical feedback devices, such as the Visi-Pitch (described in Chapter 7), in working with voice and resonance problems.

Approaches to Training

Aural/Oral Method

The aural/oral method is also called the oral approach, the auditory–global approach, and the multisensory approach. Users of this method attempt to use amplification methods such as hearing aids or cochlear implants to tap children's residual hearing.

- In this approach, children undergo intensive auditory habilitation and speech reading instruction. It is expected that they will eventually learn to speak and will fit into mainstream social, vocational, and educational settings.

Manual Approach

The manual approach is a means of nonverbal communication that involves signing and fingerspelling.

- Proponents of the manual approach believe that early in life, children who are deaf must be taught a comprehensive sign language system. The sooner the child learns this system, the better.
- The sign language system is viewed as part of the Deaf culture and is the standard means of communication in the community of people who are deaf. Therefore, children who are deaf learn not only a means of communication, but also a way of integrating into that community.

Total Communication

Total communication, advocated by some experts, involves teaching both verbal and nonverbal means of communication. Signs and speech are used simultaneously. People who are deaf are taught speech and language along with a sign system. There is no attempt to tap residual hearing through amplification.

- Although critics believe that it is unrealistic to expect children to follow signs, read lips, and sign simultaneously, total communication is a popular current teaching method for children with hearing loss in the profound–severe range (Martin & Clark, 2014).

Nonverbal Communication: Sign Language

American Sign Language

American Sign Language, or ASL, is the best known of the sign language approaches. Because there are many variations of ASL, there is no single definition.

- ASL is widely used in the United States and Canada. It is not considered a manual version of English but is viewed as a separate language.
- In ASL, signs are used to express ideas and concepts through complex hand and finger movements. Each sign expresses a different idea.
- Different signs are made in quick succession, much like spoken words are put into sentences. The syntax of ASL differs from that of spoken Mainstream American English.
- ASL is frequently the preferred mode of communication within communities of persons who are deaf; they use it for vocational, educational, and social interactions (Hulit, Fahey, & Howard, 2015).

Seeing Essential English

Seeing Essential English (SEE 1) primarily employs ASL. It breaks down words into morphemes and uses written English word order.

- SEE 1 uses some markers to help identify number and tense and also uses specific signs for some verbs and articles (e.g., *the, an*).

Signing Exact English

Signing Exact English (SEE 2) is similar to SEE 1. However, it is used more widely than SEE 1 and is more flexible about precise word order in sentences.

- SEE 2 breaks down words into morphemes that are words when they stand alone (e.g., *hot–dog*).

Fingerspelling

In fingerspelling, ideas are communicated through quick, precise movements made by the fingers.

- Fingerspelling may be used alone or in conjunction with other methods, such as ASL. Sometimes fingerspelling is used for unusual words that do not lend themselves to standard signs.

Rochester Method

The Rochester method uses a combination of oral speech and fingerspelling. Signs are not used in this method. The oral aspect of the Rochester method is traditional English.

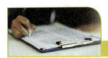

SUMMARY

- There are many approaches to the habilitation of people with hearing impairment. These people frequently have disorders of speech, language, voice, fluency, and resonance.
- People with hearing loss can be helped by amplification devices, such as hearing aids, cochlear implants, tactile aids, and various assistive devices.
- People with hearing loss may also receive communication learning, which can consist of auditory habilitation; speech reading; cued speech; oral language therapy; speech, rhythm, and voice therapy; and various verbal and nonverbal approaches to communication.

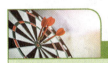

CHAPTER HIGHLIGHTS

- Audiology is the study of hearing, its disorders, and the measurement and management of those disorders. Audiologists identify, evaluate, and rehabilitate people with hearing losses due to peripheral or central auditory impairments.
- The ear consists of three basic parts: the outer, middle, and inner ear. These parts must function normally in order for sound to be converted to electrical impulses within the cochlea and then sent to the brain via the auditory nervous system. Cranial nerve VIII, the acoustic nerve, sends sound impulses to the brain, where the sound is interpreted.
- Acoustics, a branch of physics, involves the study of sound as a physical event. The human ear perceives sound in terms of pitch or frequency, and loudness or intensity. Frequency is measured in hertz, or cycles per second, while intensity is measured in decibels.
- Hearing is a miraculous ability that depends on the intricate, precise, and accurate workings of the auditory system. When the outer or middle ear malfunctions, a person may manifest conductive hearing loss. Sensorineural loss reflects malfunctioning of the inner ear, and a mixed loss reflects both conductive and sensorineural components. People with central auditory and retrocochlear disorders manifest auditory nervous system impairments, which are challenging to assess.
- Assessment of hearing impairment depends upon the nature of the problem. Standard procedures in assessment include pure-tone and speech audiometry, which can be carried out through air- or bone-conduction testing. Acoustic immittance testing, involving tympanometry or acoustic reflex testing, is used to assess middle-ear function.
- Electrophysiological audiometry and medical imaging are often employed when retrocochlear damage is suspected. This damage is usually caused by tumors, which can grow slowly and make diagnosis very challenging. New, sophisticated techniques such as electrocochleography and magnetic resonance imaging help teams of specialists assess possible pathology of the auditory mechanism.

- Hearing screenings quickly identify people with normal hearing and people who need more in-depth testing due to a possible hearing loss. Infants and children who have a hearing loss often need to be assessed with special techniques that allow for reflexive responses if necessary.
- People with hearing impairment manifest a range of communicative disorders. The severity of these disorders depends on the age of onset of the hearing loss, as well as the degree of the loss. People with hearing loss may manifest problems in one or more of the areas of articulation, fluency, voice, resonance, and language.
- Aural rehabilitation involves an educational and clinical program implemented by teams to help people with a hearing loss achieve their full potential. Aural rehabilitation usually includes several key components. Amplification, one component, can involve hearing aids, cochlear implants, tactile aids, and assistive devices.
- Communication learning, a second component of aural rehabilitation, may involve one or more of several methods. These methods include auditory habilitation; speech reading; cued speech; and oral language, speech, voice, fluency, and resonance therapy. Various approaches to therapy may include a verbal emphasis (e.g., total communication and the aural/oral approach) or a nonverbal emphasis, which involves use of a form of sign language.

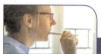

STUDY AND REVIEW QUESTIONS

1. A 51-year-old woman comes to an audiologist and states that she feels like she is losing her hearing in her left ear. The woman says that she generally feels healthy but has noticed that she now uses her right ear exclusively when talking on the telephone. She states, "Sometimes the left side of my face tingles. It doesn't bother me much, but I do notice it sometimes." She also reports that she feels slight dizziness and has noticed some mild balance problems. For example, when she is on an escalator, she has to "hang on more." She says that "sometimes my left ear rings." Her preliminary audiological results show that she has normal ability to detect pure tones and that she has normal speech recognition in a quiet room. The most probable diagnosis of this woman's problem is

    A. central auditory processing disorder.
    B. Meniere's disease.
    C. acoustic neuroma.
    D. otosclerosis.

2. A person with otosclerosis often has an audiogram reflecting Carhart's notch. Carhart's notch is

    A. a specific type of sensorineural hearing loss characterized by a "dip" at 1000 Hz.
    B. a specific loss at 4000 Hz, as indicated by both air- and bone-conduction testing.
    C. specific losses at both 2000 and 4000 Hz, as indicated by bone-conduction testing.
    D. a specific loss at 2000 Hz, as indicated by bone-conduction testing.

3. A mother brings her 3-year-old, Sasha, for a hearing screening. She shares that Sasha has had many middle-ear infections, which have been treated with antibiotics. These middle-ear infections started when Sasha was

9 months old. The mother has been told by a friend that "middle ear tubes" might be a good option for Sasha, but the mother states that she is afraid of the surgery that this would entail. After all, Sasha is only 3 years old, and her mother does not want her to be traumatized. The mother tells you, "Even though Sasha ignores me sometimes, I think everything will be okay. I just wanted her to get checked out to be sure." The audiologist assesses Sasha, with the resulting audiogram shown below. What type of hearing loss does Sasha have, based on this audiogram?

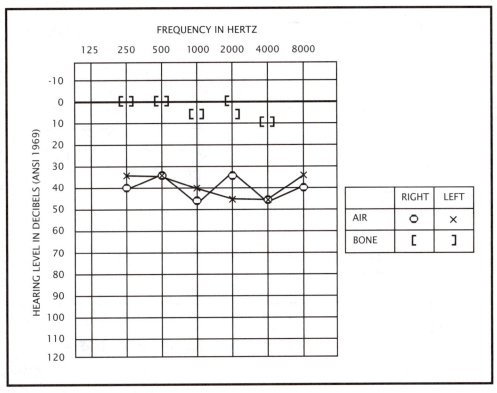

- **A.** Mixed loss
- **B.** Retrocochlear loss
- **C.** Sensorineural loss
- **D.** Conductive loss

4. Key parts of the auditory nervous system include cranial nerve VIII, which has two branches: the _____ branch and the _____ branch, which carries the electrical sound impulses from the cochlea to the brain.

- **A.** Retrocochlear, vestibular
- **B.** Vestibular, auditory–acoustic
- **C.** Auditory–acoustic, retrocochlear
- **D.** Cochlear, auditory–acoustic

5. Sensorineural hearing loss can be caused by many things. _____, a hearing impairment in older people, results in a sloping, high-frequency loss. _____, which also causes sensorineural hearing loss, is accompanied by vertigo and tinnitus.

- **A.** Presbycusis, Meniere's disease
- **B.** Meniere's disease, Otosclerosis
- **C.** Presbycusis, Otosclerosis
- **D.** Central auditory processing disorder, Presbycusis

6. A patient has her hearing tested, and the resulting audiogram has the configuration below.

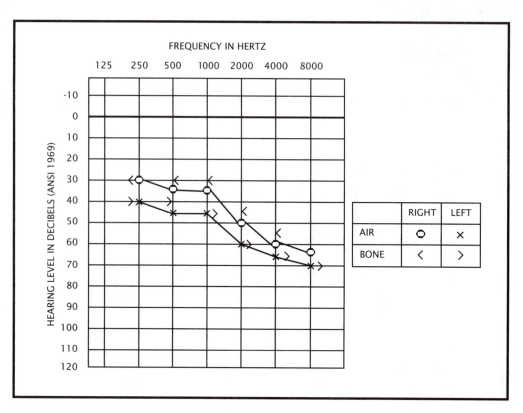

You can assume that this patient has

   A. mixed hearing loss.
   B. conductive hearing loss.
   C. sensorineural hearing loss.
   D. noise-induced hearing loss.

7. A 65-year-old man with presbycusis comes to you complaining that when he is in social situations such as parties, people don't speak loudly enough. He says that the noise creates a problem for him in hearing what people are saying. This client has difficulty with

   A. signal-to-noise ratio.
   B. auditory discrimination.
   C. figure–ground discrimination.
   D. pragmatic skills.

8. Which one of the following is a homophenous pair?

   A. *sheep–beep*
   B. *man–ban*
   C. *pan–fan*
   D. *honey–money*

9. The muscle that exerts the pull that allows the Eustachian tube to open during yawning and swallowing is the

   A. tensor veli palatini.
   B. levator veli palatini.
   C. tensor tympani.
   D. stapedius muscle.

10. An infant with cleft palate will most likely have hearing problems because of

　　A. aural atresia.
　　B. an incompletely formed cochlea.
　　C. Eustachian tube dysfunction.
　　D. malformed ossicles.

11. Jasmine D. is a fourth-grade girl who is struggling academically. She has difficulty paying attention in class, and her grades are low. She has been tested by several specialists, and there is no evidence of a learning disability or clinically significant attention issue. She has passed routine school hearing screenings every year; these screenings have been conducted at 25 dB bilaterally. However, teachers over the years keep referring her because they think that she is not hearing as well as she should. What course of action would you take?

　　A. Don't do anything; she has passed hearing screenings and probably just needs to exhibit greater self-discipline in class.
　　B. Talk to her parents and suggest ways that they can help her improve her behavior.
　　C. Talk to her teacher and suggest discipline strategies for the classroom to help Jasmine behave and focus better.
　　D. Refer Jasmine and her parents to an audiologist for a comprehensive hearing test.

12. Speech reception thresholds (SRTs) are

　　A. determined by the patient's response to a list of monosyllabic words presented at a low level of hearing.
　　B. determined by looking at the patient's pure-tone test results at the frequencies most important to speech.
　　C. the lowest or softest level of hearing at which a person can understand 100% of the words presented.
　　D. the lowest or softest level of hearing at which a person can understand 50% of the words presented.

13. Popular forms of amplification today include hearing aids and cochlear implants. Which one of the following is *not true* about these devices?

　　A. Hearing aids deliver amplified sound to the ear canal, while cochlear implants deliver electrical impulses (converted from sound) directly to the middle ear.
　　B. Digital hearing aids provide a better signal-to-noise ratio than analog aids.
　　C. Cochlear implants can help prelingual children to make substantial progress through maximizing their potential.
　　D. A consideration in fitting clients with hearing aids is whether the clients are motivated to use and properly care for the aids.

14. A father comes to you regarding his daughter, who is 8 months old. When the baby was 4 months old, he and his wife noticed that she did not respond to noise. Even when the dog barked loudly or the TV was turned up, the baby did not respond. They took her to an audiologist and found out that the baby had a bilateral hearing loss and that she was profoundly deaf. The father states that he wishes for his daughter, as she grows older, to "fit in with children with normal hearing." He is interested in any possible amplification and says that he wants his daughter to lead a life that is "as normal as possible." Which training approach would best fit this father's wishes?

A. Total communication
B. Aural/oral method
C. Manual approach
D. Rochester method

15. Spondee words are

A. polysyllabic words with at least two voiceless sounds.
B. two-syllable words with primary stress on the first syllable.
C. two-syllable words with equal stress on each syllable.
D. one-syllable words that are phonetically balanced.

References and Recommended Readings at www.advancedreviewpractice.com

STUDY AND REVIEW ANSWERS

1. C. These symptoms are typical of a patient with an acoustic neuroma.
2. D. Carhart's notch reflects specific loss at 2000 Hz, as indicated by bone-conduction testing.
3. D. This child has a conductive hearing loss.
4. B. Key parts of the auditory nervous system include cranial nerve VIII, which has two branches: the vestibular branch and the auditory–acoustic branch; the auditory–acoustic branch carries the electrical sound impulses from the cochlea to the brain.
5. A. Sensorineural hearing loss can be caused by many things. Presbycusis, a hearing impairment in older people, results in a sloping, high-frequency loss. Meniere's disease, which also causes sensorineural hearing loss, is accompanied by vertigo and tinnitus.
6. C. A sensorineural loss is usually characterized by an audiogram reflecting a sloping, high-frequency loss.
7. A. People who have difficulty separating the signal of interest (speech) from background noise have difficulty with the signal-to-noise ratio.
8. B. Homophenous pairs are those words that look the same on the lips. *Man* and *ban* begin with bilabials; thus, the words look similar to listeners with a hearing loss.
9. A. The muscle that exerts the pull that allows the Eustachian tube to open during yawning and swallowing is the tensor palatini.
10. C. Infants with cleft palate frequently have Eustachian tube dysfunction because of the oral–facial anomalies inherent within the cleft palate condition.

11. D. It is very likely that Jasmine has a mild hearing loss that is not being detected by routine public school hearing screenings that are conducted at 25 dB. In this case, referral to a professional audiologist is the best course of action.
12. D. Speech reception thresholds (SRTs) are the lowest level of hearing at which a person can understand 50% of the words presented.
13. A. Hearing aids deliver amplified sound to the ear canal, whereas cochlear implants deliver electrical impulses (converted from sound) directly to the middle ear.
14. B. The aural/oral method emphasizes (a) making use of residual hearing through amplification, and (b) helping people with hearing impairment learn to communicate so that they are comfortable in mainstream settings with hearing people.
15. C. Spondee words are two-syllable words with equal stress on each syllable.

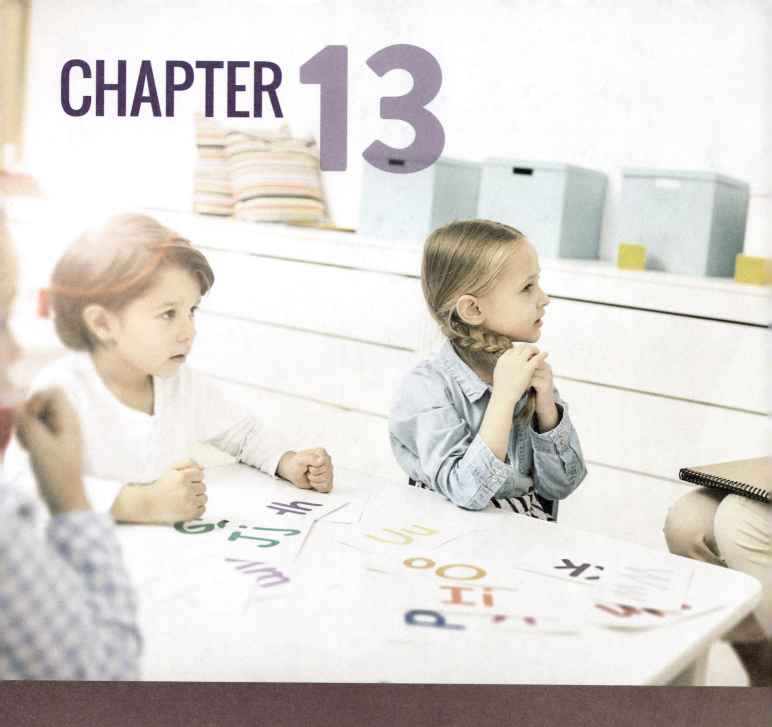

CHAPTER 13

ASSESSMENT AND TREATMENT: PRINCIPLES OF EVIDENCE-BASED PRACTICE

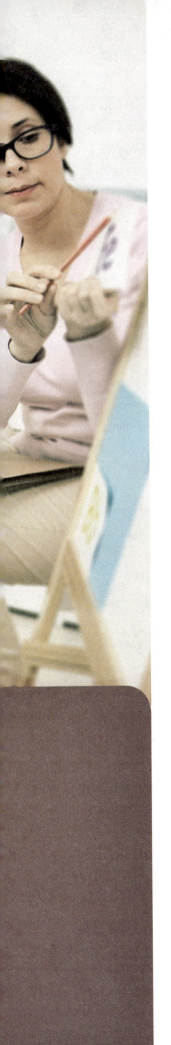

Various communication disorders discussed in different chapters offer assessment and treatment information that is unique to those disorders. In this chapter, we give an overview of assessment and treatment concepts and methods that cut across disorders.

There is a difference between assessment and diagnosis. *Assessment* (also called *evaluation*) refers to the activities designed to collect clinical data essential to make a diagnosis. A *diagnosis* is an understanding of the problem or naming a disorder by analyzing the symptoms presented and, if possible, specifying the underlying causes of the symptoms (Haynes & Pindzola, 2012; Hegde, 2018a; Hegde & Freed, 2017; Hegde & Pomaville, 2017). To assess clients and arrive at a diagnosis, clinicians use standard (common) assessment procedures and a combination of standardized, client-specific, and alternative (nonstandardized) measures that are culturally and linguistically appropriate for individual clients (Hegde & Pomaville, 2017; Roseberry-McKibbin, 2014).

Treatment in communicative disorders involves several common concepts and procedures. Although treatment is conceptualized in different ways, it essentially involves changing an existing, perhaps nonfunctional, pattern of communication (Hegde, 2018b). It requires working not only with clients, but also with the family members, other caregivers, teachers, and others who routinely interact with them. In addition, it requires sensitivity to relevant cultural and linguistic variables. Designing effective treatment procedures requires an accurate assessment of the client's problem. In this chapter, the basic assessment and treatment principles, procedures, and concepts are summarized. Consistent with the current trends in speech–language pathology, the need to select treatment procedures that are based on treatment efficacy evidence is emphasized.

EVIDENCE-BASED PRACTICE IN SPEECH–LANGUAGE PATHOLOGY

In medicine, speech–language pathology, and all health-related professions, the current emphasis is on evidence-based practice. Evidence-based practice ensures that clients receive services that are known to be based on reliable and valid research and sound clinical judgment. As currently defined (and often debated), evidence-based practice has different connotations (Dijekers, Murphy, & Krellman, 2012; Hegde, 2003; Lohr, Eleazer, & Mauskopf, 1998; Sackett, Rosenberg, Gray, Hayes, & Richardson, 1996; Sackett, Straus, Richardson, Rosenberg, & Hayes, 2000; see also the ASHA website for more information on evidence-based practice, www.asha.org/members/ebp).

- Experimentally demonstrated effects of treatment are crucial to evidence-based practice. It is unethical to use treatment procedures that have not been supported by experimental research (see Chapter 14 for details on this kind of research). Only treatment procedures that have been shown to be better than no treatment and have been replicated in different settings, with different clients, and by different investigators may be recommended for general practice (Hegde, 2003). Different levels of evidence are summarized in Chapter 14.
- Evidence-based practice requires an integration of the best research evidence for clinical methods with clinical expertise and sound judgment. Evidence-based practice is always client-centered. That is, when selecting assessment and treatment procedures, the clinician takes into consideration not only the research evidence, but also what is best for an individual client and his or her preferences (Sackett et al., 1996; Sackett et al., 2000). When treating children, the child and the family are all involved in making clinical decisions that affect them. This is because a method supported by evidence may be unacceptable to clients, their families, or both.
- Evidence-based practice also means that the clinician would not use procedures unsupported by evidence, contradicted by evidence, or known to produce negative effects (Hegde, 2003). The clinician must critically analyze the quantity and quality of evidence supporting the use of available (and often vigorously advocated) treatment techniques and consider the characteristics of the individual client seeking the services. The clinician also should critically examine his or her own training, expertise, and experience in advanced procedures before using them.
- Finally, evidence-based practice is ethnoculturally sensitive. Selection of assessment and treatment procedures should be made on the basis of not only the experimental evidence supporting them, but also the relevance of procedures to the ethnocultural and family background of the client. See Chapter 11 for more on ethnocultural issues that affect service delivery in communicative disorders.

STANDARD ASSESSMENT PROCEDURES

Certain standard assessment procedures are used across types of communication disorders. Note that the standard procedures do not exclusively refer to standardized tests but include common procedures that are necessary to assess clients of any age exhibiting any type of a disorder; common procedures may be supplemented with procedures that are unique to a given disorder, the client, or both. Standard procedures usually include a speech, language, and hearing screening, a case history, an orofacial examination, an interview, a speech and language sampling, administration of standardized tests, and a review of assessment reports from other professionals (Haynes & Pindzola, 2012; Hegde, 2018a; Hegde & Freed, 2017; Hegde & Pomaville, 2017; Roseberry-McKibbin, 2014).

Screening

- A **screening** is a brief procedure that helps determine whether a client should undergo further, more detailed, assessment.
- Clients who pass a screening are judged to be within the normal limits on the skills screened, and thus are not assessed at length. Clients who fail screening procedures are scheduled for comprehensive assessments because they may have a communication disorder.

- Screening procedures are used in many facilities, especially in public schools, to determine who should receive full assessments and who need not.

Case History

- The **case history** yields detailed information that helps the clinician understand the client and his or her communication disorder, and such related variables as the client's family, health, education, occupation, and cultural and linguistic background.
- Emphasis within a case history depends upon the age of the client and the nature of the disorder. Often, the adult and the child case history forms are different. A printed case history form and interview of the client, family, or both help obtain information.
- The clinician should get identifying information (e.g., the client's name, date of birth, address, and phone number) as well as other information summarized in the following sections.

Description of the Communication Disorder

- By asking adult clients or parents of child clients, the clinician gets detailed information on the nature of the communication problem, signs at the time of onset, and changes in the course of the disorder.
- In many cases, information on the cultural dispositions toward the disorder may also be sought.

Prior Assessment and Treatment of the Disorder

- Clinicians seek information on prior assessment, recommendations, and whether they were followed.
- Prior treatment, who offered it, and the outcome also are of interest to the clinician.

Family Constellation and Communication

- Clinicians would enquire about family history of communication disorders, the living arrangements (alone or with members of family), sibling status, and the client's communication patterns within the family.
- Clinicians find out about a child client's play activities and social communication.
- Whether the client and family members are bilingual, and if so the primary languages spoken at home would be relevant information.
- The client's literacy skills and the language in which the client reads and writes need to be described as well.

Prenatal, Birth, and Developmental History

- In the case of a child client, the clinician would ask questions about the mother's health during the pregnancy, as well as any major accidents or illnesses and drugs used or abused.
- Prematurity, any birth complications, type of delivery, and birthweight of the child need to be ascertained.
- Growth and development of the child are evaluated by asking about feeding or nursing problems, physical development and any specific problems, and evidence of hearing loss and genetic syndromes.
- Clinicians pay special attention to the child's speech and language development.

Medical History

- Clinicians need to find out about illnesses, trauma, and accidents during childhood.
- Medical or surgical treatment the client may have received and the prior and current medication need to be determined.

Educational History

- The level of education an adult has completed or the grades a child is enrolled in is useful information to be obtained. Information on any special education services received will be useful.
- Whether the client's communication problem posed any educational or occupational difficulties are also important to determine.

Occupational History

- In case of adult clients, the clinician might want to know the current occupation, the types of tasks performed on the job, and any limitations the communication problem may have created for the client.
- How the client gets along with his or her colleagues, why clinical services are being sought, and what occupational goals are set are also important to ask.

Prognosis

- A **prognosis** is a professional judgment made about the future course of a disorder or disease. It is a predictive statement about what may be expected under various future circumstances. Clients and their families want to know if treatment can be beneficial, and if so, to what extent. For example, a clinician could predict what might happen if a disorder of fluency remains untreated in a 4-year-old child versus what might happen if the child receives treatment. Or a clinician could predict whether a client who has sustained a stroke will possibly be able to return to his or her previous job.
- The American Speech-Language-Hearing Association's Code of Ethics specifies that it is unethical to promise a specific outcome, but it is acceptable to make a reasonable statement of possible outcomes under specified conditions.
- Factors influencing the prognosis for a client include
  - the severity of the disorder.
  - the client's general health and the physiological course of an underlying disease (e.g., a stable, improving, or progressively deteriorating neurological disease).
  - the time of intervention (e.g., whether therapy for aphasia is initiated soon after the onset or several years later).
  - the quality, quantity, and intensity of treatment offered and the consistency with which treatment is received.
  - family support for the client, their participation in the treatment process, and social reinforcement for maintaining gains made in treatment.
  - the client's motivation to work hard in treatment and outside the treatment setting.
  - the client and family's religious and cultural beliefs about the necessity for and efficacy of treatment.

Hearing Screening

A **hearing screening** is a quick procedure to determine whether a client can be assumed to have normal hearing or needs to be more thoroughly evaluated by an audiologist.

Speech–language pathologists should

- screen the hearing of all clients whom they assess for speech and language disorders.
- use a screening procedure adopted at their clinical sites.
- make sure the ambient noise in the screening situation does not compromise validity and reliability of screening results.
- generally, screen hearing at 20 or 25 dB HL for 500, 1000, 2000, and 4000 Hz; screen at 25 dB HL for 500 Hz.
- screen younger children at 15 dB HL for 500, 1000, 2000, 4000, and 8000 Hz.
- refer the client who fails the screening test to an audiologist for a comprehensive hearing evaluation.

Orofacial Examination

The **orofacial examination** is an evaluation of the oral and facial structures to identify or rule out obvious structural abnormalities that affect speech production, and therefore, may require medical attention or affect communication treatment.

The orofacial examination is an important standard (common) assessment procedure that is used with a variety of clients, including children and adults with speech sound disorders, cleft palate, neurological problems, and other disorders that affect speech production. (For more detailed information on the components of an orofacial examination, see Hegde, 2018c; find procedures and forms in Hegde & Pomaville, 2017 and Hegde & Freed, 2017.)

Interview

- An **interview** involves a face-to-face exchange with the client, family members, or both to obtain additional information and to clarify and expand upon the information given on the printed case history form.
- There are three basic purposes of interviewing (Haynes & Pindzola, 2012; Shipley & Roseberry-McKibbin, 2006): to obtain data or information, to inform the clients and their families, and to provide support.
- Establish rapport with the client and accompanying family members is important in an interview. The term **rapport** means respect, trust, and a harmonious relationship between the clinician and the family. Establishing trust between the clinician and the client's family involves (Shipley & Roseberry-McKibbin, 2006)

  - orienting the interviewees to the nature of the interview.
  - explaining why certain information is requested.
  - not making the client feel rushed.
  - listening.
  - using appropriate verbal and nonverbal communication.
  - assuring the client of (and maintaining) confidentiality.

- Maintaining rapport and establishing trust also involve recognizing and accounting for cultural and linguistic variables that might influence the interview. For example, the family might need an interpreter present to assist in the process, or the family might come from a culture where it is considered inappropriate to reveal personal details. Clinicians must be sensitive to these issues (Roseberry-McKibbin, 2014).
- During the interview process, it is important to occasionally reflect or summarize to clients and family members what they have been saying. In this way, clinicians can make sure that the recorded information is accurate.

Speech and Language Sample

Nature and Purposes

- The **speech and language sample** is the primary means of assessing a client's speech and language production. The sample may be audio- or video-recorded for later analysis.
- The samples are more naturalistic than standardized tests. Tests and samples complement each other.
- The goal of speech and language sampling is to obtain a representative sample of the client's speech–language production in naturalistic contexts that reflect the client's everyday communication.
- The samples can be recorded during conversation between the client and the clinician, between the client and a caregiver, or among other conversational partners. It is best to obtain the samples that reflect the client's interactions with several different interlocutors.
- Clinicians can allow the sample to be mostly unstructured. Clinicians need to manipulate contexts and materials to varying extents to evoke specific speech sounds or language skills (structures) from clients, because a completely unstructured sample may not evoke all of the language skills of interest.
- An adequate sample helps analyze a client's speech, language, voice, and fluency skills.

Procedures for Obtaining the Sample

Procedures for obtaining speech and language samples may vary across clinicians and settings, but the following recommendations help secure a representative speech and language sample (Hegde, 2018a; Hegde & Pomaville, 2017):

- Audio-record the entire sample in stereo for an optimal dynamic range. If it looks like the child is self-conscious, spend a few minutes to get the child used to the tape recorder.
- Obtain a minimum of 100 utterances. This may take more or less time, depending on the client.
- Take notes on the context of the utterances that may not be clear from the audiotaped sample. When working with a 3-year-old child, for example, the clinician may take notes on what books, toys, and other stimuli are being used at certain times when recording the sample.
- Use a quiet room and avoid noisy stimulus materials. Consider covering the table with a soft cloth when using toys to prevent additional noise on the recording.
- Select stimuli that are appropriate for the client's cultural–linguistic background, educational level, occupation, and age.

- Use only an essential number and variety of objects and pictures when evaluating children. Adults can carry on a conversation about their communication problem, topics of interest, recent events, and so forth. However, in evaluating adults with neurogenic disorders, pictures and objects may be needed.
- In the case of children, use procedures appropriate to the child's age. For most young children, it is best to have parents bring several favorite books and toys from home. Many young children react best to interesting, attractive games, toys, and books that are appropriate to their age level.
- Use age-appropriate conversational topics (e.g., movies, sports) with older children. If necessary, use pictures with older children who are reluctant to converse.
- When appropriate, especially with young children, begin by having the child interact with one or more family members, such as a parent or sibling. As the child becomes more comfortable in the clinical situation, interact alone with the child.
- Do not bombard a child or adult client with questions. Give the client opportunities to initiate the conversation and allow enough periods of silence to encourage the client to initiate speech.
- With an unintelligible client (especially a child) who is being audio-recorded, repeat what the client says so that the utterance can be accurately transcribed from the recording.
- Ask as few yes–no questions as possible. Ask primarily open-ended questions; this usually involves *wh-* questions, such as "What is . . . ?" or "Why do . . . ?"
- Obtain a home language sample if the family is willing to audio-record the client at home. The home sample would supplement the sample collected in the clinic and can give the clinician additional information about the client's speech–language skills in his or her natural setting.
- The speech and language sample may be analyzed for various aspects of language and communication. For example, production of various words, phrases, sentences, and different types of sentences may be analyzed. With younger children, the clinician can calculate the mean length of utterance. The clinicians can note such pragmatic skills as turn taking, topic initiation and maintenance, narrative skills, and eye contact during conversation. In addition, accurate and inaccurate speech sound productions, dysfluencies, and voice qualities and deviations also may be noted from the sample. Clinicians may use computer software to analyze certain aspects of language production (Nelson, 2010).

Obtaining Related Assessment Data

When working with children, clinicians should obtain information related to

- hearing evaluations.
- behavioral and psychological evaluations.
- medical evaluations and current medications and their side effects.
- regular and special education evaluations from teachers, resource specialists, psychologists, and other professionals.

When working with adults in medical settings, clinicians should obtain information related to

- the patient's current medical diagnosis, prognosis, and medications and their side effects.
- medical personnel's current and future medical treatment plans for the patient.

- brain imaging and radiologic data that might be related to diagnosis of the communication disorder (especially in older patients with neurological disorders).
- audiologic findings that might be related to or integrated with the communication assessment.
- physical rehabilitation plans that might affect treatment of the communication disorder.

Clinicians may work on teams with other professionals. Westby, Stevens-Dominguez, and Oetter (1996) have described three kinds of teams:

- **Multidisciplinary teams.** Team members represent multiple disciplines, but each member conducts his or her individual evaluation, writes a separate report, and has little interaction with other team members.
- **Transdisciplinary teams.** Multiple specialists work together in the initial assessment, but only one or two team members provide services.
- **Interdisciplinary teams.** Team members from multiple disciplines interact and use each other's suggestions and information in interpreting data. The team collaboratively writes the evaluation report and intervention plan.

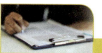

SUMMARY

- Most clinicians use certain standard (i.e., common) procedures to assess clients with a wide range of communication disorders. These procedures should be based on established evidence that demonstrates the reliability, validity, and appropriateness of procedures.
- The common procedures include screening, obtaining a case history, conducting a hearing screening and orofacial examination, conducting an interview, recording a speech and language sample, administering standardized tests (see the following section for more detail), and obtaining related assessment data.
- After these standard assessment procedures have been completed, most clinicians implement certain client- or disorder-specific procedures as the next step in the evaluation process.

PRINCIPLES OF STANDARDIZED ASSESSMENT

Standardized, norm-referenced assessment is commonly used in speech–language pathology. It offers a number of advantages to clinicians: ease of test administration, ease of test scoring, and some assurance of reliability or stability when a well-standardized test is used. For clinicians in the public schools, standardized test scores may help determine children's eligibility for treatment. Standardized tests yield quantitative scores and can be judged according to their validity and reliability.

The Nature and Advantages of Standardized Assessment

- A **standardized test** is typically standardized and normed on a specific sample drawn from a population. Standardized tests have explicit directions and strict controls about what the examiner must say and do; specific stimuli are used, and there are explicit rules for scoring the test (Hegde &

Pomaville, 2017). Controlled test administration procedures eliminates or minimizes the examiner's biases, and the measurement process will be uniform across examiners.
- The results of standardized tests yield quantitative information (scores or numbers). These scores (described later in this section) allow the client's performance to be compared to peer performance that was sampled in the standardization process.
- A standardized test is not the same as a **norm-referenced test**. A test can be standardized without being norm-referenced; however, many tests are frequently norm-referenced as well as standardized.
- In creating norm-referenced tests, the authors select tasks that they believe are valid in measuring target behaviors and administer those tasks to groups of participants who are representative of the population. The performance of the large sample is analyzed, resulting in normative data for specific age groups (Hegde & Pomaville, 2017). Thus, **norms** represent the average performance of a typical group of people (usually children), sampled at different age levels during the standardization of a test.
- The primary purpose of norm-referenced tests is to compare the individual client's score to the average score of the normative group to determine (a) if the client has a problem, (b) if the problem is clinically significant, and (c) whether the problem warrants intervention.
- Children who are similar to the client should have been represented in the normative sample. For example, if a white, middle-class, 8-year-old girl is being tested, other white, middle-class, 8-year-old girls should have been included in the normative sample.

Limitations of Standardized Tests
- Standardized tests have many limitations that are inherent to inadequate sampling of children as well as an inadequate sampling of behaviors to be assessed (Hegde & Pomaville, 2017).
- A major problem in assessing culturally and linguistically diverse (CLD) children is that such children are not well represented in the normative sample. A test standardized on middle-class, monolingual, English-speaking, white children in Utah, Arizona, and Illinois would not be invalid for use with a bilingual, Spanish-speaking child who immigrated from Cuba at age 5 years and currently lives in Louisiana. Many clinicians in the United States continue to use standardized tests to assess these children, even though this is not the best practice (Hegde & Pomaville, 2017; Roseberry-McKibbin, Brice, & O'Hanlon, 2005).
- The interactive styles of many children may not match the formal fixed visual stimulus-question-response format of many tests; this may be especially so for children from multicultural backgrounds who may not be sophisticated in test taking.
- Many standardized tests have small sample sizes. If a test has subgroups, there should be at least 100 participants per group (Haynes & Pindzola, 2012). This is frequently not the case. Very few, if any, standardized tests of speech and language are based on a national as well as *representative* sample.
- Standardized tests sample skills in such a highly structured context that the skills assessed may not be representative of any child's communicative behavior in natural environments. Such tests rarely give children opportunities to initiate conversation and do not effectively sample nonverbal means of communication.

- Standardized tests rarely give information about how clients arrived at answers or the strategies they used to complete the activities.
- Many formal tests sample behaviors inadequately, which helps keep the length of the test manageable. For example, a test may assess the production of a phoneme or a grammatical morpheme in just one or two words.
- The practice of comparing a child's performance level on a test with the performance of an average normative group to determine deficiency in the child is the most troublesome aspect of standardized testing. This practice ignores the well-documented individual differences and variations in speech and language learning (or any other skill learning).
- Formal tests do not give clinicians specific guidance for planning treatment or evaluating treatment progress. It is critical that clinicians not use formal tests for those purposes.

Prudent Use of Standardized Tests

Because of their significant limitations, standardized tests should be used with caution, and avoided when inappropriate. In prudently using standardized tests, clinicians may use the following general guidelines (Hegde & Pomaville, 2017):

- Select a test only if its standardization sample matches the client's ethnocultural background; generally, select tests that are standardized on large and diverse samples (Roseberry-McKibbin, 2014).
- Do not modify test items to suit a client, because such modifications invalidate the test's scoring and interpretation of results.
- Use only those tests that have detailed manuals and clear instructions, offer current norms, and report satisfactory reliability and validity.
- Select a test that you are well trained to administer.
- Always consider standardized test results supplemental to naturalistic and in-depth assessments that include speech–language samples, baselines, and probes.
- Take the test items the client answered incorrectly on the formal test and create informal probe measures that sample the behaviors of interest in much greater depth. For example, if the test results show a potential difficulty with the plural morpheme, the clinician can assess its production with multiple plural words and phrases she creates.
- After administering a formal test, examine incorrect items and record them. For example, "The child missed 3/4 items assessing the use of *is-* verbing, and 2/4 items assessing the use of regular past tense *-ed*."
- Use informal probe tasks to assess the production of speech or language skills in greater depth. For example, use conversational speech and structured tasks with words, phrases, and sentences to assess the child's production of phonemes or grammatical features.
- Document the accuracy of production of the skills during such probes. For example, "The child was 40% accurate in producing the /s/ in word-initial positions" or "the child was 20% accurate in producing the regular plural morpheme /s/ when shown pictures and asked 'What are these?'"

- Create treatment goals based upon these probe measures. For example, "The target is to have the child produce the regular plural /s/ with 90% accuracy when asked 'What are these?' while showing pictures or objects."
- Measure treatment progress by assessing accuracy of the child's production of the target skills using tasks similar to the probe tasks (see "Treatment of Communication Disorders" later in this chapter for more details).

Types of Scores in Standardized Assessment

- As stated earlier, the goal of standardized testing is to yield scores or quantitative measures that compare the client's performance to that of a normative group—a group in which the client is represented.
- A test administration yields a **raw score** for a client. Raw scores are the actual scores earned on a test. For example, on an aphasia test, a patient might receive a raw score of 55, indicating that he or she answered 55 items correctly. The raw score is converted so it can be viewed on a distribution.
- To compare the client's performance to that of a normative group, test makers use **distributions**. Distributions yield measures of the client's performance compared to the performance of the normative sample.
- Two statistical measures of a distribution are the mean and the standard deviation. The **mean** is the arithmetic average of the scores of the normative sample. The **standard deviation** is the extent to which scores deviate from the mean or average score in the same sample. It reflects the variability of all the measures or scores of the normative sample. The larger the standard deviation, the more variable the scores and vice versa.
- Among scores that have a normal distribution, 34.13% fall within one standard deviation above the mean and 34.13% fall within one standard deviation below the mean. In other words, if scores are normally distributed in a bell-shaped curve, 68% of the sample will have scores between 85 and 115 (assuming 100 is the average score). The standard deviation is 15 points.
- A client's score enables the clinician to evaluate the client's performance in relation to the mean. The client's score(s) may be expressed in terms of its standard deviation from the mean. Scores may also be expressed in terms of percentile ranks.
- **Percentile ranks** are converted scores that show the percentage of subjects who scored at or below a specific raw score. Percentile ranks use percentile points to express a client's score relative to the normative sample. For example, if a child's score is at the 25th percentile, 75% of children did better on the test than did that child.
- The 50th percentile is equivalent to the mean and **median**. The median is the score in the exact middle of the distribution; it divides the distribution into two parts so that an equal number of scores fall to the right and to the left of it.
- Usually, clients whose scores place them one standard deviation below the mean score slightly below the 16th percentile. People whose scores are two standard deviations below the mean score close to the 2nd percentile.

- Formal tests often yield age-equivalency and grade-equivalency scores. Scores indicating **age equivalency** show the chronological age for which a raw score is the mean or average score in the standardization sample. Scores indicating grade equivalency show the grade placement for which a raw score is the mean or average score.
- For example, a 6-year-old's score on a test might be typical of a 4-year-old's score in the normative sample. Or a fifth grader's score might be typical of the average score of the third-grade children in the normative sample.
- Because age- and grade-equivalency scores are easier for parents and clients to understand than percentile ranks and standard deviations, many clinicians use them to explain test performance. However, experts do not recommend this practice (Haynes & Pindzola, 2012).

Validity and Reliability of Standardized Tests

Validity and reliability are basically a matter of trustworthiness of measurement. Standardized tests as well as measurement of variables in research studies should meet the expectations of validity and reliability. Therefore, these two critical topics are addressed in Chapter 14.

- Research indicates that many clinicians express a low level of concern with these psychometric characteristics of tests (Huang, Hopkins, & Nippold, 1997); thus, it becomes even more important to understand and apply the concepts of validity and reliability to the evaluation of tests. In-depth discussions of validity, reliability, and test construction may be found in the classic work by Anastasi & Urbina (1997).
- Briefly, validity refers to the degree to which a measuring instrument measures what it purports to measure. For the different kinds of validity, including concurrent, construct, content, and predictive types, see Chapter 14.
- Briefly, reliability means the **consistency** or **stability** with which the same event is repeatedly measured. Scores are **reliable** if they are consistent across repeated testing or measurement of the same skill or event. For the different types of reliability, including interjudge, intrajudge, alternate form, test-retest, and split-half reliability, see Chapter 14.

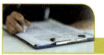

SUMMARY

- Standardized, norm-referenced tests, though commonly used to assess clients, have both advantages and disadvantages.
- Formal test results alone should never be used to establish treatment goals or measure treatment progress.
- Clinicians can analyze formal tests to determine how reliable and valid the tests are, especially for the specific populations the clinician serves.
- Clinicians use formal tests in conjunction with nonstandardized, client-specific assessment tools to obtain the most complete profile of clients' skills.

RATING SCALES, QUESTIONNAIRES, AND DEVELOPMENTAL INVENTORIES

Many clinicians supplement formal test results with other assessment measures, some of which are not standardized. These additional procedures include rating scales, questionnaires, and inventories of skills that develop over time. These procedures are less rigid and more adaptable to individual clients than standardized tests; however, the behaviors, qualities, or skills they measure may be poorly defined and subject to examiner bias. For example, vocal hoarseness may be subjectively defined and therefore rated differently by various examiners. The skill of cohesive adequacy in narratives is difficult to operationalize, thus making it subjective. A major challenge with informal assessment is to make it reliable and valid for optimal use with clients (Haynes & Pindzola, 2007).

Rating Scales

- A rating scale describes a phenomenon, a property, or a characteristic and asks the responder to suggest (rate) the quantity or severity of what is described. Rating scales are statistically based means of assessment and include **nominal** or **ordinal** scales. Clinicians often use rating scales to evaluate the severity of disorders (e.g., *mild*, *moderate*, *severe*). See Chapter 14 for details on rating scales.

Questionnaires and Interviews

- **Questionnaires** contain questions to which clients or family members respond. A questionnaire may be used as an interview template or guide. It may be administered personally or sent to the homes of clients or caregivers, who fill them out and return them to the clinician.
- With some populations, questionnaires may be more valid than formal tests. For example, with CLD children and adults, questionnaires that account for linguistic and cultural backgrounds may be more useful than standardized tests to obtain information that more validly reflects clients' actual skills in daily life settings (Roseberry-McKibbin, 2014).
- **Interviews** may stand alone or be used in conjunction with questionnaires. Interviews are generally carried out for the purpose of getting information about a particular client and family and to give information to them. Interviews have the advantage of being more personalized than questionnaires used alone.
- The use of questionnaires and interviews can yield quantitative data, qualitative data (verbal descriptions), or both. For example, persons who stutter might be asked to circle numbers on a scale reflecting attitudes toward stuttering, and a clinician also might record the client's verbal descriptions of his or her own attitudes toward stuttering.

Developmental Inventories

- Developmental inventories help track children's physical and behavioral changes over time. Some degree of standardization is necessary to construct developmental inventories. Children at different ages may be sampled to assess their typical physical and behavioral development (including speech–language development).
- The inventory helps assign observed skills or developmental levels to specific ages. This is similar to establishing developmental norms.
- Clinicians can use the inventory to conduct an interview to record a child's development across time. Such inventories save time in summarizing a child's development.

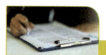

SUMMARY

- Informal, nonstandardized measures of assessment include rating scales, questionnaires, and developmental inventories.
- These measures have many advantages for use with clients. Informal measures allow clinicians to tailor assessment to individual clients, create treatment goals, and monitor treatment progress.
- Clinicians must take precautions to ensure that informal assessment measures are reliable and valid.

ALTERNATIVE ASSESSMENT APPROACHES

Because of the many limitations of standardized test-based assessment, clinicians have developed alternative methods of assessing communicative behaviors. Relying much less on standardized tests, alterative methods target naturalistic and clinically relevant measures. These approaches are especially useful in assessing clients who belong to various ethnocultural minority groups, although the approaches offer significant advantages to clients of all cultural backgrounds, including the ethnocultural majority (Hegde & Pomaville, 2017; Roseberry-McKibbin, 2014). It should also be noted that alternative approaches do not dispense with all elements of the traditional assessment. All alternative approaches need the various elements of the traditional assessment (e.g., the case history, language sampling, orofacial examination, hearing screening, etc.). For this reason, this section will not only briefly review selected alternative approaches, but will also describe an integrated approach that includes elements of major approaches (Hegde & Pomaville, 2017).

Functional Assessment

- The purpose of **functional assessment** is to evaluate a client's day-to-day communication skills in naturalistic, socially meaningful contexts. The approach does not depend on standardized test scores.
- Speech–language pathology is increasingly turning to functional assessment, because reimbursers and third-party payers are requiring documentation of functional outcomes of treatment. These should be outcomes that are meaningful in a client's everyday environment; increase a client's educational, social, or occupational participation; and enhance the client's overall quality of life.
- Many clinicians target clients' functional communication skills during traditional assessments. Functional assessment requires the clinician to make targets, procedures, and settings of assessment as naturalistic and "real life" as possible.
- To target a client's functional communication during an assessment, clinicians may (Hegde, 2018a; Roseberry-McKibbin, 2014):
  - Observe the client's communication with family members and peers, if appropriate.
  - Arrange a child–caretaker interaction that approximates their typical, everyday interaction to observe naturalistic communication rather than the limited responses the test stimuli evoke.

- Arrange for various peer interactions for children and adolescents and observe communication patterns within those situations. Talk with two or three peers about how the client communicates in social contexts.
- Obtain several home speech and language samples. Tell the family to record natural, everyday communication interactions.
- Observe the child in the classroom, in the cafeteria, on the playground, and in other settings with peers in school (educational) settings. Obtain information from teachers and other professionals about the child's communication skills as observed in everyday settings, such as the playground and classroom.
- Observe the patient's interaction with health care providers and family members while assessing clients in medical settings. Interview them as to when and how the patient communicates with such professionals as the physicians, nurses, or physical therapists.
- Interview at least one person with whom an adult client regularly interacts (e.g., colleague, significant other, friend).
- Emphasize conversational interaction. Do not make clinical judgments based solely on imitative or picture-naming tasks (although use of those tasks, in conjunction with analysis of conversational interaction, may be necessary with some clients).
- Observe and record conversational speech in naturalistic situations outside the clinic room with various conversational partners.
- Create and structure assessment tasks that are meaningful to the individual client. This is especially important with linguistically and culturally diverse clients who do not relate well to the stimuli and pictures in standardized tests that are geared toward white, monolingual, English-speaking clients.
- Use sentences that include names of family members, activities the client enjoys, interests that the client has, and so forth, when carrying out meaningful assessment tasks.
- Document variations in the disorder in natural settings. For example, in assessing the fluency of a person who stutters, document the person's degree of fluency in such naturalistic contexts as talking on the telephone, ordering in a restaurant, or purchasing items in a store.
- Examine the effect the client produces when he or she attempts to communicate. For example, whether a patient with Alzheimer's dementia can communicate his or her basic needs effectively may be more important than the syntactic structures of that patient's speech.

Client-Specific Assessment

- **Individualized** or **client-specific procedures** are a preferred alternative to standardized tests. Client-specific procedures generate data that are helpful in developing client-specific treatments. These procedures use the evocation of speech–language samples over time, by means of culturally appropriate client-specific materials instead of standard stimuli. Baselines before starting treatment are another valid client-specific pretreatment measure of communication skills.
- **Establishing reliable baselines** regardless of how the skills were initially assessed is a hallmark of the client-specific approach. Baselines are extended measures of target behaviors in the absence of planned treatment. For instance, the production of a phoneme or a grammatical morpheme may be

baserated with 20 client-specific stimulus items each, instead of just one or two items that are typical of standardized tests.
- Clinicians can establish baselines of targeted communicative behaviors just before they are taught; this kind of measurement is always current and helps establish the need for treatment. Because they are extended and repeated, baselines provide more reliable assessment data than tests and other procedures.
- Baselines, being pretreatment measures, provide a reliable means for evaluating changes in skills (or lack thereof) under treatment.

Criterion-Referenced Assessment

- **Criterion-referenced testing** is another form of assessment that minimizes the role of standardized test scores in assessing skills. It is so named because the performance assessed through any means—including even standardized tests—is evaluated not against the statistical norms, but against a standard of performance, called a **criterion**, selected by the clinician.
- The clinician may use standardized test items to evoke certain skills (e.g., phonemic or morphologic productions). Alternatively, and preferably, the clinician may develop her own stimulus material and evoke the target skills. In either case, the client's performance (the recorded responses) is evaluated against such commonly accepted criterion as either 80% or 90% accuracy level. In other words, some level of performance is viewed as minimal and acceptable.
- When using this approach, the clinician will have to determine the level of acceptable phonologic, morphologic, syntactic, and pragmatic skills necessary to consider the client of a particular characteristic to be within the normal limits. Those acceptable levels (the standard of performance) are somewhat similar to the norms that help evaluate normal or typical performance. Nonetheless, the approach gives greater flexibility to the clinician to set the criterion that may be educationally and clinically meaningful, thus avoiding a more rigid comparative evaluation against the test norms.
- Criterion-referenced measures may prove to be especially helpful when the norms of standardized tests do not apply to a particular client (e.g., a CLD client) or when the available standardized tests do not assess specific client skills of interest to the clinician (McCauley, 1996). Criterion-referenced assessment also allows for more in-depth evaluation of the client. For instance, the clinician may increase the number of stimuli to assess phonemic or morphemic productions.

Authentic Assessment

- Emphasizing naturalistic observation of skills, **authentic assessment** samples speech and language skills in everyday settings and thus avoids contrived or formal test situations. Skills are assessed in the context of realistic learning situations and demands. Speech samples collected in classrooms, homes, and other naturalistic settings constitute the primary assessment data (Udvari & Thousand, 1995).
- A variation of authentic assessment is based on the concept of **minimal competency core** (Stockman, 1996). Taking age and specific context into account, the least amount of linguistic skill or knowledge that a typical speaker is expected to display is the minimal competency core. Whether a client exhibits such a minimal competency is the concern of assessment.

- Another variant of authentic assessment is **contrastive analysis**. Appropriate for establishing whether a speech pattern is a part of a speaker's cultural background or is a disorder, contrastive analysis requires a knowledge of the speaker's dialect and a naturalistic language sample to determine whether the differences found in the sample are disorders or culturally appropriate communication patterns (McGregor, Williams, Hearst, & Johnson, 1997).

Dynamic Assessment

- **Dynamic assessment**, another alternative to standardized-test–based assessment, seeks to evaluate a child's ability to learn when provided with instruction (Kohnert, 2008; Roseberry-McKibbin, 2014).
- Dynamic assessment uses a test-teach-retest format. Clients (usually children) are tested, and their skills are measured. Then the children are taught the skills that they did not manifest during testing. Finally, the child is retested to assess how quickly and well the child learned the material presented. A unique feature of dynamic assessment is the incorporation of intervention into the assessment process.
- Dynamic assessment helps demonstrate modifiability of deficient skills; children who learn the skills are at a lesser degree of risk than those who do not learn the skill in the dynamic test-teach-retest format. The problem with this approach is that it is not clear when the clinician can finally determine that a child's skills are not modifiable, and therefore, the child has a disorder. A more basic problem is that the clinician has to treat before diagnosing the problem.

Comprehensive and Integrated Assessment

- While standardized-test–based assessment has its limitations, no single alternative approach has replaced it, mostly because each alternative, too, has its limitations. Furthermore, the traditional approach has several indispensable elements. Therefore, what is needed is a comprehensive approach that integrates the most useful elements of major approaches, including the traditional approach. Such an approach will be applicable to clients of all backgrounds, not just to those with ethnocultural minority backgrounds (Hegde & Pomaville, 2017).
- In a **comprehensive and integrated assessment**, the clinician will retain the necessary elements of the traditional approach (case history, interview, language sampling, orofacial examination, and hearing screening). Standardized tests may not be used, but if necessary, the clinician will prudently select ethnoculturally appropriate tests and interpret all test results cautiously.
- The clinician will use client-specific stimulus materials, sample communication in natural settings, and evaluate each skill in depth. Targets of assessment will always be functional and meaningful communication in social contexts. The clinician will consider standardized test results, if obtained, as supplemental to other, more naturalistic and client-specific assessment results.
- The clinician might expand the traditional clinical file to include such additional materials as drawing and writing samples, copies of other academic records, reports or notes from teachers or other professionals, parents' notes or comments, video of the child's conversation with peers or family members, and so forth. Results of brief experimental treatment sessions may be included (Hegde & Pomaville, 2017).
- In essence, the comprehensive approach includes elements of the functional, client-specific, criterion-referenced, authentic, and dynamic assessments along with the essential elements of the

traditional approach. It uses standardized tests in a prudent and limited manner, totally avoiding their use when considered inappropriate for a given client (Hegde & Pomaville, 2017).

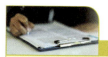

SUMMARY

- Alternative approaches that help overcome the limitations of normative tests include functional, client-specific, criterion-referenced, authentic, dynamic, portfolio, and integrated assessments.
- The integrated assessment allows clinicians to tailor assessment to individual clients, create treatment goals, and monitor treatment progress.
- Clinicians must take precautions to ensure that informal assessment measures are reliable and valid.

TREATMENT OF COMMUNICATION DISORDERS: BASIC CONCEPTS

Treatment, remediation, intervention, and therapy are all terms used to refer to ways of modifying impaired or deficient communication to achieve patterns of normal, functional, or socially more acceptable patterns of communication. Treatment follows a comprehensive assessment, which results in a diagnosis of a communication disorder. Treatment procedures specific to given disorders were summarized in their respective chapters. Therefore, we summarize treatment principles and procedures that are common to treating any disorder of communication.

Treatment: Definition

- **Treatment** in communicative disorders includes teaching, training, any type of remedial or rehabilitative work, and all attempts at helping people by changing their behaviors or teaching new skills.
- Treatment also involves working with family members of the client, teachers, peers, and institutional caretakers (e.g., the staff at a rehabilitation facility) to support and sustain communication and swallowing skills in natural and institutional settings.
- A technical definition of treatment is that it is a procedure in which contingent relations between antecedents, responses, and consequences are managed by a clinician to effect desirable changes in communication.
- Communicative behaviors are considered disorders when they create difficulty in social interactions and when an individual's speech and language skills fail to effectively influence the behavior of others. Communication disorders also create academic, social, and occupational limitations for the individual.
- The clinician rearranges listener–speaker relations by first organizing his or her interaction with the client. Eventually, as the client learns new behaviors, the clinician rearranges the communicative relations between the client and the client's family, friends, colleagues, and other important people in the client's environment.
- Success in treating communication disorders depends upon how effectively the clinician changes the way speakers and their listeners react to each other.

- Historically, speech–language pathologists have focused upon the clinician–client relationship within the therapy room. Because the communicative behaviors mastered in the clinic may not generalize to the environment, clinicians take additional steps to have the client produce clinically learned skills in natural environments.
- That goal can be accomplished in several ways. Clinicians can spend increased time working with the client in interactions with significant others as well as in situations outside the therapy room. In public schools, for example, clinicians can collaborate with classroom teachers and carry out therapy in classroom settings (Nelson, 2010; Roseberry-McKibbin, 2014).

A Treatment Paradigm for Communication Disorders

- Clinicians identify target behaviors for a client, arrange stimulus conditions for those behaviors, select materials and procedures to evoke the responses, evoke the responses, and apply consequences to the responses. In this way, clinicians arrange optimal learning conditions for their clients to acquire desirable speech–language skills.
- Ideally, treatment procedures should be objective, measurable, empirical, and reliable. Clinical procedures should include methods that help document the effectiveness of treatment.
- Unfortunately, many treatment concepts and procedures are not empirically validated. They are based upon speculation, anecdotal evidence, or opinions of "experts" who have not empirically tested their ideas. Many mistakes are made when clinicians "jump on a bandwagon" and vigorously use and promote treatment ideas that have never been subjected to scientific scrutiny.
- It is the clinician's responsibility to search evidence for their treatment procedures. The American Speech-Language-Hearing Association's website includes information on evidence-based practice and summary statements on treatment efficacy for various disorders. Clinicians may check the evidence for treatment procedures of their choice.

Basic Treatment Terms

There are some common terms that most clinicians use in describing general treatment and specific techniques (Hegde, 2018b). An understanding of these terms helps clarify the treatment of specific disorders described in other chapters.

- **Antecedents** or **treatment stimuli**—various objects, pictures, instructions, modeling, prompts, and other stimuli the clinician uses to evoke target responses from clients.
- **Aversive stimuli**—events people describe as unpleasant and, hence, work hard to avoid. For example, a person who stutters might try to avoid speaking on the telephone when possible; speaking on the telephone is aversive to the person.
- **Avoidance**—an action that results in not coming in contact with an aversive event and, hence, is repeated in the future when such contact seems imminent (e.g., avoiding an aversive person by not going to a place at a time when he or she is likely to be there). Avoidance is a behavior exhibited by many clients (e.g., a person who stutters may avoid specific speaking situations). It is a behavior that needs to be reduced; contrasted with **escape**.
- **Baselines**—measured response rates in the absence of treatment; the natural rate of a response when nothing special is done to affect its frequency. Baselines help prove that treatment was necessary by

establishing that the client did not produce the target behaviors. Baselines also help compare the initial and final response rates under treatment. Reliable baselines are a part of evidence-based practice.

- **Booster treatment**—treatment given any time after the client was dismissed from the initial treatment. It is an important maintenance strategy and may involve the original or a new form of treatment.
- **Consequences (of target responses)**—clinician reactions when the client gives a correct or incorrect response or simply fails to respond; include positive reinforcement and corrective feedback; contrasted with **antecedents**.
- **Constituent definitions**—definitions of target behaviors in dictionary terms; defining concepts with the help of other conceptual (not procedural) terms (e.g., **language** is the mental capacity to communicate); not helpful in measuring what is being defined; contrasted with operational definitions.
- **Corrective feedback**—information given to the client on incorrect or unacceptable responses in an effort to decrease those responses (e.g., saying "no" or "wrong" when an incorrect response is given).
- **Criteria**—guidelines for making such clinical decisions as when to judge whether a response has been learned, when to move on to another target, and when to dismiss the client from treatment.
- **Direct methods of response reduction**—reducing behaviors by immediately providing a corrective feedback (e.g., saying "no" or "that's not correct" when a client gives a wrong response); contrasted with indirect methods of response reduction.
- **Discrete trials**—treatment methods in which each opportunity to produce a response (e.g., individual words in learning correct speech sound production) is counted separately. Each opportunity is a trial and all trials are clearly separated in time (e.g., by pausing for a few seconds after each attempt and scoring each response as correct or incorrect). Discrete trials are more efficient in establishing target behaviors but are less efficient than naturalistic methods in promoting generalization.
- **Escape**—a behavior that reduces or terminates an aversive event after having come in contact with that event; a behavior that increases in frequency because it helped to reduce or terminate an aversive event (e.g., a person who stutters may respond to a hostile listener by terminating a conversation). Escape is a behavior to be reduced in some clients; contrasted with **avoidance**.
- **Evoked response**—spontaneous responses given to natural stimuli (e.g., "what is this?"); response given without modeling; contrasted with **modeled response**.
- **Evoked trial**—clinical procedure in which no modeling is given to the client; pictures, questions, and other stimuli are used to provoke a response (e.g., asking the client to name a picture or asking such questions as "Johnny, what is this?" while showing a picture or an object). Evoked trials follow modeled trials; contrasted with modeled trial.
- **Exemplar**—a specific target response that illustrates a broader target behavior. Exemplars are individual items trained in therapy sessions (e.g., the word *soup* in teaching the /s/ is an exemplar of that phoneme production; the phrase *two cups* in teaching the regular plural morpheme is an exemplar of that morpheme).
- **Extinction**—withholding such reinforcers as attention to reduce a response; appropriate in reducing such behaviors as crying and interfering questioning in treatment.
- **Fading**—a treatment procedure in which the controlling power of a stimulus is gradually reduced while the response is maintained (e.g., making modeling less and less audible to the client until finally only an articulatory posture is modeled and then withdrawn).

- **Follow-up**—a posttreatment assessment procedure designed to find out if clients have maintained their treatment gains; involves recording a conversational speech sample to evaluate the continued use of clinically established communicative behaviors. Follow-up may involve a regular schedule (e.g., semiannual or annual assessments following dismissal from treatment).
- **Functional outcomes**—effects of treatment that are generalized, broader, and socially and personally meaningful to clients, their families, caregivers, and others. Functional outcomes are qualitative effects (e.g., posttreatment improvements in social communication for a person who had a stuttering problem) that go beyond quantitative changes in traditionally measured behaviors (e.g., reduction in the number of stuttering behaviors); related to quality of life.
- **Generality of treatment**—evidence that a treatment found effective in one situation, by one clinician, with some clients, is effective in other situations, when used by other clinicians, with other clients. Generality is important in recommending a treatment for broader application.
- **Generalized production**—production of a clinically established behavior in natural settings with no particular or systematic reinforcement; may be temporary unless reinforced.
- **Imitation**—a process of learning in which the learner reproduces what is modeled by an instructor or clinician.
- **Indirect methods of response reduction**—reducing undesirable behaviors by positively reinforcing, and thus increasing, desirable behaviors. For example, reinforcing quiet sitting and other cooperative behavior during treatment with verbal praise but ignoring uncooperative behaviors. Note that nothing is done directly to decrease the undesirable behaviors; contrasted with **direct methods of response reduction**.
- **IEPs**—individual educational programs for children with disabilities or special needs; legally mandated in public school settings.
- **IFSPs**—individualized family service plans that are legally mandated for infants and toddlers with disabilities or special needs and their family members. The goal is to involve the family members in the treatment process.
- **Informative feedback**—telling clients how well they are doing in treatment sessions; giving specific quantitative information on performance to motivate the client (e.g., telling the client, "During the last sessions, you were 70% correct; this time, you are 85% correct.").
- **Initial response**—the first, simplified component of a target response the client can imitate while shaping a target response (e.g., putting the lips together for production of the word *mom*).
- **Intermediate response**—a response that helps move toward the final target in a shaping procedure (e.g., vocalizing the /m/, opening the mouth while vocalizing, and closing the mouth in saying the word *mom*); a response that should not be stabilized by excessive reinforcement.
- **Intermixed probes**—assessment of generalized production of trained responses by alternating trained and untrained stimulus items; contrasted with **pure probes**.
- **Maintenance strategy**—various methods used to help maintain treatment gains in natural settings; include training family members and others in evoking and reinforcing target behaviors and the client's self-monitoring of communicative skills.
- **Manual guidance**—the use of physical guidance in a shaping process (e.g., moving a client's tongue with a tongue blade to a correct articulatory position; taking a child's hand and pointing to the correct picture).

- **Mode of responses**—manner or method of a response; typical modes include imitation, oral reading, and conversational speech.
- **Modeled trial**—a discrete opportunity to imitate a response when the clinician models it. A modeled trial is typically preceded by a question (e.g., "What is this? Say . . . "); contrasted with **evoked trial**.
- **Modeling**—the clinician's production of the response the client is expected to learn. Modeling is used to teach imitation and is effective in establishing target behaviors. It is used in the initial stages of treatment and faded out as soon as possible.
- **Operational definitions**—definitions that describe how what is defined is measured (e.g., **morphologic skills** include production of plural morphemes in words, phrases, and sentences with 90% accuracy); helpful in quantitatively measuring changes in target behaviors during treatment; contrasted with **constituent definitions**.
- **Peer training**—training peers of clients to identify, prompt, evoke, reinforce, and record target behaviors in natural settings; a response maintenance strategy.
- **Physical setting generalization**—production of clinically established responses in such extraclinical environments as the home, school, and office.
- **Physical-stimulus generalization**—production of clinically established responses to stimuli that were not used in training but are similar to training stimuli.
- **Post-reinforcement pause**—absence of responses following the delivery of a reinforcer; commonly observed under fixed-interval schedules of reinforcement.
- **Posttests**—procedures designed to measure target behaviors after treatment to document changes from the pretests.
- **Pretests**—procedures to measure target behaviors before starting treatment; necessary to justify the need for treatment and to document changes under treatment, compared to the results of posttests.
- **Probes**—procedures to assess generalized production of responses without reinforcing them; involve a criterion to be met before shifting training to a more complex level or to another target behavior.
- **Procedures of treatment**—methods of treatment (e.g., modeling, instructions, verbal praise, prompting, reinforcing); what the clinician does to teach target behaviors in clients.
- **Prompts**—additional verbal or nonverbal (e.g., "The word starts with a *t* . . . " in teaching a person with aphasia to name *table* or showing an articulatory posture in the absence of voicing) that increase the probability of a target response; should eventually be faded out.
- **Punishment**—procedures of reducing undesirable behaviors by response-contingent presentation or withdrawal of stimuli; includes corrective feedback, time-out, and response cost.
- **Pure probes**—procedures for assessing generalized production when only untrained stimulus items are presented; contrasted with **intermixed probes**.
- **Response cost**—a method of reducing responses by withdrawing reinforcers contingent on each response (e.g., taking a token away from the client for every incorrect production of a phoneme).
- **Response generalization**—production of new (untrained) responses that are functionally similar to those that have been trained.
- **Response-mode generalization**—production of new (untrained) responses in a mode not involved in training (e.g., spontaneous production of untrained words after correct and reinforced imitation training).
- **Satiation**—an internal body state that renders primary reinforcers (such as food) temporarily ineffective; for example, a child might feel full and thus not desire the food reinforcers offered.

- **Self-control**—deliberately maintaining, increasing, or decreasing specific behaviors of oneself; useful in a response-maintenance strategy and includes such procedures as self-monitoring correct responses and self-recording undesirable behaviors.
- **Shaping**—a method of teaching nonexistent responses that are not even imitated; the target response is broken down into initial, intermediate, and terminal components and those are then taught in an ascending sequence; also known as **successive approximation**.
- **Stimulus generalization**—evocation of clinically established responses by stimuli not involved in training; for example, a child learned to produce /s/ correctly in the words *see*, *sun*, and *saw* might correctly name the word sock, a stimulus not used in training; this is stimulus generalization.
- **Targets of treatment**—skills and behaviors a client is taught; contrasted with **procedures of treatment**.
- **Terminal response**—the final target behavior in a shaping procedure; for example, with a nonverbal child, the final target might be production of selected words in conversational speech the child produces in the home or other situations; the words themselves will have been shaped.
- **Time-out**—a brief period of silence, inactivity, averted eye contact, and lack of reinforcement imposed on a response to be reduced (e.g., a silent period of five seconds imposed on every instance of stuttering).
- **Tokens**—objects that are given for correct responses and later exchanged for one of a several backup reinforcers; help minimize the satiation effect.
- **Trial**—a structured and discrete opportunity to produce a response; may involve showing various kinds of stimuli, asking questions, modeling, or prompting; the response given to each trial is scored separately.

Reinforcers and Reinforcement

Clinicians shape and change clients' behavior through procedures, such as reinforcement. Reinforcement is a key component of treatment programs and is essential in treating clients of all ages and all disorders of communication.

Reinforcement

Reinforcement is a method of selecting and strengthening behaviors by arranging immediate consequences under specific stimulus conditions. In speech and language treatment sessions, target behaviors are the ones selected for strengthening. Reinforcement, however, may be withdrawn or arranged in specific ways to weaken and reduce an undesirable response. Types of reinforcement or the different ways in which they may be delivered include the following:

- **Continuous reinforcement**—all correct responses in treatment sessions are reinforced; contrasted with **intermittent reinforcement**; needed to establish the target skills.
- **Intermittent reinforcement**—reinforcing some responses while others go unreinforced; in a fixed ratio 2, for example, every second response is reinforced; such **stretching the reinforcement** is essential to strengthen and generalize the target responses.
- **Differential reinforcement**—teaching a client to give different responses to different stimuli (e.g., teaching the plural response to plural stimuli and the singular response to singular stimuli); reinforcing the correct response while ignoring the incorrect response to the same stimuli.

- **Differential reinforcement of alternative behaviors (DRA)**—reinforcing a specified, desirable alternative to an undesirable behavior; replacing undesirable behaviors with desirable behaviors that give the client access to the same effects or consequences (e.g., teaching a child to verbally request, instead of whining, to get something desired).
- **Differential reinforcement of low rates of responding (DRL)**—decreasing undesirable behaviors gradually by reinforcing progressively lower frequencies of that behavior (e.g., reinforcing a child for asking progressively fewer interfering questions during treatment until the frequency is reduced to zero or near zero).
- **Differential reinforcement of incompatible behaviors (DRI)**—reinforcing a desirable behavior that cannot coexist with the undesirable behavior to be reduced (e.g., heavily reinforcing a child to sit quietly when the target is to reduce restless in-seat behavior or off-seat behavior during treatment).
- **Differential reinforcement of other behaviors (DRO)**—specifying one behavior that will not be reinforced (e.g., leaving the chair in a group treatment session) while reinforcing many unspecified desirable behaviors (e.g., quiet sitting, coloring, reading, writing), any one of which is accepted and reinforced.
- **Negative reinforcement**—strengthening of behaviors by the termination of an aversive event; involved in aversive conditioning (e.g., a person who stutters avoids speaking situations because this avoidance is reinforced by the termination of aversive listener reactions); typically not used by the clinician to increase desirable behaviors, but observed in the clinic as in the case of a child who crawls under the table because the target skills is difficult for the child and the therapy is therefore aversive; the child avoids it by exhibiting that undesirable response; the clinician should simplify the target skill and *positively* reinforce its production.
- **Reinforcement withdrawal**—prompt removal of reinforcers to decrease a response; includes such procedures as extinction, time-out, and response cost.

Reinforcers

Reinforcers are events that follow behaviors and thereby increase the future probability of those behaviors. Note that reinforcement is the method of increasing target skills, but reinforcers are the actual events or object used in that method. Reinforcers may be verbal or nonverbal and are essential to establish target behaviors. Descriptions of types of reinforcers follow:

- **Automatic reinforcer**—sensory consequences of a behavior that reinforce that behavior (e.g., the sensation associated with an autistic child's head banging that increases its frequency).
- **Backup reinforcer**—reinforcer given at the end of a treatment session in exchange for tokens the client earned in the treatment session. For example, if a child earns 10 happy face chips during the session, he or she might get a sticker at the end of the treatment session.
- **Conditioned generalized reinforcer**—reinforcer whose effect does not depend on a particular motivational state of the client. These reinforcers are effective in a wide range of situations and include tokens and money.
- **Conditioned** or **secondary reinforcers**—events, such as praise, smiles, and approval, that strengthen a person's response because of past experience.
- **Negative reinforcers**—events that are aversive and thus reinforce a response that terminates, avoids, or postpones them. For example, an aversive event might be teasing endured by a boy who

stutters. The boy learns to be silent in the presence of his peers because silence helps avoid teasing; in this case, silence is **negatively reinforced**.

- **Positive reinforcers**—events that follow a response and thereby strengthen them. Positive reinforcers are necessary in teaching any kind of skill to any client. They may be verbal (e.g., verbal praise) or nonverbal (e.g., the presentation of a token).
- **Primary reinforcers**—events whose reinforcing effects do not depend on past learning or conditioning. Primary reinforcers are biologically determined because of their survival value (e.g., food and water). They are useful for establishing target responses, not for promoting generalized productions. Also known as unconditioned reinforcers, they are especially useful in teaching infants and toddlers or those with severe intellectual disability; they are essential to reinforce verbal mands (requests for food and drink) in any client of any age.
- **Secondary reinforcers**—social or conditioned reinforcers whose effects depend on past learning (e.g., social praise and tokens).

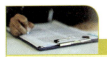

SUMMARY

- Treatment involves teaching new skills to people who manifest disorders of communication; the clinician manages contingent relations between antecedents, responses, and consequences to teach those skills.
- Ideally, selected treatment procedures are supported by experimental evidence for their effectiveness; there is plenty of evidence to show that the behavioral methods of reinforcing target sills in the context of various stimuli are effective in teaching communication skills to children and adults.
- Many terms are used in describing treatment. Some of these terms are used to describe treatment stimuli, reinforcement, and types of reinforcers.

AN OVERVIEW OF THE TREATMENT PROCESS

Clinicians select treatment targets with either the normative strategy, client-specific strategy, functional communication strategy, or the integrated approach. The clinician can then teach the skills in a certain sequence, follow-up the client, and offer booster treatment if necessary.

Selection of Treatment Targets

The clinician may select one of the following approaches to target behavior selection:

Normative Strategy

- This strategy is based on the notion that, especially for children, norms provide the best basis for selecting target behaviors. Within this approach, age-based norms dictate the selection of speech and language targets for children. For example, target responses for a 4-year-old child with a language delay would be those language behaviors that are considered appropriate for a typically developing 4-year-old child. Similarly, phonemes selected for treatment in the case of a child with a speech sound disorder would be the age-appropriate sounds based on speech sound acquisition norms.

- Published norms are often limited to speech–sound and language-structure acquisition. The normative strategy is of little help in selecting treatment targets for most adults and for those with fluency and voice disorders.

Client-Specific Strategy
- Within this strategy, behaviors that will improve the client's communication and help meet the social, academic, and other demands made on the client will be selected for teaching. Some of these behaviors may be consistent with the normative strategy, but others may not be. For example, in selecting language treatment targets for a 10-year-old child with developmental disabilities, one might select the educational terms she needs to learn in her special education class, instead of what might be appropriate for a typical 10-year-old.
- The client-specific strategy is suitable for selecting target behaviors that are appropriate for clients of varied ethnocultural backgrounds. Because the approach emphasizes the individual's needs and uniqueness, it allows the selection of target skills that are relevant to the particular cultural and linguistic background of the client.

Functional Communication Strategy
- Similar to the client-specific approach, the target behaviors selected are the most useful skills that enhance communication and help meet the demands of daily living. More than grammatical accuracy or articulatory accuracy, effective communication (e.g., verbal requests, gestures, writing) is the target; most useful for clients with severe aphasia, apraxia of speech, dysarthria, and other neurogenic communication disorders in adults.
- Functional communication targets help improve naturalistic communication. Any mode of response is accepted, provided it results in effective communication.

Integrated Approach to Target Behavior Selection
- Within this approach, treatment targets are appropriate for the client's age, ethnocultural background, individual uniqueness, and communication requirements. The targets should be functional and useful and should enhance natural communication in everyday situations, including the school, occupational settings, home, and other social situations.
- The approach places a greater emphasis on the client and effective communication and does not negate the importance of age-appropriate targets, especially for children.

Treatment Sequence
Treatment has a typical sequence that is usually modified to suit an individual client. The sequence may be based on response complexity, degree of structure, response modes, multiple targets, training and maintenance, and shifts in treatment contingencies.

- **Response complexity.** Generally, treatment starts at a simple level and proceeds to more complex levels. At each level, a performance criterion must be met before the client advances to the next level of response complexity. Typical levels of response complexity include the simpler level of syllables and moves through, words, phrases, and sentences, the most complex level; it is neither necessary nor desirable to always start at the simplest level. Clinicians are free to start at a more complex level to see if the client would still learn. For instance, one child may need training at the sound or syllable level whereas another child might learn the sound at the word or even phrase level to begin with.

- **Degree of structure**. Treatment is more structured in initial stages when the target skills are established and less structured in later stages when generalization is promoted; after establishing the target behaviors in the clinic, informal therapy may be conducted outside the clinic.
- **Response modes**. Different response modes used in training create a sequence; in most cases, the treatment starts with imitation of modeled responses; modeling is then withdrawn on evoked trials; eventually, teaching progresses to spontaneous productions under more or less structured environments; reading and writing, if they are a part of the training, might introduce additional sequences.
- **Multiple targets**. Multiple targets that most clients need create a sequence; multiple phonemes may be taught with a certain sequence to a child with speech sound disorders; airflow management, gentle phonatory onset, and slow speech may be taught in that sequence to a person who stutters; conversational turn taking and topic maintenance cannot be taught until the client has mastered certain words, phrases, and sentences that make it possible for the client to talk on a topic.
- **Training and maintenance**. A well-known sequence is based on initial training (establishment of target behaviors) and eventual maintenance of those behaviors in natural settings and over time.
- **Shifts in treatment contingencies**. Initially, the client is reinforced for every correct response. Soon, the reinforcement schedule is changed from continuous to intermittent. With children, initial reinforcers may be tangible, but later ones may be social.

Maintenance Program

Clinically established speech–language skills may not necessarily be maintained over time in natural settings. Fluency of a speaker or the naming skills of a person with aphasia, reliably produced in the clinic may be extinguished over time. To help client maintain their skills, the clinician needs to take additional steps:

- Select target behaviors that are more likely to be produced in natural settings (i.e., functional skills that help meet daily communication needs).
- Use a variety of stimuli and stimuli from home to teach skills.
- Give sufficient treatment with varied exemplars, as inadequate treatment with limited exemplars is a major reason for lack of maintenance.
- Before dismissal, reinforce the skills in more naturalistic conversational speech.
- Teach the client self-monitoring skills (e.g., have the clients chart their own target response productions in the clinic; have them stop when they make mistakes and correct themselves; delay reinforcement or corrective feedback to encourage self-evaluation).
- Fade the initial continuous reinforcement to an intermittent schedule; toward the end, use only social reinforcers (except for requests for food and drink).
- Teach family members to stimulate, prompt, and reinforce correct responses at home and other settings; train teachers and others to do the same.
- Teach the client to prime others for reinforcement (e.g., teach the child to draw attention to his or her newly established fluency when parents are too busy to notice and reinforce it).
- Follow up with the client and give booster treatment when needed.

Follow-Up

Follow-up is a procedure of finding out whether the client has maintained the target communicative skills, and whether there is a need for additional treatment. Follow-up involves the following procedures:

- Record an extended conversational speech sample to analyze the continued production of communicative behaviors that were initially established; the need for treating additional targets may also be assessed.
- Determine a follow-up schedule, which tends to vary across clinics and may depend on the type of disorder; some may need more frequent assessments than others. For example, successfully treated clients with fluency disorders need to be followed up for more than 2 years, whereas similarly treated children with speech sound disorders may need to be followed up only for a year or less. A general follow-up schedule is as follows:
  - First follow-up assessment: 3 months postdismissal
  - Second follow-up assessment: 6 months postdismissal
  - Third follow-up assessment: 1 year postdismissal
  - Subsequent assessments as necessary

Booster Treatment

Booster treatment, important for maintenance and loose in structure, is treatment offered any time after the initial dismissal from services. Some disorders need booster treatment more than the others. For example, successfully treated adults who stutter need more frequent booster treatments than similarly treated children with speech sound disorders. Booster treatment may be

- identical to the original and effective treatment.
- a modified version of the original treatment.
- a different form of treatment known to be more effective than the original.
- much less extended than the original.

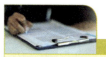

SUMMARY

- Clinicians may select treatment targets using the normative, client-specific, functional communication, or integrated approach.
- Response complexity, degree of structure, response modes, multiple targets, training and maintenance, and shifts in treatment contingencies create sequences in treatment.
- A maintenance program, follow-up, and booster treatment are essential to ensure that clients sustain skills taught in therapy.

A GENERAL OUTLINE OF A TREATMENT PROGRAM

The general outline specifies the steps involved in developing and implementing a treatment program. All clients are assessed before starting treatment. Therefore, the outline begins with the selection of target behaviors and ends with maintenance and potential booster treatment.

Seven Steps of All Treatment Programs

Step 1. Select target behaviors that are empirical response classes that are functional and useful to the client. When taught or modified, the behaviors will reduce or eliminate the disorder. Select short-term and long-term target behaviors. Make these target behaviors objective, measurable, functional, and ethnoculturally relevant for each client.

Step 2. Before initiating treatment, establish baselines, the measured response rates in the absence of treatment, for all relevant response modes: conversational, modeled, and evoked speech, as well as oral reading if appropriate.

Step 3. Plan a comprehensive treatment program that specifies what the client will be required to do, what the clinician will do, and how the two will interact. Ideally, the program should be written after baselines are established and before treatment is started.

Step 4. Implement the treatment program. Precisely manage the behavioral contingencies that will decrease undesirable responses and those that will increase desirable responses.

Step 5. Implement a maintenance program even if some generalization of target behaviors takes place, because the behaviors may not be maintained. Teach the client to self-monitor and train the key people in the client's environment to prompt and reinforce those responses. Arrange for booster treatment.

Step 6. Follow up with the client to assess response maintenance over time and in the natural environment. Measure the responses in the absence of treatment variables. Schedule follow-ups as specified earlier.

Step 7. Conduct booster treatment sessions if necessary to help promote maintenance of target behaviors taught in treatment.

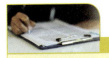

SUMMARY

- Based on the results of an assessment, the clinician selects both short-term and long-term target behaviors for training. Before treatment is initiated, the clinician gathers baselines or measures response rates in the absence of treatment.
- After baselines are established, the clinician plans and implements a comprehensive treatment program by managing contingencies that decrease undesirable responses and those that increase desirable responses.
- The clinician implements a maintenance program and follows up on the client's progress and, when necessary, arranges for booster treatment.

CULTURAL-LINGUISTIC CONSIDERATIONS IN ASSESSMENT AND TREATMENT

Due to the increasing numbers of culturally and linguistically diverse (CLD) clients with communication disorders, clinicians must be aware of special considerations that apply to CLD populations (Battle, 2002; Brice, 2002; Hegde & Pomaville, 2017; Kohnert, 2008; Roseberry-McKibbin, 2014). The issues and research that affect service delivery to ethnoculturally diverse populations are described in Chapter 11. Here, we will briefly summarize the need for individualized assessment and treatment of ethnoculturally diverse children and adults.

The Need for Individualized Assessment and Treatment

While it is important to keep general ethnocultural and linguistic information in perspective, all clinicians should also be aware of individual factors that might affect service delivery to CLD clients and families. Carefully, the clinicians should

- explore to what extent a member of a cultural group is different from the majority of that group (e.g., an African American who does not speak African-American English or a southern rural white person who does); see Chapter 11 for details.
- understand how refugee or immigrant status affects CLD people and how CLD people born and raised in the United States differ from immigrants and refugees of the same cultural background (Roseberry-McKibbin, 2014).
- select standardized tests that have, in their standardization process, sampled the ethnocultural group to which the client belongs; if no such tests are available, use alternative assessment tools described in this chapter and get additional information from Chapter 11.
- avoid testing information about practices or events that may be culturally inappropriate (e.g., Christmas for Muslims); still, avoid stereotypes; some non-Christians may celebrate Christmas as a social holiday.
- consider the client's home environment and past experiences (e.g., exposure to certain kinds of television shows, books, or toys) before selecting assessment or treatment stimuli.
- consider the client's bilingual or multilingual status; use trained interpreters to assess CLD clients who speak two or more languages.
- determine whether an underlying communication disorder exists that affects English, the primary language, or both (Hegde & Pomaville, 2017; Roseberry-McKibbin, 2014).
- avoid diagnosing a communication disorder based solely on English production influenced by the primary language (e.g., labeling a Yugoslavian client who makes a d/th substitution in all word positions as having a disorder).
- be aware of the great heterogeneity of language patterns and dialects among members of the same general language group (e.g., the Hmong language includes the different dialects of Green Hmong and White Hmong).
- have parents participate in target behavior selection to pick out treatment targets that are appropriate and specific for the client's ethnocultural and linguistic background.
- discuss potential treatment procedures with the client, the family, or other caregivers.
- note that what may be inappropriate for assessment may be appropriate for treatment; for instance, pictures that depict objects or situations that are unfamiliar to a client who is a recent immigrant may not be appropriate to assess the production of words or phonemes they evoke, yet the same pictures and the words they evoke may be appropriate for treatment, because the client's new home and school environment may demand the production of such words and phonemes. Parental consultation and approval would still be necessary.

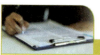

SUMMARY

- The increasing numbers of CLD clients in society make it important for assessment and treatment to reflect sensitivity to the needs of those clients.
- It is critical to individualize assessment and treatment for each client and family served.

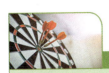

CHAPTER HIGHLIGHTS

- The standard assessment procedures clinicians use include a general screening, a case history, a hearing screening, an orofacial examination, an interview, a speech and language sample, and related assessment data. Assessment procedures must be evidence-based to be valid.
- The vast majority of clinicians assess their clients through standardized, norm-referenced tests that include systematic procedures for administration and scoring. Norm-referenced test results may be used to compare the client's performance with that of the normative group.
- In addition to formal tests, clinicians also use rating scales, questionnaires, and developmental inventories.
- Formal tests can be evaluated according to their reliability and validity for use with specific client populations. Reliability is replicability, and validity is the degree to which a test measures what it purports to measure.
- Because of the limitations of standardized tests, clinicians have developed such alternative assessments as client-specific, criterion-referenced, authentic, and dynamic procedures. An integrated approach that selects the most useful elements of all available approaches, including the essential elements of the traditional approach, will best serve most clients.
- Treatment involves changing a nonfunctional communication pattern to one that is functional and requires systematic work with clients and their families. Although there are many approaches to treating communication disorders, a mastery of certain common concepts, principles, and procedures will help clinicians effectively treat clients with varied disorders of communication.
- Treatment targets may be selected on the basis of the normative, client-specific, functional communication, or an integrated approach.
- Treatment is sequenced based on response complexity, the degree of treatment structure, response modes, multiple targets, training and maintenance, and shifts in treatment contingencies. Based on these factors, various sequences are created: simpler responses are treated before complex responses, initial sessions are more structured than later sessions, imitation is used before spontaneous productions, certain targets are taught before certain other targets, certain maintenance procedures are implemented only in later stages of training, and reinforcers are initially continuous and subsequently intermittent.
- Follow-up is designed to assess maintenance of clinically established behaviors and the need for additional treatment. Typically a 3-, 6-, and 12-month follow-up schedule may be used; additional follow-up may be scheduled as necessary.
- Booster treatment, which may be the same as the original treatment, a modified version, or a different form of treatment, may be essential for maintenance of communicative skills when performance deteriorates.
- When working with culturally and linguistically diverse (CLD) clients, clinicians must be fully knowledgeable about their ethnocultural and linguistic backgrounds, family values and views, and their disposition to disorders and their treatment.

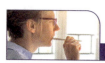

STUDY AND REVIEW QUESTIONS

1. If a test is being evaluated to see whether responses to the items on the first half of the test correlate with responses to the items on the second half, then that test is being evaluated for

   A. test–retest reliability.
   B. interjudge reliability.
   C. split-half reliability.
   D. parallel form reliability.

2. If this test has adequate construct validity, then

   A. several judges have agreed that the test has been constructed appropriately and measures what it purports to measure.
   B. the test items are relevant to measuring what the test purports to measure.
   C. the test accurately predicts future performance on a related task.
   D. the test scores are consistent with theoretical concepts.

3. Which one of the following would NOT be a feature of this norm-referenced, standardized test?

   A. Generation of information that can be used to create treatment goals and assess treatment progress
   B. The comparison of a client's score to that of a normative sample
   C. Ensuring of consistency of administration and scoring across examiners
   D. The provision of systematic procedures for administration and scoring of the test

4. A clinician was working with a 4-year-old boy, Emile, who stuttered. During treatment, the clinician found that every time she asked Emile to imitate a long phrase or sentence, he got out of his chair, tried to wander around the room saying, "That's too hard!" To control Emile's undesirable behaviors, the clinician simplified the target skill; she modeled simpler, shorter sentences with the goal of increasing the utterance length more gradually and slowly than she had done previously. Consequently, Emile's undesirable behaviors decreased and were eventually eliminated. This shows that Emile's undesirable behaviors were

   A. being effectively punished.
   B. being positively yet indirectly reinforced during treatment sessions.
   C. being reinforced on an intermittent, variable ratio schedule.
   D. being negatively reinforced in treatment sessions.

5. Among the traditional and alternative assessment approaches, the one that requires the clinician to offer some treatment before making a full diagnosis and test again to make a final decision is known as

   A. dynamic assessment.
   B. authentic assessment.
   C. criterion-referenced and client-specific approach.
   D. standardized-test–based assessment.

6. You are offering language treatment to a 7-year-old boy, Cameron. Among other things, you are working on the goals of helping Cameron accurately produce the regular plural *-s* and regular past tense *-ed*. You need to measure the generalized production of those skills when you withhold reinforcement for correct responses. The procedure you would use to achieve this is

A. the pre- and posttest results of a standardized test administered at the beginning and conclusion of treatment.

B. probes.

C. dynamic assessment.

D. baserates.

7. Baselines

A. help establish the initial (natural) level of clients' behaviors.

B. help measure responses that are generalized to natural settings.

C. may replace probes.

D. are not necessary for evidence-based practice.

8. A clinician in a hospital setting is informed that insurance companies have begun to demand specific evidence that the clients with neurologically based disorders are taught functional communication skills. These skills are

A. age- and norm-based skills that are appropriate for the client.

B. useful only for adult clients.

C. behaviors that promote communication in natural settings.

D. useful only for clients with language disorders.

9. Negative reinforcement

A. decreases the behaviors.

B. is the same as punishment.

C. does not involve aversive events.

D. increases the frequency of behaviors.

10. You are observing treatment session in which a clinician is treating a 65-year-old man who has aphasia. In the previous sessions, the client had been reinforced for correctly naming several pictures. In the current session, the clinician shows 10 untrained stimuli and asks, "What is this?" for each picture/stimulus item. However, the does not reinforce correct responses. In this latter procedure, the clinician is

A. fading the reinforcers but differentially applying indirect reinforcement.

B. measuring generalized production with a probe.

C. fading the reinforcers.

D. assessing whether the client has learned to name the treatment stimuli.

11. The difference between modeling and imitation is that

A. imitation is a treatment procedure, and modeling is a treatment target.

B. imitation is usually superior to modeling as a treatment strategy.

C. modeling is clinician's behavior, and imitation is client's behavior.

D. modeling is necessary at all stages of treatment, but imitation is necessary only in the initial stage of treatment.

12. In assessing the language skills of Rica, an 8-year-old speaker of Cantonese and English, the clinician, with the help of a Cantonese interpreter, obtained extensive samples of both the languages. After consulting with Rica's teacher and interviewing her parents, the clinician selected additional vocabulary items and common expressions to be included in systematic assessment. This type of assessment is known as

A. functional and criterion-referenced assessment.

B. norm-referenced and criterion-referenced assessment.

C. standardized assessment without being norm-referenced.

D. functional and standardized assessment without being norm-referenced.

13. A clinician working with a 3-year-old girl, Josie, who has a severe speech sound disorder, found the child very uncooperative. She hid under the table, threw therapy materials, and cried. Ignoring the behaviors and admonishing her to sit quietly did not work. The clinician then began to praise Josie for sitting quietly for one minute and naming pictures; she also gave Josie a sticker for being a "good girl" during the preceding one minute. In gradual steps, the clinician extended the duration between verbal praise and presentation of stickers and eventually praised Josie only occasionally. The clinician has just used a procedure known as

A. corrective feedback.

B. differential reinforcement of incompatible behavior.

C. time-out.

D. extinction.

14. A clinician administers the *Language Achievement Test* (LAT) to Bret, who is described as "low" in oral and written language skills. On LAT, Brett's overall score falls in the 25th percentile rank. This means that

A. out of 100 children, 75 did better than Brett on the LAT and 25 children did worse.

B. 75% of the children in the LAT's normative sample did better than Brett.

C. of children in the LAT's normative sample performed about the same as Brett did, but they scored 2–3 points higher on the test overall.

D. Brett scored about the same as 75% of fifth graders in the LAT's normative sample.

15. Various objects, pictures, instructions, modeling, prompts, and other stimuli the clinician uses to evoke target responses from clients are called

A. antecedents or treatment stimuli.

B. reinforcing stimuli.

C. procedural probes.

D. baselines.

References and Recommended Readings at www.advancedreviewpractice.com

STUDY AND REVIEW ANSWERS

1. **C.** If a test is being evaluated for internal consistency and whether responses to the items on the first half of the test correlate with responses to the items on the second half, then that test is being evaluated for split-half reliability.
2. **D.** The concept of adequate *construct validity* means that test scores are consistent with theoretical concepts or constructs.
3. **A.** Norm-referenced, standardized tests are NOT meant to provide information that can be used to create treatment goals and assess treatment progress.
4. **D.** Emile's undesirable behaviors were being negatively reinforced in treatment sessions.
5. **A.** Dynamic assessment, which requires teaching of some deficient skills before making a final diagnosis.
6. **B.** The best way to measure generalized productions is to administer probes.
7. **A.** Baselines help establish the initial level of clients' behaviors
8. **C.** Functional communicative behaviors are behaviors that promote communication in natural settings.
9. **D.** Negative reinforcement increases the frequency of behaviors.
10. **B.** The clinician is measuring generalized production with a probe.
11. **C.** Differences between modeling and imitation are that modeling is clinician's behavior, and imitation is client's behavior; also, modeling is a treatment procedure, and imitation is a target behavior.
12. **A.** The clinician is using functional and criterion-referenced assessment.
13. **B.** The clinician has used the differential reinforcement of incompatible behavior.
14. **B.** Brett's overall score falls in the 25th percentile rank. This means that 75% of the children in the LAT's normative group did better on that test than Brett did.
15. **A.** Various objects, pictures, instructions, modeling, prompts, and other stimuli the clinician uses to evoke target responses from clients are called antecedents or treatment stimuli.

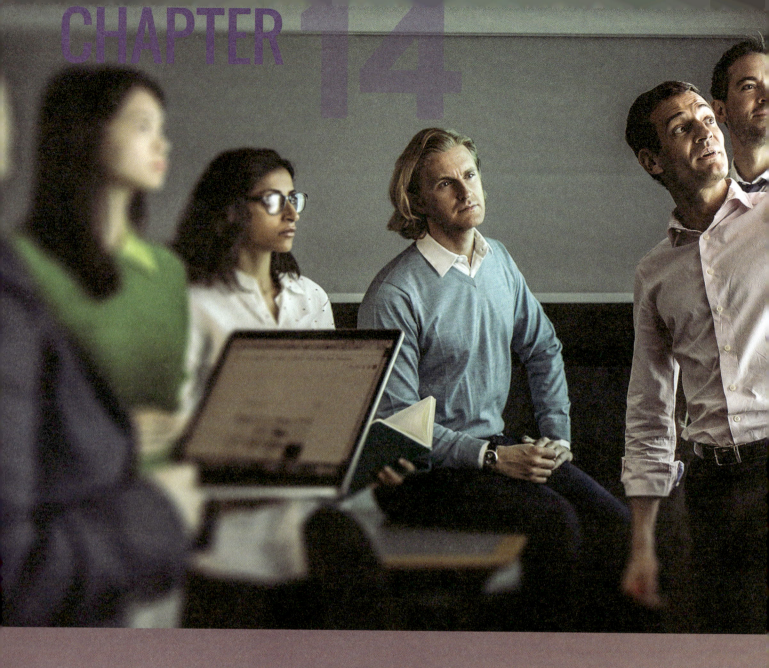

CHAPTER 14

RESEARCH DESIGN AND STATISTICS: A FOUNDATION FOR CLINICAL SCIENCE

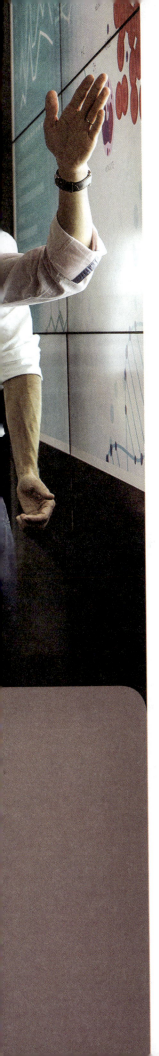

All professional practices are built upon a foundation of basic and applied research. The current emphasis on evidence-based practice in speech–language pathology requires an understanding of the philosophy of science, methods of basic and applied research, techniques of data analysis, and the constraints on drawing valid conclusions from data. Speech–language pathology and audiology are clinical sciences that build upon research evidence gathered by scientists in several disciplines. Today's clinicians are expected to be critical consumers of research so that they may select methods of assessment and intervention that are based on scientifically replicated evidence for their usefulness and effectiveness.

Because most readers will have completed coursework on research designs, statistics, and evidence-based practice, the information presented in this chapter serves to refresh readers' knowledge and strengthen their understanding of critical concepts.

ESSENTIALS OF THE SCIENTIFIC METHOD

Scientists use objective, experimental methods to systematically investigate research questions. Being the means of answering such questions, the research methods involve observation, measurement, and manipulation of some variables to produce valid and reliable data from which objective conclusions may be drawn.

The Philosophy of Science: Basic Concepts

Science developed out of curiosity and a need to understand the world around us. The beginnings of science were based in the philosophical inquiry into truth. Therefore, philosophy, especially empirical philosophy, is the basis of modern science.

- **Science** is a philosophy of events and nature that values evidence more than opinions. The scientist uses objective, experimental methods to systematically investigate research questions and produce valid and reliable results that help answer them.
- **Research** is what scientists do as they practice science; it is science in action. Research is the process of asking and answering questions; it includes steps scientists take as they search for uniformity and order in nature. Science is conceptual and philosophical whereas research is methodological.
- The two philosophical hallmarks of science are empiricism and determinism. **Empiricism** is the philosophical position that statements must be supported by experimental or observational evidence; this evidence is typically sensory

experience (the touching, seeing, tasting, smelling, and hearing of phenomena) must be objectively verifiable. In other words, events must be experienced in such a way as to permit *observation* and *measurement* because sensory experience is the basis of scientific knowledge.

- **Determinism** means that events do not happen randomly or haphazardly; they are caused by other events. Scientific activity based on determinism is a search for causes of events. The goals of science are to (Clark-Carter, 2009; Hegde, 2003; Maxwell & Satake, 2006)

  - *describe* natural events or phenomena.
  - *understand* and *explain* natural phenomena, especially in terms of cause–effect relationships.
  - *predict* occurrences of events.
  - *control* natural phenomena by understanding the causes of events and predicting their occurrence.

- Scientists frequently conduct research with the goal of explaining events and effects. An explanation of an event specifies its causes, and an event is scientifically explained when the scientist experimentally demonstrates its cause(s). To explain events, scientists may use one of two approaches: the inductive method or the deductive method.

  - The **inductive method** is an experiment-first-and-explain-later approach. The researcher first observes the phenomenon, conducts a series of experiments on it, and then proposes a theory based on the results of those experiments.
  - The **deductive method** is an explain-first-and-verify-later approach. In this method, based on initial observations, the investigator explains an event by proposing a theory and then attempts to verify the theory by conducting experiments. Hypothesis-testing is a deductive method.

- Scientists use inductive and deductive reasoning to build theories. A **theory** is a systematic body of information concerning a phenomenon, describing an event, explaining why the event occurs, and specifying how the theory can be verified. A theory specifies causal variables; a theory states that X causes Y.

- A **hypothesis** is a proposed answer to a research question, but verifiable through additional research. A hypothesis is concerned with a more specific prediction stemming from a theory. For example, a hypothesis might state, "When people who stutter are put in highly stressful speaking situations, their amount of stuttering will increase." In other words, the hypothesis is that *stressful speaking situations will cause the effect of increased stuttering.*

- Hypotheses may be **null** or **alternative**. *Null* means zero, and a **null hypothesis** states that two variables are not related. An **alternative hypothesis** states that the two variables are indeed related; perhaps one is the cause of the other.

- In the example just given, the null hypothesis would be that stressful situations and stuttering are *not* related, that when people who stutter are placed in highly stressful speaking situations, stuttering does not increase. The alternative hypothesis is that there is indeed a cause–effect relationship between stressful situations and stuttering. That is, highly stressful speaking situations do cause an increase in stuttering.

- The researcher hopes to *reject the null hypothesis* and *accept the alternative hypothesis*, because the researcher usually believes in the alternative hypothesis. The alternative hypothesis holds that there is a specific relationship between the variables specified.

- **Data** are the result of systematic observation, and in many cases, experimentation. To test their hypotheses, or to answer questions with no particular hypothesis, scientists gather data. Scientists observe events and record some measured values of those events (in our earlier example, the actual number of dysfluencies when stress was increased). Scientific data are empirical, meaning that they are based upon actual events that resulted in some form of sensory contact.
- *Qualitative data are verbal descriptions* of attributes of events, whereas *quantitative data are numerical descriptions* of attributes of events. Qualitative data are stated in words; quantitative data are given in numbers (Clark-Carter, 2009). For example, a clinician might state, "The client has a severe articulation disorder characterized by multiple omissions of phonemes" (qualitative data). The clinician might further state, "In a 5-minute spontaneous speech sample, the client omitted word-final phonemes in 75% of the contexts" (quantitative data).
- Scientific data should meet two criteria of **validity** and **reliability**. Validity and reliability are critical aspects of any type of scientific measurement, including measurement through standardized tests. Measures in speech–language pathology, whether they apply to research studies, clinical measurement of clients' skills, or standardized and nonstandardized tests, need to be valid and reliable, as defined in the next section.

Validity of Measurements

Validity is the degree to which an instrument measures what it purports to measure. For example, a valid child language test should measure language skills, not auditory memory. In research studies, the skills or behaviors measured should be relevant to the research question asked. For example, in an investigation of stuttering treatment, stuttering, not the self-concept of the participants, should be measured.

- There are different kinds of validity:

  - **Predictive validity**, also called **criterion validity**, is the accuracy with which a measure predicts future performance on a related task. The concept applies to both standardized tests and research study results (measures). For example, the performance on the Graduate Record Examination (GRE) should predict the GPA or other measures in graduate programs. Measures reported in a research study on language development in children should be able to predict the developmental stages in children not sampled in the study.
  - **Concurrent validity**, considered a form of criterion-related validity, is the degree to which a new measure correlates with an established measure of known validity; the concept applies most forcefully to standardized tests. For example, a new test of language skills might be correlated with a well-established test of known validity to demonstrate the concurrent validity of the new test. A moderate, positive correlation is good for the new test; if the correlation is too high, however, there may be a question of the need for the new test.
  - **Construct validity** is the degree to which measures are consistent with theoretical constructs or concepts. For instance, a test of language development in children should meet the theoretical expectation that as children grow older, their language skills improve. Similarly, a study on speech sound development may meet certain theoretical expectations (e.g., systematic increase in sound learning across age groups).

- **Content validity** is derived from an examination of the measuring instrument to determine if this instrument samples the full range of skills that it purports to measure. More relevant to standardized tests, content validity is based on expert judgment that a particular test measures what it purports to measure.

Reliability of Measurements

Reliability is the **consistency** with which the same event is measured repeatedly. Scores are reliable if they are consistent across repeated testing or measurement. A standardized test given to the same individual on two occasions should result in similar scores. A clinician who measures stuttering in a client on two consecutive days should record similar rates of dysfluencies. The number of misarticulations baserated by a researcher before administering an experimental treatment should be comparable. Measures will not be trustworthy without that kind of consistency across two or more measures.

- Most measures of reliability are expressed in terms of a **correlational coefficient**. The correlational coefficient is a number or index that indicates the relationship between two or more independent measures. It is usually expressed through Pearson Product Moment r (often referred to as r).

- An r value of 0.00 indicates that there is no relationship between two measures. The highest possible positive value of r is 1.00. Conversely, the lowest possible negative value of r is -1.00.

- The closer the r is to 1.00, the greater the reliability of the test or measurement. There are several types of reliability of a measure or a test:

  - **Test–retest reliability** refers to consistency of measures when the same test is administered to the same people twice. When the two sets of scores are positively correlated, the stability of the scores over time is assumed.

  - **Alternate-form reliability** (also known as **parallel form reliability**) is based on the consistency of measures when two parallel forms of the same tests are administered to the same people.

  - **Split-half reliability** is a measure of internal consistency of a test. Responses to items on the first half of a test are correlated with responses given on the second half. Or the responses to even-numbered items may be correlated with responses to odd-numbered items. Split-half reliability generally overestimates reliability because it does not measure stability of scores over time.

  - **Interobserver** or **interjudge reliability** refers to the extent to which two or more observers agree in measuring an event. For example, if three judges independently rate the fluency of a speaker, there is high interjudge reliability if there is good agreement between judges. Optimally, good agreement results in an interjudge reliability coefficient of 0.90 or more.

  - **Intraobserver** or **intrajudge reliability** refers to the extent to which the same observer repeatedly measures the same event consistently. For example, if the same clinician rates a child's intelligibility over several sessions, those ratings should be consistent to assure acceptable level of intraobserver reliability (assuming, of course, the child's speech intelligibility has not changed).

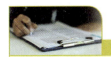

SUMMARY

- Science is based on certain philosophical assumptions including **empiricism** (knowledge based on sensory experience or objective observations) and **determinism** (events have causes, nothing happens without a cause).
- People who use the scientific method may use either inductive or deductive reasoning to create theories and test hypotheses.
- Validity and reliability of measurements are important aspects of good scientific measurement.

EXPERIMENTAL RESEARCH

Experimental research investigates cause–effect relationships. Experimenters manipulate independent variables to assess the effect of these variables upon dependent variables. Group designs, the most popular type of experimental design in medicine and speech–language pathology, usually involve control and experimental groups. Single-subject experimental designs (SSDs) are often used in treatment evaluations in behavioral and clinical sciences. SSDs usually involve 6 to 10 participants and help establish cause-effect relations based on individual performance as opposed to group averages.

Definitions of Terms

- An **experiment** is a means of establishing **cause–effect** relationships. Experiments test *if–then* relationships. For example, *if* a man who stutters is put into a highly stressful situation, *then* will he stutter more? Does the highly stressful situation *cause* the *effect* of increased stuttering?
- An **independent variable** is directly manipulated by the experimenter to produce changes in a dependent variable. In treatment research, for example, all treatments are independent variables.
- A **dependent variable** or **effect** is the variable that is affected by manipulation of the independent variable. In treatment research, all disorders are dependent variables. Manipulation of treatment (independent variable) changes the dependent variable (disorder or a particular skill). Dependent variables must be defined very specifically so that they are measurable. Table 14.1 contains examples of independent and dependent variables.
- **Extraneous** or **confounding** variables should be ruled out in experiments. Study conditions are carefully controlled to eliminate the influence of unwanted variables. To establish a cause–effect relationship in clinical treatment research, the experimenter should rule out the influence of extraneous variables that may also affect the disorder or the skill. For instance, in demonstrating that a child language treatment is effective, the investigator must rule out the influence of maturation and the teachers' or parents' work on the child's language skills.
- Group designs and single-subject designs (SSDs) are the two types of experimental designs used in speech–language pathology.

Table 14.1

Examples of Independent and Dependent Variables

Independent variable	Dependent variable
Stressful situation	Amount of stuttering
Amount of noise in environment	Amount of difficulty understanding spoken speech
Length and complexity of reading passage	Number of errors client with aphasia makes while reading it
Number of times client uses hard glottal attack	Amount of hoarseness present when client is speaking
Number of toys and games present in clinic room	Length of child's MLU as he or she interacts with clinician
Clinician's modeling of a target skill	Client's imitation of the skill
Clinician's verbal praise for correct articulation	Increase in client's correct phoneme production

Note. All things that cause disorders, and all things that are treatment procedures, may be classified as independent variables. All disorders themselves, and target skills that are treated, may be classified as dependent variables.

Group Designs of Research

In the group designs, the average performance of one group is analyzed or those of two groups are compared.

- Research involving a group design may be experimental or nonexperimental. If it is nonexperimental, it will consist of only one group; the research is then observational, or a case study if it is clinical. If it is experimental, it will consist of two or more groups.
- **Experimental designs** using groups to rule out the influence of confounding (extraneous) variables through the use of experimental and control groups.
- **Experimental group** receives treatment and thus shows significant changes in behaviors treated.
- **Control group** does not receive treatment and does not show significant improvement. The goal of having these two groups is to demonstrate that the treatment is better than no treatment—an essential condition to show that the treatment was effective.
- **Randomization** is one method of forming two or more groups for a study. The researcher first randomly selects a sample from the population. The selection is random when each potential participant in the population has an equal chance of being selected for the study.
- A **population** is a large, defined group (e.g., patients scheduled for laryngectomy surgery, people who stutter) identified for the purpose of a study.
- A **sample** is a smaller set that is representative of the population.
- Randomly selected sample participants are then **randomly assigned** to treatment and control groups. The assignment is random when each selected participant has the same chance of being selected to one or the other group.
- Experimental and control groups are equal when random selection and random assignment are done properly. The two levels of randomization reduce experimenter bias in selecting participants and ensure that the sample is representative of the population.

- **Matching** is an alternative to random selection and assignment. In an experimental group–control group design, researcher will first identify two participants who are similar on relevant variables and then assign one to the experimental group and the other to the control group. This ensures that those who receive treatment and those who do not are similar kinds of participants. When individual-to-individual matching is impractical, groups may be matched on the basis of the statistical mean. For instance, the mean dysfluency rates in the experimental and control group in a treatment efficacy study may be comparable (e.g., 15% vs. 14.5%).

Pretest–Posttest Control Group Design

There are several group experimental designs. Many advanced designs are variations of the basic designs. We will describe one basic design that helps evaluate the effects of a single treatment and the other basic design that helps evaluate more than one treatment.

- The **pretest–posttest control group design** is the basic experimental group design to establish causality. It has two groups: an experimental group and a control group. This design helps evaluate the effects of a single treatment.
- The participants should be randomly selected and assigned to groups, although in practice randomization is compromised at various levels. Each participant in each group undergoes a pretest and a posttest.
- **Pretests** are participants' existing behaviors or skills measured before starting an experimental treatment or teaching program. **Posttests** are measures of behaviors established after completing the treatment program. A comparison of pre- and posttest measures helps demonstrate the effects of treatment while ruling out the influence of confounding variables by showing that only the treated group changed and the control group remained at or close to the pretest. The participants are selected and assigned to the two groups randomly. Ideally, the pretest measures of the two groups are similar, and if the treatment was effective, the posttest measures will be significantly different.

Experimental group	Pretest	Treatment	Posttest
Control group	Pretest	—	Posttest

- For example, an investigator seeks to study the effects of enriched maternal speech on infant language development. She forms a control and an experimental group of infant–mother pairs by randomization or matching, most likely matching. The investigator must match the mothers on such characteristics as age, socioeconomic status, language background, and educational level. The experimental group of mothers is taught specific strategies for enriching their infants' language; the control group of mothers is not taught those strategies. The vocalizations of babies in the experimental and control groups are measured before the experiment (pretest) and after the experiment (posttest). If vocalizations increased only in the babies of the experimental group then the enriched maternal speech is the cause of that increase, because in its absence, the vocalizations of babies in the control group did not increase.

Multigroup Pretest–Posttest Design

- The multigroup pretest–posttest design helps evaluate the relative effects of two or more treatments. A question of **relative effects** asks: Of the two or more, which treatment is more effective? Each treatment requires an experimental group, as shown below. The illustrated design helps evaluate relative effects of three treatments. The participants are selected and assigned randomly. Each group receives a different treatment. The control group in this design is optional; hence, it is shown in parentheses.

Experimental group 1	Pretest	Treatment 1	Posttest
Experimental group 2	Pretest	Treatment 2	Posttest
Experimental group 3	Pretest	Treatment 3	Posttest
(Control group)	Pretest	—	Posttest

- In evaluating the relative effects of three treatments that are known to be effective, for example, the investigator randomly selects a sample from the population and randomly assigns them to one of three groups. Each group receives a different treatment. If an optional control group is included, the investigator will know whether treatments are better than no treatment and whether one treatment is better than the other. If no control group is included, the investigator can only answer the question: Which treatment is better?

Advantages and Disadvantages of Group Experimental Designs

- True experimental designs are the most powerful of the group design strategies. They are useful in isolating cause–effect relationships between variables.
- Well-conducted experimental group designs have strong internal validity (described later in this chapter, in the section dealing with evaluation), in that extraneous or confounding variables are ruled out. Thus, the experimenter can be confident that it was indeed the manipulation of the independent variable (treatment) that caused the change in the dependent variable (improvement).
- A major limitation of group experimental designs is that it is not always possible to randomly draw participants from specific clinical populations to which clinicians do not always have access.
- Another limitation of group experimental designs is that the results may be extended to groups but not individual clients. Most practitioners wish to extend treatment study results to their individual clients; SSDs fare better in this respect.

Single-Subject Designs of Research

Single-subject designs compare the performance of the same participant under different conditions of an experiment.

- **Single-subject designs** (SSDs) are playing an increasing role in establishing efficacy of communication treatment procedures. These designs help establish cause–effect relations based on **differential** performances under different conditions of an experiment.

- Unlike group designs, SSDs allow extended and intensive study of individuals and do not involve comparisons based on group performances.
- Instead of the pre- and posttests of group designs, SSDs measure the dependent variables continuously and repeatedly to establish their reliability. Participants are not necessarily randomly selected, and the results of SSDs are not always analyzed statistically.
- Most SSDs do not necessarily have a single participant; most have multiple participants. Each participant's data are analyzed separately and displayed graphically; no group averages are used.
- Most SSDs are experimental. However, as in the group design strategy, there is a single-subject design, called an AB design, which is not experimental and is similar to the **case study** that is used also in group design strategy. The routine clinical work in which the baselines are established (A), treatment is offered (B), and the progress is summarized at the end is a case study. Based on a case study's results, the clinician can claim improvement but not effectiveness for the procedure.
- The SSD experimental strategy demonstrates treatment effects by contrasting conditions of no treatment, treatment, withdrawal of treatment, and other control procedures. All of these conditions are applied to all participants; there are no control participants who do not receive treatment.
- There are many types of SSDs (Hegde, 2003); three designs—the ABA design, the ABAB design, and the multiple-baseline design—are used most often.

ABA and ABAB Designs

- The **ABA design** is the basic experimental SSD. The **ABAB design** is an extension of the basic design. Both are useful in establishing treatment efficacy. In both designs, the first A condition refers to baselines, the next B condition refers to treatment, and the third A condition refers to treatment withdrawal. In the ABAB design, the fourth B condition refers to the reinstatement of treatment.
- The ABA design consists of three conditions:

  - During the first, A condition, the skills to be treated (the dependent variables) are baserated.
  - During the second, B condition, treatment (independent variable) is applied to the skills.
  - In the final, A condition, the treatment is withdrawn and the skills are measured.

- If the study demonstrates that the baserated skills were stable in the first A condition, increased when the treatment was applied in the B condition, and decreased when the treatment was withdrawn in the second and final A condition, then it may be concluded that it was the treatment, and no other variable, that was responsible for the increase in skill levels during B treatment condition (see Figure 14.1 for a graphic representation of hypothetical results from an ABA design study). Although the design helps establish treatment efficacy, it ends with no treatment, and hence no benefit to the participants. The next design avoids this problem.
- The ABAB designs consists of four conditions:

  - During the first A condition, the target skills are baserated without treatment.
  - During the second B condition in which the new treatment is offered.
  - During the third A condition, the treatment is withdrawn.
  - During the fourth and final B condition, the same treatment is reinstated.

- The ABAB design, by adding the final treatment reinstatement condition, ends with treatment; clients benefit from the experiment. The final phase may be continued as long as it is necessary to stabilize the newly established skills. By showing that the baserated stable and low-level skills (A) increased markedly under the new treatment (B), but decreased when the treatment was withdrawn (A) and increased again when the treatment was reapplied (B), we demonstrate that treatment was indeed effective (see Figure 14.2 for a graphic representation of the results of a hypothetical study using the ABAB design).

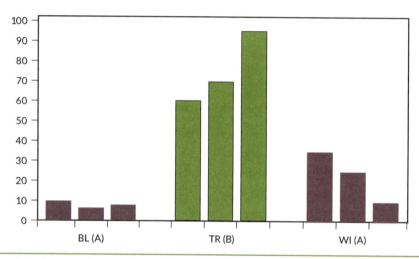

Figure 14.1 Hypothetical results of an ABA single-subject experimental study. A target behavior that is stable under the A condition (BL for baseline), increases in the A condition when treated (TR), and decreases in the final A condition when the treatment is withdrawn (WI). From *Clinical Research in Communicative Disorders: Principles and Strategies* (3rd ed., p. 328), by M. N. Hegde, 2003, Austin, TX: PRO-ED. Copyright 2003 by PRO-ED, Inc. Reprinted with permission.

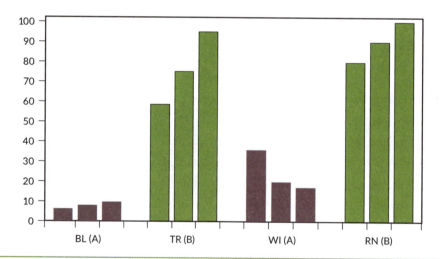

Figure 14.2 Hypothetical results of an ABAB single-subject experimental study. A target behavior that is stable under the A condition (BL for baseline), increases in the A condition when treated (TR), decreases in the final A condition when the treatment is withdrawn (WI), and increases again when the treatment is reinstated in the final condition (RN for reinstatement). The results demonstrate that the treatment was effective. From *Clinical Research in Communicative Disorders: Principles and Strategies* (3rd ed., p. 332), by M. N. Hegde, 2003, Austin, TX: PRO-ED. Copyright 2003 by PRO-ED, Inc. Reprinted with permission.

Multiple-Baseline Designs

- A single-subject design that avoids the disadvantage of treatment withdrawal is the **multiple baseline design**, in which the effects of treatment are demonstrated by showing that untreated skills did not change and only the treated skills did. The three variations of the multiple-baseline design are across subjects, across settings, and across behaviors (Hegde, 2003).

- A **multiple baseline across subjects design** involves several participants who are taught one or more behaviors sequentially (in a staggered fashion) to show that only the behaviors of treated participants change; those of untreated participants do not change. This outcome, too, demonstrates that the treatment was effective. The researcher

  - selects a target behavior to be taught to three or more participants.
  - baserates the target behaviors in all participants before treatment is applied.
  - treats one participant while repeating the baserates on the untreated participants.
  - treats the second participant while repeating the base rates on the untreated participants.
  - alternates treatment and base rates until all participants receive treatment.

- A **multiple baseline across settings design** involves a single behavior being sequentially taught in different settings to demonstrate that the behavior changed only in a treated setting, and thus treatment was effective. The researcher

  - baserates a target behavior in three or more settings (e.g., the hospital room, hospital lobby, parking lot, and home).
  - teaches the behavior in one setting.
  - repeats the base rates in the remaining untreated settings.
  - teaches the behavior in another setting.
  - continues to alternate base rates and teaching in different settings until the behavior is taught in all settings.

- A **multiple baseline across behaviors design** involves several behaviors that are sequentially taught to show that only treated behaviors change, untreated behaviors show no change, and thus the treatment was effective. The researcher

  - selects three or more target behaviors.
  - baserates those target behaviors.
  - teaches the first behavior to a training criterion (e.g., 80% accuracy over three sessions).
  - repeats the baserates on the remaining untreated behaviors.
  - teaches the second behavior while repeating base rates on the remaining untreated behaviors.
  - continues to alternate baserates and treatment until all the behaviors are taught.

Advantages of Single-Subject Designs

- First, clinicians can integrate research and clinical service by using the clients they serve as participants in experiments that attempt to answer significant clinical questions. Except for the ABA design, clients who participate in a study receive treatment; they are not denied treatment as clients in a control group might be if a group design is used.

- SSDs help generalize from research studies to individual clients. Detailed descriptions of individual client characteristics and treatment effects can help establish generalizability of treatments across a wide variety of clients.
- SSDs are much more easily replicated than group design studies, because the difficulty of randomly selecting and assigning a large number of people is avoided.

Disadvantages of Single-Subject Designs

- The results of a single or few SSD studies cannot be generalized to the population. However, the results may be extended to individual clients who have the same profile as those in the research study. However, generality may be achieved by replicating the experiments with different participants in different settings by different investigators.
- SSD studies are not efficient in predicting the behaviors of groups of individuals; they are good at intensively studying individuals.
- To extend the conclusion of SSD studies, investigators need to replicate studies in different settings with different participants. Replications are needed to extend conclusions to the population even when group designs are used, however.

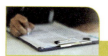

SUMMARY

- The goal of experimental research is to establish cause–effect relationships.
- Investigators assess the effects of an independent variable on a dependent variable and rule out confounding variables that might affect the dependent variable.
- To establish efficacy of new treatment procedures, it is necessary to use experimental research.
- Researchers may use group or single-subject designs to achieve that goal.

VARIETIES OF DESCRIPTIVE RESEARCH

While the goal of experimental research is to *explain the effects* by finding their causes, the goal of descriptive research is to *describe* phenomena. There is no manipulation of variables (e.g., offering treatment) in descriptive research; hence, it cannot demonstrate cause–effect relationships. Varieties of descriptive research include ex post facto research (retrospective research), survey research, comparative research (standard-group comparisons), developmental (normative) research, correlational research, and ethnographic research (Hegde, 2003; Nelson, 2017; Schiavetti, Metz, & Orlikoff, 2011).

Basic Concepts

- In **descriptive research**, researchers observe phenomena of interest and records their observations. The researchers do not want their presence to interfere with the natural phenomena that are being observed (Clark-Carter, 2009; Schiavetti et al., 2011).
- Unlike experimental research, no variety of descriptive research can lead to cause–effect statements.

- There are two types of variables in some kinds of descriptive research. The **classification variable** is analogous to the independent variable in experimental research, although unmanipulated, and the **criterion variable** is analogous to the dependent variable in experimental research.
- For example, people with dementia might be compared to people without dementia on cognitive and linguistic measures. The classification variable would be group status (*dementia* as opposed to *without dementia*) and the criterion variable would be the performance on the cognitive and linguistic measures.
- Descriptive research is useful when it would be unethical to use experimental methods. For example, to find out the effects of maternal drinking on the baby's eventual language skills, researchers would not tell one group of pregnant women to drink alcohol daily and tell a second group of pregnant women not to drink alcohol. However, researchers can observe and measure the language skills of babies born to women who consumed notable quantities of alcohol during pregnancy and *describe* those language skills. Children of a second group of women who never drank alcohol during their pregnancy may provide comparative data.
- Descriptive research is also useful in understanding a phenomenon. For instance, descriptive research helps us understand the nature of language disorders. It also helps us understand what are the typical behaviors of children on the autism spectrum, what behaviors are commonly manifested after a stroke, and so forth. In essence, descriptive research helps us understand what already exists. Experimental research permits us to actively manipulate conditions to change what exists.

Ex Post Facto (Retrospective) Research

- **Ex post facto research** is after-the-fact research. Because the investigator makes a retrospective search for causes of events that have occurred, it is also called **retrospective research**. In most clinical disciplines, ex post facto studies also may be called **causal–comparative studies**. Researchers begin by defining the effect as it currently exists. They then look backward in an effort to describe potential cause or causes.
- Investigations into *potential* causes of disorders or diseases are typically ex post facto. For example, one might investigate the potential causes of hearing loss in a child. In this case, both the causes and the effects have occurred in the past. A detailed history of the child may reveal that the mother, while carrying the child, had an infection that is suspected to cause fetal ear damage. Potential causes of many diseases, including cancer or stroke, are investigated only through ex post facto case studies.
- In contrast to retrospective research, one might design a study that is **prospective**. Smokers who do not have lung cancer may be followed up for a decade to see how many develop that type of cancer.
- Retrospective cases studies also help study rare, individual cases of diseases and disorders in depth. For example, a child with Russell-Silver syndrome (a type of dwarfism) would be an ideal subject for a case study because the syndrome is rare and almost no literature exists that describes communication disorders in that population.
- The most significant limitation of ex post facto research is that it can only suggest, but not confirm, causes of disorders and diseases
- Usefulness of retrospective studies is that they help investigate phenomena that are not amenable to experimental manipulation at the human level. For example, researchers would not ask some people

to smoke and others not to and then observe over the years to see if those who smoked developed lung cancer. Thus, in many cases, ex post facto research is the only option that is ethically possible.

Survey Research

- **Surveys** assess some characteristics of a group of people or a particular society. Surveys attempt to discover how variables such as attitudes, opinions, or certain social practices are distributed in a population (Hegde, 2003).
- Because researchers cannot assess an entire population, they survey a randomly selected, representative sample of that population. Each person in the sample is asked a set of questions of interest designed to evoke answers.
- The two most common types of survey research tools are **questionnaires** and **interviews**, although the two may be combined. Personal interviews help obtain in-depth answers from survey participants. Questionnaires filled out by survey participants may yield a greater quantity of responses, but those responses may not contain the depth of those given in interviews.
- An advantage of surveys is the wide range of data that can be obtained. For example, one can literally sample thousands of people through a survey. The problems of surveys are that (a) they cannot be used to illustrate cause–effect relationships, and (b) their samples are often biased because those who return surveys may not be comparable to those who do not.
- TV shows on dance or music competition that ask viewers to vote illustrate both the strengths and weaknesses of survey research. Thousands of votes are generated, but those who vote tend to be people who are very strongly biased toward one performer or another. People who have a neutral stance toward the performers and their success or failure generally do not cast votes.

Comparative Research

- The purpose of **comparative research**, also known as standard-group comparison, is to measure the similarities and differences of groups of people with defined characteristics.
- Attention and memory skills of people with head injury, for example, may be compared and contrasted with those of individuals without head injury.
- A difficulty with comparative research is that the similarities and differences found between groups of individuals might be due to variables other than the classification variable. For instance, in the above example, clients with head injury might perform differently than non-head-injured clients due to premorbid educational or socioeconomic differences, not the presence or absence of head injury (classification variable).

Developmental (Normative) Research

- The purpose of **developmental research** is to measure changes in individuals over time as they mature or get older. In developmental research, the presumed independent variable is maturation, which implies that *age* is the cause of changes seen in people, especially developing children. Developmental research has been used extensively to create developmental norms. Therefore, developmental research is also known as **normative research**.
- Normative research methods have been used extensively to establish age-based norms on children's speech sound and language skills. The method has also been used to study the cognitive skills of

older adults as they continue to age. Three methods are used in this type of research: longitudinal, cross-sectional, and semilongitudinal.

- In **longitudinal research**, the same participants are studied over time to observe the changes that occur *within* them as they get older. An advantage of longitudinal research is that the investigator can directly observe changes in such behaviors as language skills or fluency in the same participants as they get older. Disadvantages are that it is (a) time consuming, (b) expensive, and (c) vulnerable to subject attrition. Thus, longitudinal studies often have small numbers of participants, limiting the generalizability of the results.
- In the **cross-sectional method**, researchers select participants from various age levels and simultaneously or within a short duration of time sample the behaviors or characteristics of the groups formed on the basis of age. The cross-sectional method is cheaper, faster, and more practical than longitudinal research. A problem with cross-sectional studies is that what is observed for a particular age group in the study may not hold good for others of the same age who were not in the study.
- In the **semi-longitudinal procedure**, the total age range to be studied is divided into several overlapping age spans. The participants selected are those who are at the lower end of each age span, and they are followed until they reach the upper end of their age span. For example, researchers might select three groups of participants and study the language development of those groups for 1 year. The groups might be as follows: 3-year-olds followed until the age of 4; 4-year-olds followed until the age of 5; and 5-year-olds followed until the age of 6. By the end of the study, the researcher would have made observations both *between* and *within* participants as time passed.

Correlational Research

- Correlational research tries to find relationships or associations between variables. Like descriptive research, correlational research cannot uncover cause–effect relations. Correlation suggests that events studied are related, but whether there is a cause–effect relation would not be clear.
- A correlation is a statistical method of data analysis suggesting that two or more events are somehow associated or related. It suggests the direction (positive or negative) and the strength (high or low) of the relationship.
- A positive correlation is found when high values of one variable predict high values of the other variable; when one event increases, the other event increases. For example, as the temperature rises on a hot July day, local grocery stores sell increased quantities of ice.
- A negative correlation is found when high values of one variable are associated with low values of the other variable. When one event increases, the other event decreases. For example, increased pressure to communicate may decrease a speaker's fluency.
- As previously stated, to express the strength and direction of correlational relationships, the Pearson product moment correlation coefficient is used. This is usually abbreviated *Pearson r*. Pearson *r* is a number ideally ranging from −1.0 to +1.0. Positive and negative correlation coefficient 1 in relation to 0, as shown below.

```
- . . . . . . . . . . . . . 0 . . . . . . . . . . . . +
-1.0                                              +1.0
```

- The closer a number is to +1.0, the stronger and more positive the relationship. The closer a number is to −1.0, the stronger and more negative the relationship. The closer a number is to 0, the weaker the relationship. An *r* of 0.35 suggests a weaker relation between two events than an *r* of 0.95.

Ethnographic Research

- **Ethnographic research** involves observation and description of naturally occurring phenomena; thus, it is included under the aegis of descriptive research (albeit somewhat artificially). It is not an experimental type of research.
- Ethnographic research was originally designed by anthropologists as a means of conducting in-depth analytical descriptions of cultural scenes. The most common method of ethnographic research is for investigators to immerse themselves in the situation being studied to gain a deeper understanding of it. Ethnographic researchers study existing phenomena without altering them.
- The investigators conduct detailed observations, making copious notes and sometimes video and audio recordings of phenomena and people being studied. Without formulating hypotheses, investigators take an inductive approach in which observations eventually lead to conclusions. Unlike experimental research, ethnographic research is qualitative. Extensive verbal descriptions are generated, but quantitative analyses are uncommon.
- In speech–language pathology, ethnographic research is advantageous for detailed study of clients, situations, and cultural groups when experimentation is not ideal or possible. Disadvantages of ethnographic research are that it is time consuming, often expensive, yields data that are difficult to quantify, and lacks the objectivity of experimental research. Ethnographic research is still relatively new in speech–language pathology.

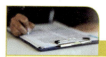

SUMMARY

- A variety of descriptive research studies are used when investigators want to observe and describe phenomena that are naturally occurring in the environment. No cause–effect relationships can be inferred in descriptive research.
- Common descriptive research varieties include ex post facto (retrospective or case studies), survey, comparative or standard-group comparisons, developmental or normative, correlational, and ethnographic research.

EVALUATION OF RESEARCH

Research studies can be evaluated according to the parameters of internal and external validity. Internal validity is the degree to which the extraneous variables were ruled out and the cause–effect relations revealed in an experiment are trustworthy. External validity is the degree to which the results of an experiment may be extended to specific populations.

Internal Validity

- **Internal validity** is the degree to which data in a study reflect a true cause–effect relationship. A study with strong internal validity is one in which the dependent variable was affected only by manipulation of the independent variable. No confounding variable was present. In a treatment study, for example, an internally valid study can claim that *it was the treatment, and no other variable, that produced the positive changes in the clients who received it.*
- Certain factors can reduce the internal validity of a study. These **threats to internal validity** include instrumentation, history, statistical regression, maturation, attrition, testing, subject selection biases, and interaction of factors (Hegde, 2003; Schiavetti et al., 2011).

Instrumentation

- Instrumentation refers to problems with such measuring devices as mechanical and electrical instruments, pencil-and-paper instruments (e.g., questionnaires and tests), and human observers.
- Mechanical instruments (e.g., audiometers) that are not properly calibrated may negatively affect the internal validity of a study in which the hearing loss is measured before and after the administration of a drug to improve hearing.
- Standardized tests administered to inappropriate samples also affect internal validity of a study. For example, administering a test standardized on monolingual, English-speaking, white children to Vietnamese refugee children who speak English as a second language to distinguish language differences from language disorders would pose a serious threat to the internal validity of the study.
- Observers used in a study also act as instruments. Like bad instruments, biased or inexperienced observers negatively affect the internal validity of a study. Individuals who observe glottal fry, for example, on pretests and posttests in a voice treatment study may render invalid scores because they lacked experience in measuring the behavior at the pretest and gained it by the posttest. Observers also may become bored during the posttest and fail to observe and score as vigilantly. Finally, criteria used by individual judges may become more or less stringent over the course of a study. Different judges may render vastly different judgments on the same phenomenon.
- Threats from instruments is controlled by frequent calibration of mechanical equipment and adequate training of human observers.

History

- History includes the participant's life events that occur during the course of an experiment that may be partially or totally responsible for changes recorded in the dependent variable after the independent variable is introduced. For example, a child who receives therapy for a speech disorder and shows significant improvement may have received pressure-equalizing tubes in her ears during the course of therapy. Any improvement noted in speech intelligibility may be partly or wholly due to the aural intervention, not speech therapy.
- Generally, relevant events that occur outside the experimental setting, and thus outside the experimenter's control, have a greater chance of occurring in long-term studies.
- Control groups in group designs and treatment reversal and other measures in SSDs adequately control for history.

Statistical Regression

- **Statistical regression**, also called **statistical regression to the mean**, refers to a behavior that goes from an extreme high or low point to an average level.
- In clinical research, many clients seek treatment when their problem is at its worst. For example, clients who abuse their voices may seek treatment when they are the most hoarse after cheering at a ball game. However, the voice will eventually (in most cases) sound less hoarse (regression to the mean). Improvement in hoarseness shown by the participants in a voice treatment research may be confounded by such regression.
- Control groups in group designs and treatment reversal and staggered treatments in SSDs help control the effects of regression to mean.

Maturation

- **Maturation** refers to biological and other kinds of changes within participants themselves; such changes can have an effect on the dependent variable.
- For example, a study on the effect of a language stimulation program on kindergarten children, conducted over a period of one year, runs the risk of maturation confounding the results. Improved language skills in the children may be due to maturation to an unknown extent.
- Control groups in group designs and treatment reversal in SSDs help control the effects of maturation.

Attrition

- Also called **mortality**, **attrition** refers to the problem of losing participants as the course of an experiment and thus affecting the final results of the study.
- Group designs, which depend heavily on analysis of results based on group averages, are very vulnerable to attrition. Attrition is a serious problem when the investigator uses statistical analysis based on group means and the attrition is **differential** in the experimental and control groups. For example, if more severely affected participants drop out of the experimental group and less severely affected participants drop out of the control group, the pre- and posttest scores of the two groups may differ in favor of treatment, even if the treatment was ineffective.
- Attrition is not a threat in SSDs that include one or more participants. Participants who drop out of those studies are typically replaced. Also, there are no statistically compared participant groups.

Testing

- **Testing** refers to **reactive measures**, changes that occurs in a dependent variable simply because it has been measured more than once (e.g., the administration of pre- and posttests). In such cases, the investigator may incorrectly conclude that the treatment variable was responsible for the change recorded. For example, attitude questionnaires participants fill out before and after treatment are highly reactive. The clients may show significant attitude changes when they fill out the posttreatment questionnaire, even though their attitudes have not changed much.
- The effects of testing may be minimized by measuring behaviors directly, instead of through questionnaires and interviews.

Subject Selection Biases

- **Subject selection biases** are subjective factors that influence the selection of who participates in a study. A key feature of internally valid experiments is that differences found between experimental and control groups on posttests are attributable only to the treatment. However, if the two groups were different to begin with, the initial differences in the participants themselves may account for the differences in posttest measures.
- To control for subject selection biases, it is best to use randomly selected and assigned groups. Another solution is to use groups that have very carefully matched participants—that is, participants who are similar on important variables. As the SSDs do not use group comparisons, selection bias is not significant in them.

Interaction of Factors

- Results of a study may be confounded by a combination of factors described so far. For example, a study involving the use of questionnaires to evaluate attitudes of spouses of people with aphasia might suffer from both testing and attrition.
- Interpretation of data may especially be confounded by the interaction between participant selection and some other factor, such as maturation.

External Validity

- **External validity** refers to **generalizability** of research findings. It is the extent to which an investigator can generalize the study's results to other individuals and situations (Hegde, 2003).
- Threats to **external** validity **limit the degree** to which well-established cause–effect relations, that is, internally valid results, can be generalized. Results of a single study—regardless of the design used—cannot be generalized to a wide variety of settings and people.
- For example, a study on the language skills of Spanish-speaking Mexican children living in California cannot be generalized to Spanish-speaking Puerto Rican children living in New York or to Spanish-speaking Cuban children living in Florida.
- External validity of a study can be threatened by several factors. These include the Hawthorne effect, multiple-treatment interference, and reactive or interactive effects of pretesting.

Hawthorne Effect

- The **Hawthorne effect** is the extent to which a study's results are affected by participants' knowledge that they are taking part in an experiment or that they are being treated differently than usual (Hegde, 2003).
- People who take part in research studies may know what is expected of them; this knowledge alone may influence how they respond under different study conditions. For instance, individuals who completed an experimental treatment for their stuttering may be asked to fill out a questionnaire to assess their satisfaction with the treatment. Because they know they are part of a research project, the participants might want to please the experimenters and state high satisfaction. The experimenters' conclusion that the treatment was highly satisfactory may be questionable. Such results cannot be generalized to people at large who stutter.

Multiple-Treatment Interference

- **Multiple-treatment interference** refers to the positive or negative effect of one treatment over the other when two or more treatments are evaluated in a single study and all participants receive all the treatments.
- For example, when people who stutter receive both counseling and time-out for stuttering, administered in a certain order, the overall outcome may be a result of one treatment influencing the other and one treatment following the other (called the **order effect**). The results may be generalized only to those clients who receive both the treatments, administered in the same order, not to any one treatment administered by itself.

Pretest and Posttest Sensitization to Treatment

- Both the pre- and posttests might sensitize the study participants so that the treatment effect is enhanced (Hegde, 2003). Unlike **testing** that directly changes behaviors as discussed under internal validity, sensitization makes the participants more *receptive* to treatment; the final outcome is partly determined by this sensitization. Sensitization itself does not change the behavior, but makes it more likely to change with the treatment.
- For example, before participating in a voice therapy program to reduce vocally abusive behaviors, the participants might fill out a questionnaire that assessed how often they abused their vocal mechanism. This pretest may not have changed their vocally abusive behaviors (hence no **testing** effect), but they may have become more receptive (sensitized) to treatment. When they take a posttest, they may simply recall some of the suggestions on reducing vocally abusive behaviors that were offered during treatment. Study results may be generalized only to those who take similar pre- and posttests.

Levels of Evidence for Evidence-Based Practice

- A critical examination of research evidence is the heart of evidence-based practice (see Chapter 13 for a description of evidence-based practice). Clinicians are expected to systematically gather and integrates information on treatment procedures from such sources as treatment research evidence, client preferences, and prior knowledge to arrive at a decision. After examining the internal and external validity of treatment research evidence, clinicians may choose techniques that are supported by well-designed and well-executed treatment efficacy studies (Dollaghan, 2007). Evidence to support a treatment procedure is often not categorical; it varies on a continuum. In medicine, evidence is classified into three major classes.

  - **Class I evidence**. Class I evidence is based on a randomized group experimental design study, often referred to as a **randomized clinical trial**; this is the best evidence supporting a procedure. To be classified as Class I, the evidence must come from at least one larger clinical trial with experimental and control groups as described earlier.
  - **Class II evidence**. Class II evidence is based on well-designed studies that compare the performance of groups that are not randomly selected or assigned to different groups. Because of lack of randomization, the groups may or may not be equal to begin with. Therefore, there is no assurance that differences noted on posttests are due to treatment.

- **Class III evidence.** Class III evidence is based on expert opinion and case studies. As noted, case studies can claim improvement, but not effectiveness. Case studies do not include control groups. This is the weakest of the levels of evidence. Nevertheless, evidence based on case studies is preferable to that based on expert opinion.

■ For these levels of evidence and any updated information, see the American Speech-Language-Hearing Association's website (www.asha.org).

■ One problem with the levels of evidence just described is that they ignore the SSDs that have produced significant evidence supporting procedures used to treat communication disorders. Also, the levels equate expert opinion with uncontrolled case studies. With all their limitations, the results of case studies still offer better guidelines for treatment selection than are expert opinions. An alternative way of classifying evidence for clinical procedures accepts all valid research designs and is based on research that is uncontrolled, controlled, and replicated by the same or different investigators. This hierarchy of evidence moves from the least desirable to the most desirable evidence (Hegde, 2003).

- **Level 1. Expert advocacy.** There is no evidence supporting a treatment; the procedure is advocated by an expert. Such a procedure is good only for research, not for routine clinical practice.
- **Level 2. Uncontrolled unreplicated evidence.** A case study with no control group or such single-subject control conditions as baseline, withdrawal, reinstatement, or multiple baselines has shown the procedure to produce improvement; there is no assurance of effectiveness. The procedure is acceptable only if one with better evidence is not available.
- **Level 3. Uncontrolled directly replicated evidence.** A case study without controls has been replicated by the same investigator in the same setting and has obtained the same or similar levels of improvement. While there is better evidence than that in the previous two levels, still there is no assurance of effectiveness (we do not know if it is better than no treatment).
- **Level 4. Uncontrolled systematically replicated evidence.** A case study has been replicated by another investigator in another setting with different clients and has obtained the same or similar levels of improvement reported by the original investigators. Although still uncontrolled, the evidence is getting stronger and is likely to show effectiveness in a controlled study.
- **Level 5. Controlled unreplicated evidence.** The first level at which efficacy is substantiated for a treatment procedure. One of the group or single-subject designs has been used to show that treatment is better than no treatment and that extraneous variables (such as maturation or family's work at home) are not responsible for the positive changes observed. Not only improvement, but also effectiveness has been demonstrated for the procedure.
- **Level 6. Controlled directly replicated evidence.** The same investigator who demonstrated the effectiveness for the first time has replicated the study with new clients and has obtained similar results to document effectiveness. The technique is now known to reliably produce the effects, at least in the same setting.
- **Level 7. Controlled systematically replicated evidence.** This is the highest level of evidence. The effectiveness of a treatment technique has been replicated by other investigators, in different settings, with different clients, to show that the technique will produce effects under varied conditions. A technique that reaches this level may be recommended for general practice.

- It is the responsibility of the clinician to evaluate treatment techniques in terms of the level of evidence they have attained. Generally, it is unethical to select a technique with a lower level of evidence when one that is supported by a higher level of evidence is available. This is why it is important to understand the research methods used in generating scientific evidence.

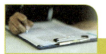

SUMMARY

- Investigators who conduct studies must control for threats to both the internal and the external validity of those studies.
- Threats to internal validity include instrumentation, history, statistical regression, maturation, attrition, testing, subject selection biases, and interaction of two or more of those factors.
- Threats to external validity include the Hawthorne effect, multiple-treatment interference, and pre- and posttest sensitization.
- Critically examining research evidence for particular treatment procedures, clinicians should choose techniques that are supported by well-designed and well-executed treatment efficacy studies.

DATA ORGANIZATION AND ANALYSIS: PRINCIPLES OF STATISTICS

Group design studies conducted in any discipline use statistics to help organize, summarize, and analyze data. Dozens of statistical techniques are available. Commonly used techniques include measures of variability and measures of central tendency. Measurement scales are often involved, as they are closely related to statistical scaling techniques.

Basic Concepts
- Statistical techniques help organize, analyze, and draw conclusions from research data.
- **Statistics** in its singular form refers to the field of study involved with the art and science of data analysis. Statistics deals with **probability**, or the chance of something occurring. For example, if the probability of rain is 0.75, there is a 75% chance that it will rain.
- When used in the plural form, **statistics** refers to specific pieces of data that will be or have been gathered. For example, baseball statistics might include a baseball player's number of home runs and strikeouts.
- The singular **statistic** is a **measure** or a number calculated from a sample. This differs from a **parameter**, which refers to a characteristic of a population. Examples of statistics, or summaries of samples, include percentages, means, variances, standard deviations, and other measures calculated from samples.
- There are several major purposes for statistics. The first purpose is to take large quantities of data and reduce them to manageable form. For example, if there are 100 individual scores on an examination, it is easier to calculate an average than to look at and remember 100 individual scores.
- The second purpose of statistics is to aid the researcher in making inferences. An **inference** is a conclusion one arrives at through reasoning. Statistical inferences are frequently made from samples

to populations. That is, researchers make observations on a sample, or small group of people, to make a decision about a larger group.
- For example, investigators who have studied the effects of exercise on cholesterol levels in samples of participants have discovered that the individuals who increased their level of exercise had a decrease in their cholesterol levels. Thus, the investigators *inferred* that people not in the study, the larger population of people with high cholesterol, might benefit from increased levels of exercise.

Statistical Techniques for Organizing Data
- Three measures help organize and summarize data: measures of central tendency, measures of variability, and measures of association.
- Measures of association (also called **correlation**) have been described already. Thus, measures of variability and measures of central tendency will be briefly discussed.

Measures of Variability
- **Variability** refers to the dispersion or spread in a set of data. Common measures of variability include the range, interquartile range, semi-interquartile range, and standard deviation. For example, if an instructor administers an examination to 50 students and the highest score is 100 and the lowest score is 40, there is great variability in that set of scores. But if the lowest grade is 90 and the highest grade is 100, the variability in that set of scores is minimal.
- The **range** is the difference between the highest and the lowest scores in a distribution or set of scores. For example, a test on which the highest score is 100 points and the lowest score is 40 points, the range is 60 points. One hundred (highest score) minus 40 (lowest score) yields the range in that set of scores.
- The range can be deceptive, however, because extremely high and low scores can make the range appear greater or more variable than it really is. For example, let us assume 1 student received a score of 40 on the examination. The next highest score was 70, and 49 out of the 50 students received scores between 70 and 100. The 1 student scoring 40 caused the class to have a 60-point range in scores instead of a 30-point range.
- To deal with such problems, the interquartile range and semi-interquartile range may be used. The interquartile range "cuts off" the highest and lowest 25% of the scores in a distribution. Thus, what is left is the middle 50% of the scores. The semi-interquartile range is the interquartile range divided by 2. For example, if 100 students take an examination and the 25 highest scores range from 75 to 100 and the 25 lowest scores range from 0 to 25, the interquartile range of those scores is 50, because the lowest 25 scores and the highest 25 scores are disregarded. The semi-interquartile range is 25:50 (the interquartile range divided by 2).
- The **standard deviation** (SD) is the extent to which scores deviate from the mean or average score. SD reflects the variability of all measures or scores in a distribution. The larger the standard deviation, the more variable the scores, and vice versa.
- For example, if on an instructor's test, the highest score is 100 and the lowest score is 50, that 50-point difference in the highest and lowest scores results in a large standard deviation. If on another test, the highest score is 100 and the lowest score is 85, that 15-point difference between the highest and lowest scores results in a relatively small standard deviation.

Measures of Central Tendency

- The **central tendency** of a distribution or set of scores is an index of the **average** or **typical** score for that distribution. There are three measures of central tendency: mean, median, and mode.

- The **mean** is the most commonly used measure of central tendency. To calculate a mean, the investigator adds up the scores and divides the total by the number of scores that were added together. For instance, 60 + 50 + 40 + 80 = 230. Next, 230 ÷ 4 = 57.5. Thus, the mean for this set of scores is 57.5.

- The **median** is the score in the exact middle of the distribution. The median divides the distribution into two parts so that an equal number of scores fall above and below it, as shown:

  38   42   51   57   63   **69**   78   85   88   90   97

  The *median* score is 69 because five scores fall below it, and five scores fall above it.

- The **mode** is the most frequently occurring score in a distribution. This is illustrated as follows:

  22   29   34   46   57   **63**   **63**   **63**   78   85   100

  The *mode* is 63, because 63 is the most frequently occurring score in this distribution.

- If distributions are relatively symmetrical, the three measures of central tendency should be the same, and results in a **normal distribution** or **bell-shaped curve**.

Types of Measurement Scales

- Psychological and social scientists typically describe what they term **levels of measurement**. Some of these levels of measurement are closely related to statistical scaling techniques. The four commonly used levels of measurement are represented by nominal, ordinal, interval, and ratio scales.

- In a **nominal scale**, a category is present (e.g., hypernasality) or absent (normal nasality). Items or observations are classified into named groupings or discrete categories that do not have a numerical relationship to one another. For example, in a survey of clinical practices, respondents might be asked if they "never," "sometimes," or "always" engage in a certain clinical practice. Or, a researcher might label diagnostic categories in a nominal way as "aphasia," "specific language impairment," "dementia," "dysphagia," and others.

- An **ordinal scale** is a numerical scale that can be arranged according to rank orders or levels. Ordinal scales use relative concepts, such as **greater than** and **less than**. The numbers in an ordinal scale and their corresponding categories do not have mathematical meaning. Also, the intervals between numbers of categories are unknown and probably not equal. Examples of ordinal scales of measurement are

  1 = strongly agree   2 = agree   3 = neutral   4 = disagree   5 = strongly disagree

  1 = little hoarseness   3 = moderate hoarseness   5 = great hoarseness

- An **interval scale** of measurement is a numerical scale that can be arranged according to rank orders or levels; the numbers on the scale must be assigned in such a way that the intervals between them are equal with regard to the attribute being scaled. For example, the attribute of distance is equal between one number and another.

    1-----2-----3-----4-----5-----6-----7-----8-----9-----10

- A **ratio scale** has the same properties as an interval scale, but numerical values must be related to an **absolute zero point**. The **zero** suggests an absence of the property being measured. An example of a ratio scale is one that involves frequency counts in stuttering; it is possible to have zero instances of stuttering in a speech sample. A ratio scale for the attribute of distance is shown below.

    0-----1-----2-----3-----4-----5-----6-----7-----8-----9-----10

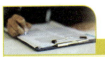

SUMMARY

- Statistical techniques enable investigators to organize, summarize, and analyze data. These techniques include measures of variability and measures of central tendency.
- Measures of variability include the range, interquartile range, semi-interquartile range, and standard deviation from the mean.
- Measures of central tendency include the mean, median, and mode.
- Measurement scales used in research include nominal, ordinal, interval, and ratio scales.

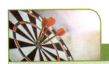

CHAPTER HIGHLIGHTS

- Science, a philosophy based on empiricism and determinism, uses objective experimental methods to systematically investigate research questions and produce valid and reliable results. Scientists may use either inductive or deductive reasoning to create theories and test hypotheses. Hypothesis testing is a major goal of science.
- A rigorous method of hypothesis testing is experimental research. An experiment is a means of establishing cause–effect relationships between variables. An independent variable is directly manipulated by the experimenter to cause changes in the dependent variable being studied. Ideally, confounding variables are ruled out as potential causes of changes in the dependent variable.

- There are many experimental group designs. In the basic experimental group design, there is at least one experimental group that receives treatment, and one control group that does not. These groups constitute the sample, a small number of participants drawn from the population. The sample should be randomly selected and representative of the population.
- The pretest–posttest design is a prototype of experimental group designs. In this design, the experimental and control groups are similar to begin with. They are different only after the experimental group receives treatment. Both groups are given a pretest, only the experimental group receives the treatment, and then both groups are given a posttest. This arrangement allows the researcher to evaluate the effect of the independent variable (treatment) on the behavior of the experimental group. This basic design may be extended to include additional groups to evaluate multiple treatments.
- Single-subject designs are experimental designs that demonstrate cause–effect relationships in small numbers of participants whose performance is recorded individually. ABA and ABAB designs are commonplace in SSD research. The A phase is the no-treatment phase, and the B phase is the treatment phase. Multiple-baseline designs are another common type of single-subject research designs.
- Sometimes experimental research is not possible or desirable, so investigators use descriptive research strategies instead. In descriptive research, there is no demonstration of cause–effect relationships. Common types of descriptive research include ex post facto (retrospective or case study), survey, comparative or standard-group comparison, developmental or normative, correlational, and ethnographic research.
- Research may be evaluated in terms of its internal and external validity. Internal validity refers to the degree to which data in a study reflect a true cause–effect relationship. External validity refers to the generalizability of a study's results.
- Possible threats to a study's internal validity include instrumentation, history, statistical regression, maturation, attrition, testing, subject selection bias, and interaction of two or more of those factors. Possible threats to external validity include the Hawthorne effect, multiple-treatment interference, and reactive or interactive effects of pretesting.
- When clinicians choose treatment techniques to use with their clients, they should ideally choose techniques that are supported by well-designed and well-executed treatment efficacy studies. This will help the clinicians to use evidence-based practice, or practice that is supported by research.
- Statistics may be defined as the field of study involved with data organization, summary, and analysis. Statistics is based on the theory of probability. Two foundational types of statistical analysis used for data organization and summary include measures of variability and measures of central tendency.
- Levels of measurement used by scientists are related to statistical scaling techniques. Four commonly used levels of measurement include nominal, ordinal, interval, and ratio scales.

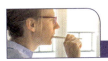

STUDY AND REVIEW QUESTIONS

1. A new test of morphological skills, the *Morphological Estimate of Students' Skills* (MESS), correlates very well with a test of morphological skills that has been used nationally for the last 15 years. One could say that the MESS has good

   A. content validity.
   B. concurrent validity.
   C. construct validity.
   D. predictive or criterion validity.

2. Reliability means that a test or measure

   A. measures what it purports to measure.
   B. has scores that are consistent across repeated testing or measurement.
   C. has items that adequately sample the full range of the skill being tested.
   D. correlates well with an established test of known validity.

3. A researcher investigates the effect of rate of speech upon stuttering during sibling interaction. She gathers conversational samples from children who stutter and their siblings. She asks the siblings in the control group to speak as they normally would at home. Siblings in the experimental group are asked to speak much more quickly than they would at home. The investigator wishes to answer the question whether increased rate of sibling speech causes children to stutter more. In this study, the dependent variable is

   A. the amount of stuttering done by the children who stutter before and after the siblings increase their rate of speech.
   B. the rate of speech of the siblings in the experimental group.
   C. the rate of speech of the siblings in the control group.
   D. the combined amount of stuttering done by the children in both the experimental and the control groups.

4. An experimental design involving only a few participants and focusing on individual performance would be called a

   A. case study design.
   B. ex post facto design.
   C. single-subject design.
   D. single correlational design.

5. In a single-subject design, the following are true:

   I. The A phase is the no-treatment or baseline phase.
   II. The B phase is the treatment phase.
   III. The A phase is the treatment phase.
   IV. The B phase is the no-treatment or baseline phase.
   V. There is no control group.

A. III	**C.** I, II
B. III, IV, V	**D.** I, II, V

6. A type of research involving the effect of independent variables that have occurred in the past and the investigator is making a retrospective search for causes of events is called

- **A.** single-subject design research.
- **B.** ex post facto research.
- **C.** survey research.
- **D.** ethnographic research.

7. A difficulty with cross-sectional studies is that

- **A.** what is observed for a particular age group in the study may not hold good for others of the same age who were not in the study.
- **B.** observations are made of differences *within* participant groups of different ages to generalize about developmental changes that would occur *between* participants as they mature.
- **C.** the same participants are studied over time, and this is expensive, time consuming, and difficult because participants might drop out of the study.
- **D.** the total age span of children to be studied is divided into several overlapping age spans, and it is difficult to follow participants from the lower to the upper end of each age span.

8. A researcher teaches a new book reading program to caregivers of low-income children and evaluates the language skills of the children one year later to evaluate whether or not there is a relationship between caregivers' implementation of the program and children's language skills. The researcher finds that there is an $r = 0.10$ correlational relationship between caregivers' reported implementation of the program and children's language skills. The researcher can safely conclude that

- **A.** there is a strong positive correlation between the caregivers' implementation of the program and children's language skills.
- **B.** there is a strong negative correlation between the caregivers' implementation of the program and children's language skills.
- **C.** there is a moderately significant cause–effect relationship between the caregivers' implementation of the program and children's language skills.
- **D.** there is no significant relationship between the caregivers' implementation of the program and children's language skills.

9. A group of clinicians wishes to conduct research in a hospital setting. These clinicians work with clients who have voice disorders. Many of the clients are hoarse because they work in noisy factories where they shout a great deal during the work week. The clinicians devise a rating scale to evaluate the hoarseness of these clients during evaluation sessions. The scale looks like this:

1	2	3	4
almost no hoarseness	slight hoarseness	moderate hoarseness	great amount of hoarseness

This type of scale would be called a(n)

A. ratio scale.
B. nominal scale.
C. ordinal scale.
D. logarithmic scale.

10. The *range* in a distribution can be defined as

A. the difference between the highest and the lowest scores in a distribution.
B. the middle 50% of scores of a distribution.
C. the middle 50% of scores in a distribution divided by 2.
D. the variance plus the difference between the highest and lowest scores in a distribution.

11. Studying the speech of a group of children who have developmental apraxia of speech, the researcher finds that the faster the children speak, the less intelligible they are. The researcher obtains a Pearson *r* correlational relationship of –0.92. One could say that this shows that there is _____ between rate of speech and intelligibility.

A. a positive correlational relationship
B. a strong negative (or inverse) correlational relationship
C. a canonical correlational relationship
D. a cause–effect relationship

12. Single-subject design strategy

A. allows extension of the results to others in the population as long as the study was done properly.
B. does not allow extension from a single study.
C. can never allow extension of results.
D. can allow extension through replications.

13. A speech–language pathologist who has been working on improving speech intelligibility of non-native speakers of English wanted to collect objective evidence that his client's speech intelligibility was improving. She recruits four speech–language pathology graduate students at the local university to watch "before-and-after" videos of his accent clients and independently rate each client's speech intelligibility. He finds that for the same client, the intelligibility ratings varied from a 30% to 60% across the four students. In this situation, one can say that

A. there is low interjudge reliability.
B. there is high interjudge reliability.
C. there is low intrajudge reliability.
D. there is high intrajudge reliability.

14. A hospital-based clinician is conducting an experiment to assess the efficacy of the new, exciting Newton Aphasia Program (NAP) in increasing the word-retrieval skills of her people with aphasia. The experimental and control groups have been carefully matched on all variables. Halfway through the experiment, the clinician finds that many of the experimental participants attend church each Sunday and go to Sunday school after church. In Sunday school, there is bible study and a great deal of discussion. None of the control participants attends church or Sunday school. At the end of the experiment, the clinician finds that the experimental group of participants who received the NAP have improved significantly in their word-retrieval skills compared to the control participants, who have been treated with more traditional word-retrieval therapy techniques. What can the researcher safely conclude from her study?

   A. The NAP was more successful in helping the experimental patients improve their word retrieval skills than were the traditional methods in helping patients in the control group improve their word retrieval skills.
   B. The NAP was not successful in helping the patients in the experimental group improve their word-retrieval skills; the improvement was due to weekly church and Sunday school attendance.
   C. The experimental group's Sunday school and church attendance on a weekly basis was a possible confounding variable in the study, making it impossible to firmly conclude that the NAP alone caused the difference in the performance of the experimental and control groups.
   D. The NAP was only moderately successful in helping experimental group patients improve their word-retrieval skills.

15. A clinician in private practice often administers the *Word Abilities Keystone Evaluation–Upper Portion* (WAKE-UP) test to the children with language disorders. One day, she becomes curious about the "typical score" of the children to whom she administers the WAKE-UP. The clinician takes the WAKE-UP scores of 17 children and lines them up in order from lowest to highest score:

33   33   46   48   51   55   60   69   73   82   85   89   91   93   95   95   95

The clinician identifies a number below and above which the same number of scores existed. That number is called a

   A. mean.
   B. mode.
   C. median.
   D. standard deviation.

16. The highest level of evidence supporting a treatment procedure comes from

   A. controlled research, systematically replicated.
   B. controlled research, directly replicated.
   C. an experimental study with a large number of participants.
   D. a multiple baseline design study.

17. A clinical researcher, who has been using Van Riper's fluent stuttering approach to treating stuttering in adults, realizes that its effectiveness is unknown. He plans to design a study to find out if the method is effective. To make a valid conclusion, the researcher must use

   A. the survey method in which he would seek the opinions of other clinicians who use the method.
   B. one of the experimental designs.
   C. the case study method.
   D. the retrospective research method.

18. The belief that vocally abusive behaviors in humans lead to vocal nodules and the resulting voice disorder is supported by

   A. experimental research.
   B. prospective research.
   C. ex post facto or retrospective research.
   D. experimental group control-group research.

19. An investigator is interested in evaluating the relative effects of three treatments on the production of grammatical morphemes in children with autism spectrum. The investigator also wishes to see if each treatment is effective in its own right. The most appropriate experimental design for this study is

   A. a group design with four groups.
   B. a pretest–posttest control group design.
   C. multiple baseline design across subjects.
   D. an ABAB design.

20. Too many treatment procedures to treat a single communication disorder is one of the perplexities clinicians face. To survive this perplexity and to select a treatment procedure for a given disorder, the clinician should

   A. find out the most well-established procedure.
   B. read the survey research reports to find out the most popular technique.
   C. consult the manuals of various treatment procedures.
   D. select a technique with the highest level of evidence available.

References and Recommended Readings at www.advancedreviewpractice.com

STUDY AND REVIEW ANSWERS

1. B. The MESS has good concurrent validity because it is a new test that correlates well with an established test of known validity.
2. B. *Reliability* means that a test or measure has scores that are consistent across repeated testing or measurement. The other answers in this item relate to validity, not reliability.
3. A. The dependent variable is the amount of stuttering done by the children who stutter before and after the siblings increase their rate of speech. The rate of speech of siblings in both groups is the independent variable, which is manipulated by the investigator.
4. C. Single-subject designs are experimental and may involve few participants. Case study designs are descriptive.
5. D. In a single-subject design, the A phase is the no-treatment or baseline phase, the B phase is the treatment phase, and there is no control group.
6. B. A type of research involving the effect of independent variables that have occurred in the past and the investigator is making a retrospective search for causes of events is called ex post facto research.
7. A. A problem with cross-sectional studies is that what is observed for a particular age group in the study may not hold good for others of the same age who were not in the study.
8. D. The researcher can safely conclude that there is no significant relationship between the caregivers' implementation of the program and their children's language skills.
9. C. An ordinal scale of measurement would be represented by numbers that can be arranged according to rank orders or levels, but the intervals between the numerals are unknown and probably not equal.
10. A. The *range* in a distribution can be defined as the difference between the highest and lowest scores in a distribution.
11. B. The faster the children speak, the less intelligible they are; Pearson r is -0.92 is a strong negative (or inverse) relationship between speed and intelligibility; high values of one variable (speed) are associated with low values of the other variable (intelligibility).
12. D. Single-subject designs allow extension through replications; generality is achieved by replicating the experiments with different participants in different settings by different investigators.
13. A. If judges who are measuring the same event markedly disagree with one another, then one can say there is low interjudge reliability.
14. C. The experimental participant's weekly attendance at church and Sunday school was a possible confounding variable, making it impossible to firmly conclude that the NAP alone caused the difference in the performance of the experimental and control groups.
15. C. The clinician has just calculated the median score, which is the score in the exact middle of the distribution. An equal number of scores fall above and below it.
16. A. The highest level of evidence supporting a treatment procedure comes from controlled systematically replicated research.

17. B. An investigator trying to find if a treatment is effective for a disorder should use one of the experimental designs.
18. C. The belief that vocally abusive behaviors in humans lead to vocal nodules and the resulting voice disorder is supported by ex post facto or retrospective research; experimentation is neither feasible nor ethical.
19. A. The investigator needs four groups, three groups to evaluate the relative effects of three treatments and one control group to assess whether each treatment is better than no treatment.
20. D. The clinician should always select a technique that has been supported by the highest level of evidence available.

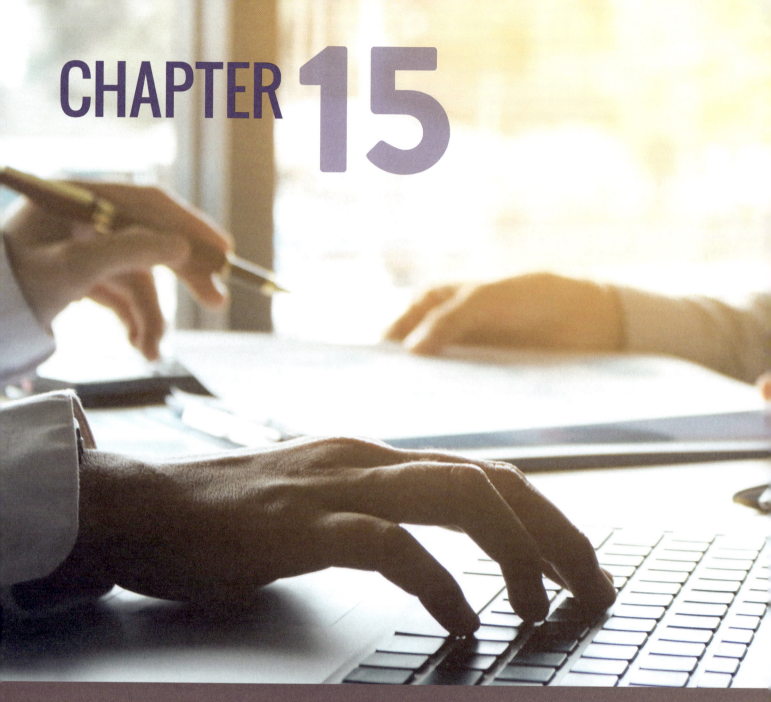

CHAPTER 15

PROFESSIONAL ISSUES

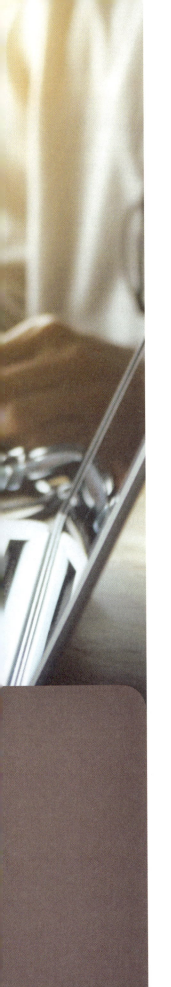

At the beginning of the 20th century, there were no professionally trained speech–language pathologists or audiologists in the United States. There were no educational or professional training programs in the country. In Europe, the treatment of speech disorders was a domain of medicine. In the United States, it was the public schools that took a leading role in providing special teaching programs for children with communicative disabilities. By 1910, Chicago public schools began to hire specialists to work with children with disorders of speech. These specialists, called speech correction teachers, worked mostly with children who stuttered or had disorders of articulation. Other disorders of communication began to be treated only later. In the early 1920s, the University of Wisconsin and the University of Iowa began to offer doctoral programs with an emphasis on speech disorders. Soon other universities across the country, such as Northwestern University, instituted degree programs in speech disorders.

Today, in the 21st century, the profession of communicative sciences and disorders continues to undergo rapid changes and expansion. Such expansion is due in large part to a phenomenal growth in the amount of research information on communication and its disorders. In this chapter, an overview of the American Speech-Language-Hearing Association (ASHA) and the professions of speech–language pathology and audiology is given. Issues related to certification and licensure and legislative matters in regulation of the professions are also discussed.

ASHA AND THE PROFESSIONS

The American Speech-Language-Hearing Association is the national professional organization for speech–language pathologists (SLPs) and audiologists. It fulfills many functions, including research in the field, legislation that affects the profession, regulation of the profession, academic training, and public information. Most SLPs and audiologists are members of ASHA. SLPs and audiologists are professionals who deal with typical development and disorders of communication (including hearing) and swallowing. ASHA and the professions of speech–language pathology and audiology are continually expanding to serve greater numbers of clients who have communicative disorders.

In this chapter, we give a brief historical introduction to ASHA, discuss how the national organization regulates academic training and clinical certification, and describe how it takes steps to ensure that clinicians practice their profession ethically. The chapter also describes how federal legislation affects professional practice in speech–language pathology and audiology.

The American Speech-Language-Hearing Association

The American Speech-Language-Hearing Association has undergone several name changes. In 1925, when it was established by a handful of people at the University of Iowa, it was called the American Academy of Speech Correction. In 1927, it was renamed the American Society for the Study of Speech Disorders. In 1934, the name was changed to the American Speech Correction Association.

- In 1947, the organization was renamed the American Speech and Hearing Association (ASHA). The addition of "hearing" to the name was significant, recognizing the intertwined nature of speech–language pathology and audiology.
- In 1978, the name was changed to the American Speech-Language-Hearing Association to reflect the field's deeper involvement in language and its disorders. This name stands today, although the acronym is still ASHA.
- All the statistical information that follows is taken from ASHA's website (http://www.asha.org/).
- Most members of ASHA are speech–language pathologists and audiologists living in the United States, but ASHA is also open to international membership. In 2016, ASHA had 504 international affiliate members in 60 countries. It is the leading international organization of speech–language pathologists and audiologists.
- ASHA has grown dramatically in recent decades. In 1935, the organization had fewer than 100 members; at the year-end 2017, membership exceeded 191,500 speech–language pathologists, audiologists, speech–language and hearing scientists, and other professionals. About 13,000 ASHA members are audiologists. In addition, approximately 40,000–50,000 speech–language pathologists, many of whom work in public schools, are not members of ASHA.
- By the end of 2016, only 4.7% of ASHA members were males, compared to 4.8% in 2015. Only 7.9% of ASHA members belong to an ethnic or racial minority group. This percentage is far below the distribution of minorities in the general population (27.6%). Hispanic or Latino membership stands at 5% (16.3% in the general population).
- Both the professional organization and the range of professional services offered to the public are growing. In 2016, 74.1% of audiologists were employed in health care facilities, including 47.4% that worked in nonresidential health care settings, 25.8% in hospitals, and 1.0% in residential health care facilities; 15.2% were in educational settings (schools and colleges) and 30.4% in private practice.
- In 2016, 55% of speech–language pathologists worked in schools, preschools, and grade schools; 2.7% worked in colleges or universities; 39.5% worked in health care facilities, and 20.1% in private practice.
- ASHA membership-related statistical data, summarized here, change annually. To get the latest data, visit www.asha.org.
- ASHA's office is located in the Washington, DC, metropolitan area (in Rockville, Maryland). As a scientific and professional organization, ASHA plays a major role in promoting awareness of communicative disorders in the public and the government.

The American Speech-Language-Hearing Association (2017) has several goals, including the following:

- Encourage basic scientific study of human communication, with special emphasis on speech, language, and hearing

- Promote high standards for academic and clinical preparation of individuals who will serve people with communication disorders and promote the maintenance of current knowledge and skills of those within the discipline
- Promote the acquisition of new knowledge and skills in the members
- Promote investigation, prevention, and the diagnosis and treatment of communication and related disorders
- Foster improvement of clinical services and intervention procedures for communication and related disorders
- Stimulate exchange of information among persons and organizations and help disseminate such information
- Inform the public about communication sciences and disorders, related disorders, and the professionals who offer services
- Advocate on behalf of persons with communication disorders
- Promote the individual and collective professional interests of the members of the association

To fulfill its goals, ASHA (2017) does the following:

- Sponsors various scientific and professional conferences and conventions, institutes, and workshops each year as part of its continuing professional education program
- Maintains programs related to research, education, and delivery of clinical services
- Maintains a national career information program, a governmental affairs program, and a public information program
- Carries out a continuing program of data collection related to professional training, human resource needs, and membership characteristics and activities
- Sponsors a voluntary continuing education program that approves providers of continuing education activities and offers an Award for Continuing Education to certified individuals and members
- Publishes several professional journals and other professional materials that provide technical support to practitioner members on issues affecting the delivery of services
- Maintains a computerized database that provides information about federal and private funding sources in the United States and Canada
- Protects the public interest by maintaining high standards for members, certificate holders, accredited clinics, and accredited graduate educational programs

ASHA (2014) has several membership categories:

- **Certified Membership** is open to those who have a master's degree from an ASHA-accredited university program with a major emphasis in speech–language pathology or audiology and have completed all requirements for the Certificate of Clinical Competence (described under "Clinical Certification" later in the chapter). To continue in this category, a member must meet the mandatory continuing education requirements.
- **Membership without Certification** is open to U.S. residents who have a master's degree in speech–language pathology, audiology, or speech, language, and hearing sciences but are not involved in providing clinical services or clinical supervision.

- **Membership without Certification (research or allied professional)** is open to individuals who hold a graduate degree and are involved in human communication research but do not provide clinical services.
- **International Affiliation** is open to those who hold a graduate degree and reside abroad. These members are not eligible for clinical certification.
- **Certificate holders only** are those who maintain their clinical certification but do not become members of the association; they do not enjoy membership benefits.
- **Life Membership** is open to those who are 65 years or older and have been members of the association for 25 consecutive years.

Students who have declared their major as speech–language pathology or audiology may become members of the National Student Speech-Language-Hearing Association (NSSLHA), which is recognized by ASHA. Benefits of membership in NSSLHA include reduced fees for conventions and scientific journals. Many colleges and universities have active local chapters of NSSLHA that sponsor professional and social events.

ASHA has a number of **special interest groups** (SIGs) for members who wish to interact with other members who have similar interests. Each division sponsors special presentations at ASHA, and many hold their own national conferences. Any ASHA member may join one or more SIGs for an additional annual fee. As of 2017, there are 19 special interest groups:

Division 1. Language Learning and Education
Division 2. Neurogenic Communication Disorders
Division 3. Voice and Voice Disorders
Division 4. Fluency and Fluency Disorders
Division 5. Craniofacial and Velopharyngeal Disorders
Division 6. Hearing and Hearing Disorders: Research and Diagnostics
Division 7. Aural Rehabilitation and Its Instrumentation
Division 8. Audiology and Public Health
Division 9. Hearing and Hearing Disorders in Childhood
Division 10. Issues in Higher Education
Division 11. Administration and Supervision
Division 12. Augmentative and Alternative Communication
Division 13. Swallowing and Swallowing Disorders (Dysphagia)
Division 14. Cultural and Linguistic Diversity
Division 15. Gerontology
Division 16. School-Based Issues
Division 17. Global Issues in Communication Sciences and Related Disorders
Division 18. Telepractice
Division 19. Speech Science

Until the end of 2013, ASHA maintained a Clinical Specialty Recognition (CSR) program, in which ASHA members who met additional requirements in a particular area of practice could obtain specialist status. Beginning January 1, 2014, this program transitioned to a new Clinical Specialty Certification

(CSC) program. In 2014, ASHA offered specialty certifications in Child Language, Fluency Disorders, Swallowing and Swallowing Disorders, and Intraoperative Monitoring. ASHA may expand this program at any time and establish new specialty certifications; you can visit asha.org to find out the currently available specialty certification programs. Neither the old specialty recognition nor the new certification is necessary to assess and treat clients with a given disorder. Each certification requires ASHA members to fulfill additional requirements. See www.asha.org for details.

The Professions of Speech–Language Pathology and Audiology

Speech–language pathology is the scientific profession concerned with normal development and disorders of human communication (speech and language) and the assessment and treatment of those disorders.

- The term **speech–language pathologist** is preferred among members of the profession. However, some people use the terms **speech therapist** and **speech–language clinician**.
- Audiologists are specialists concerned with hearing, its disorders, and the assessment and rehabilitation of persons with hearing loss. Educational audiologists work in public schools, and industrial audiologists work in the industrial sector.
- Speech–language pathologists and audiologists work in a variety of professional settings, including hospitals, public and private schools, private practices, rehabilitation facilities, skilled nursing and long-term care facilities, home health agencies, colleges and universities, research institutes, private medical clinics, behavioral and mental health facilities, armed forces, correctional facilities, and corporate and industrial settings.
- Speech–language and hearing scientists generally work in research laboratories and university departments of speech–language pathology and audiology. Their primary task is to generate new knowledge through research and to teach students in undergraduate and graduate programs.

The Scope of Practice: Speech–Language Pathology

ASHA is the main regulatory body that develops policies on the scope of practice of the profession (ASHA, 2007). The scope-of-practice document specifies what clinicians can and cannot do; it is a guideline for ethical practice of the profession. When scientific evidence and expertise of the profession warrant it, the scope of practice may be expanded, as in the case of swallowing disorders and literacy skills. Students and clinicians should be fully aware of the most current version of this document, as it restricts practice to certain domains while opening possibilities for new services. In all cases, however, the scope-of-practice statement should be interpreted within the extent of existing state licensure laws; the laws supersede the statement. A few highlights of the document include the following:

- It is presumed that one can practice the profession with only required qualifications, certification, licensure, and credential, when necessary.
- Speech–language pathologists are independent professionals whose clinical services are not prescribed by other professionals.
- All clinical decisions should be made on the basis of best available evidence.
- The domain of practice includes human communication behaviors and disorders, as well as swallowing disorders and upper aerodigestive disorders.

- Speech–language pathology practice involves offering prevention, screening, consultation, assessment, diagnosis, treatment, management, counseling, and follow-up services for disorders of

  - speech sound production, including articulation, apraxia of speech, dysarthria, ataxia, and dyskinesia.
  - resonance and voice (of, e.g., phonation quality, pitch, loudness, and respiration).
  - fluency (stuttering and cluttering).
  - language (disorders of language, literacy problems, pre- and paralinguistic communication).
  - cognition (attention, memory, sequencing, etc.); feeding and swallowing and upper aerodigestive disorders (e.g., infant feeding); and orofacial myology.

- Speech–language pathology practice also involves

  - developing and implementing augmentative and alternative forms of communication (AAC) and prescribing AAC devices and systems.
  - screening hearing and offering auditory training and speech–language services to the deaf and the hard of hearing.
  - using such instruments as videofluoroscopy, EMG, nasendoscopy, stroboscopy, and computerized instruments to observe, collect, and analyze data relative to communication and swallowing functions.
  - selecting, fitting, and training in the use of prosthetic devices for communication and swallowing; this excludes the prescription of hearing aids.
  - collaborating in the assessment and treatment of central auditory disorders associated with communication disorders.
  - educating and counseling individuals, families, co-workers, educators, and other professionals about communication disorders and swallowing.
  - promoting community awareness about communication disorders and their assessment and treatment and about removing barriers to individuals with such disorders.
  - working with other professionals and making referrals when they are in the best interests of individuals being served.
  - serving ethnoculturally diverse populations with communication and swallowing disorders with procedures that are suited or modified for their cultural background (ASHA, 2007).

The settings in which speech–language pathology may be practiced consist of a variety of educational and health care facilities, as previously noted. Therefore, clinicians should follow not only ASHA's practice guidelines but also its guidelines for the professional work setting.

ASHA Accreditation

ASHA has established standards of scientific and professional education in speech–language pathology and audiology. The standards include the kinds and variety of academic courses that must be offered and the amount and quality of supervised clinical practice that student clinicians must complete.

- Through its Council on Academic Accreditation in Audiology and Speech–Language Pathology (CAA), ASHA accredits master's degree programs in speech–language pathology and audiology that

meet its minimum standards. A national team visits graduate degree programs in audiology and speech–language pathology and evaluates their quality.
- Through its Council for Clinical Certification, ASHA evaluates and approves clinical certification standards (described in the next section of this chapter).

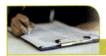

SUMMARY

ASHA, the national professional and scientific organization of communicative disorders professionals, has an interesting history, which includes phenomenal growth and change.

- With an ever-expanding membership base, ASHA continually works to promote high ethical standards, pertinent legislation, and regulation of the professions of speech–language pathology and audiology. ASHA accredits graduate academic programs that meet its standards and certifies individuals who complete its clinical requirements.
- ASHA offers various kinds of memberships with and without clinical certification.
- Students may join the ASHA-affiliated NSSLHA, the national student organization, which provides many benefits.
- Members of ASHA include speech–language pathologists and audiologists who work in a variety of professional settings to provide comprehensive services to individuals with disorders of language, speech, and hearing.

ISSUES IN CERTIFICATION AND LICENSURE

ASHA-administered certification helps ensure the quality of services provided to individuals with communication disorders. Each state also has licensing and educational credentialing requirements for clinicians. The necessity of holding a state license, state credential, ASHA certificate, or all three, depends upon (a) the individual state, and (b) the professional setting in which the clinician works. In this section, we discuss ASHA certification, state regulation of the professions, and issues regarding support personnel.

Clinical Certification

To ensure the quality of speech–language and hearing services offered to the public, ASHA has developed two clinical certificates that are issued to members who meet the respective academic and clinical standards of the association. The standards are developed by the members of ASHA's Council for Clinical Certification in Audiology and Speech–Language Pathology (CFCC).

ASHA certifies speech–language pathologists and audiologists separately, although the requirements are parallel. The **Certificate of Clinical Competence in Speech–Language Pathology** (CCC-SLP) is issued to those individuals who have achieved the following:

- Earned their master's degree or its equivalent in speech–language pathology at an ASHA-accredited institution and fulfilled clinical practicum and fellowship requirements. A minimum of 75 semester hours of coursework must be completed in speech–language pathology and related disciplines; a minimum of 36 of the 75 hours must be at the graduate level.

- Demonstrated the acquisition of knowledge and clinical skill adequate for entry into professional practice. Required knowledge pertains to basic scientific understanding of communication and its disorders, feeding and swallowing disorders, research methods and evaluation of research evidence, the code of ethics, and professional issues and credentials. The students should acquire clinical skills, as well as oral and written presentation skills.
- Completed their clinical practicum with a minimum of 400 hours of supervised clinical work, out of which 25 hours are set aside for preclinical observation of clinical work; 375 hours must be spent in direct client or patient contact; 325 of the 400 clock hours must be completed during graduate study. All hours must be supervised by an individual holding the CCC. Supervised practicum should include clients or patients with diverse linguistic and ethnocultural backgrounds.
- Obtained a passing score on the National Examination in Speech–Language Pathology and Audiology (Praxis). See the Appendix for information on the Praxis.
- Completed a supervised clinical fellowship (CF) within 4 years of the date the academic coursework and clinical practicum were completed. The fellowship may be completed in a full-time job of 35 hours per week for 36 weeks, totaling a minimum of 1,260 hours, with 80% of the time involving direct client or patient contact. Part-time work is acceptable, but the clinical fellow must work for a minimum of 5 hours per week. The CF must be monitored by an individual holding the CCC.

The **Certificate of Clinical Competence in Audiology** (CCC-A) has similar requirements, with the academic coursework, clinical practicum, and clinical fellowship completed in audiology with appropriate supervision for the clinical practicum and mentoring or monitoring of the fellowship by an ASHA-certified audiologist.

- The clinical certificates are renewable every 3 years. To maintain clinical certification, all certificate holders must accumulate 30 contact hours of professional development (continuing education units) over the 3-year period.
- ASHA's certificates are not legal documents comparable to a state license. However, they are recognized by most employers, including hospitals, clinics, public school districts, and universities throughout the country. Many employers consider the certificates favorably in promotion and salary increases. Many state licensure laws are modeled after the ASHA requirements.
- Individuals who hold ASHA membership and clinical certification are committed to uphold the highest standards of clinical services. Treating people with communicative disorders is an ethical and socially responsible activity. Speech–language pathologists and audiologists who hold a certificate from ASHA are committed to its Code of Ethics.

ASHA's Code of Ethics contains extensive guidelines on practicing the profession in an ethical and responsible manner (ASHA, 2016; Purtilo, 2005). All student clinicians, too, are held to the ethical code. The code specifies what a clinician can and cannot do. The Code of Ethics was recently revised in 2016.

ASHA's Board of Ethics interprets, administers, and enforces its code, which contains four **principles of ethics** and several **rules of ethics**. The main points of each principle and the rules under it follow:

- *Principle of Ethics I*: states that clinicians shall hold the welfare of persons they serve paramount by making sure that they (a) are well prepared to serve their clients; (b) make appropriate referrals when necessary; (c) do not discriminate on such bases as race, gender, ethnicity, national origin, disability, or sexual orientation; (d) do not misrepresent the credentials of speech–language pathology assistants (SLPAs), students, research assistants, or clinical fellows and inform those working with them of their credentials; (e) SLPAs or other support services may perform tasks related to clinical services only if they are properly qualified and supervised by an SLP with their CCC; (f) SLPs with their CCC may not delegate work to SLPAs or other support personnel that requires skills beyond the assistant's scope of practice; (g) students may only perform tasks that require unique clinical skills and knowledge only is they are properly trained and supervised by an SLP with their CCC, who hold the responsibility and welfare of those being served; (h) obtain informed consent on all aspects of service delivery and research and seek appropriate consent from caregivers or legal guardians from those who are unable to represent themselves/make appropriate judgments; (i) research participation must be voluntary and not coerced; (j) do not misrepresent the purpose of a service or research study; (k) SLPS with their CCC should evaluate the effectiveness of their services and the technology they are using, and they should only provide services that they expect to benefit an individual; (l) do not guarantee the effects of treatment but make only reasonable statements of prognosis; (m) offer treatments that are evidence-based; (n) do not offer services solely by correspondence, although they may engage in telehealth or e-health; (o) and (p) maintain the confidentiality of their clients and research participants; (q) enter accurate records for billing and do not bill for services that were not provided; (r) seek professional help and, if appropriate, withdraw from practice if clinical skills are negatively affected by substance abuse, addiction, or other health-related conditions; (s) if it is known that a colleague is unable to provide clinical services with appropriate skill and safety, individuals should report their colleague to an appropriate authority; and (t) provide information for alternative care if unable to provide professional services.
- *Principle of Ethics II*: states that clinicians shall maintain the highest level of professional competence by (a) offering services that are within the scope of practice and their own education, training, and experience; (b) those who are in the process of obtaining their CCC should provide services consistent with state laws and ASHA's certification requirements; (c) comply with regulations set by the institution, state, and federal government when performing research involving human and animal participants; (d) obtaining continuing education (lifelong learning); (e) not requiring or allowing persons working under their supervision to perform activities for which they are not qualified in research and (f) in clinical activities; (g) meeting appropriate guidelines when using technology and instrumentation and making appropriate referrals when necessary technology is not available; and (h) maintaining all research, clinical assessment, and treatment instruments in proper working order.
- *Principles of Ethics III*: states that clinicians shall honor their responsibility to the public by (a) not misrepresenting their qualifications; (b) avoiding conflicts of interest; (c) avoiding any

misrepresentation of clinical services or their effects; (d) avoiding schemes to defraud in connection with obtaining payment, reimbursement, grants, research, or products dispensed; (e) providing accurate information to the public about the profession's services and products; (f) adhering to professional standards in advertising and promotion; and (g) avoiding knowingly releasing false financial or nonfinancial statements.

- *Principles of Ethics IV*: states that clinicians shall honor their responsibilities to their profession, colleagues, students, and members of related professionals by (a) collaborating with other professional colleagues to enhance the quality of care; (b) using professional judgment (not extraneous considerations) in offering services; (c) making professional statements to colleagues about research and clinical services; (d) upholding the standards of the profession; (e) not committing fraud, deceit, or negligence; (f) maintaining honesty; (g) not engaging in harassment of any form; (h) not engaging in sexual activities with persons with which a professional or authoritative relationship exists; (i) taking adequate supervisory responsibilities, (j) crediting only those who have contributed to a project; (k) giving clinical or authorship credits to others when they are due; (l) being nondiscriminatory; (m) working to resolve violations to the Code of Ethics, or informing the Board of Ethics if necessary; (n) reporting fellow professionals who violate the Code of Ethics; (o) reporting to the Board of Ethics only on the basis of professionalism, not as a means of personal gain or retaliation; (p) complying by all necessary policies when reporting to the Board of Ethics; (q) reporting only truthful information to the Board; (r) abiding by local, state, and federal government regulations when conducting research; (s) notifying ASHA within 30 days if convicted or found guilty of a misdemeanor or felony; and (t) informing ASHA within 30 days if revoked of a license or professional credential.

Violation of the code has serious consequences, including revocation of the clinical certificate and cancellation of membership in ASHA. Professional practice periodically may pose ethical dilemmas to all clinicians. It is essential for the clinician to understand not just the ethical rules but also their broader implications and deeper meanings. Clinicians should seriously study the code and consult additional sources to fully understand and uphold it (ASHA, 2016; Irwin, Pannbacker, Powell, & Vekovius, 2007; Lubinski, Golper, & Frattali, 2007).

Speech–Language Pathology Assistants

The American Speech-Language-Hearing Association (ASHA, 2013) supports the use of speech–language pathology assistants (SLPAs) who have received training according to its guidelines, but it does not require their use. SLPs should not be expected to use any kind of support personnel (assistants, aides, associates) if they, the SLPs, judge that the support personnel are not well qualified. ASHA may impose sanctions on SLPs who use unqualified support personnel, because such use violates the Code of Ethics and the scope-of-practice guidelines. The Code of Ethics applies not to the SLPAs (though they are expected to be knowledgeable in it) but to the supervising SLP.

- The goal of support personnel is not to reduce the caseload of SLPs but to assist them in managing their caseloads. SLPs should inform consumers when services are to be provided by support personnel.
- ASHA's current position is not to require SLPAs to register with ASHA and not to review their academic and clinical program to give approval. ASHA recommends that assistants complete an

approved training program that includes coursework and fieldwork; on-the-job training may be acceptable. SLPAs should be supervised by ASHA-certified clinicians. ASHA has established an Associate's Affiliation Program for qualified support personnel, working under the supervision of a certified audiologist or SLP, who are in compliance with any state requirement, who may then join the organization as associates (ASHA, 2013).

Minimum qualifications required for SLPAs include the following:

- An associate's degree in an SLPA program, *or*
- A bachelor's degree in SLP, *and*
- A minimum of 100 hours of supervised clinical experience or fieldwork, *and*
- Demonstration of competence in the skills required of an SLPA.

ASHA specifies that SLPAs may perform the following:

- Assist with screenings and assessments without administering tests or interpreting the results; serve as interpreters; perform clerical duties (scheduling and record keeping); assist in conducting research, in-service training, and public relations programs; implement treatment plans developed and supervised by speech–language pathologists
- Document client performance (prepare charts, records, and graphs)
- Check and maintain equipment
- Collect and document data for quality improvement

SLPAs should not do any of the following:

- Represent self as an SLP
- Administer standardized or nonstandardized tests or interpret the results
- Screen or diagnose patients for feeding or swallowing disorders
- Participate in parent or case conferences or counsel parents or clients unless supervised by a speech–language pathologist
- Write or modify treatment plans; offer treatment that is not developed by a speech–language pathologist; offer any treatment without supervision; or sign treatment plans or assessment reports
- Select, refer, or discharge clients
- Disclose confidential information
- Demonstrate swallowing strategies or precautions
- Design or select augmentative and alternative communication systems

The 2016 ASHA document cited at the beginning of this section specifies the roles and responsibilities of the SLP in supervising SLPAs. Clinicians who plan to have SLPAs work under their supervision should be thoroughly familiar with this document.

State Regulation of the Profession

State governments have laws and regulations that affect the work of speech–language pathologists and audiologists.

- State departments of education give credentials to their speech–language pathologists and audiologists working in the public schools. Generally, the requirements are similar to those of ASHA, except some states require coursework in education.
- A few states also combine a teaching credential with a credential in speech–language pathology, resulting in more coursework in education, because the professional in this case is both a teacher and a speech–language pathologist. State credentials may or may not transfer to another state's public schools. State public school credentials are specific to the public school setting only. They do not allow private practice, work in a hospital or clinic, or supervision of clinical practice in university speech and hearing centers.
- Most state governments issue licenses to practice speech–language pathology or audiology. Most state licensure requirements are similar to those of ASHA. Professional settings other than public schools (e.g., hospitals and private clinics) usually require either the ASHA Certificate of Clinical Competence, state licensure if it exists, or both. However, in many states, public school districts are also beginning to require, or at least strongly encourage, speech–language pathologists to possess, in addition to the required education credential, state licensure and ASHA certification.
- In 2011, the state of California (through its Department of Education) began offering a type of special education credential called the Language and Academic Development Credential (LAD). Holders of this credential would be authorized to offer instruction in academic communication and language, but they could not offer speech, language, or hearing services that fall within the scope of practice of SLPs and audiologists. The training was to be offered in departments of education in colleges and universities, although as of 2014, there were no such programs (Moore, 2012).
- By meeting the ASHA requirements, graduates in most states also meet the requirements for a credential to work in schools and a license to practice speech–language pathology or audiology in non-school settings.
- An important difference between a license and an ASHA certificate is that only the license carries the force of law. State licensure is administered by a board or committee created by the state legislature.

SUMMARY

ASHA regulates the quality of services offered to the public through its clinical certifications.

- States regulate the quality of services offered in different professional settings through their education credentials and state licensure.
- ASHA has specific guidelines on what speech–language pathology assistants can and cannot do; they always should work under the supervision of a certified clinician.

LEGISLATIVE REGULATION OF THE PROFESSION

Both state and federal laws affect the services offered in various professional settings. In this section, we summarize some of the key national laws that have affected service delivery in the public schools, employment, and health care settings.

Federal Legislation Affecting School Settings

Public Law 94-142

Enacted in 1975, the Education of the Handicapped Act (later retitled the Individuals With Disabilities Education Act) mandated free and appropriate education for disabled students from ages 3 to 21. Basic tenets of this law included the following:

- Disabled children and youth from ages 3 to 21 years were guaranteed free and appropriate public education in the "least restrictive environment," including special education and related services. (In some states, due to conflicts with state laws and court orders, children under age 5 and over age 18 were excluded.)
- All students receiving special education services were to have Individualized Education Programs (IEPs), determined by parents and professionals, that served as written records of commitments to meet students' goals.
- Students and parents were guaranteed protection of their rights through due legal process, including the right to an impartial due process hearing and the right to examine all relevant records.
- The federal government was to provide funds for local and state agencies to carry out prescribed programs and to monitor and evaluate those programs.

Public Law 99-457

Public Law 99-457, enacted in 1986, contained amendments to P.L. 94-142 that were intended to provide early intervention that would reduce the number of children requiring special education services in later years.

- P.L. 99-457 increased federal monetary support for states to provide services for disabled children between the ages of 3 and 6 years. It also created a new program that provided funds for services to infants and toddlers (up to 2 years) with disabilities.
- An important tenet of P.L. 99-457 is that all school service providers must meet their state's highest requirements for their discipline (in many states, that meant a master's degree, which fulfilled the academic criteria for state licensing).

P.L. 99-457 established mandated development of Individualized Family Service Plans (IFSPs), requiring, among other things, the following:

- The child's current level of development
- The family's needs and strengths relating to the child's development
- The major goals for the child and family, and services to be provided
- A review of the plan at 6-month intervals or more frequently if needed

A major provision of P.L. 99-457 is multidisciplinary programming for infants and toddlers with disabilities and their families. This includes involvement of agencies outside the education setting (e.g., community programs).

- Under P.L. 99-457, states were no longer required to report preschool children by disability category (e.g., hearing loss, mental retardation, learning disability). At-risk preschool children, including children who had experienced traumatic life events, depression, child abuse, and substance abuse, also became eligible for special education services.

Individuals With Disabilities Education Act

The Individuals With Disabilities Education Act (IDEA; P.L. 101-476), enacted in 1990, reauthorized P.L. 94-142 and P.L. 99-457 and altered the language used in referring to its beneficiaries. Specifically, the term *disability* replaced the word *handicap*.

- The IDEA also expanded the number of categories of disabilities. Originally, P.L. 94-142 included 11 disability categories; the IDEA created 13 categories, newly including autism and traumatic brain injury.
- The definition of **special education** was expanded to include instruction in all settings (not just the school), including training centers and workplaces.

The Amendments of 1997, Public Law 105-17, constitute the reauthorization of the IDEA. This reauthorization was signed into law by President Bill Clinton on October 22, 1997, and included the following (California Speech-Language-Hearing Association, 1997; Miller & Hoffman, 2002):

- Increased, meaningful parental involvement in evaluations, including parental access to reports, test instruments, and other interpretative materials that contain personally identifiable information
- Improved educational results for children with disabilities
- Increased participation of special educators in the general classroom setting, including involvement with curriculum
- Increased participation of children with learning problems in regular classroom activities
- Prevention of inappropriate identification and mislabeling of children who are ethnically, linguistically, or racially diverse
- Improved use of alternative assessments for children who cannot participate in standard assessments

On December 3, 2004, President George W. Bush signed into law the new IDEA reforms, officially known as Public Law 108-446, or the Individuals With Disabilities Education Improvement Act of 2004 (U.S. Department of Education, 2004a). The signing marked the end of a 3-year reauthorization process and represented the first update to the country's special education law in 7 years. The effective date for most changes to the law was July 1, 2005.

- Foundational to this new law are the findings of the 2002 President's Commission on Excellence in Special Education, which recommended special education reforms based on paperwork reduction, parental choice, early intervention, and academic results for students.
- The new IDEA puts a greater emphasis on using pre-referral services to prevent unnecessary referrals to special education. Under the new IDEA, states are required to provide coordinated,

comprehensive, and early-intervention programs for children in groups that are overrepresented in special education. Part C of IDEA provides early intervention services to eligible children from birth to two years old and their families through an Individualized Family Service Plan (IFSP). An IFSP is a document that details the intervention plan so the family and early intervention providers can work together as a team to meet the needs of the child (Center for Parent Information & Resources, 2016).

- The U.S. Department of Education periodically issues new regulations under the scope of the law. Clinicians are encouraged to visit the department's website (idea.ed.gov).

Every Student Succeeds Act (ESSA)

Every Student Succeeds Act (ESSA) was signed by President Barack Obama in 2015. It governs the U.S. K–12 public education policy. This law replaces the No Child Left Behind Act (NCLB). Under ESSA, students still take yearly tests between 3rd and 8th grade and once again during the junior year of high school; however, individual states, rather than the federal government determine standards, choose short- and long-term goals for proficiency on exams, English language proficiency, and rates for high school graduation. One of the goals of ESSA is to prepare all students, regardless of ethnicity, English proficiency, income, race, or disability, for success in college. Under ESSA, schools are required to offer college and career counseling as well as advanced placement courses to all students.

- During an English-language learner's (ELL) second year in a U.S. school, his or her score counts toward the school's proficiency rating; however, it can take between 5 and 10 years for an ELL to achieve cognitive–academic language proficiency (CALP) that is equivalent to native English-speaking students. SLPs, therefore, must be able to advocate for their culturally and linguistically diverse students and educate teachers and administrators about typical CALP development, so that CLD students are not unnecessarily referred for special education intervention.

Federal Legislation Affecting Employment Settings

The Americans With Disabilities Act (ADA; P.L. 101-336), enacted in 1990, provides civil rights protection relative to employment, state and local government services, telecommunications, and public accommodations to all individuals with disabilities.

- The ADA bars employment discrimination against qualified people with mental or physical disabilities or disabilities that substantially limit one or more of the basic activities of life, such as talking or walking.
- The ADA requires that employers make "reasonable accommodations" for workers with disabilities. This includes making existing facilities such as public buildings and mass transportation accessible and arranging modified or part-time work schedules.
- Employers must also provide special equipment for workers with disabilities. Examples include relay stations for users of telecommunication devices for the deaf (TDDs), ramps for people in wheelchairs, and auditory signals to visual signs to assist people who are blind (e.g., an auditory signal that alerts them to an open elevator door).
- According to the ADA, employers do not have to provide accommodations that impose an "undue hardship" on business operations. The meaning of the term "undue hardship" has been the subject of much discussion and some lawsuits.

Federal Legislation Affecting Health Care Settings

Health care legislation is under constant revision in the United States. One reason is that millions of Americans do not receive adequate health care. Statistics show that groups that are especially affected are children, low-income people, and people from culturally and linguistically diverse backgrounds.

- A major effort to overhaul the American health care system is the Affordable Health Care Act, signed into law by President Barack Obama on March 23, 2010. This law is designed to cover many Americans with no health insurance. It established the Health Insurance Marketplace, where individuals and families can choose and enroll in health insurance plans. Among its many significant provisions, the law prohibits insurance companies from denying health insurance based on preexisting conditions and requires insurance companies to cover preventive services.
- This extensive and complex law is still undergoing executive modifications. State participation in providing services under the law is variable; some states have opted out. Although the law does affect the services of SLPs, it is not the purpose of this chapter to give details on this law.
- Each year, the federal government announces new changes. These changes and updates are routinely announced by the U.S. Department of Health and Human Services (HHS).
- Clinicians may obtain specific and up-to-date information from www.hhs.gov/healthcare. Another source that clinicians may check as often as necessary is the website of the American Speech-Language-Hearing Association (www.asha.org). On either website, clinicians can conduct a search with the key words "affordable health care act." *The ASHA Leader,* a professional issue-oriented magazine that all ASHA members receive as a membership benefit, is another source for reliable and up-to-date information on health care acts and policies that affect the services of SLPs. As each professional setting (hospitals, public schools, private clinics) will have specific policies that affect speech–language pathology service delivery and reimbursement, it is the responsibility of SLPs to understand and comply with the rules and policies of their workplace.

Social Security Act (SSA)

Passed in 1935, during the Great Depression, the SSA expanded the federal government's grant-in-aid assistance to the states. It was the federal government's first major step toward involvement in a widespread program of living and medical assistance to the population at large.

- The SSA provided the foundation for Medicaid and Medicare. It also provided for the general welfare of the public by establishing federal benefits for older people. Further, it helped states provide more services for public health, maternal and child welfare, people who are blind, and children who are dependent or have a disability.
- The SSA undergoes periodic amendments. The amendments of 1983 had a significant effect on speech–language pathology and audiology services. They offered incentive reimbursements for hospitals to provide more "efficient" and "cost-effective" treatment for patients.
- Unfortunately, although inpatient rehabilitation units and rehabilitation hospitals were exempt from some of the flat-payment regulations imposed on other services, cost limits were placed on services provided. These limits have resulted in fewer speech–language pathology and audiology services being offered to patients.

Health Insurance Portability and Accountability Act (HIPAA)

In 1996, Congress called on the U.S. Department of Health and Human Services to issue patient privacy protections as part of the Health Insurance Portability and Accountability Act (HIPAA). Health care providers were mandated to comply with these protections starting April 14, 2003. HIPAA involves a set of rules followed by doctors, health plans, hospitals, and health care providers. It is the first-ever set of federal privacy standards to protect patients' medical records and other health information provided to health plans, hospitals, doctors, and other health care providers (covered entities).

- These new standards represent a uniform set of federal privacy protections for American consumers by limiting the ways that pharmacies, health plans, hospitals, and other covered entities can use and share patients' personal medical information. HIPAA's regulations protect medical records and other individually identifiable health information in any form—information communicated on paper, electronically, or orally. A description of the key provisions of HIPAA's privacy standards follows (U.S. Department of Health and Human Services, 2004):

  - Patients generally should have access to their medical records. If there are mistakes, patients should be able to request corrections. Doctors, hospitals, clinics, nursing homes, health plans, and other covered entities generally must provide access to these records within 30 days; they may charge patients for the cost of copying and sending the records.
  - Health care providers and all covered entities must provide a notice to their patients about how providers may use personal medical information as well as patients' rights under the new privacy regulation. This generally should happen on the patient's first visit. Patients are asked to initial, sign, or otherwise acknowledge that they have received this notice.
  - Limits are set on how covered entities may use personally identifiable health information. Covered entities may share information with each other related to patients' treatment. For example, a doctor may talk with a clinician about swallowing treatment for a patient with dysphagia. However, these entities may not share personal health information for purposes unrelated to health care unless the patient specifically signs an authorization. For example, without signed authorization from the patient, a hospital could not release the patient's medical information to a marketing firm, bank, or life insurance agency for purposes not related to the patient's health care.
  - Patients may request that covered entities take reasonable steps to make sure that their communications with patients are confidential. For example, a man with mild aphasia who has been discharged from treatment can ask the doctor or speech–language pathologist to call him at home, not at work. The patient's request should be reasonably accommodated. Consumers may file a formal complaint regarding the privacy practices of a covered provider such as a doctor, speech–language pathologist, hospital, or clinic. Such complaints may be made directly to the covered provider or to the Department of Health and Human Services' Office for Civil Rights (OCR). The OCR is charged with investigating complaints and enforcing the privacy regulation.
  - If covered entities misuse personal health information, civil and criminal penalties may be imposed. For civil violations of the standards, the OCR can fine a covered entity up to $25,000 a year. If a covered entity knowingly obtains protected health information in violation of the law, criminal penalties can range between $50,000 and $250,000, accompanied by 1–10 years in prison,

depending upon the nature and extent of the violation. Speech–language pathologists and audiologists must be sure to follow HIPAA regulations in all their dealings with clients and their families.

Future Trends

Health care policy and special education policies that affect speech–language pathology and audiology services are constantly evolving. There is an increased emphasis on showing that services offered to children and adults with communication disorders make a difference in the lives of the individuals who receive them.

- This means that there will be an increased emphasis on documentation of treatment outcomes and evidence-based practice. ASHA's *National Outcome Measurement System* (NOMS; https://www.asha.org/noms/national-outcomes-measurement-system/) will play an increasingly important role in selecting and evaluating treatment procedures.
- Limited financial resources will call for collaborative efforts, resulting in cost savings and improved outcomes for the clients. In the public schools, emphasis on literacy skills of children will make additional demands on speech–language pathologists. Children with varied ethnocultural backgrounds provide both challenges and exciting opportunities to serve them.
- An aging population in the United States will escalate demands for services that specialize in geriatric communication disorders. Doing all this in a cost-effective manner will be a pervasive theme.
- ASHA has an increased emphasis on telepractice. Telepractice refers to the application of telecommunications technology to delivering speech–language pathology and audiology services from a geographical distance. For example, a speech–language pathologist might provide remote treatment to a client who lives 100 miles away and cannot come to see the clinician in person. This is done by linking the clinician to the client or patient for consultation, assessment, or intervention (ASHA, 2014).
- Those clinicians who use telepractice must still adhere to the ASHA Code of Ethics, ASHA scope of practice (in speech–language pathology and audiology), ASHA policy, and state and federal laws (e.g., HIPAA, licensure). Services must comply with national, state, institutional, and professional regulations and policies.

Telepractice venues include the following (ASHA, 2014):

- Community health centers
- Schools
- Medical centers and hospitals
- Rehabilitation hospitals
- Patients' homes
- Universities
- Child care centers
- Corporate settings
- Residential health care facilities
- Outpatient clinics

SUMMARY

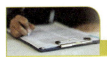

State and federal legislation has a major effect on speech–language pathology and audiology services provided in public school, employment, and health care settings. Such legislation can expand or limit the services provided to clients with communicative disorders.

- The Health Insurance Portability and Accountability Act (HIPAA) is a new set of federal privacy regulations that protect patients' personal medical information and help ensure confidentiality.
- Future trends affecting health care settings include increased accountability for documenting functional gains and providing measurable outcomes of services provided. Telepractice is becoming increasingly common.

CHAPTER HIGHLIGHTS

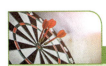

- The American Speech-Language-Hearing Association (ASHA) is a national professional and scientific organization that regulates the quality of service offered, promotes relevant legislation, encourages research, and facilitates exchange of information. Most speech–language pathologists and audiologists are members of ASHA.
- ASHA awards national certification when its members meet certain requirements. Many states also have credentialing and licensing requirements that clinicians must meet, depending upon the professional setting in which they work.
- ASHA supports the use of speech–language pathology assistants (SLPAs) who have received training according to its guidelines. ASHA recommends that these assistants complete an approved training program that includes coursework and fieldwork; on-the-job training may be acceptable.
- State and federal laws regulate service provision in public schools, employment settings, and health care settings. All communicative disorders professionals and clients are affected by those laws, which are primarily influenced by the availability of funding. A recently enacted law affecting speech–language pathologists and audiologists is HIPAA, the Health Insurance Portability and Accountability Act of 1996, which took effect April 14, 2003.
- Because of legislation and resulting budget cuts, speech–language pathology and audiology services are often curtailed in many settings. Clinicians increasingly need to make the public aware of their specialty and the services they offer. This can be done through marketing research and advertising. ASHA provides educational opportunities to teach its members about those areas. The new area of telepractice expands clinicians' opportunities to provide services to those who need them.

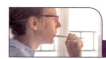

STUDY AND REVIEW QUESTIONS

1. The Health Insurance Portability and Accountability Act (HIPAA) includes, among other mandates,

   A. a requirement that each state develop standards for protecting the privacy of medical patients, to be reviewed and approved by the federal government.
   B. a uniform federal standard for protecting the privacy of patients, to be followed by all medical, nonmedical, and allied health personnel in the country.
   C. a stipulation that different health care entities involved in providing services to a patient cannot share information about that patient.
   D. a requirement that when a request is received, health care providers have 90 days to provide access to the patient's medical (and related) records.

2. Public Law 99-457

   A. increased federal support for services to disabled children 3–6 years of age and provided funding for infants and toddlers.
   B. was enacted in 1986.
   C. restricts special education services to children with documented disabilities.
   D. requires states to report the number of preschoolers served under different categories of disabilities.

3. In most states, to work in the public schools, speech–language pathologists and audiologists are required to possess

   A. a state license.
   B. ASHA certification.
   C. a state-issued credential from an agency such as the Department of Education.
   D. state license and ASHA certification.

4. Which one of the following is *not true*?

   A. Many state licensure laws are modeled after ASHA's requirements.
   B. Violation of ASHA's Code of Ethics can have major consequences, including revocation of ASHA's clinical certificate and cancelation of ASHA membership.
   C. A Certificate of Clinical Competence and state license are not necessarily required to practice in public school settings.
   D. To receive a Certificate of Clinical Competence in speech–language pathology or audiology, a speech–language pathologist or audiologist needs only to have a state-granted credential to work in public schools.

5. P.L. 94-142, the Education of the Handicapped Act, was later reauthorized and retitled as

   A. the Americans With Disabilities Act.
   B. the Education of Disabled Individuals Act.

C. the Handicapped Individuals Education Act.

D. the Individuals With Disabilities Education Act.

6. Activities that may be carried out by a trained SLPA (according to ASHA) include

  A. implementing treatment plans developed by the supervising SLP, checking and maintaining equipment, and collecting and documenting data for quality improvement.
  B. demonstrating swallowing strategies or precautions, collecting and documenting data for quality improvement, and assisting with speech–language and hearing screenings.
  C. writing and modifying treatment plans, assisting with clerical duties and in-service training, and checking and maintaining equipment.
  D. signing treatment plans or assessment reports when the SLP is not available, assisting with speech–language and hearing screenings, and assisting with clerical duties.

7. Parents in a local school district have asked a clinician to give an in-service on the IDEA (1997). The parents are interested in the content of the IDEA regarding their parental rights, and so forth. Which one of the following *would not* be accurate for the clinician to tell the parents at the in-service?

  A. The IDEA discourages serving children with disabilities in general education classroom settings; rather, it encourages school districts to create more specialized pull-out programs for such children to best serve their needs.
  B. The IDEA promotes increased, meaningful parental involvement in evaluations, including access to reports and test instruments.
  C. The IDEA mandates the development of alternative assessments for children who cannot participate in standard assessments.
  D. One goal of the IDEA is to promote increased participation of special educators in general classroom settings, including involvement with curriculum.

8. Which statement is true about ASHA's special interest groups (SIGs)?

  A. Membership in SIGs is free to all ASHA members.
  B. Clinical Specialty Recognition is available only in a few specialty areas.
  C. A Clinical Specialty Recognition is essential to assess and treat clients with a specified disorder.
  D. Each SIG is concerned with a specific disorder of communication.

9. According to ASHA standards, which one of the following activities *would not* be within the scope of practice of a speech–language pathologist?

  A. Assessing and treating swallowing and upper aerodigestive disorders (e.g., infant feeding).
  B. Developing and implementing augmentative and alternative forms of communication (AAC) and prescribing AAC devices and systems.
  C. Prescribing hearing aids for children and adults with hearing losses.
  D. Screening hearing and offering auditory training and speech–language services to the deaf and the hard of hearing.

10. P.L. 99-457 established mandated development of Individualized Family Service Plans (IFSPs). Which one of the following is *not* required to be included in a child's IFSP?

    A. The child's present level of development.
    B. The family's needs and strengths relating to the child's development.
    C. The major goals for the child and family, and services to be provided.
    D. A review of the plan at 12-month intervals or more frequently if needed.

11. The law stating that employers must provide special equipment for workers with disabilities (e.g., relay stations for users of TDDs) is

    A. the Americans With Disabilities Act.
    B. HIPAA.
    C. P.L. 94-142.
    D. No Child Left Behind.

12. ESSA stands for

    A. Elementary Student Success Act.
    B. Every Student Succeeds Act.
    C. English Speaking Student Act.
    D. English Studies Success Act.

13. Which of the following is *not* true regarding ESSA?

    A. Under ESSA, the federal government creates short- and long-term goals for academic proficiency.
    B. Under ESSA, the individual states create short- and long-term goals for academic proficiency.
    C. ESSA was signed by President Barack Obama.
    D. During an English-language learner's (ELL) second year in a U.S. school, his or her score counts towards the school's proficiency rating.

14. Passed in 1935, the federal government's first major step toward involvement in a widespread program of living and medical assistance to the population at large is known as the

    A. Americans With Disabilities Act (ADA)
    B. Health Insurance Portability and Accountability Act (HIPPA)
    C. Social Security Act (SSA)
    D. Individuals With Disabilities Education Act (IDEA)

15. A minimum of how many hours of supervised clinical experience is needed for an individual to be an SLPA?

    A. 150
    B. 250
    C. 100
    D. 200

References and Recommended Readings at www.advancedreviewpractice.com

STUDY AND REVIEW ANSWERS

1. B. The HIPAA mandates a uniform federal standard for protecting the privacy of patients, to be followed by all medical, nonmedical, and allied health personnel in the country.
2. A. P.L. 99-457 increased federal support for services to disabled children three to six years of age and provided funding for infants and toddlers.
3. C. In most states, public school systems require only a state-issued credential. Licensure and certification are required by many other settings, such as hospitals and clinics.
4. D. To receive a Certificate of Clinical Competence in speech–language pathology or audiology, a speech–language pathologist or audiologist needs only to have a state-granted credential to work in public schools.
5. D. In 1990, the Individuals With Disabilities Education Act (IDEA) reauthorized and retitled P.L. 94-142 and made some changes in it.
6. A. According to ASHA, SLPAs may be involved in implementing treatment plans developed by the supervising SLP, checking and maintaining equipment, and collecting and documenting data for quality improvement.
7. A. It is not true that the IDEA discourages serving children with disabilities in general education settings and encourages school districts to create more specialized pull-out programs for such children to best serve their needs. It is the reverse; the IDEA encourages districts to serve children with disabilities in general classroom settings.
8. B. Clinical Specialty Recognition is available only in a few specialty areas. It is not required to practice the profession. ASHA's SIGs hold their own conferences, membership has a fee, and not all of them are related to specific disorders.
9. C. According to ASHA standards, prescribing hearing aids for children and adults with hearing losses *would not* be within the scope of practice of a speech–language pathologist.
10. D. P.L. 99-457 requires a review of the plan at 6-month intervals or more frequently if needed, not at yearly intervals.
11. A. The law stating that employers must provide special equipment for workers with disabilities (e.g., relay stations for users of TDDs) is the Americans With Disabilities Act.
12. B. ESSA stands for Every Student Succeeds Act.
13. A. Under ESSA, the individual states, rather than the federal government, create short- and long-term goals for academic proficiency. It was enacted by President Barack Obama, and during an ELL's second year in school, his or her score counts toward the school's proficiency rating.
14. C. Passed in 1935, the federal government's first major step toward involvement in a widespread program of living and medical assistance to the population at large is known as the Social Security Act (SSA).
15. C. A minimum of 100 hours of supervised clinical experience is needed for an individual to be an SLPA.

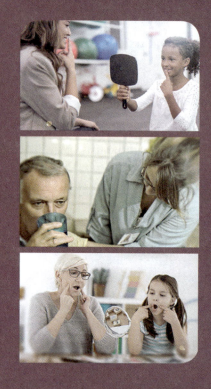

APPENDIX

STUDY AND TEST-TAKING TIPS FOR THE PRAXIS

Most readers of this book are preparing for the Praxis examination in speech–language pathology. The purpose of this appendix is to provide a brief orientation to the Praxis and to give study and test-taking tips to help pass the Praxis. (*Note*: Some of these suggestions may also be applied to studying for and passing comprehensive examinations in graduate programs; readers may apply the information to their individual programs as needed.)

The Nature and Purpose of the Praxis

- Essentially, the purpose of the Praxis is to ask questions in all areas of speech–language pathology to assess whether examinees are prepared to competently serve as speech–language pathologists in a variety of clinical settings (American Speech-Language-Hearing Association [ASHA], 2017).
- The development of the exam is commissioned by ASHA and facilitated by the Educational Testing Service (ETS) to provide a system of fair, thorough, carefully validated assessments.
- According to ASHA (2017), the Praxis Examinations in Speech–Language Pathology and Audiology make up a major component of ASHA certification, as well as most state licensing requirements. The Praxis Series Specialty Area tests in Speech–Language Pathology and Audiology are owned by ETS. Speech–language pathologists take the Praxis-II Subject Assessments in the area of speech–language pathology.
- In September 2014, the previous version of the Praxis was discontinued and replaced with test #5331, which is administered via computer only. The paper-and-pencil format is no longer an option. See Tables A.1–A.3 for specifics about test #5331. For helpful information about the Praxis examination go to: www.ets.org/praxis. See also: www.asha.org/Certification/Praxis/About-the-Speech-Language-Pathology-Praxis-Exam/.
- There are several versions of each Praxis examination in speech–language pathology and audiology. Test takers in both speech–language pathology and audiology who have not earned a passing score can retake the Praxis an unlimited number of times over the next 2 years.

Table A.1

Praxis Test at a Glance

Test aspect	Speech–Language Pathology
Test code	5331
Number of questions	132
Time	150 minutes
Test delivery	Computer-delivered
Format	Selected-response questions

Note. This portion of the *Praxis®* Study Companion is reprinted by permission of Educational Testing Service, the copyright owner. All other information contained within this publication is provided by PRO-ED Inc., and no endorsement of any kind by Educational Testing Service should be inferred. Copyright © 2015 Educational Testing Service. www.ets.org.

Table A.2

Praxis Exam Content Categories

Category	Approximate number of questions	Approximate percentage of exam
I. Foundations and professional practice	44	33⅓%
II. Screening, assessment, evaluation, and diagnosis	44	33⅓%
III. Planning, implementation, and evaluation of treatment	44	33⅓%

Note. Copyright © 2015 Educational Testing Service. www.ets.org. Portion of the *Praxis*® Study Companion is reprinted by permission of Educational Testing Service, the copyright owner. All other information contained within this publication is provided by PRO-ED Inc. and no endorsement of any kind by Educational Testing Service should be inferred.

- If a person does not pass the Praxis within a 2-year period, his or her certification file will be closed. If the person passes the Praxis after the 2-year period, he or she must reapply for certification under the standards in effect at the time of reapplication.
- Results of the exam submitted for initial certification must come directly to ASHA from ETS and must have been obtained no more than 5 years prior to the submission of the application for certification. Scores that are more than 5 years old will not be accepted for certification.
- ASHA (2017) recommends that students take the Praxis *no earlier* than at the completion of their graduate clinical practicum and graduate coursework or during their clinical fellowship year. (*Note*: It is the authors' experience that students who take the Praxis before these timelines almost invariably fail the exam. Though the exam can be retaken, it is expensive and time consuming, and the authors heartily agree with ASHA's recommendation based upon experience working with students at several universities.)
- Questions on the Praxis are gathered from courses in undergraduate and graduate programs in speech–language pathology. The questions cover all age levels of clients, from newborns to geriatric patients.
- ASHA nominates subject matter experts to serve on Praxis committees that work with ETS to develop the exams (ASHA, 2017).
- Passing the Praxis is one of the requirements for obtaining a Certificate of Clinical Competence issued by the American Speech-Language-Hearing Association. Individual states may use the Praxis as part of their licensing requirements. Some graduate programs may use the Praxis as part of the requirements to obtain a master's degree.
- A passing score on the new Praxis for purposes of ASHA certification is 162 (on a 100- to 200-point scale).
- If you are applying for ASHA certification and you have a disability that impairs your ability to take the examination under standard conditions, contact ETS directly to arrange for appropriate accommodations. Write to The Praxis Series, Educational Testing Service, 660 Rosedale Rd., Princeton, NJ 08541. You can also go to www.ets.org/praxis/register/disabilities.

Table A.3

Topics Covered in the Praxis Examination

Area I: Foundations and professional practice

A. Foundations
1. Typical development and performance across the lifespan
2. Epidemiology and characteristics of common communication and swallowing disorders
3. Factors that influence communication, including feeding and swallowing

B. Professional practice
1. Prevention and wellness
2. Linguistically and culturally appropriate service delivery
3. Collaboration, teaming, and counseling
4. Ethics
5. Documentation
6. Research methodology and evidence-based practice
7. Legislation and client advocacy

Area II: Screening, assessment, evaluation, and diagnosis

A. Screening
1. Communication disorders
2. Feeding and swallowing disorders

B. Approaches to assessment and evaluation
1. Developing case histories
2. Selecting appropriate assessment materials, procedures, and instruments
3. Assessing factors that influence communication and swallowing disorders
4. Assessment of anatomy and physiology

C. Assessment procedures and assessment
1. Fluency
2. Voice, resonance, and motor speech
3. Speech sound production
4. Expressive and receptive language
5. Cognitive aspects of communication
6. Social aspects of communication, including pragmatics
7. Hearing
8. Feeding and swallowing
9. Augmentative and alternative communication

D. Etiology
1. Developmental
2. Genetic
3. Disease processes
4. Auditory problems
5. Psychogenic
6. Neurological
7. Structural and functional

(continues)

Table A.3 (continued)

Area III. Planning, implementation, and evaluation of treatment

A. **Treatment planning**
 1. Evaluating factors that can affect treatment
 2. Initiating and prioritizing treatment and developing goals
 3. Determining appropriate treatment details
 4. Generating a prognosis
 5. Communicating recommendations
 6. General treatment principles and procedures

B. **Treatment evaluation**
 1. Establishing methods for monitoring treatment progress and outcomes to evaluate assessment and/or treatment plans
 2. Follow-up on post-treatment referrals and recommendations

C. **Treatment**
 1. Fluency
 2. Speech sound production
 3. Expressive and receptive language
 4. Voice, resonance, and motor speech
 5. Social aspects of communication, including pragmatics
 6. Treatment involving augmentative and alternative communication
 7. Communication impairments related to cognition
 8. Swallowing and feeding
 9. Hearing and aural rehabilitation

Note. Copyright © 2015 Educational Testing Service. www.ets.org. Portion of the *Praxis*® Study Companion is reprinted by permission of Educational Testing Service, the copyright owner. All other information contained within this publication is provided by PRO-ED Inc., and no endorsement of any kind by Educational Testing Service should be inferred.

- If you speak English as a second or foreign language, you may be able to obtain extended time to take the Praxis. For information regarding accommodations (in addition to the above address), visit the ETS website at http://www.ets.org/.
- If you request nonstandard testing arrangements (e.g., extended time), you must complete and submit to ETS the following items (available from http://www.ets.org/praxis): (a) exam registration form, (b) eligibility questionnaire, and (c) Certification of Documentation Form. Appropriate forms and additional information regarding the requirements for nonstandard testing accommodations can be found in the examination Registration Bulletin, as well as on the ETS website.

Study Tips for Preparing for the Praxis

- Many test takers, being human, attempt to memorize a great deal of information right before the examination. Research indicates that ideal learning does not occur under those conditions.
- It is best to start studying at least several months before you take the Praxis. Ideally, you should try to study a little bit each day. Many examinees attempt to study for several hours only on weekends. It is optimal to study a little bit daily rather than try to "cram in" studying on weekends only.

- If you studied 15 minutes a day, 6 days a week, that would equal 1.5 hours of study a week. If you did that for 3 months, you would have studied for 18 hours total.
- When it comes to studying, more is usually better. However, reality dictates that 15 minutes of studying a day for several months is the most many people can manage. When you do a little studying each day, you learn more than if you cram your study into large blocks of time right before the examination.
- Many adults learn best in a multimodal fashion. That is, they retain information best if they read it, write it, say it aloud, and discuss it with others, as opposed to just passively reading it. Thus, it is ideal to study both alone and with other people if possible. You should try to form study groups that meet once or twice a week. Many adults learn best in a study group format.
- It is very helpful, in trying to retain information, to write the information down. You might want to make flash cards with pertinent information. Carry them around with you and review them often.
- It is extremely helpful to take practice Praxis examinations. We recommend you use the online practice program *An Advanced Review of Speech–Language Pathology: Preparation for Praxis and Comprehensive Examination—Practice Tests: Fifth Edition*, www.advancedreviewpractice.com.
- It is best to set aside 2.5 hours and take a practice examination with no interruptions. While it is challenging for many busy people to find a 2.5-hour uninterrupted time block, we have found that this is the very best way to prepare to take the Praxis.
- Many students have told us over the years, after taking the examination, that they ran out of time at the end because they worked too slowly. Thus, taking a practice examination in an uninterrupted 2.5-hour time block helps you prepare for the actual situation ahead.
- Many examinees stay up late the night before an examination. They spend those late hours "cramming" for the examination the next day. For many people, this does not work well when taking the Praxis. The Praxis questions do not necessarily require rote, pre-memorized answers. Rather, many questions require a great deal of reading, careful thought, and subjective clinical judgment decisions.
- Such higher-level thought questions are usually most accurately answered if you have had a good night's sleep before the examination. In our opinion, the night before the Praxis is best spent sleeping and attempting to wake up refreshed to answer challenging questions the next day.
- For more suggestions, see "Tips to Pass the Praxis" at www.advancedreviewpractice.com.

General Tips for Taking the Praxis

- Right before taking the examination, it is best to go to the bathroom. If you take 10 minutes during the Praxis to go to the bathroom, that is 10 minutes lost during the exam. In other words, if the Praxis is administered from 8:00 to 10:30 in the morning, you do not get to take 10 minutes in the bathroom during the examination and then continue taking the test until 10:40. Time spent in the bathroom is time lost in test taking!
- When you go to the bathroom during the test, you will need to sign out with the proctor. When you come back in, you will need to sign back in, be "wanded" by the proctor again, and turn out your pockets, as well.

- It is best to wear loose, comfortable clothing during the examination. It is recommended that you wear a long-sleeved T-shirt, even if it's hot outside. Sometimes the air conditioning can make the room uncomfortably cold. You may not be allowed to bring a sweater or jacket into the testing room.
- Be sure to bring photo identification with you.
- You will be given four pages of scratch paper to use during the exam. Pencils will be provided. After you have finished taking the test, you must hand your scratch paper to the test proctor to be destroyed.
- You will be restricted from bringing in the following items: handbags, briefcases, water bottles, canned or bottled beverages, study materials, electronic devices, and food. Some testing centers have storage places, such as lockers; others do not. Test centers assume no responsibility for your personal items.
- You may not wear a watch of any kind, and most jewelry and hair clips are unacceptable. No scarves, hats, or bowties are allowed. If you wear glasses, you must remove them for close inspection by testing staff.
- You will be "wanded" (as at airport security) and asked to turn out your pockets when you enter the testing room. This will occur if you re-enter the room after taking a break. We recommend that if possible, you wear clothing without pockets as this can save time.
- If you must have a cough lozenge, you will be asked to unwrap it and put it in your mouth in front of the test proctor before you enter the testing room. Unwrapped cough lozenges, candies, and gum are not permitted inside the testing room. If you need tissues, the test proctor will supply preapproved ones for you; you may not bring in your own.
- Many examinees feel very nervous. Deep breathing is an excellent way to deal with nervousness. Deep breathing also enhances concentration by providing increased oxygen to the brain.
- Be constantly mindful of time. As stated earlier, many examinees' greatest problem was running out of time at the end. It is quite upsetting to realize you have only 10 minutes left and 35 questions still to answer. *Keep moving along*, even if you are unsure of each answer. The on-screen clock, positioned in the upper right-hand corner, will tell you how much time you have left.
- Occasionally, you will encounter a question that seems deceptively simple and quick, as in the following example:

Which is the primary cranial nerve involved in innervation of the muscles of the larynx?

    A.   Cranial nerve VIII   **C.**   Cranial nerve II
    B.   Cranial nerve IX   **D.**   Cranial nerve X

The answer is D, cranial nerve X.

- There are very few such questions on the Praxis. Answer them as best you can and use the time you save on those questions to answer the questions that require more reading.

- Some Praxis questions require a great deal of reading. They often involve cases in which a clinical decision is necessary. Examinees have shared with us that they were unhappily surprised by the sheer number of these complicated questions. Knowing that such questions exist is very helpful. An example of a complicated clinical scenario follows:

A 6-year-old child with a repaired posterior cleft palate has been referred to you by her teacher. The child's speech is hypernasal with numerous articulatory errors, including glottal stops, distortions of sibilants, and substitutions of w/r and j/l. During phonation of /u/, a palatopharyngeal gap exceeding 15 millimeters is observed. The cleft palate team, consisting of an orthodontist, plastic surgeon, pediodontist, and oromaxillofacial surgeon, is consulting with you in this case. The parents are eager for their child to get as much assistance as possible and have indicated their willingness to provide as much support as is necessary. Given this information, which of the following will be your first priority in clinical management of this case?

- **A.** Therapy beginning with the easy initiation /u/ blended with stop consonants to lower tongue position, reduce nasality, and eliminate glottal stops
- **B.** Blowing exercises to strengthen velopharyngeal valving
- **C.** Therapy to remediate the w/r and j/l substitutions
- **D.** Referral to the appropriate specialists to determine physical management of the palatopharyngeal gap

The answer is D.

- Read all choices before you decide on the best answer. Reading all choices increases the chances of answering the question accurately.
- Never leave any questions blank. Always answer each question. You are never penalized for guessing incorrectly, but you are always penalized for leaving items blank and unanswered, in that you have no chance to get an unanswered question right.
- If you do not know the answer to a question, guess. Your first guess is usually the right one. We have heard dozens of times over the years that examinees changed their answers, only to find later that the first guess was actually the right one.
- If you are unsure of your answer on an item, answer it as best you can and, if time permits, come back to it after you have completed the examination. In this way, you keep moving forward.
- Today's new computerized version of the Praxis allows you to mark items that you are unsure about. So, for example, if you are unsure about question 56, you can answer it and then click on "Mark" at the top of the screen.
- At any time, you can click on Review (also at the top of the screen) for a view of the entire exam where you can see which questions you have marked. This helpful and efficient tool will guide you immediately to questions you want to come back to.

- Try to relax as much as possible. This is easier said than done, but the more relaxed you are, the higher your likelihood of passing the examination. Remember that if you should fail the Praxis, you can take it again. (*Note*: Policies on the number of retakes change occasionally, so check into the latest available information about this at www.ets.org/praxis.)
- At the end of the exam, you will be given two choices: (a) Cancel, or (b) Report. If you click Cancel, you will not find out your score, and it will not be reported anywhere. If you click Report, your score will be reported to the institutions you have designated.
- If you click on Report, you can immediately find out your test score. You will also be shown your raw score for each of the three previously mentioned areas.
- Some may wish to take the Praxis twice and plan to click Cancel the first time. Although this option is available, the exam costs $120 and will have to be retaken and the score reported in order for ASHA to accept it.
- All those who take the Praxis can access their test scores through My Praxis Account online free of charge for one year from the posting date. This process replaces the mailing of a paper score report. Just log into My Praxis Account at www.ets.org/praxis and click on your score report. You must create a Praxis account to access your scores, even if you have already registered by phone or mail.
- You will need to wait for 12 days before receiving formal notice of your test score (however, you already know what it is). When you receive an email notifying you formally of your score, print out several copies to have available just in case there is ever a question. It is ideal to have at least one hard copy of your score and other test information.

Understanding Computer-Generated Questions

- All questions on the Praxis are multiple choice. The previous versions of the Praxis had five choices (A–E). The new, current edition has four choices (A–D). The examinee clicks on a button to indicate his or her choice of answer.
- At the time of this writing, the most recent edition of the Praxis is 2017. The Praxis is updated every several years. Though the vast majority of questions are in A–D format, there are just a few questions that are different. Several require you to click on the correct answer and drag it into a box. A few questions have five options, and you must click on the three best ones.
- As previously indicated, some questions are short and simple. Other questions are based on lengthy, involved case studies. For example, you may be given case studies that are three or four paragraphs long and have three or four questions to answer on a single case study.
- It is optimal to do your best to read each case carefully, as three or four questions are based upon it. But do not linger too long on these types of questions. It is ideal to "mark" these questions and come back to them after you have finished the entire examination.
- It is also ideal to use your scratch paper to help you process these kinds of questions. Using a pencil to write ideas and thoughts on paper can help you think through long questions analytically and accurately.
- You can find the link to the computer-delivered testing demonstration at www.ets.org/praxis/prepare/video

Conclusion

The newest edition of the Praxis exam is a computer-based test. This test must be taken and passed in order to receive ASHA certification. Most states require the Praxis as part of licensing requirements, as well. With extensive studying, preparation, and taking of practice exams such as those on our website, you stand an excellent chance of passing the Praxis the first time. Good luck!

References and Recommended Readings at www.advancedreviewpractice.com

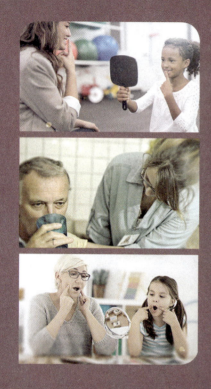

INDEX

A

AA. *See* Anomic aphasia (AA)
AAC. *See* Augmentative and alternative communication (AAC)
AAE. *See* African American English (AAE)
ABAB design, 605–606
ABA design, 605–606
ABCD. *See* Arizona Battery for Communication Disorders of Dementia (ABCD)
AB design, 605
Abdomen, 6
Abdominal muscles of expiration, 8
Abducens nerve (cranial nerve VI), 34, 35
Abductor spasmodic dysphonia, 319
ABR. *See* Auditory brainstem response (ABR)
Absolute zero point, 621
Abuse, language problems related to, 158–159
Abusive behaviors, and phonation disorders, 304
Academic language, 175
Academic performance and speech sound disorders, 206
Acceleration, 93
Acceleration–deceleration head injuries, 381
Accreditation, 636–637
Acculturation, 463
Acetylcholine, 31
Achalasia, 419
Acoustic analysis of speech, 95–96, 287–289
Acoustic branch, 513
Acoustic highlighting, 542
Acoustic immitance, 533
Acoustic nerve (cranial nerve VIII), 34, 37, 513
Acoustic neuroma, 527, 530
Acoustic phonetics, 73, 74
Acoustic reflex, 511, 533
Acoustics
    defined, 90
    frequency and intensity, 517
    measurements, 291
    sound pressure level and hearing level, 518
    sound waves, 516–517
    source of sound, 515–516
Acquired immune deficiency syndrome (AIDS)
    as cause of strokes, 492
    dementia complex, 368
Acquired stuttering. *See* Neurogenic stuttering (NS)

Acronyms
    SCERTS, 153
    STORCH, 526–527
    TOSS, 279
Active sentence, 105
ACTS. *See* Auditory Comprehension Test for Sentences (ACTS)
Acute otitis media, 523
ADA. *See* Americans With Disabilities Act (ADA)
Adam's apple. *See* Thyroid notch
Adaptation as stimulus control in stuttering, 249
Addenbrooke's Cognitive Function–Revised, 372
Adductor spasmodic dysphonia, 319–320
Adenoidectomy, 295
ADHD. *See* Attention-deficit/hyperactivity disorder (ADHD)
Adjacency effect as stimulus control in stuttering, 249
Admittance of sound, 533
Adolescents
    assessment, 171–174
        guidelines and procedures, 172–173
        standardized tests, 174
    language assessment, 162
    language impairments, 489–490
    stuttering treatment for, 259
    voice changes, 280–281
Adopted children, second-language acquisition of, 478–479
ADP. *See* Aphasia Diagnostic Profiles (ADP)
Adults
    with neurologically based communication disorders, 492–494
    stuttering in, 248
        treatment, 260
    voice changes, 281
Aerodynamic measurements, 290
Afferent nerves, 34
Affordable Health Care Act, 646
Affricates, 82–83
Affrication, 204
African American English (AAE), 465–468
    articulation and phonology characteristics, 466–468, 470
    background, 395
    bias against AAE speakers on tests, 467
    examples of acceptable utterances, 468, 471
    misconceptions about, 466
    morphology and syntax characteristics, 466–468, 469

African American Language. *See* African American English (AAE)
African Americans, medical conditions and communication disorders, 491
Age-equivalency scores, standardized test, 572
Agnosia, 360
Agrammatic speech, 340
Agraphia, 359
AIDS. *See* Acquired immune deficiency syndrome (AIDS)
Air–bone gap, 536
Air conduction of sound, 519
Air-conduction testing, 532
Alaryngeal speech, 301–303
Alcohol abuse
    as cause of strokes, 492
    language problems related to, 159–160
Alexia, 359
Allomorph, defined, 104
Allophones, defined, 74, 196
ALS. *See* Amyotrophic lateral sclerosis (ALS)
Alternate-form reliability, 600
Alternative assessment, 163–164
Alternative hypothesis, 598
Alveolar arch, 23
Alveolar ducts, 3
Alveolar process, 23
Alzheimer's disease, 361–363, 369–370
American Congress of Rehabilitation Medicine, 382
American English, dialects, 464–465
American Psychiatric Association (APA), 361
    DSM-V. *See Diagnostic and Statistical Manual of Mental Disorders–Fifth Edition* (DSM-V)
    intellectual disability definition, 149
American Sign Language (ASL), 183, 552
American Speech-Language-Hearing Association (ASHA)
    accreditation, 636–637
    Certificate of Clinical Competence, 656
    certification, 637–640
    Code of Ethics, 564, 638–640
    functions, 631
    goals, 632–633
    history of, 632
    membership, 632, 633–634
    multicultural issues, 463–464
    National Outcome Measurement System (NOMS), 648
    orofacial myofunctional disorders, 209
    scope-of-practice document, 635–636

special interest groups, 634
speech–language pathology
   assistants, 640–641
stuttering, 239
telepractice, 648
Americans With Disabilities Act (ADA), 645
Amnesia, 56
Amplification aids for hearing
   impairment, 542–547
   assistive devices, 547
   cochlear implants, 545–547
   hearing aids, 542–545
Amplitude, 90, 94, 517
Amplitude perturbation (shimmer), 283
Amsterdam-Nijmegen Everyday Language Test (ANELT), 350
Amyloid plaques, and dementia, 362
Amyotrophic lateral sclerosis (ALS), 320–321, 403, 411
Analog hearing aid, 543
ANELT. *See Amsterdam-Nijmegen Everyday Language Test* (ANELT)
Angelman Syndrome (AS), 444
Angular gyrus, 55
Ankyloglossia (tongue-tie), 208
Ankylosis, 317
Anomia, 340, 347
Anomic aphasia (AA), 347–348
Anosognosia, 344
ANS. *See* Autonomic nervous system (ANS)
Antecedents, 579, 580
Anterior belly of digastric muscle, 24
Anterior cerebral artery, 66
Anterograde amnesia, 56
Aorta, 63
AOS. *See* Apraxia of speech (AOS)
APA. *See* American Psychiatric Association (APA)
Aperiodic vibrations, 93, 515, 516
Aperiodic waves, 90
Apert syndrome, 444–445
Aphasia, 337–360
   agnosia, 360
   agraphia, 359
   alexia, 359
   assessment, 349–353
      functional communication tests, 350–351
      outline, 351–353
      screening tests, 349
      standardized tests, 349–350
   in bilingual populations, 348–349
   classification, 340
   crossed, 348
   defined, 337, 340
   fluent, 344–348
      anomic aphasia, 347–348

   conduction aphasia, 346–347
   transcortical sensory aphasia, 345–346
   Wernicke's aphasia, 56, 344–345
incidence and prevalence of, 337–338
key terms, 339–340
neuropathology of, 338–339
nonfluent, 340–344
   Broca's aphasia, 340–341
   global aphasia, 343–344
   mixed transcortical aphasia, 342–343
   transcortical motor aphasia, 342
subcortical, 348
treatment, 354–359
   auditory comprehension, 354–355
   bilingual speakers, 359
   compensatory approach, 354
   experimental approaches, 359
   group treatment, 358
   reading skills, 357
   restorative approach, 354
   social approaches, 354, 358
   types of, 337
   verbal expression, expanded utterances, 356–357
   verbal expression, naming, 355–356
   writing skills, 357–358
Aphasia Diagnostic Profiles (ADP), 350
Aphasia Rapid Test, 349
Applied (clinical) phonetics, 74
Apraxia of speech (AOS), 393–398
   Apraxia Battery for Adults–Second Edition (ABA–2), 397
   assessment, 211, 396–397
   causes of, 211
   characteristics, 211
   communication deficits in, 395–396
   defined, 393
   differentiating from dysarthria, 412
   distinctions, 393–394
   neuropathology of, 394
   primary progressive apraxia of speech, 394
   pure apraxia, 394
   symptoms, 395
   treatment, 212, 397–398
Arachnoid, 62
Arcuate fasciculus, 61, 347
Arizona Battery for Communication Disorders of Dementia (ABCD), 372
Arteries feeding the larynx, 275
Arteriosclerosis, and strokes, 492
Articulation
   African American English, 466–468, 470
   Asian-influenced languages, 475
   bunched articulation, 84

   coarticulation, 88
   Deep Test of Articulation, 224
   defined, 1, 18, 196
   disorder, defined, 195
   errors, 207
   foundations of, 195–197
   functional articulation disorder, 205
   fundamentals of, 18–30
      face (lips and cheeks), 27–29
      hard palate, 22–23
      mandible, 23–24
      pharynx, 19–20
      soft palate (velum), 20–22
      teeth, 24–25
      tongue, 25–27
   glottal articulation, 81, 204
   Iowa Pressure Articulation Test, 439
   lateral, 84
   manner of, 79, 81–84
   place of, 79, 80–81
   rapid-fire articulation, 410
   skills development, 197–205
      in children, 201, 202
      in infants, 199–200
      intelligibility, 201–203
   skills development theories
      behavioral theory, 197–198
      generative phonology theory, 198
      linear *vs.* nonlinear phonology theories, 199
      natural phonology theory, 198
      optimality theory, 199
   Spanish-influenced English, 468, 472
   Templin Darley Test of Articulation, 439
Articulatory errors, 207
Articulatory phonetics, 74
Articulatory problems, 146
Artificial larynx, 302
Aryepiglottic folds, 13, 275, 277
Arytenoid adduction, 319
Arytenoid cartilage, 10, 274, 275, 277, 278
AS. *See* Angelman Syndrome (AS)
ASD. *See* Autism spectrum disorder (ASD)
ASHA. *See* American Speech-Language-Hearing Association (ASHA)
Asian Americans, medical conditions and communication disorders, 491
Asian-influenced languages
   articulation, 475
   background, 471
   characteristics, 471–475
   language differences, 474
ASL. *See* American Sign Language (ASL)
Asperger, Hans, 151

Asperger's syndrome, 151, 152–153
Assessment
    aphasia, 349–353
    apraxia of speech, 211, 396–397
    children with clefts, 437–439
    cluttering, 264
    criterion-referenced, 163
    defined, 561
    dementia, 372–373
    dynamic, 163, 486–487
    Dynamic Evaluation of Motor Speech Skill (DEMSS), 211
    dysarthrias, 412–414
    of EL students, multicultural population communication disorders, 481–488
    evidence-based practice. *See* Evidence-based practice
    hearing impairment, 531–538
    of information processing skills, 163
    language disorders, 162–174
    need for individualized assessment, 590
    neurogenic stuttering, 262
    portfolio assessment, 163
    right hemisphere disorder, 376–377
    speech sound disorder, 213–219
    standardized. *See* Standardized assessment
    stuttering, 252–254
    swallowing disorders, 419–420
    traumatic brain injury, 382–383
        associated with communicative deficits, 383–384
    voice disorders, 285–294
Assessment of Intelligibility of Dysarthric Speech, 414
Assessment of Living with Aphasia, 350
Assimilation, 88, 463
Assimilation patterns, 204
Assimilative nasality, 296
Associated motor behaviors, and stuttering, 246
Association fibers, 61
Associative play, 168
Astrocytes, 30
Ataxia, 51, 404
Ataxic cerebral palsy, 155
Ataxic dysarthria, 51, 399, 404–405
    ataxic–spastic dysarthria, 411
Atherosclerosis, 338
Athetoid cerebral palsy, 155
Attention-deficit/hyperactivity disorder (ADHD), 160–162
Attention to task deficits, 148
Attrition, 614
Audience size effect as stimulus control in stuttering, 249
Audiologists, 507, 541, 635

Audiology. *See also* Hearing impairment
    defined, 507
    doctorate in audiology (AuD), 507
    education and training for, 507
    as a profession, 507
Audiometer, 531–532
Audiometry, 531–533, 534
    auditory brainstem response, 535
    behavioral observation, 535
    electrophysiological, 534
    localization, 457
    play, 535
    pure-tone x, 532
    speech, 533
    visual reinforcement, 535
Auditory agnosia, 360
Auditory association cortex, 55
Auditory attention, 131
Auditory brainstem response (ABR), 534
    audiometry, 535
Auditory branch, 513
Auditory comprehension
    assessment, 352
    treatment, 354–355
Auditory Comprehension Test for Sentences (ACTS), 351
Auditory development, 519
Auditory discrimination/perceptual training, 222
Auditory discrimination skills, 131
    as factor in speech sound disorders, 206–207
Auditory-evoked potentials, 534
Auditory–global approach. *See* Aural/oral training method
Auditory habilitation, 548–549
Auditory memory, 131
Auditory nervous system, 513–514
    impairments, 528–531
        central auditory disorders, 528–529
        retrocochlear disorders, 529–531
Auditory phonetics, 74
Auditory rate, 131
Auditory sequencing, 131
Auditory tube. *See* Eustachian tube
Auditory verbal agnosia, 360
Augmentative and alternative communication (AAC), 181–184
    basic principles, 181–183
    dysarthria, 414
    gestural (unaided), 183
    gestural-assisted (aided), 183–184
    neuro-assisted (aided), 184
    spasmodic dysphonia, 320
Aural atresia, 521
Aural/oral training method, 551
Aural rehabilitation, 541–542
Auricle of the outer ear, 508

Auricular muscle, 37
Authentic assessment, 576–577
Autism spectrum disorder (ASD), 151–153
    Asperger's syndrome, 151, 152–153
    background of term, 151
    characteristics, 151–152
    language problems, 152
    manifestations, 151
    treatment, 152
Autistic psychopathy, 151
Automated speech and singing assessment, 353
Automatic language, 340
Automatic reinforcer, 584
Autonomic nervous system (ANS), 43
Average score, 620
Aversive stimuli, 579
Avoidance
    defined, 579
    escape *vs.*, 580
    stuttering and, 247, 251
Axon, 31

B

BA. *See* Broca's aphasia (BA)
Backing, 204
Backup reinforcer, 584
Back vowels, 84, 86–87
BAHA. *See* Bone-anchored hearing aids (BAHA)
Basal ganglia, 48, 49–50
Baselines, 575–576, 579–580
Base morpheme, 104
Basic Interpersonal Communication Skills (BICS), 479–481
Basilar artery, 63
Basilar membrane, 513
BDAE-3. *See* Boston Diagnostic Aphasia Examination–Third Edition (BDAE-3)
Bedside Western Aphasia Battery, 349
Behavioral observation audiometry, 535
Behavioral theory
    articulatory skills development, 197–198
    language development, 125–126
Behavioral variant of frontotemporal dementia (bvFTD), 363, 364
Behavioral voice therapy, 319, 322–327
    chest resonance, 324
    coughing and throat clearing, 326–327
    hard glottal attack, 326
    integrated implicit–explicit approach, 325–326
    Lessac-Madsen Resonant Voice Therapy, 324
    Lombard effect, 327

rhythmic breathing, 327
singhale (inhalation phonation), 326
stretch and flow, 325
twang, 325
vocal function exercises, 325
yawn–sigh method, 324
Behavior assessment batteries, 253
Behavior Assessment Battery for Adults who Stutter, 253
Behavior Assessment Battery for School-Age Children Who Stutter, 253
Behavior Inattention (BIT), 377
Behind-the-ear hearing aids, 542
Bel, 90–91, 94
Bell-shaped curve, 620
Bernoulli effect, 14–15
BICS. See Basic Interpersonal Communication Skills (BICS)
Bicultural immigrants, 463
Bifid (cleft) uvula, 435
Bilabials, 81
Bilateral paralysis of vocal folds, 318
Bilingual populations with aphasia
 assessment, 353
 Bilingual Aphasia Test (BAT), 353
 generally, 348–349
 treatment, 359
Biofeedback, for treating hypernasality, 297
Birth defects as cause of hearing loss, 526
Birth history, 563
Birth order as factor in speech sound disorders, 206
BIT. See Behavior Inattention (BIT)
Black Dialect. See African American English (AAE)
Black English. See African American English (AAE)
Black English Vernacular. See African American English (AAE)
Blade of the tongue, 26
Blast (multisystem) head injury, 381
Blends. See Consonant clusters
Blom-Singer tracheoesophageal puncture, 302–303
Blood supply, cerebral, 62–66
Bolus, 417
Bone-anchored hearing aids (BAHA), 544
Bone-conduction hearing aids, 544
Bone conduction of sound, 519
Bone-conduction testing, 532
Bony growths, 521
Booster treatment, 580, 588
Boston Diagnostic Aphasia Examination–Third Edition (BDAE-3), 349, 353
Botox injections, 319
Bound morpheme, 104, 150
Brachycephaly, 445

Brain, 44
 connecting fibers, 60–61
 damage. See Right hemisphere disorder (RHD); Traumatic brain injury (TBI)
 injury
  as cause of cerebral palsy, 155
  stuttering prevalence and, 244
  traumatic brain injury, 153–154
 left hemisphere, 375
 protective layers, 62
 right hemisphere, 375
 speech, language, hearing areas of, 52
Brain dysfunction hypotheses for stuttering, 251
Brainstem, 44–48
 functions, 44
 medulla, 47–48
 midbrain, 44, 46
 pons, 46–47
 structures, 44, 47
Breastbone (sternum), 5
Breathing
 abnormalities and stuttering, 246–247
 clavicular, 293
 diaphragmatic–abdominal, 293
 rhythmic, 327
 thoracic, 293
Breathy voice, 284
Brief Test of Head Injury (BTHI), 382
Broad phonetic transcription, 75
Broca's aphasia (BA), 340–341
Broca's area, 16, 53, 54, 340–341
Broken words, 240
Bronchi, 2–3
Bronchioles, 2
BTHI. See *Brief Test of Head Injury* (BTHI)
Buccal branches, 27
Buccinator muscle, 27, 28, 37
Bunched articulation, 84
Burden of Stroke Scale (BOSS), 350
Burns Brief Inventory, 377
bvFTD. See Behavioral variant of frontotemporal dementia (bvFTD)

C

CA. See Conduction aphasia (CA); Crossed aphasia (CA)
CAA. See Council on Academic Accreditation in Audiology and Speech–Language Pathology (CAA)
CADL-3. See *Communicative Abilities in Daily Living–Third Edition* (CADL-3)
CALP. See Cognitive Academic Language Proficiency (CALP)
Camperdown Program, 257

Cancer of the larynx, 299
Canonical babbling stage of sound development, 200
CAPE-V. See Consensus Auditory–Perceptual Evaluation of Voice (CAPE-V)
Carcinoma and laryngectomy, 299–304
 alaryngeal speech, 301–303
 basic principles, 299
 medical treatment, 299–300
 physiology of head and neck before and after laryngectomy, 301
 rehabilitation issues, 300
 surgical modifications and implants, 302–303
Caregivers
 impact on language development, 109–110
 infant–caregiver interaction, assessment of, 168
 parental impact on language development, 132
Carhart's notch, 523
Carotid arteries, 65–66
CAS. See Childhood apraxia of speech (CAS)
Case history
 communication disorder description, 563
 educational history, 564
 family constellation and communication, 563
 function of, 563
 medical history, 564
 multicultural population communication disorders, 485
 occupational history, 564
 prenatal, birth, and developmental history, 563
 prior assessment and treatment, 563
 prognosis, 564
 research history, and validity, 613
 speech sound disorder assessment, 214
 voice disorders, 285
CAT. See *Comprehensive Aphasia Test* (CAT)
Cauda equina, 43
Caudate nucleus, 50
Causal–comparative studies, 609
Cause–effect relationships, 601
CAVS. See Cephalometric Assessment of Velopharyngeal Structures (CAVS)
CCC-A. See Certificate of Clinical Competence in Audiology (CCC-A)
CCC-SLP. See Certificate of Clinical Competence in Speech–Language Pathology (CCC-SLP)
CDS. See Child-directed speech (CDS)
Central auditory disorders, 528–529

Central auditory processing, 528
Central electroauditory prosthesis (CEP), 547
Central nervous system (CNS), 44–66
 basal ganglia, 48, 49–50
 basic principles, 44
 brainstem, 44–48
  functions, 44
  medulla, 47–48
  midbrain, 44, 46
  pons, 46–47
  structures, 47
 cerebellum, 49, 50–51
 cerebral blood supply, 62–66
 cerebral ventricles, 61
 cerebrum, 51–56
  basic principles, 51–52
  frontal lobe, 52, 53–54
  occipital lobe, 55
  parietal lobe, 54–55
  temporal lobe, 55–56
 connecting fibers in brain, 60–61
 diencephalon, 49
 extrapyramidal system, 57, 60
 nerve cells, 30–31
 protective layers of the brain, 62
 pyramidal system, 56–57, 58
  basic principles, 56
  corticobulbar tract, 57, 59
  corticospinal tract, 56, 58
 reticular activating system, 48
Central sulcus (fissure of Rolando), 51
Central tendency, 620
Central vowels, 86
CEP. See Central electroauditory prosthesis (CEP)
Cephalometric analysis, 438
Cephalometric Assessment of Velopharyngeal Structures (CAVS), 438
Cerebellopontine angle, 514
Cerebellum, 16, 49, 50–51
Cerebral aqueduct, 61
Cerebral blood supply, 62–66
 aorta, 63
 carotid arteries, 65–66
 circle of Willis, 66
 vertebral arteries, 63
Cerebral palsy (CP)
 ataxic, 155
 athetoid, 155
 causes of, 155
 defined, 155
 paralysis manifestations, 155
 spastic, 155
 speech and language problems, 155
 treatment, 155
Cerebral ventricles, 61
Cerebrovascular accident (CVA), 338
 and dementia, 371

Cerebrum (cerebral cortex), 51–56
 basic principles, 51–52
 frontal lobe, 52, 53–54
 lobes of, 52
 occipital lobe, 55
 parietal lobe, 54–55
 temporal lobe, 55–56
Certificate of Clinical Competence in Audiology (CCC-A), 638
Certificate of Clinical Competence in Speech–Language Pathology (CCC-SLP), 637–638
Certification, 637–640, 656
Cerumen, 508
Cervical vertebrae, 5
CETI. See *Communicative Effectiveness Index* (CETI)
CFCC. See Council for Clinical Certification in Audiology and Speech–Language Pathology (CFCC)
Cheek. See Face muscles
Chemotherapy, 300
Chest, 5–6
Chest resonance, 324
Chewing (mastication), 24
Child-directed speech (CDS), 110
Childhood apraxia of speech (CAS), 210–212
Children. See Adolescents; Elementary-age children; Infants; Preschoolers; Toddlers
Chomsky, Noam, 126–127
Chomsky-Halle distinctive features of English consonants, 79
Chondroglossus muscle, 27
Choroid plexus, 61
Chronic otitis media, 523
Cilia, 513
Circle of Willis (circulus arteriosus), 66
Circulus arteriosus (circle of Willis), 66
Circumlocution, 340
Citation form of sound, 88
Classes of evidence for evidence-based practice, 616–618
Classification of speech sounds, 78–80
 distinctive feature analysis, 79
 place-voice-manner analysis, 79–80
Classification variable, 609
Classroom-based intervention, 176
Clause, independent (main), 105
Clavicular breathing, 293
Cleft, defined, 431
Cleft lip, 431–432
Cleft palate, 432–443
 assessment of children with clefts, 437–439
 as cause of hypernasality, 295
 classification of, 434–435
 congenital palatopharyngeal incompetence, 435

 embryonic growth of facial structures, 433
 etiology of, 433–434
  environmental factors, 434
  genetics, 434
  mechanical factors, 434
 hearing loss and, 435–436
 language disorders, 437
 laryngeal and phonatory disorders, 437
 speech sound disorders, 436
 treatment, 297, 439–443
  language disorders, 443
  resonance disorders, 443
  speech sound disorders, 441–443
  surgical, 440–441
Client-specific assessment, 575–576
Client-specific treatment strategy, 586
Clinical certification, 637–640
Clinical science. See Scientific method
Closed-captioning on television, 547
Closed-head (nonpenetrating) injury, 380–381
Closed syllables, 78
CLQT. See *Cognitive Linguistic Quick Test* (CLQT)
Cluttering, 237, 263–264. See also Fluency
 assessment, 264
 defined, 263
 description of, 263–264
 treatment, 264
Cluttering Severity Instrument, 264
CNS. See Central nervous system (CNS)
Coarticulation, 88, 224
Cocaine-exposed-children, effects of enriched environment on, 160
Coccyx, 4
Cochlea, 512
Cochlear implants, 545–547
Coda of syllables, 78
Code of Ethics (ASHA), 564, 638–640
Code-switching, 478
Cognate pairs, 81
Cognitive Academic Language Proficiency (CALP), 479–481
Cognitive connectionism, 128
Cognitive deficits, 144
Cognitive definitions of aphasia, 340
Cognitive Linguistic Quick Test (CLQT), 382
Cognitive processing deficits, 148–149
Cognitive processing skills, 181
Cognitive rehabilitation, 384
Cognitive theory of language development, 127–128, 129–130
Cohesion, and pragmatics, 108
CO_2 laser surgery
 for papilloma, 314
 for spasmodic dysphonia, 319

Collaboration in treatment, 175–176
Collaborative play, 169
Coloboma, 450
Coma Recovery Scale–Revised (CRS-R), 382
Commenting, 108
Commissural fibers, 61
Common Core State Standards
  achievement by students with language impairments, 176
  goals, 124
  teaching literacy skills, 180
Communication Attitude Test for Preschool and Kindergarten Children Who Stutter, 253
Communication training for dementia, 373–374
Communication training for the hearing impaired, 547–552
  auditory habilitation, 549
  aural/oral training method, 551
  cued speech, 549–550
  FM system, 549
  general guidelines, 547–548
  manual training approach, 551
  sign language, 551, 552
  speech, rhythm, and voice training, 550–551
  speech–language communication, 550
  speech reading, 549
  total communication, 551–552
Communicative Abilities in Daily Living–Third Edition (CADL-3), 350, 353
Communicative disorders, 337–385
  agnosia, 360
  agraphia, 359
  alexia, 359
  aphasia, 337–360
    assessment, 349–353
    in bilingual populations, 348–349
    crossed aphasia, 348
    definition and classification, 340
    fluent aphasias, 344–348
    incidence and prevalence, 337–338
    key terms, 339–340
    neuropathology of, 338–339
    nonfluent aphasias, 340–344
    subcortical aphasia, 348
    treatment, 354–359
  case history, 563
  clefts and, 435–437
    hearing loss, 435–436
    language disorders, 437
    laryngeal and phonatory disorders, 437
    speech sound disorders, 436
  dementia, 360–374
    Alzheimer's disease, 361–363
    assessment, 372–373
    cerebrovascular accidents, 371
    clinical management, 373–374
    definition and classification, 361
    frontotemporal dementia, 363–366
    Huntington's disease, 367–368
    infectious dementia, 368, 370–371
    Lewy body, 371
    Parkinson's disease, 366–367
    Pick's disease, 363
    primary progressive aphasia, 363, 364–366
    traumatic brain injury, 371
    vascular dementia, 371
    Wernicke-Korsakoff syndrome, 371
  genetic syndromes associated with, 444–452
    Angelman syndrome, 444
    Apert syndrome, 444–445
    Cri du chat syndrome, 445
    Crouzon syndrome, 445
    Down syndrome, 445–446
    Fragile X syndrome, 446
    Hurler's syndrome, 446–447
    Landau-Kleffner syndrome, 447
    Marfan syndrome, 447
    Moebius syndrome, 447–448
    Pierre-Robin syndrome, 448
    Prader-Willi syndrome, 448–449
    Russell-Silver syndrome, 449
    Tourette syndrome, 449–450
    Treacher Collins syndrome, 450
    Trisomy 13, 450
    Turner syndrome, 451
    Usher syndrome, 451
    velocardiofacial syndrome, 451–452
    Williams syndrome, 452
  hearing impairment, 539–541
  in multicultural populations. *See* Multicultural population communication disorders
  right hemisphere disorder, 375–379
    assessment, 376–377
    symptoms, 375–377
    treatment, 378–379
  traumatic brain injury, 379–385
    assessment, 382–384
    causes of, 380
    consequences of, 380–382
    definition and incidence, 379–380
    dementia, 371
    treatment, 384–385
  treatment paradigm, 579
Communicative Effectiveness Index (CETI), 350
Communicative potency, 220
Communicative temptations, 175
Comparative research, 610
Competence of language, 125
Completely-in-the-canal hearing aids, 543
Complex sentence, 106
Complex tone, 93, 515
Compound sentence, 105
Comprehension
  auditory, treatment, 354–355
  of sentences, paragraphs, and discourse assessment, 352
  of single words
    assessment, 352
    treatment, 355
  of spoken sentences, treatment, 355
Comprehensive and integrated assessment, 577–578
Comprehensive Aphasia Test (CAT), 350
Comprehensive Test of Phonological Processing Skills–Second Edition (CTOPP-2), 487
Compression, 90, 93, 516
Computer axial tomography, for hearing impairment assessment, 534
Computers, 165
  -assisted, language therapy, 175
  Computerized Profiling computer software, 165
  Computer Speech Laboratory, 289
  -generated questions, Praxis examination, 662
  hearing aid technology, 544
  Lingquest 1 computer software, 165
  sampling program software, 165
  Speech Intelligibility Test for Windows, 414
  swallowing disorder treatment applications, 423
  Systemic Analysis of Language Transcripts (SALT), 165
Conceptual scoring, 486
Concordance/concordance rate of stuttering in twins, 243
Concrete operations, cognitive development, 130
Concurrent validity, 599
Concussion. *See* Mild traumatic brain injury
Condensation, 90
Conditioned generalized reinforcer, 584
Conditioned reinforcers, 584
Conduction aphasia (CA), 346–347
Conductive hearing loss, 520–524
Confounding variables, 601
Congenital hearing loss, 539
Congenital laryngeal stridor, 312
Congenital palatopharyngeal incompetence (CPI), 435
Consensus Auditory–Perceptual Evaluation of Voice (CAPE-V), 291

Consequences of target responses, 580
Consistency effect as stimulus control in stuttering, 249
Consistency (core vocabulary) treatment approach, 226–227
Consonant clusters, 84
Consonant-cluster simplification or reduction, 204
Consonants, 80
   Chomsky-Halle distinctive features, 79
   harmony, 204
   place-voice-manner analysis, 80–84
   syllable as a unit, 77–78
   voicing of, 196
Constituent definitions, 580, 582
Construct validity, 599
Contact ulcers, 308, 316
Content validity, 600
Content words, 340
   and stuttering, 248
Context
   effect on speech production
      dynamics of speech production, 88
      suprasegmentals, 88–89
   of language, 108
   naturalistic, 485
Context utilization approaches, 223–224
Continuous reinforcement, 583
Contralateral motor control, 53
Contralateral pathways, 514
Contrastive analysis, 577
Control group, 602
Conus medullaris, 43
Conversational speech samples for assessment, 215
Conversion aphonia, 321–322
Cooing or gooing stage of sound development, 200
Cooperative play, 169
Coprolalia, 449
Core vocabulary (consistency) treatment approach, 226–227
Corniculate cartilage, 10, 277
Cornu, 10
Corona radiata, 60
Corpus callosum, 61, 62
Corpus of the sternum, 5
Corpus striatum, 50
Corrective feedback, 580
Correlational coefficient, 600
Correlational research, 611–612
Cortex, brain, 51
Cortical areas, 16
Corticobulbar tract, 57, 59
Corticospinal tract, 56, 58
Costal cartilages, 6
Coughing, 326–327
Council for Clinical Certification in Audiology and Speech–Language Pathology (CFCC), 637
Council on Academic Accreditation in Audiology and Speech–Language Pathology (CAA), 636–637
Counseling
   in dementia treatment, 374
   personal adjustment, 548
   in psychogenic voice disorders treatment, 321
   in stuttering treatment, 255, 256, 259
Countercoup injury, 381
Country of birth, and communication disorders, 463
Coup injury, 381
Coupling of nasal and oral cavities, 17
Cover-body theory of phonation, 274
CP. *See* Cerebral palsy (CP)
CPI. *See* Congenital palatopharyngeal incompetence (CPI)
Cranial nerves, 34–40
   abducens nerve (cranial nerve VI), 34, 35
   acoustic nerve (cranial nerve VIII), 34, 37, 513
   damage, flaccid dysarthria caused by, 406–407
   facial nerve (cranial nerve VII), 16, 24, 34, 37, 38, 275
   functions, 34
   glossopharyngeal nerve (cranial nerve IX), 34, 37–39
   hypoglossal nerve (cranial nerve XII), 24, 34, 40, 41
   motor nerves, 34
   nuclei, 44
   oculomotor nerve (cranial nerve III), 34, 35
   olfactory nerve (cranial nerve I), 34, 35
   optic nerve (cranial nerve II), 34, 35
   peripheral nervous system, 33–43
   sensory nerves, 34
   spinal accessory nerve (cranial nerve XI), 19, 34, 40, 41
   structure, 34
   trigeminal nerve (cranial nerve V), 24, 34, 35, 36, 37
   trochlear nerve (cranial nerve IV), 34, 35
   vagus nerve (cranial nerve X)
      functions, 34, 39–40
      neuroanatomy, 16
      structure, 19, 39–40
      vocal anatomy and physiology, 275
   vocal mechanism, 16
Craniocerebral trauma. *See* Traumatic brain injury (TBI)
Craniofacial anomalies, 431–443
   cleft lip, 431–432
   cleft palate, 432–443
Craniosynostosis, 445
Creutzfeldt-Jakob disease, 368, 370–371
Cricoarytenoid joint, 277, 278
Cricoid cartilage, 10, 277
Cricopharyngeal myotomy, 423
Cricothyroid artery, 275
Cricothyroid muscle, 11, 12
Cri du chat syndrome, 445
Criteria, defined, 580
Criterion-referenced assessment, 163, 576
Criterion validity, 599
Criterion variable, 609
Crossed aphasia (CA), 348
Cross-sectional research, 611
Crouzon syndrome, 445
CRS-R. *See* Coma Recovery Scale-Revised (CRS-R)
CSG system, 91
CTOPP-2. *See* Comprehensive Test of Phonological Processing Skills–Second Edition (CTOPP-2)
Cubitus valgus, 450
Cued speech, 549–550
Cul-de-sac resonance, 296–297
Culture
   acculturation, 463
   assessment and treatment considerations, 589–590
   assimilation, 463
   bicultural immigrants, 463
   cultural competence, 462
   culturally and linguistically diverse (CLD) people. *See* Multicultural population communication disorders
   cultural sensitivity, 462
   defined, 462
   pragmatics and, 109
   stereotyping, 462
   variables influencing individual behavior, 462–463
Cuneiform cartilage, 10, 278
CVA. *See* Cerebrovascular accident (CVA)
Cycles of vibration, 93, 515
Cysts, 306–307
Cytomegalovirus as cause of hearing loss, 527

D

DAF. *See* Delayed auditory feedback (DAF), for stuttering treatment
DAS. *See* Developmental apraxia of speech (DAS)

Data
- defined, 599
- organization and analysis, 618–621
  - basic concepts, 618–619
  - measurement scales, 620–621
  - statistical techniques, 619–620
- qualitative, 599
- quantitative, 599
- reliability of, 599
- validity of, 599

Deaf, defined, 520
Deaffrication, 204
Deceleration, 93
Decibel (dB), 91, 94, 517
Deciduous teeth, 24
Declarative sentence, 105
Deductive method of research, 598
Deep Test of Articulation, 224
Deficiencies, language disorders, 144
Definitions
- acoustics, 90–92
- experimental research, 601–602
- phonetics, 73–74
- reinforcement, 583–584
- reinforcers, 584–585
- stuttering, 238–239
- treatment terms, 579–583

Deglution disorders. *See* Swallowing disorders (dysphagia)
Degree of treatment structure, 587
Delayed auditory feedback (DAF), for stuttering treatment, 257–258
Delayed echolalia, 152
Delayed hard palate closure surgery, 441
Deletions, 207
Demands and capacities model of stuttering, 251
Dementia, 360–374
- assessment, 372–373
- classification of, 361
- clinical management of, 373–374
- defined, 361
- Dementia of the Alzheimer Type, 361–363
- frontotemporal, 363–366
- Huntington's disease, 367–368
- infectious dementia, 368, 370–371
- Lewy body dementia, 371
- mild cognitive impairment, 361
- multiple cerebrovascular accidents, 371
- Parkinson's disease, 366–367
- Pick's disease, 363
- primary progressive aphasia, 363, 364–366
- traumatic brain injury, 371
- vascular dementia, 371
- Wernicke-Korsakoff syndrome, 371

DEMSS. *See* Dynamic Evaluation of Motor Speech Skill (DEMSS)

Denasality, 296
Dendrites, 31
Density, 91
Density of matter, 91
Dental deviations, 208
Dental malocclusion, 208
Depalatization, 204
Dependent clause, 106
Dependent variable (effect), 601, 602
Depressor anguli oris (triangularis) muscle, 28, 37
Depressor labii inferioris muscle, 28, 37
Depressors (infrahyoid muscles), 12, 13, 24, 279
Derivational morpheme, 104
Descriptive phonetics, 74
Determinism, 598
Developmental apraxia of speech (DAS), 210
Developmental history, 563
Developmental inventories, 573
Developmental (normative) research, 610–611
Developmental Sentence Scoring (DSS), 165
Development of language. *See* Language development in children
Devoicing, 207
Diabetes, and stroke, 492
Diacritical marks (diacritics), 75, 77
Diadochokinetic rate, 208
Diadochokinetic test, 396
Diagnosis, defined, 561
Diagnostic and Statistical Manual of Mental Disorders–Fifth Edition (DSM-V)
- ADHD characteristics, 160
- autism spectrum disorders, 151
- language disorder, defined, 143

Dialogic reading, 178–179
Diaphragm, 3, 6, 7
Diaphragmatic–abdominal breathing, 293
Diary studies, 197
Dichotic listening tasks, 529
Diencephalon, 49
Differential reinforcement, 583
Differential reinforcement of alternative behaviors (DRA), 584
Differential reinforcement of incompatible behaviors (DRI), 584
Differential reinforcement of low rates of responding (DRL), 584
Differential reinforcement of other behaviors (DRO), 584
Diffuse polyposis. *See* Reinke's edema
Digastric muscle, 12, 13, 24, 37
DiGeorge sequence, 451
Digital devices used for treatment, 359
Digital hearing aid, 543, 544
Diminutization, 204

Diphthongs, 87, 197
Diplegia, and cerebral palsy, 155
Diplophonia, 284, 306
Direct laryngoscopy, 286
Direct methods of response reduction, 580, 581
Direct selection for augmentative and alternative communication, 182
Direct speech acts or requests, 108
Direct stuttering reduction treatment, 258–259
Disability Rating Scale (DRS), 382
Disability *vs.* handicap, 644
Disconnection syndromes, 61
Discourse, 108
- comprehension
  - assessment, 352
  - treatment, 355
- skills, assessment, 352
Discrete trials, 580
- procedure, 176–177
Disorders. *See* Autism spectrum disorder (ASD); Communicative disorders; Impairments; Language disorders; Multicultural population communication disorders; Organically based disorders; Speech sound disorders (SSDs); Swallowing disorders (dysphagia)
Displacement, 91
Displays for augmentative and alternative communication, 182
Distinctive feature analysis, 79
Distinctive features paradigm, 197
Distributions of test scores, 571
Dodd, B., 226
Dominant hemisphere hypothesis for stuttering, 251
Dopamine, 31, 50
Dorsum of the tongue, 26
Double voice. *See* Diplophonia
Down syndrome
- cause of, 150, 445
- characteristics, 446
- stuttering prevalence and, 244
DRA. *See* Differential reinforcement of alternative behaviors (DRA)
DRI. *See* Differential reinforcement of incompatible behaviors (DRI)
DRL. *See* Differential reinforcement of low rates of responding (DRL)
DRO. *See* Differential reinforcement of other behaviors (DRO)
DRS. *See* Disability Rating Scale (DRS)
Drug abuse
- as cause of strokes, 492
- language problems related to, 159–160
Drug treatment, for aphasia, 359
Dry spirometers, 290

DSM-V. *See* Diagnostic and Statistical Manual of Mental Disorders–Fifth Edition (DSM-V)
DSS. *See* Developmental Sentence Scoring (DSS)
DTTC. *See* Dynamic Temporal and Tactile Cueing (DTTC)
Dual diathesis stressor model of stuttering, 251
Dual Iceberg Model of specific language impairment, 146
Dura mater, 62
Dynamic assessment, 163, 486–487, 577
Dynamic Evaluation of Motor Speech Skill (DEMSS), 211
Dynamic Temporal and Tactile Cueing (DTTC), 212
Dyne, 91, 94
Dysarthria, 50, 398–416
   assessment, 412–414
   ataxic dysarthria, 399, 404–405
   cerebral palsy and, 155
   characteristics, 210
   communicative disorders of, 403–404
   defined, 210, 398, 403
   differentiating apraxia of speech from, 412
   flaccid dysarthria, 399–400, 405–408
     caused by cranial nerve damage, 406–407
   hyperkinetic dysarthria, 400, 408–409
   hypokinetic dysarthria, 401, 409–410
   mixed dysarthrias, 411
   neuropathology of, 403
   spastic dysarthria, 410–411
   treatment, 210, 414–416
   types of, 399–402
   unilateral upper motor neuron dysarthria, 402, 411–412
Dysfluency
   broken words, 240
   defined, 237
   definition of stuttering, 239
   incomplete sentences, 240
   interjections, 240
   pauses, 240
   prolongations, 239–240
   repetitions, 239
   revisions, 240
   theoretical and clinical significance of, 240–241
Dyskinesias, 50
   Dyslexia, 359
     Dysmetria, and ataxic dysarthria, 404
       Dysphagia. *See* Swallowing disorders (dysphagia)

E

Eardrum (tympanic membrane), 435, 436, 508
Ear training, for hypernasality treatment, 297
Ebonics. *See* African American English (AAE)
Echolalia, 150
Ecological validity of formal tests, 483
Economics
   poverty, language problems related to, 156–158
   socioeconomics. *See* Socioeconomic status (SES)
Education
   case history, 564
   and culture, 463
   educator of the deaf, 542
   language problems and, 157
   records of multicultural students, 486
   special education, 644
Eucation of the Handicapped Act, 643
Effect (dependent variable), 601, 602
Efferent nerves, 34
Efferent neurons. *See* Motor neurons
Effortful swallow, 423
EGG. *See* Electroglottography (EGG)
Elasticity, 91
Electrocochleography, 534
Electroglottography (EGG), 289
Electrolarynx, 302
Electropalatography (EPG), 442–443
Electrophysiological audiometry, 534
Elementary-age children
   articulation development, 201, 202
   assessment of, 169–171
     guidelines and procedures, 169–171
     language disorder description, 169
     response to intervention, 171
     standardized tests, 171
   cognitive development, 129
   hearing loss assessment, 535
   language assessment, 162
   language development and education, 124
   language impairments, 489–490
   morphology
     5–6 years, 121
     6–7 years, 122
     7–8 years, 123
   pragmatics
     5–6 years, 121–122
     6–7 years, 123
     7–8 years, 123–124
   semantics
     5–6 years, 121
     6–7 years, 122
     7–8 years, 123
   stuttering in, 248
     treatment, 259
   syntax
     5–6 years, 120
     6–7 years, 122
     7–8 years, 123
   voice changes, 281
Elevators (suprahyoid muscles), 12, 13, 24, 280
Elfin-face syndrome, 452
Embolus, 338
Emergent literacy skills, 124
Emotional control deficits, 148
Emotions, and stuttering, 247
Empiricism, 597–598
Employment legislation, 645
Empty speech, 340
Endolymph, 512
Endoscopy, with videostroboscopy, 286–287
English Language Arts Common Core State Standards, 124
English learners (ELs). *See* Multicultural population communication disorders
Environmental factors of clefts, 434
Ependymal cells, 30
Epenthesis, 204
EPG. *See* Electropalatography (EPG)
Epiglottis, 10, 274, 275, 277, 278
Episodic paroxysmal laryngospasm, 317
Epithelium, 13
Epithelium lamina propria, 15, 274
Escape behavior, 579, 580
Esophageal phase and its disorders (swallow), 418–419
   treatment, 421
Esophageal speech, 302
Esophagostomy, 424
ESSA. *See* Every Student Succeeds Act (ESSA)
Estill voice training model, 326
Estrogen, 328
Ethnocultural status and stuttering prevalence, 244
Ethnographic research, 612
Ethnolinguistic theory, 466
Etiology
   clefts, 433–434
   hearing loss, 519–531
   of stuttering, 261–262
   swallowing disorders, 416–417
Eustachian tube, 508, 511
   dysfunction, 436
Evaluation. *See* Assessment
Every Student Succeeds Act (ESSA), 482, 645
Evidence-based practice, 561–590
   authentic assessment, 576–577
   client-specific assessment, 575–576

communication disorder treatment, 578–585
   paradigm, 579
   reinforcement, 583–584
   reinforcers, 584–585
   terms, 579–583
   treatment, defined, 578–579
comprehensive and integrated assessment, 577–578
criterion-referenced assessment, 576
cultural-linguistic considerations, 589–590
   need for individualized assessment and treatment, 590
developmental inventories, 573
dynamic assessment, 577
functional assessment, 574–575
levels of evidence, 616–618
overview, 561–562
procedures, 562–568
   case history, 563–564
   hearing screening, 565
   interview, 565
   obtaining related assessment data, 567–568
   orofacial examination, 565
   screening, 562–563
   speech and language sample, 566–567
questionnaires and interviews, 573
rating scales, 573
standardized assessment, 568–572
   limitations of standardized tests, 569–570
   nature and advantages of standardized assessment, 568–569
   prudent use of standardized tests, 570–571
   standardized test, defined, 568
   types of scores, 571–572
   validity and reliability of, 572
treatment process, 585–588
   booster treatment, 588
   follow-up, 588
   maintenance program, 587
   treatment sequence, 586–587
   treatment targets, selection of, 585–586
treatment program outline, 588–589
Evoked response, 580
Evoked speech samples for assessment, 216
Evoked trial, 580, 582
Exclamatory sentence, 105
Executive functioning
   attention-deficit/hyperactivity disorder, 160
   deficits of SLI, 148–149
   defined, 148
   targeting treatment, 181

Exemplars, 224, 580
Exhalation, 1, 2
Exner's writing area, 359
Expanded utterances, 356–557
Expansion, 177
Expansion stage of sound development, 200
Experimental design, 602
Experimental group, 602
Experimental phonetics, 74
Experimental research, 601–608
   definition of terms, 601–602
   experiment, defined, 601
   group designs, 602–604
   single-subject designs, 604–608
Ex post facto (retrospective) research, 609–610
Expressive language delay, and abuse, 158
Extension, 177
External auditory canal/external auditory meatus, 508
External carotid artery, 65
External intercostals, 6, 7
External otitis, 521
External validity, 615–616
Extinction, 580
Extracerebral ruptures, 338
Extraneous variables, 601
Extrapyramidal system, 50, 57, 60
Extrinsic laryngeal muscles, 12–13, 14, 279–280
Extrinsic tongue muscles, 26, 27
Eye contact used for language development, 110

F

Face muscles, 27–29
Facial nerve (cranial nerve VII), 16, 24, 34, 37, 38, 275
   damage, and flaccid dysarthria, 406
Facial structure embryonic growth, 433
FACS. *See* Functional Assessment of Communication Skills for Adults (FACS)
FACT. *See* Functional Auditory Comprehension Task (FACT)
Fading, 580
FAE. *See* Fetal alcohol effects (FAE)
Faithfulness constraints, 199
Falsetto, 322
False vocal folds, 13, 274
Family
   case history, 563
   dementia and, 374
   and rehabilitation, 493
   stuttering and, 249–250
      prevalence, 243
      treatment, 260

Fasciculus, 60
FASD. *See* Fetal alcohol spectrum disorder (FASD)
Fast mapping, 107
FDA-2. *See* Frenchay Dysarthria Assessment–Second Edition (FDA-2)
Feedback, 581
Feeding disorders, 417
FEES. *See* Flexible Endoscopic Evaluation of Swallowing (FEES)
Fetal alcohol effects (FAE), 159
Fetal alcohol spectrum disorder (FASD), 159
Fetal alcohol syndrome, 150
Fibers in the brain, 61
Filum terminale, 43
FIM. *See* Functional Independence Measure (FIM)
Final-consonant deletion, 204
Final-position errors, 207
Fingerspelling, 552
Fissure of Rolando (central sulcus), 51
Fissures, 51
Flaccid dysarthria, 399–400, 405–408
   caused by cranial nerve damage, 406–407
   flaccid–spastic dysarthria, 411
Flexible Endoscopic Evaluation of Swallowing (FEES), 420
Flexible endoscopy with videostroboscopy, 286–287
Fluency. *See also* Dysfluency; Neurogenic stuttering (NS)
   aphasia. *See* Aphasia
   characteristics, 237
   cluttering. *See* Cluttering
   description of, 238–239
   disorders, 237
   fluency reinforcement stuttering treatment, 257
   fluency shaping stuttering treatment (speak-more-fluently), 256–257
   fluent stuttering treatment method (stutter-more-fluently), 255–256
   hearing impairment and, 541
   neurogenic stuttering, 237
   stuttering. *See* Stuttering
Fluent aphasia, 344–348
   anomic aphasia, 347–348
   conduction aphasia, 346–347
   transcortical sensory aphasia, 345–346
   Wernicke's aphasia, 344–345
FM system, 549
Focused stimulation, 177
Focusing for hyponasality treatment, 298
Follow-up, 581, 588
Foramen magnum, 47

Foramina, 34
Force, 91
Formal operations, cognitive development, 130
Formant frequency, 91
Fourth ventricle, 61
Fragile X syndrome, 446
Free morpheme, 104
Frenchay Dysarthria Assessment–Second Edition (FDA–2), 414
Frequency
    acoustics, 517
    defined, 91, 93, 515
    formant, 91
    fundamental, 91, 95, 282
    mean fundamental frequency, 280–281
    natural, 91
    phonation, 93–94
Frequency perturbation (jitter), 283
Fricatives, 82, 207
Friedreich's ataxia, 411
Frontalis muscle, 37
Frontal lisp, 207
Frontal lobe, 52, 53–54
Fronting, 207
Frontonasal process, 433
Frontotemporal dementia (FTD), 363–366
    behavioral variant of, 363, 364
    Pick's disease, 363
    primary progressive aphasia, 363, 364–366
Frontotemporal lobar degeneration. *See* Frontotemporal dementia (FTD)
Front vowels, 84, 86
FTD. *See* Frontotemporal dementia (FTD)
Functional articulation disorder, 205
Functional assessment, 574–575
Functional Assessment of Communication Skills for Adults (FACS), 350
Functional Auditory Comprehension Task (FACT), 351
Functional Communication Profile–Revised, 373
Functional communication skills assessment, 352
Functional communication treatment strategy, 586
Functional Independence Measure (FIM), 350
Functional Linguistic Communication Inventory, 372
Functional outcomes, 581
Function words, 150, 340
    and stuttering, 248
Fundamental frequency, 91, 95, 282

G

GA. *See* Global aphasia (GA)
Galveston Orientation and Amnesia Test (GOAT), 382
Games for language development, 110
Gargoylism, 446–447
Gastroesophageal reflux disease (GERD), 316
Gastrostomy, 424
Gastrostomy tube (G-tube), 448
Gates-MacGinitie Reading Test (GMRT), 351
Gender
    as factor in speech sound disorders, 206
    stuttering prevalence and, 242
    transgender voice issues, 327–328
Generality of treatment, 581
Generalizability, 615
Generalization of stuttering treatment, 260
Generalized production, 581
General neuronal atrophy, and dementia, 362
Generative phonology theory of development, 198
Genetics
    clefts, 434
    hypothesis for stuttering, 250
    syndromes, 150, 444–452
        Angelman syndrome, 444
        Apert syndrome, 444–445
        Cri du chat syndrome, 445
        Crouzon syndrome, 445
        defined, 444
        Down syndrome, 445–446
        Fragile X syndrome, 446
        Hurler's syndrome, 446–447
        Landau-Kleffner syndrome, 447
        Marfan syndrome, 447
        Moebius syndrome, 447–448
        Pierre-Robin syndrome, 448
        Prader-Willi syndrome, 448–449
        Russell-Silver syndrome, 449
        Tourette syndrome, 449–450
        Treacher Collins syndrome, 450
        Trisomy 13, 450
        Turner syndrome, 451
        Usher syndrome, 451
        velocardiofacial syndrome, 451–452
        Williams syndrome, 452
Genioglossus muscle, 12, 13, 27
Geniohyoid muscle, 12, 13, 24
GERD. *See* Gastroesophageal reflux disease (GERD)
Geriatric voice, 281–282
German measles as cause of hearing loss, 526

Gestural-assisted (aided) augmentative and alternative communication, 183–184
Gestural (unaided) augmentative and alternative communication, 183
Gestures, assessment, 353
Glasgow Coma Scale, 382
Glial cells, 30
Glides
    defined, 83
    onglide, 83
    substitution processes, 204
Global aphasia (GA), 343–344
Global Deterioration Scale, 372
Global Disability Action Plan, 491
Globus pallidus, 50
Glossopharyngeal nerve (cranial nerve IX), 34, 37–39
    damage, and flaccid dysarthria, 406
Glossoptosis, 448
Glottal articulation
    place-voice-manner analysis, 81
    replacement, 204
Glottal fry, 284
Glottis, 12, 274
GMRT. *See Gates-MacGinitie Reading Test* (GMRT)
GOAT. *See Galveston Orientation and Amnesia Test* (GOAT)
Government binding theory, 127
Grade-equivalency scores, standardized test, 572
Graduate Record Examination (GRE), 599
Grammar, deficient, 144
Grammatical morpheme, 104
Granuloma, 307
Granulovacuolar degeneration, and dementia, 362
Gray matter, 51. *See also* Brainstem
GRE. *See* Graduate Record Examination (GRE)
Group designs, 602–604
    advantages and disadvantages of, 604
    control group, 602
    experimental group, 602
    multigroup pretest–posttest design, 604
    pretest–posttest control group design, 603
Group treatment for aphasia, 358
G-tube. *See* Gastrostomy tube (G-tube)
Gyrus, 51

H

Handicap *vs.* disability, 644
Hard glottal attack, 326
Hard palate, 22–23

Harmonics, 95
Harshness, vocal quality, 284
Hawthorne effect, 615
HD. *See* Huntington's disease (HD)
Health care
  Affordable Health Care Act, 646
  Health Insurance Marketplace, 646
  legislation affecting health care settings, 646–648
  limited access and language development, 157
Health Insurance Marketplace, 646
Health Insurance Portability and Accountability Act (HIPAA), 647–648
Hearing
  acoustics, 515–518
    frequency and intensity, 517
    sound pressure level and hearing level, 518
    sound waves, 516–517
    source of sound, 515–516
  anatomy and physiology, 508–514
    auditory nervous system, 513–514
    inner ear, 511–513
    middle ear, 508–511
    outer ear, 508
Hearing aids, 542–545
Hearing impairment, 519–552. *See also* Audiology
  air and bone conduction of sound, 519
  assessment, 531–538
    acoustic immitance, 533
    audiometry, 531–532
    electrophysiological audiometry, 534
    hearing screening, 534–535
    infants and children, 535
    interpretation of test results, 535–538
    medical imaging, 534
    pure-tone audiometry, 532
    screening, 565
    speech audiometry, 533
  assessment result interpretation, 535–538
    audiograms, 536, 537–538
    bilateral losses, 536
    conductive hearing loss, 536, 537
    levels of hearing loss, 536
    mixed hearing loss, 536, 538
    noise-induced hearing loss, 536, 538
    sensorineural loss, 536, 537
    unilateral losses, 536
  auditory development, 519
  auditory nervous system impairments, 528–531
  clefts and, 435–436
  conductive hearing loss, 520–524
  deaf, 520
  defined, 520
  hard of hearing, 520
  management of, 539–552
    amplification, 542–547
    aural rehabilitation, 541–542
    communication disorders, 539–541
    communication training, 547–552
    language disorders, 540
    speech disorders, 540
    voice, fluency, and resonance disorders, 541
  mixed hearing loss, 528
  nature of, 520
  normal hearing, 519
  range and categories of, 521
  sensorineural hearing loss, 525–528
Hearing level (HL), 94, 518
Hearing loss. *See also* Hearing impairment
  and speech sound disorders, 209–210
  and stuttering, 244
Hearing screening, 215
Helm Elicited Language Program for Syntax Stimulation, 357
Hemangioma, 307–308
Hemilaryngectomy, 300
Hemiplegia, and cerebral palsy, 155
Hemorrhagic strokes, 338–339
Herpes simplex as cause of hearing loss, 527
Hertz (Hz), 93, 517
Heschl's gyri, 55
High-amplitude sucking paradigm, 199
High-technology devices for augmentative and alternative communication, 182
High vowels, 84
HIPPA. *See* Health Insurance Portability and Accountability Act (HIPAA)
Hippocampus, 56
Hispanics. *See also* Spanish-influenced English
  articulation differences, 468, 472
  background, 468
  characteristics, 468, 472–473
  language differences, 473
  medical conditions and communication disorders, 490
  and rehabilitation, 493
History. *See* Case history
HIV. *See* Human immunodeficiency virus (HIV)
HL. *See* Hearing level (HL)
Hoarseness, vocal quality, 283
Hodson and Paden's cycles treatment approach, 226
Holophrastic speech, 112, 113
Holoprosencephaly, 450
Hormonal therapy, 328

Human immunodeficiency virus (HIV)
  encephalopathy, 368
  infectious dementia, 368
Huntington's disease (HD), 367–368, 369–370
Hurler's syndrome, 446–447
Hyoglossus muscle, 12, 13, 27
Hyoid bone
  structure, 9
  vocal anatomy and physiology, 275, 277
Hyperfunctional voice disorders, 303
Hyperkeratosis, 311
Hyperkinetic dysarthria, 400, 408–409
Hypernasality
  causes of, 295
  defined, 295
  resonance assessment, 293
  treatment, 297–298
Hypertension, 338
  and strokes, 492
Hypodontia, 435
Hypofunctional voice disorders, 303–304
Hypoglossal nerve (cranial nerve XII), 24, 34, 40, 41
  damage, and flaccid dysarthria, 407
Hypokinetic dysarthria, 401, 409–410
Hyponasality
  causes of, 296
  defined, 296
  resonance assessment, 293
  treatment, 298
Hypothalamus, 49
Hypothesis. *See also* Theory
  alternative, 598
  defined, 598
  null, 598
Hypotonia, 405, 449
Hysterical aphonia, 321–322

I

ICF-CY. *See International Classification of Functioning, Disability, and Health–Children and Youth* (ICF-CY)
Iconic symbols for augmentative and alternative communication, 182
IDEA. *See* Individuals with Disabilities Education Act (IDEA) of 1990
IEP. *See* Individualized Education Program (IEP)
IFSP. *See* Individualized Family Service Plans (IFSPs)
Illocutionary behavior, 112
Imitation
  defined, 581
  evoked speech samples, 216
Immediate echolalia, 150
Immigrants, 463

Impairments. *See* Disorders; Hearing impairment; Language disorders; Specific language impairment (SLI)
Impedance, 91
    acoustic, 533
Impedance bridge, 533
Impedance meter, 533
Imperative sentence, 105
Incidence
    aphasia, 337–340
    culturally and linguistically diverse clients, 490–491
    defined, 490
    stuttering
        defined, 241
        in general population, 241–242
    traumatic brain injury, 379–380
Incidental teaching, 178
Incisors, 22
Incomplete sentences, 240
Inconsistent speech sound disorder (ISSD), 226
Incus, 511
Independent analysis of assessment data, 217
Independent clause, 105, 106
Independent variable, 601, 602
Indirect laryngoscopy, 286
Indirect methods of response reduction, 580, 581
Indirect speech acts or requests, 108
Individualized assessment, 575
Individualized Education Program (IEP), 581, 643
Individualized Family Service Plans (IFSPs), 581, 643, 645
Individuals with Disabilities Education Act (IDEA) of 1990, 166, 644–645
Individuals with Disabilities Education Improvement Act of 2004, 482, 644
Indole-3-carbinol, for papilloma, 314
Inductive method of research, 598
Infants. *See also* Preschoolers; Toddlers
    articulatory and phonological skills
        development, 199–200
        perception, 199–200
        production, 200
    assessment of, 164–169
        guidelines and procedures, 167
        infant–caregiver interaction, 168
        language comprehension, 168
        language-related skills, 168
        late talkers, 167
        play activities, 168–169
        prelinguistic behavioral deficiencies, 166–167
        risk factors for language disorders, 166
        verbal communication, 168
    bilinguality, 480

cognitive development, 129
hearing loss assessment, 535
language developmental milestones, 112–114, 115
pragmatics, 113
semantics, 113, 115
syntax, 112–113
voice changes, 280
Infectious dementia, 368, 370–371
Inference, 618–619
Inferior cerebellar peduncles, 50
Inferior cornua, 10, 275
Inferior laryngeal artery, 275
Inferior longitudinal muscle, 27
Inferior peduncles, 47, 50
Inferior pharyngeal constrictor
    cricopharyngeus muscle, 20
    thyropharyngeus muscle, 20
Inferior (lower) temporal gyrus, 55
Inflectional morpheme, 104–105
Information processing. *See* Working memory
Information-processing theory of language development, 128, 130–131
Informative feedback, 581
Infrahyoid muscle (depressors), 12, 13, 24, 279
Inhalation, 1, 2
Inhalation method of esophageal speech, 302
Inhalation phonation, 326
Initial-position errors, 207
Initial response, 581
Injection method of esophageal speech, 302
Inner ear, 511–513
Innermost intercostal, 7
Inspiration, 6–7
Instructional discourse, in classrooms, 176
Instrumentation, and internal validity, 613
Intact repetition skill, 342
Integrated implicit–explicit approach to voice training, 325–326
Integrated treatment approach, 586
Intellectual disability
    causes of, 150
    characteristics, 149–151
    defined, 149
    stuttering prevalence and, 244
Intelligence as factor in speech sound disorders, 206
Intelligibility, 201–203
Intensity of sound, 89, 90, 517
Intensity threshold, 532
Interaction of threat factors, and internal validity, 615
Interarytenoid muscle, 277, 278
Intercostal muscles, 6

Interdisciplinary teams, 568
Interference, and second-language acquisition, 478
Interhemispheric fibers, 60
Interjections, 240
Interjudge reliability, 600
Intermediate response, 581
Intermittent reinforcement, 583
Intermixed probes, 581, 582
Internal auditory meatus, 514
Internal capsule, 48, 60
Internal carotid artery, 65
Internal intercostals, 6, 7
Internal oblique abdominis, 8
Internal thyroarytenoid, 11
Internal validity of research, 613–615
International Classification of Functioning, Disability, and Health–Children and Youth (ICF-CY), 195
Internationally adopted children, second-language acquisition of, 478–479
International Phonetic Alphabet (IPA), 75, 76, 218
Interneurons, 31, 33
Interobserver reliability, 600
Interpreters for assessment of EL students, 487–488
Interrogative sentence, 105
Interval scale, 621
Intervention for children in poverty to enrich language skills, 157–158
Interviews, 565, 573, 610
Intervocalic errors, 208
In-the-canal hearing aids, 543
In-the-ear hearing aids, 543
Intracerebral ruptures, 338
Intrahemispheric fibers, 60
Intrajudge reliability, 600
Intralexical pauses, 240
Intraobserver reliability, 600
Intrinsic laryngeal muscles, 11–12, 13, 278–279
Intrinsic tongue muscles, 26–27
Involuntary movement disorders, 60
Iowa Pressure Articulation Test, 439
IPA. *See* International Phonetic Alphabet (IPA)
iPad, 175, 182, 423
Ipsilateral pathways, 514
Ischemic core, 338, 339
Ischemic infarct, 338, 339
Ischemic penumbra, 338
Ischemic strokes, 338, 339
Isolation and language skill development delays, 158
ISSD. *See* Inconsistent speech sound disorder (ISSD)
Iteration, and stuttering, 245

J

Jitter (frequency perturbation), 283
Joint book reading, 178–179
Joint reference, 112
Juncture (vocal punctuation), 89
Juvenile papillomas, 313

K

Kanner, Leo, 151

L

Labeling, 108
Labialization, 207
Labial muscles, 37
Labiodentals, 81
Labyrinths, 511
LAD. *See* Language acquisition device (LAD); Language and Academic Development Credential (LAD)
Laminae, 10
Lamina propria, 13, 274
Landau-Kleffner syndrome (LKS), 447
Language
　automatic, 340
　Basic Interpersonal Communication Skills, 479–481
　Cognitive Academic Language Proficiency, 479–481
　context, 108
　defined, 73, 103, 143, 196, 476
　development. *See* Language development in children
　differences *vs.* impairments, 476–477
　functions, 103, 108
　loss, 478
　preserved, 340
　sampling, 164–166
　second-language acquisition, 477–479
　spoken within a culture, 463
Language acquisition device (LAD), 126
Language and Academic Development Credential (LAD), 642
Language Assessment, Remediation, and Screening Procedure (LARSP), 165
Language comprehension assessment
　elementary-age children, 170–171
　infants and toddlers, 168
Language development in children, 103–132
　developmental milestones, 109–125
　　birth–1 year, 110–112
　　1–2 years, 112–114, 115
　　2–3 years, 114–117
　　3–4 years, 117–119
　　4–5 years, 119–120
　　5–6 years, 120–122
　　6–7 years, 122–123
　　7–8 years, 123–124
　　caregiver roles, 109–110
　　literacy development, 124
　　school-age education, 124
　as factor in speech sound disorders, 206
　morphology, 103–105
　pragmatics, 108–109
　semantics, 106–107
　syntax, 105–106
　theories, 125–132
　　behavioral theory, 125–126
　　cognitive theory, 127–128, 129–130
　　information-processing theory, 128, 130–131
　　nativist theory, 126–127
　　social interactionism theory, 131–132
　variables, 109
Language disorders, 143–184
　assessment, 162–174
　　adolescents, 171–174
　　alternative assessment, 163–164
　　elementary-age children, 169–171
　　general principles and procedures, 162–166
　　infants and toddlers, 164–169
　　language sampling, 164–166
　　preschool children, 169–171
　　screening, 162–163
　　standardized assessment, 163
　attention-deficit/hyperactivity disorder, 160–162
　characteristics
　　cognitive processing/executive functioning deficits, 148–149
　　subtle brain abnormalities, 146
　clefts and, 437, 439, 443
　culturally and linguistically diverse clients, 489–490
　description of, 144
　DSM-V definition, 143
　hearing impairment and, 540
　infants and toddlers, 164–169
　kinds of deficiencies, 144
　language differences *vs.*, 476–477
　multicultural populations. *See* Multicultural population communication disorders
　physical and sensory disabilities, 149–156
　　autism spectrum disorders, 151–153
　　brain injury, 153–156
　　cerebral palsy, 155–156
　　intellectual disability, 149–151
　　traumatic brain injury, 153–154
　risk factors, 144–145
　service delivery models, 489–490
　SLI characteristics, 145–149
　　generally, 145–146
　　speech and language deficits, 146–148
　　subtle brain abnormalities, 146
　social-environmental factors, 156–160
　　neglect and abuse, 158–159
　　parental drug and alcohol abuse, 159–160
　　poverty, 156–158
　treatment, 174–184
　　augmentative and alternative communication, 181–184
　　cognitive processing skills, 181
　　discrete trial procedure, 176–177
　　executive functioning skills, 181
　　expansion, 177
　　extension, 177
　　focused stimulation, 177
　　general principles, 174–176
　　gestural (unaided) AAC, 183
　　gestural-assisted (aided) AAC, 183–184
　　joint book reading (dialogic reading), 178–179
　　milieu teaching, 177–178
　　narrative skills training, 179
　　neuro-assisted (aided) AAC, 184
　　parallel talk, 179
　　recasting, 180
　　self-talk, 180
　　teaching literacy skills, 180–181
　　working with interpreters, 487–488
Language Sampling, Analysis, and Training procedure (LSAT), 165
LARSP. *See Language Assessment, Remediation, and Screening Procedure* (LARSP)
Laryngeal disorders, and clefts, 437
Laryngeal dysfunction hypothesis for stuttering, 250
Laryngeal dyskinesia, 317
Laryngeal electromyography (LEMG), 289
Laryngeal keel, 315
Laryngeal trauma, 315
Laryngeal web, 314–315
Laryngectomy, 299–304
Laryngitis, 308
Laryngomalacia, 312
Laryngopharyngeal reflux, 316
Laryngopharynx, 19
Larynx (voice box), 2, 8–9
　anatomy and physiology, 273–280
　　structures and cartilages, 275–280
　　vocal folds, 273–275
　defined, 273

extrinsic muscles, 12–13, 14
   functions, 273
   intrinsic muscles, 11–12, 13
   structures and cartilages, 9–10
Lateral articulation, 84
Lateral cerebral fissure (Sylvian fissure), 51
Lateral cricoarytenoid, 11, 12, 277, 278
Lateral lisp, 207
Lateral (external) pterygoid muscle, 24
Lateral ventricles, 61
Late talkers, 167
Latinos. *See* Hispanics
Latissimus dorsi, 8
L-dopa (levodopa) for Parkinson's treatment, 321
Leading-edge hypothesis of stuttering, 251
Lee Silverman Voice Treatment (LSVT), 321, 416
Left hemisphere (LH), 375
Left inferior frontal gyrus. *See* Broca's area
Left neglect, 376
Legislation. *See* Regulations
LEMG. *See* Laryngeal electromyography (LEMG)
Length of vowels and consonants, 88
Lessac-Madsen Resonant Voice Therapy (LMRVT), 324
Leukoplakia, 311–312
Levator anguli oris muscle, 28
Levator costarum brevis muscles, 6, 7
Levator costarum longis muscles, 6, 7
Levator labii superioris alaeque nasi muscle, 28
Levator labii superioris muscle, 28
Levator scapulae, 7
Levator veli palatini muscle, 21, 22, 511
Level of measurement, 620
Levels of evidence for evidence-based practice, 616–618
Lewy bodies, 371
Lewy body dementia, 371
Lexicon, 106
LH. *See* Left hemisphere (LH)
Lidcombe Program, 257
Limited bilingualism, 481
Linear phonology theories of development, 199
Line of regard, 110
Linguest 1 computer software, 165
Lingua-alveolars, 80
Linguadentals, 80
Lingual frenulum of tongue, 26, 207
Lingual sweep, 421
Linguapalatals, 80
Linguavelars, 80
Linguistics, defined, 103

Linguistic treatment approaches, 224–226
   assessment and treatment considerations, 589–590
   Hodson and Paden's cycles approach, 226
   minimal pair contrast therapy, 225
   overview, 224–225
   phonological pattern approach, 225–226
   service delivery barriers, 491–492
Lip position for vowels, 85
Lipreading. *See* Speech reading
Lips. *See* Face muscles
Lip surgery for clefts, 440
Liquids, 84
Lisp, 207
Literacy skills
   deficiency, 144
   development, in school-age years, 124
   reading skills, 353, 357
   speech and language treatment, 175
   teaching, 180–181
   writing skills, 353, 357–358
Literal paraphasia, 339
LKS. *See* Landau-Kleffner syndrome (LKS)
LMN. *See* Lower motor neurons (LMNs)
LMRVT. *See* Lessac-Madsen Resonant Voice Therapy (LMRVT)
Loci of stuttering, 247–248
Locutionary stage, 112
Logarithmic scale for measuring sound, 517
Logopenic primary progressive aphasia (lvPPA), 364, 365
Logorrhea, 340, 344
Lombard effect, 327
Longitudinal fiber tracts, 44
Longitudinal fissure, 51
Longitudinal research, 611
Loudness (volume) of sound, 283
   amplitude and, 89, 94
   assessment, 291
   defined, 94
   intensity, 517
Lou Gehrig's disease, 320–321
Lower motor neurons (LMNs), 57, 405
Low-technology devices for augmentative and alternative communication, 182
Low vowels, 84
LSAT. *See Language Sampling, Analysis, and Training* procedure (LSAT)
LSVT. *See* Lee Silverman Voice Treatment (LSVT)
Lumbar vertebrae, 5

Lungs, 3
lvPPA. *See* Logopenic primary progressive aphasia (lvPPA)

M

MAE. *See* Mainstream American English (MAE); *Multilingual Aphasia Examination–Revised Edition* (MAE)
Magnetic resonance imaging (MRI), for hearing impairment assessment, 534
Magnitude, 94
Main clause, 106
Mainstream American English (MAE)
   dialects, 464–465
   influence of dialects and languages, 464
Maintenance of target behaviors, 587
Maintenance program, 587
Maintenance strategy, 581
Malingered stuttering, 265
Malleus, 510–511
Malocclusions, 25, 208
Mandible, 23–24
Mandibular branch, 37
Mandibular marginal branch, 27
Mandibular processes, 433
Manner of articulation, 79, 81–84
Manometric devices, 290
Manual guidance, 581
Manual training approach, 551
Manubrium, 5
Marfan syndrome, 447
Markedness constraints, 199
Marked sounds, 196
Masako maneuver, 422
Masking, 532
   as stuttering treatment, 257–258
Masseter muscle, 24
Mastication (chewing), 24
Matching of groups, 603
Maturation, 614
Maxillary bones, 22
Maxillary branch, 37
Maxillary processes, 433
Maximal contrast therapy, 225
Maximal opposition treatment approach, 225
Maximum phonation time (MPT), 281, 293
McDonald's sensorimotor approach, 223–224
MCI. *See* Mild cognitive impairment (MCI)
Mean fundamental frequency (MFF), 280–281
Meaning of language. *See* Semantics
Mean length of utterance (MLU), 165
Mean of test scores, 571, 620

Measurement
   levels of, 620–621
   scientific, 598
   validity of, 599–600
Measures of association, 619
Measures of central tendency, 620
Measures of correlation, 619
Measures of variability, 619
Mechanical factors of clefts, 434
Medialization laryngoplasty, 319
Medial-position errors, 207
Medial (internal) pterygoid muscle, 24
Median of test scores, 571, 620
Medical history, 564
Medical imaging, 534
Mediums for sound waves, 515
Medulla, 47–48
Medulla oblongata, 1
Memory wallets, 373
Mendelsohn maneuver, 423
Meniere's disease, 527
Meninges, 62, 63
Menstruation, and pitch disorders, 328
Mentalis muscle, 28
Mental retardation. See Intellectual disability
Mesencephalon. See Midbrain
Mestizos, 468
Metalinguistic awareness, 227
Metathesis, 204
Metencephalon. See Pons
MFF. See Mean fundamental frequency (MFF)
Microdontia, 449
Microforms, 435
Microglia, 30
Micrognathia, 451
Microtia, 521
Midbrain, 44, 46
Middle carotid artery, 65
Middle cerebellar peduncles, 50
Middle ear, 508–511
   effusion. See Otitis media with effusion (OME)
   muscles and reflexes, 511
   ossicular chain, 508, 510–511
   tympanic membrane (eardrum), 508
Middle peduncles, 47
Middle pharyngeal constrictor muscle, 20
Middle temporal gyrus, 55
   posterior, 346
Mild cognitive impairment (MCI), 361
Mild traumatic brain injury, 381
Milestones. See Language development in children, developmental milestones
Milieu teaching, 177–178
Mini Inventory of Right Brain Injury–Second Edition (MIRBI-2), 377
Minimal competency core, 576

Minimalist Program, 127
Minimal pair contrast therapy, 225
Minimal pairs, 225
Mini-Mental State Examination–Second Edition, 372, 377
Minnesota Test for Differential Diagnosis of Aphasia (MTDDA), 349
MIRBI-2. See *Mini Inventory of Right Brain Injury–Second Edition* (MIRBI-2)
Mirror laryngoscopy, 286
Mismatch hypotheses for stuttering, 251
Mississippi Aphasia Screening Test, 349
Mixed dementia, 371
Mixed dysarthrias, 411
Mixed hearing loss, 528
Mixed nerves, 34
Mixed transcortical aphasia (MTA), 342–343
MLU. See Mean length of utterance (MLU)
MoCA. See Montreal Cognitive Assessment (MoCA)
Modeled trial, 580, 581
Modeling, 582
Mode of response, 582
Mode of test scores, 620
Moebius syndrome, 447–448
Monoplegia, and cerebral palsy, 155
Montreal Cognitive Assessment (MoCA), 382
   Version 3, 372
Morpheme
   assessment of elementary-age children, 169
   base, 104
   bound, 104
   defined, 103–104
   derivational, 104
   free, 104
   function of, 104
   grammatical, 104
   inflectional, 104–105
   intellectual disability difficulties, 150
   root, 104
   rules for counting, 164
Morphological awareness, 124, 180–181
Morphologic skills, 582
Morphology
   African American English, 466–468, 469
   allomorphs, 104
   assessment of elementary-age children, 170
   defined, 103
   developmental milestones
      2–3 years, 115–116
      3–4 years, 118
      4–5 years, 120
      5–6 years, 121
      6–7 years, 122
      7–8 years, 123

   intellectual disability and, 150
   morphemes, 103–104
   specific language impairment problems, 147
Mortality, and internal validity, 614
Motherese, 110
Motor-based treatment approaches, 222–224
   context utilization approaches, 223–224
   Van Riper's traditional treatment approach, 222–223
Motor behaviors, and stuttering, 237
Motor cortex, 53
Motor fibers, 37
Motor impulses, 33
Motor nerves, 34
Motor neurons, 31, 33, 57
Motor programming disorder, 210
Motor speech area. See Broca's area
Motor speech disorders
   apraxia of speech, 393–398
      assessment, 396–397
      communication deficits, 395–396
      definition and distinctions, 393–394
      differentiating from dysarthria, 412
      neuropathology of, 394
      symptoms, 395
      treatment, 397–398
   dysarthrias, 398–416
      assessment, 412–414
      ataxic dysarthria, 399, 404–405
      communicative disorders of, 403–404
      defined, 398, 403
      differentiating apraxia of speech from, 412
      flaccid dysarthria, 399–400, 405–408
      hyperkinetic dysarthria, 400, 408–409
      hypokinetic dysarthria, 401, 409–410
      mixed dysarthrias, 411
      neuropathology of, 403
      spastic dysarthria, 410–411
      treatment, 414–416
      types of, 399–402
      unilateral upper motor neuron dysarthria, 402, 411–412
Motor strip, 53
Motor units, syllables as, 77
MPT. See Maximum phonation time (MPT)
MRI. See Magnetic resonance imaging (MRI), for hearing impairment assessment
MS. See Multiple sclerosis (MS)

MTA. *See* Mixed transcortical aphasia (MTA)
MTD. *See* Muscle tension dysphonia (MTD)
MTDDA. *See Minnesota Test for Differential Diagnosis of Aphasia* (MTDDA)
Mucosal wave action, 15, 274
Multicultural population communication disorders, 461–494
  ASHA guidelines, 463–464
  assessment
    sociocultural considerations in rehabilitation, 493–494
    working with interpreters, 487–488
  assessment of EL students, 481–488
    alternatives to standardized tests, 485–487
    legal considerations, 482
    standardized tests, 482–485
  Basic Interpersonal Communication Skills (BICS), 479–481
  Cognitive Academic Language Proficiency (CALP), 479–481
  cultural considerations, 462–463
  language differences *vs.* language impairments, 476–477
  second-language acquisition, 477–479
  speech-language characteristics, 464–475
    African American English, 465–468, 469–471
    American English dialects, 464–465
    Asians, 471–475
    Spanish-influenced English, 468, 472–473
  treatment, 488–494
    adults with neurological based disorders, 492–494
    language impairments in children, 489–490
    linguistic barriers to, 491–492
    medical conditions and communication disorders, 490–491
    sociocultural barriers to, 491–492
    sociocultural considerations in rehabilitation, 493–494
Multidisciplinary teams, 568
Multigroup pretest–posttest design, 604
Multilingual Aphasia Examination–Revised Edition (MAE), 353
Multiple-baseline-across-behaviors design, 607
Multiple-baseline-across-settings design, 607
Multiple-baseline-across-subjects design, 607

Multiple cerebrovascular accidents, and dementia, 371
Multiple sclerosis (MS), 320
Multiple-treatment interference, 616
Multisensory training. *See* Aural/oral training method
Muscles
  Eustachian tube, 511
  middle ear, 511
  of respiration, 6–8
Muscle tension dysphonia (MTD), 322
Muscular process, 10
Musculus uvulae, 21, 22
Mutational falsetto, 322
Myasthenia gravis, 320
Myelencephalon. *See* Medulla
Myelin sheath, 31
Mylohyoid muscle, 12, 13, 24
Myoelastic–aerodynamic theory, 14–15
Myoswitches, 184
Myringoplasty, 523
Myringotomy, 523

N

Naming
  evoked speech samples, 216
  skills
    assessment, 351
    treatment, 355–356
Narratives
  assessment of multicultural populations, 485
  defined, 108, 179
  macrostructure, 179
  microstructure, 179
  narrative skills
    assessment, 351
    training, 179
Narrow phonetic transcription, 75
Nasalance, 297, 438
Nasal cavity, 17, 19
Nasal cul-de-sac resonance, 296
Nasal-glide stimulation, 298
Nasalis muscle, 37
Nasalization, 207
Nasals, 81
Nasogastric feeding, 424
Nasogastric tube, 448
Nasometer, 295, 297, 438, 443
Nasopharyngoscopy, 437
Nasopharynx, 19
National Outcome Measurement System (NOMS), 648
National Student Speech-Language-Hearing Association (NSSLHA), 634
Native Americans, medical conditions and communication disorders, 491
Nativist theory of language development, 126–127

Natural frequency, 91
Naturalistic contexts, 485
Naturalness, 196
Natural phonology theory of development, 198
Natural recovery from stuttering, 244–245
NCCEA. *See Neurosensory Center Comprehensive Examination for Aphasia* (NCCEA)
NDRT. *See Nelson-Denny Reading Test* (NDRT)
Negative reinforcement, 584
Negative reinforcers, 584–585
Neglect, language problems related to, 158–159
Nelson-Denny Reading Test (NDRT), 351
Neologism, 339
Neologistic paraphasia, 339
Nerve cells, anatomy and physiology of, 30–31, 32
Nerve fibers, 31
Nerve–muscle pedicle reinnervation, 319
Nervous system, 30–66
  auditory nervous system, 513–514
  auditory nervous system impairments, 528–531
    central auditory disorders, 528–529
    retrocochlear disorders, 529–531
  autonomic nervous system, 43
  central nervous system, 44–66
    basal ganglia, 48, 49–50
    basic principles, 44
    brainstem, 44–48
    cerebellum, 49, 50–51
    cerebral blood supply, 62–66
    cerebral ventricles, 61
    cerebrum, 51–56
    connecting fibers in brain, 60–61
    diencephalon, 49
    extrapyramidal system, 57, 60
    protective layers of brain, 62
    pyramidal system, 56–57, 58
    reticular activating system, 48
  defined, 31
  neurons and neural transmission, 30–33
  peripheral nervous system, 33–43
Neural transmission, 31, 33
Neuritic plaques, and dementia, 362
Neuroanatomy
  defined, 30
  vocal mechanism, 16
Neuro-assisted (aided) augmentative and alternative communication, 184
Neurochemical changes, and dementia, 362
Neurofibrillary tangles, and dementia, 362

Neurogenic stuttering (NS), 237, 260–262. *See also* Fluency
  assessment, 262
  characteristics, 262
  defined, 261
  description of, 262
  etiology of, 261–262
  treatment, 262–263
Neuroglia, 31
Neurological diseases
  communication disorders, 492–494
  voice, 320–321
Neurology, defined, 30
Neuromuscular electrical stimulation (NMES), 423
Neuromuscular rehabilitation for swallowing disorders, 423
Neuronal loss, and dementia, 362
Neurons, 30, 31, 32
Neuropathologies, 210–212
  aphasia, 338–339
  apraxia of speech, 210–212, 394
  Creutzfeldt-Jakob disease, 370
  Dementia of the Alzheimer Type, 362
  dysarthria, 210, 403
  frontotemporal dementia, 363
  Huntington's disease, 367–368
  Parkinson's disease, 366
  primary progressive aphasia, 364, 365
Neurophysiological hypotheses for stuttering, 250–251
Neurophysiology, defined, 30
Neurosensory Center Comprehensive Examination for Aphasia (NCCEA), 350
Neurotransmitter, 31
Newton (unit), 94
Newton's Law of Motion, 91–92
NMES. *See* Neuromuscular electrical stimulation (NMES)
Noise as cause of hearing loss, 525–526
Nominal scale, 573, 620
NOMS. *See* National Outcome Measurement System (NOMS)
Nonacceleration injuries, 381
Nonfluent aphasia, 340–344
  Broca's aphasia, 340–341
  global aphasia, 343–344
  mixed transcortical aphasia, 342–343
  transcortical motor aphasia, 342
Nonfluent primary progressive aphasia (nvPPA), 364–365
Noniconic symbols for augmentative and alternative communication, 182
Non-invasive brain stimulation, 359
Nonlinear phonology theories of development, 199
Nonphonemic diphthongs, 87
Nonreduplicate babbling stage of sound development, 200

Nontypological definitions of aphasia, 340
Nonverbal communication
  manual training, 551
  sign language, 551, 552
  skill, deficiency, 144
Noonan syndrome, 450
Normal distribution, 620
Normative (developmental) research, 610–611
Normative treatment strategy, 585–586
Norm-referenced test, 569
NS. *See* Neurogenic stuttering (NS)
NSSLHA. *See* National Student Speech-Language-Hearing Association (NSSLHA)
Nucleus, 31
Nucleus of syllables, 77
Null hypothesis, 598
nvPPA. *See* Nonfluent primary progressive aphasia (nvPPA)
Nystagmus, and ataxic dysarthria, 404

O

OAE. *See* Otoacoustic emissions (OAE)
OASES. *See* Overall Assessment of the Speaker's Experience of Stuttering (OASES)
Oblique arytenoid muscle, 11, 12
Observation, scientific, 598
Occipital lobe, 55
Occlusion, 25
Occult cleft palate, 435
Occult submucous cleft, 435
Occupational history, 564
Octave, 91
Ocular hypertelorism, 445
Oculomotor nerve (cranial nerve III), 34, 35
Offglide, 87
Olfactory nerve (cranial nerve I), 34, 35
Oligodendroglia, 30
Oller, D. K., 200
OME. *See* Otitis media with effusion (OME)
Omissions, 207
Omohyoid muscle, 12, 13
Onglide, 83, 87
On Old Olympus' Towering Top, A Finn And German Viewed Some Hops, 34
Onset of syllables, 77
Open-head (penetrating) injury, 380
Open syllables, 78
Operant audiometry, 535
Operant behavior hypothesis of stuttering, 251
Operational definitions, 580, 582
Ophthalmic branch, 35
Optic nerve (cranial nerve II), 34, 35

Optimality theory of development, 199
Oral approach. *See* Aural/oral training method
Oral cavity
  functions, 17
  major structures, 21
  structure, 19
Oral cul-de-sac resonance, 296
Oral–motor control exercises, 422
Oral–motor coordination skills, 208–209
Oral myofunctional therapy, 209
Oral phase and its disorders (swallow), 418
  treatment, 421
Oral preparatory phase and its disorders (swallow), 417
  treatment, 420–421
Oral resonance, 17
Oral structure variables in speech sound disorders, 208–209
  ankyloglossia (tongue-tie), 208
  dental deviations, 208
  oral-motor coordination skills, 208–209
  orofacial myofunctional disorders (tongue thrust), 209
Orbicularis oculi muscle, 37
Orbicularis oris muscle, 27, 37
  inferioris and superioris muscles, 28
Order effect, 616
Order of mention, 148
Ordinal scale, 573, 620
Organically based disorders, 208–212
  hearing loss, 209–210
  neuropathologies, 210–212
    apraxia, 210–212
    dysarthria, 210
  oral structure variables, 208–209
    ankyloglossia (tongue-tie), 208
    dental deviations, 208
    oral-motor coordination skills, 208–209
    orofacial myofunctional disorders (tongue thrust), 209
Organizational deficits, 148
Organ of Corti, 513
Orientation, hearing aid, 548
Orofacial examination for speech sound disorders, 214–215, 565
Orofacial myofunctional disorders (tongue thrust), 209
Oropharynx, 19
Orthographic symbols, 75
Oscillation, 91
Ossicular chain, 435, 436, 508, 510–511
Ossicular discontinuity, 523, 524
Otitis media, 528
Otitis media with effusion (OME), 435, 436, 522

Otoacoustic emissions (OAE), 535
Otologists, 541
Otosclerosis, 523, 524
Otoscope, 508
Otospongiosis, 523
Ototoxic drugs, and hearing loss, 525
Outer ear, 508
Outmarriage, 463
Output constraints, 198
Oval window, 511, 512
Overall Assessment of the Speaker's Experience of Stuttering (OASES), 253
Overbite, 208
Overextended words, 147
Overextension, 107
Overjet, 208
Overtones, 95

P

PACE. See Promoting Aphasics' Communicative Effectiveness (PACE)
Palatal cleft. *See* Cleft palate
Palatal surgery for clefts, 440
Palatine bone, 23
Palatine process, 23
Palatoglossus muscle, 21, 22, 27
Palatopharyngeus muscle, 21, 22
Pantomime, 183
  assessment, 353
Papilloma, 313–314
Paradoxical vocal fold motion disorder (PVFMD), 317, 327
Paragraph comprehension, assessment, 352
Parallel form reliability, 600
Parallel play, 168
Parallel talk, 179
Paralysis of vocal folds, 317–319
Parameters, 618
Paraphasia, 339
  neologistic, 339
  perseverative, 340
  phonemic (literal), 339
  semantic, 339
Paraplegia, and cerebral palsy, 155
Parasympathetic branch, 43
Parental drug and alcohol abuse, 159–160
Parietal lobe, 54–55
Parkinsonism, 366
Parkinson's disease (PD), 321, 366–367, 369–370, 403
Part-word repetition, 239
Pascals (pa), 94, 518
Passive sentence, 105
Patterns of sound, 203
Pause-and-talk (time-out) stuttering treatment method, 258, 259
Pauses, 240

PCC. *See* Percentage of consonants correct (PCC)
PD. *See* Parkinson's disease (PD)
PE. *See* Pressure equalizing (PE) tubes
Pearson r, 600, 611
PECS. *See* Picture Exchange Communication System (PECS)
Pectoralis major, 7
Pectoralis minor, 7
Pediatric Voice Handicap Index (pVHI), 294
Pediatric Voice Related Quality of Life (PVQROL) scale, 294
Pedunculated polyps, 306
Peer training, 582
Percentage of consonants correct (PCC), 218
Percentile ranks, 571
Perception of sounds, 73, 89
Perceptual problems of specific language impairment, 147
Performance of language, 125
Perilymph, 511
Perinatal brain injury, 155
Periodic vibrations, 93, 515, 516
Periodic waves, 90
Period of sound, 93
Peripheral hearing problems, 528
Peripheral nervous system, 33–43, 45
  basic principles, 33–34
  cranial nerves, 33–40
  defined, 33
  spinal nerves, 40–43
Perlocutionary behavior, 112
Perseveration, 339–340
Perseverative paraphasia, 340
PES. *See* Pharyngoesophageal segment (PES)
PEW Research Center, 157
Pharmacological stuttering treatment, 260
Pharyngeal branch, 40
Pharyngeal cul-de-sac resonance, 296
Pharyngeal flap surgery, 441
Pharyngeal fricative, 207
Pharyngeal phase and its disorders (swallow), 418
  treatment, 421
Pharyngeal plexus, 19, 39
Pharyngoesophageal segment (PES), 302
Pharyngoplasty, 441
Pharyngostomy, 424
Pharynx (throat, pharyngeal cavity)
  functions, 19–20
  muscles, 28
  structure, 17, 19, 19–20
Phonation, 8–17
  acoustic analysis of speech, 95–96
  amplitude and loudness, 94

assessment, 293
context and speech sound production, 88–89
  dynamics of speech production, 88
  suprasegmentals, 88–89
defined, 1
disorders, and clefts, 437, 439
extrinsic laryngeal muscles, 12–13, 14
frequency and pitch, 93–94
hearing level, 94
intrinsic laryngeal muscles, 11–12, 13
larynx, 8–9
  structures and cartilages, 9–10
mucosal wave action, 15
myoelastic–aerodynamic theory, 14–15
neuroanatomy of vocal mechanism, 16
  cerebellum, 16
  cortical areas, 16
  cranial nerves, 16
physiology of, 14–15
  Bernoulli effect, 14–15
segmentals, 77–87
  classification systems, 78–80
  consonants, 77–84
  syllables, 77–78
  vowels, 84–87
sound pressure level, 94
sound wave generation and propagation, 92–93
speech science, 90–92
vocal folds, 13–14
Phonation stage of sound production development, 200
Phoneme, defined, 73, 196
Phoneme isolation, teaching, 181
Phoneme segmentation, 227
Phonemic, defined, 74, 196
Phonemic diphthongs, 87
Phonemic paraphasia, 339
Phonemic transcriptions, 75
Phonetics, 71–96
  context, 88
  defined, 73, 74, 196
  definitions, 73–74
  environment, 223
  placement, 222–223
  transcription, 75–77
Phonological awareness, 124, 181
  treatment, 227–228
Phonological disorder, defined, 195
Phonological error patterns, 207
Phonological patterns, 146
  approach, of treatment, 225–226
  categories, 203
Phonological problems, 146
Phonological processing, 130

Phonology
    African American English, 468, 470
    defined, 73, 196
    foundations of, 195–197
    skills development
        assimilation patterns, 204
        categories of patterns, 203
        in children, 200
        foundational concepts, 203
        in infants, 199–200
        intelligibility, 201–203
        substitution processes, 203–204
        syllable structure patterns, 204
    skills development theories
        behavioral theory, 197–198
        generative phonology theory, 198
        linear *vs.* nonlinear phonology theories, 199
        natural phonology theory, 198
        optimality theory, 199
Phonotrauma, 304, 310
Phrase interjections, 240
Phrase repetition, 239
Physical exercises for aphasia treatment, 359
Physical setting generalization, 582
Physical-stimulus generalization, 582
Physiological phonetics, 73, 74
Piaget, 128, 129–130, 132
Pia mater, 62
PICA-R. *See* Porch Index of Communicative Ability–Revised (PICA-R)
Pick's disease (PiD), 363
Picture Exchange Communication System (PECS), 184
PiD. *See* Pick's disease (PiD)
Pierre-Robin syndrome, 448
Pinna of the outer ear, 508
Pitch (perception)
    assessment, 291
    defined, 89, 94, 517
    frequency perturbation (jitter), 283
    fundamental frequency, 282
    monopitch, 291
Place of articulation
    defined, 79
    place-voice-manner analysis, 80–81
Place-voice-manner analysis, 79–80, 197
    consonant clusters, 84
    manner of articulation, 79, 81–84
    place of articulation, 79, 80–81
    voicing, 79, 81
Planning deficits, 148
Platysma muscle, 28, 37
Play
    assessment of, 168–169
    associative, 168
    collaborative/cooperative, 169

    parallel, 168
    solitary, 168
Play audiometry, 535
Plethysmograph, 290
Polypoid corditis. *See* Reinke's edema
Polypoid degeneration. *See* Reinke's edema
Polyps, 305–306
Pons, 46–47
Ponto hearing implants, 544
Population, defined, 603
Porch Index of Communicative Ability–Revised (PICA-R), 350
Portfolio assessment, 163, 485
Positive reinforcement, 584
Positive reinforcers, 585
Postcentral gyrus, 54
Posterior belly of digastric muscle, 24
Posterior cerebral arteries, 63
Posterior cricoarytenoid muscle, 12, 277, 278
Posterior middle temporal gyrus, 346
Posterior thoracic muscles, 7
Postlingual deafness, 539
Postnatal brain injury, 155
Post-reinforcement pause, 582
Posttest, 582
    defined, 603
    multigroup pretest–posttest design, 604
    pretest–posttest control group design, 603
    sensitization to treatment, 616
Postvocalic errors, 207
Poverty, language problems related to, 156–158, 476
PPA. *See* Primary progressive aphasia (PPA)
PPAOS. *See* Primary progressive apraxia of speech (PPAOS)
Prader-Willi syndrome (PWS), 448–449
Pragmatics
    assessment
        adolescents, 173
        elementary-age children, 169, 170
    autism spectrum disorders, 153
    children with SLI, 148
    cultural influences, 109
    defined, 108
    developmental milestones
        birth–1 year, 112
        1–2 years, 113
        2–3 years, 116–117
        3–4 years, 118–119
        4–5 years, 120
        5–6 years, 121–122
        6–7 years, 123
        7–8 years, 123–124
    direct *vs.* indirect speech acts, 108

    discourse, 108
    function of, 106
    intellectual disability and, 150
    language context and function, 108
Praxis examination
    certification requirements, 656
    computer-generated questions, 662
    content categories, 656
    general tips for taking, 659–662
    nature and purpose of, 655–658
    nonstandard testing arrangements, 658
    overview, 655
    study tips, 658–659
    test retakes, 655, 656
    topics covered, 657–658
Precentral gyrus, 53
Predictive validity, 599
Prefix, defined, 104
Prelingual deafness, 539
Prelinguistic behavioral deficiencies in infants and toddlers, 166–167
Preliteracy skills, 124
Premaxilla, 22
Prenatal brain injury, 155
Prenatal causes of hearing loss, 525
Prenatal history, 563
Preoperational cognitive development, 129
Presbycusis, 527
Presbylaryngis, 281
Presbyphonia, 281
Preschool Amendments to the Education of the Handicapped Act, 166
Preschoolers. *See also* Infants; Toddlers
    articulation development, 200, 202
    assessment of, 169–171
    cognitive development, 129
    hearing loss assessment, 535
    language developmental milestones, 117–119
    morphology, 118, 120
    pragmatics, 118–119, 120
    semantics, 117–118, 119–120
    stuttering in, 248
        treatment, 259
    syntax, 114, 119
    voice changes, 280–281
Preserved language, 340
Pressure, 91
Pressure equalizing (PE) tubes, 522
Presuppositions, 113
Pretest
    defined, 582, 603
    multigroup pretest–posttest design, 604
    pretest–posttest control group design, 603
    sensitization to treatment, 616

Prevalence
    aphasia, 337–340
    culturally and linguistically diverse clients, 490–491
    defined, 490
    stuttering
        concordance rates in twins, 243
        defined, 241
        ethnocultural variables, 244
        familial prevalence, 243
        gender ratio, 242
        in general population, 241–242
        in people with brain injuries, 244
        in people with developmental or intellectual disabilities, 244
        socioeconomic variables, 244
Prevocalic errors, 207
Primary auditory area, 514
Primary auditory cortex, 55
Primary language impairment. *See* Specific language impairment (SLI)
Primary motor cortex, 16, 53
Primary palate, 433
Primary progressive aphasia (PPA), 363, 364–366
Primary progressive apraxia of speech (PPAOS), 394
Primary reinforcers, 585
Primary stress of syllables, 88
Primary visual cortex, 55
Print knowledge, 124
Prion (proteinaceous infectious particle), 370
Probability of statistics, 618
Probes, 582
Procedures of treatment, 582, 583
Procerus muscle, 37
Processes of sound, 203
Processing speed deficits, 148
Production of sounds
    defined, 73
    in infants, 200
Professional issues, 632–648
    ASHA. *See also* American Speech-Language-Hearing Association (ASHA)
        accreditation, 636–637
        functions, 631
        goals, 632–633
        history of, 632
        membership, 632
        membership categories, 633–634
        special interest groups, 634
    audiology, 635
    scope of practice, 635–636
    speech–language pathology, 635
Prognosis, 564
Program for Infants and Toddlers with Disabilities, The, 166
Progressive Aphasia Severity Scale, 373

Progressive assimilation, 204
Projection fibers, 60
Prolongations, 239–240
Promoting Aphasics' Communicative Effectiveness (PACE), 357
PROMPT. *See* Prompts for Restructuring Oral Muscular Phonetic Targets (PROMPT)
Prompts, 582
Prompts for Restructuring Oral Muscular Phonetic Targets (PROMPT), 212
Prosody, 88
Protesting, 108
Psychoacoustics, 90, 515
Psychogenic stuttering, 265
Psychogenic voice disorders, 321–322
Psychological methods of stuttering treatment, 255
Psychotherapy, for treating stuttering, 255
Pterygoid muscle, 24
Puberphonia, 322
Puberty, voice changes during, 281
Public Law 94-142, 643, 644
Public Law 99-457, 166, 643–644
Public Law 101-336, 645
Public Law 101-476, 644
Public Law 105-17, 644
Public Law 108-446, 644
Punishment, 582
Pure apraxia of speech, 394
Pure alexia, 359
Pure probes, 581, 582
Pure tone, 93, 515
Pure-tone audiometry, 532
Pure word deafness. *See* Auditory verbal agnosia
Purkinje cells, 50–51
Putamen, 50
PVFMD. *See* Paradoxical vocal fold motion disorder (PVFMD)
pVHI. *See* Pediatric Voice Handicap Index (pVHI)
PVQROL. *See* Pediatric Voice Related Quality of Life (PVQROL) scale
PWS. *See* Prader-Willi syndrome (PWS)
Pyramidal system, 56–57
    basic principles, 56
    corticobulbar tract, 57, 59
    corticospinal tract, 56, 58
    defined, 56
Pyramidal tracts, 48

Q

Quadratus lumborum, 8
Quadriplegia, and cerebral palsy, 155
Qualitative data, 599

Quality of life evaluation, 293–294
Quantitative data, 599
Questionnaires, 485, 573, 610
Question (interrogative) sentence, 105
Quick Assessment for Dysarthria, 414
Quick incidental learning, 107

R

Radiation therapy, 300
Radical neck dissection, 300
Rancho Los Amigos Levels of Cognitive Function, 382
Randomization of groups, 602
Randomized clinical trial, 616
Range, defined, 619
Rapid-fire articulation, 410
Rapport during interviews, 565–566
Rarefaction, 90, 93, 516
RAS. *See* Reticular activating system (RAS)
Rate of speech, 89
Rating scales, 573
Ratio scale, 621
Raw score, 571
RCBA-2. *See Reading Comprehension Battery for Aphasia–Second Edition* (RCBA-2)
Reading. *See* Literacy skills
Reading Comprehension Battery for Aphasia–Second Edition (RCBA-2), 351
Reading skills. *See also* Literacy skills
    assessment, 353
        adolescents, 173
    treatment, 357
Rebuses, 184
Recasting, 180
Recruitment as hearing loss symptom, 525
Rectus abdominis, 8
Recurrent laryngeal nerve (RLN)
    functions, 40
    neuroanatomy, 16
    resection for spasmodic dysphonia, 319
    vocal anatomy and physiology, 275, 276
Reduplicated babbling stage of sound development, 200
Reduplication, 204
Reflection, 91
Refraction, 91
Regressive assimilation, 204
Regulations, 166
    Affordable Health Care Act, 646
    Americans With Disabilities Act (ADA), 645
    employment settings, 645
    Every Student Succeeds Act (ESSA), 645

future trends, 648
health care settings, 646–648
Health Insurance Portability and
  Accountability Act (HIPAA),
  647–648
Individuals with Disabilities
  Education Act (IDEA) of 1990,
  644–645
Individuals with Disabilities
  Education Improvement Act of
  2004, 482
Preschool Amendments to the
  Education of the Handicapped Act,
  166
Public Law 94-142, 644
Public Law 99-457, 643–644
Public Law 101-336, 645
Public Law 101-476, 644
Public Law 105-17, 644
Public Law 108-446, 644
school settings, 643–644
Social Security Act (SSA), 646–647
state regulation, 641–642
Reinforcement, 583–584
Reinforcement withdrawal, 584
Reinforcers, 584–585
Reinke's edema, 309
Reinke's space, 15
Reissner's membrane, 513
Relational analysis of assessment data, 217
Relative effects, 604
Reliability
  alternate-form (parallel form), 600
  correlational coefficient, 600
  of data, 599
  defined, 600
  interobserver (interjudge), 600
  intraobserver (intrajudge), 600
  of measurements, 600–601
  split-half, 600
  of standardized tests, 572
  test–retest, 6060
Religion, and rehabilitation, 494
Repeatable Battery for the Assessment of Neuropsychological Status Update, 372
Repetition, 239
  skills, assessment, 351
Representative sample, 569
Research. *See also* Scientific method
  defined, 597
  descriptive, 608–612
    basic concepts, 608–609
    comparative research, 610
    correlational research, 611–612
    developmental (normative)
      research, 610–611
    ex post facto (retrospective)
      research, 609–610

survey research, 610
ethnographic research, 612
evaluation, 612–618
  evidence levels for evidence-based
    practice, 616–618
  external validity, 615–616
  internal validity, 613–615
experimental, 601–608
  definition of terms, 601–602
  group designs, 602–604
  single-subject designs, 604–608
Resonance
  assessment, 293
  defined, 91
  disorders, 294–298
    assimilative nasality, 296
    clefts, 439, 443
    cul-de-sac resonance, 296–297
    hypernasality, 295
    hyponasality, 296, 298
    treatment, 297–298
  hearing impairment and disorders
    of, 541
Resonation
  defined, 1, 17
  fundamentals of, 17–18
Respiration, 1–8
  assessment, 293
  defined, 1
  framework, 2–6
    bronchi, 2–3
    lungs, 3
    rib cage, 5–6
    spinal column, 4–5
    sternum, 5
    trachea, 3
  muscles, 6–8
    abdominal muscles of expiration, 8
    thoracic muscles of inspiration, 6–7
  patterns during speech production,
    1–2
Response complexity, 586–587
Response cost
  defined, 582
  stuttering treatment method,
    258–259
Response Elaboration Training (RET), 357
Response generalization, 582
Response-mode generalization, 582
Response modes, 587
Response to intervention (RtI), 171, 487
RET. *See Response Elaboration Training* (RET)
Reticular activating system (RAS), 48
Reticular formation, 44
Retrocochlear disorders, 529–531
Retroflex, 84
Retrograde amnesia, 56

Retrospective (ex post facto) research,
  609–610
Revised Token Test, 351
Revisions, 240
RH. *See* Right hemisphere (RH)
RHBD. *See* Right-hemisphere brain
  damage (RHBD)
RHD. *See* Right hemisphere disorder
  (RHD)
RHLB-2. *See Right Hemisphere
  Language Battery–Second Edition*
  (RHLB-2)
Rhomboideus major, 7
Rhomboideus minor, 7
Rhotic sounds, 84
Rhyme, 78
Rhyming skills, teaching, 181
Rhythmic breathing, 327
Rhythm training, 550–551
Rib cage (thoracic cage), 5–6, 7
RICE-3. *See RIC Evaluation of
  Communication Problems in Right
  Hemisphere Dysfunction–Third Edition*
  (RICE-3)
*RIC Evaluation of Communication Problems
  in Right Hemisphere Dysfunction–Third
  Edition* (RICE-3), 377
Right hemisphere (RH), 375
Right-hemisphere brain damage
  (RHBD). *See* Right hemisphere
  disorder (RHD)
Right hemisphere disorder (RHD),
  375–379
  affective deficits, 376
  assessment, 376–377
  attentional and perceptual deficits,
    376
  communication treatment of,
    378–379
  communicative deficits, 376–377
  symptoms, 375–377
*Right Hemisphere Language Battery–Second
  Edition* (RHLB-2), 377
Right-hemisphere syndrome. *See* Right
  hemisphere disorder (RHD)
Rigid endoscopy with
  videostroboscopy, 286–287
Risorius muscle, 28
RLN. *See* Recurrent laryngeal nerve
  (RLN)
Rochester method of communication,
  552
Root morpheme, 104
Root of the tongue, 26
Rounded vowels, 84
Round window, 512
RtI. *See* Response to intervention
  (RtI)
Rubella as cause of hearing loss, 526

Rule of 10s, 439
Russell-Silver syndrome, 449

S

SA. *See* Subcortical aphasia (SA)
Sacrum, 5
Safety alerting devices, 547
Safety behaviors, and stuttering, 247
Saint-Louis University Mental Status Examination, 372
Salpingopharyngeus muscle, 20
SALT, *Systematic Analysis of Language Transcripts* (SALT) computer software
Sample, defined, 603
Sampling
    conversational speech, 215
    evoked speech, 216
    multicultural population
        communication disorders, 485
    procedures for obtaining, 566–567
    representative sample, 569
    speech and language, 566–567
Satellite cells, 31
Satiation, 582
Scalenes, 7
Scales of Cognitive Ability for Traumatic Brain Injury (SCATBI), 382
Scales of Cognitive and Communicative Ability for Neurorehabilitation (SCCAN), 383
Scanning used in augmentative and alternative communication, 182
SCATBI. *See Scales of Cognitive Ability for Traumatic Brain Injury* (SCATBI)
SCCAN. *See Scales of Cognitive and Communicative Ability for Neurorehabilitation* (SCCAN)
SCERTS model of treatment, 153
School. *See* Education
School-age children. *See* Elementary-age children
School settings, federal legislation affecting, 643–644
Schwann cells, 31
Science
    deductive method, 598
    defined, 597
    determinism, 598
    empiricism, 597–598
    hypotheses, 598
    inductive method, 598
    philosophy, 597–599
    qualitative data, 599
    quantitative data, 599
    of speech, 90–92
Scientific method, 597–621
    data organization and analysis, 618–621

basic concepts, 618–619
        measurement scales, 620
        statistical techniques, 619–620
    descriptive research, 608–612
        basic concepts, 608–609
        comparative research, 610
        correlational research, 611–612
        developmental (normative) research, 610–611
        ethnographic research, 612
        ex post facto (retrospective) research, 609–610
        survey research, 610
    experimental research, 601–608
        definition of terms, 601–602
        group designs, 602–604
        single-subject designs, 604–608
    philosophy of science, 597–599
    reliability of measurements, 600
    research evaluation, 612–618
        evidence levels for evidence-based practice, 616–618
        external validity, 615–616
        internal validity, 613–615
    validity of measurements, 599–600
Scores in standardized assessment, 571–572
Screening
    defined, 562
    evidence-based practice, 562–563
    hearing, 215, 534–535, 565
    of language skills, 162–163
    speech sound disorders, 213
Secondary reinforcers, 584
Secondary stress of syllables, 88
Secondary stutterings, 246
Second-language acquisition, 477–479
    in internationally adapted children, 478–479
    typical processes of, 478
SEE 1. *See* Seeing Essential English (SEE 1)
SEE 2. *See* Signing Exact English (SEE 2)
Seeing Essential English (SEE 1), 552
Segmentals, 77–87
    classification systems, 78–80
    consonants, 77–84
    syllables, 77–78
    vowels, 84–87
Self-control, 583
Self-repairs, 395
Self-talk, 180
Semantic feature analysis (SFA), 356
Semantic paraphasia, 339
Semantics
    assessment
        adolescents, 173
        elementary-age children, 170
    categories, 107

defined, 106
    developmental milestones
        1–2 years, 113, 115
        2–3 years, 115
        3–4 years, 117–118
        4–5 years, 119–120
        5–6 years, 121
        6–7 years, 122
        7–8 years, 123
    overextension, 107
    quick incidental learning, 107
    semantic PPA (svPPA), 364, 365
    semantic relations (utterances), 113, 114, 115
    underextension, 107
    vocabulary, 106–107
    word knowledge, 107
    world knowledge, 108
Semicircular canals, 512
Semilongitudinal procedure of research, 611
Semivowels, 83
Sensorimotor cognitive development, 129
Sensorineural hearing loss, 525–528
Sensory cortex, 54
Sensory fibers, 35
Sensory nerves, 34
Sensory neurons, 31, 33
Sensory strip, 54
Sentence
    completion, evoked speech samples, 216
    comprehension
        assessment, 352
        treatment, 355
    production, assessment, 351
    syntax, 105
Sequence of treatment, 586–587
    degree of structure, 587
    multiple targets, 587
    response complexity, 586–587
    response modes, 587
    shifts in treatment contingencies, 587
    training and maintenance, 587
Sequential bilingual acquisition, 480
Serous otitis media, 522–523
Serratus anterior, 7
Serratus posterior inferior muscles, 7
Serratus posterior superior muscles, 6, 7
SES. *See* Socioeconomic status (SES)
Sessile polyps, 306
SFA. *See* Semantic feature analysis (SFA)
Shaping, 583
Shimmer (amplitude perturbation), 283
Shprintzen syndrome, 451
Sibling status as factor in speech sound disorders, 206
Sickle cell anemia, and stroke, 492

SIG. *See* Special interest groups (SIGs), ASHA
Signal-to-noise (S/N) ratio, hearing aid, 544, 549
Signing Exact English (SEE 2), 552
Sign language, 183, 551, 552
Silent period, 476
Silent prolongations, 240
Simple harmonic motion, 90, 93, 515
Simultaneous bilingual acquisition, 480
Singhale, 326
Singing, assessment, 353
Single-subject design (SSD), 604–608
    ABAB design, 605–606
    ABA design, 605–606
    advantages of, 607–608
    defined, 604
    disadvantages of, 608
    multiple-baseline designs, 607
Sinusoidal motion or wave, 90, 93, 515
Skeletal malocclusion, 208
Skinner, B. F., 125
SLI. *See* Specific language impairment (SLI)
SLN. *See* Superior laryngeal nerve (SLN)
SLPA. *See* Speech–language pathology assistants (SLPAs)
Social anxiety, and stuttering, 249–250
Social approaches to treating aphasia, 358
Social communication deficiency, 144
Social interactionism theory of language development, 131–132
Social language, 175
Social Security Act (SSA), 646–647
Sociocultural barriers to service delivery, 491–492
Sociocultural considerations, in rehabilitation, 493–494
Socioeconomic status (SES)
    as factor in speech sound disorders, 206
        language development and, 156–158
        and rehabilitation, 493
        stuttering prevalence and, 244
Soft palate. *See* Velum (soft palate)
Solitary play, 168
Soma (cell body), 31
Somatic sensations, 54
Somatosensory cortex, 16
Sona-Graph, 289
Sonorants, 83, 84
Sound
    acoustic analysis of speech, 95–96
    acoustics, 515–518
    amplitude and loudness, 94
    defined, 90
    frequency and pitch, 93–94
    interjections, 240
    patterns, 203
    processes, 203
    prolongations, 239
    sound pressure level and hearing level, 94, 518
    sound waves
        cause of, 516
        defined, 90
        generation and propagation, 92–93
        single cycle, 516
        source of, 515–516
        spectrograph, 95, 287–288
        study of, 92–96
Sound blending, teaching of, 181
Sound pressure level (dB SPL), 94, 518
Sound production treatment (SPT), 398
Source-filter theory, 17
Spanish-influenced English
    articulation differences, 468, 472
    background, 468
    characteristics, 468, 472–473
    language differences, 473
Spasmodic dysphonia, 319–320
Spastic cerebral palsy, 155
Spastic dysarthria, 410–411
    ataxic-spastic dysarthria, 411
    flaccid-spastic dysarthria, 411
Special education, 644
Special interest groups (SIGs), ASHA, 634
Specific language impairment (SLI), 145–149
    cognitive processing deficits, 148
    executive functioning deficits, 148
    general characteristics, 145–146
    normal variation, 145
    speech and language deficits, 146–148
    subtle brain abnormalities, 146
    underlying deficits, 145
Spectrogram, 92, 95, 287–288
Speech, defined, 1
Speech audiometry, 533
Speech correction teachers, 631
Speech fluency assessment, 352
Speech Intelligibility Test for Windows, 414
Speech–language clinician, 635
Speech–language communication, 550
Speech–language pathologists, 542, 635
Speech–language pathology, 561–562, 635
Speech–language pathology assistants (SLPAs), 640–641
Speech phobia, and stuttering, 249–250
Speech-range masking, 327
Speech reading, 549
Speech reception threshold, 533
Speech science, 73, 90–92
Speech sound disorders (SSDs), 146
    articulatory errors, 207
    assessment, 213–219
        components, 215–217
        conversational speech samples, 215
        evoked speech samples, 216
        objectives, 213–214
        procedures, 214–215
        scoring and analysis, 217–219
        screening, 213, 215
        standardized tests, 216–217
        stimulability, 216
    clefts and, 436, 438–439, 441–443
    defined, 195, 205
    factors related to, 205–207
        auditory discrimination skills, 206–207
        birth order and sibling status, 206
        gender, 206
        intelligence, 206
        language development and academic performance, 206
        socioeconomic status, 206
    hearing impairment and, 540
    organically based disorders, 208–212
        ankyloglossia (tongue-tie), 208
        apraxia, 210–212
        dental deviations, 208
        dysarthria, 210
        hearing loss, 209–210
        neuropathologies, 210–212
        oral-motor coordination skills, 208–209
        oral structure variables, 208–209
        orofacial myofunctional disorders (tongue thrust), 209
    speech sound differences *vs.*, 221
    treatment, 220–228
        complexity approach (least knowledge approach), 221
        context utilization approaches, 223–224
        core vocabulary (consistency) approach, 226–227
        developmental approach, 221
        general considerations, 220–222
        Hodson and Paden's cycles approach, 226
        linguistic approaches, 224–226
        minimal pair contrast therapy, 225
        motor-based, 222–224
        phonological awareness, 227–228
        phonological pattern approach, 225–226
        Van Riper's traditional approach, 222–223
Speech therapist, 635
Speech therapy, 297
Speech training, 550–551
Speed of processing information, 148

Spinal accessory nerve (cranial nerve XI), 19, 34, 40, 41
    damage, and flaccid dysarthria, 407
Spinal column, 4–5
Spinal cord
    nerves, 42
    with vertebrae nerves, 46
Spinal nerves, 40–43
Split-half reliability, 600
Spondee words, 533
Spontaneous recovery from stuttering, 244–245
SPT. *See* Sound production treatment (SPT)
SSA. *See* Social Security Act (SSA)
SSD. *See* Single-subject design (SSD); Speech sound disorders (SSDs)
SSI-4. *See* Stuttering Severity Instrument–Fourth Edition (SSI-4)
Stages of cognitive development, 128, 129–130
Stampe, D., 198
Standard deviation
    defined, 619
    of test scores, 571
Standard-group comparison. *See* Comparative research
Standardized assessment
    adolescents, 174
    elementary-age children, 171
    multicultural population
        communication disorders, 482–485
        administration of tests, 484
        formal test assumptions, 482–483
        foundational concepts, 482
        interpretation of tests, 484–485
        selection of tests, 484
        test development in primary languages, 483–484
        translation of tests, 483
    nature and advantages of, 568–569
    overview, 163
    prudent use of, 570–571
    speech sound disorders, 216–217
    types of scores, 571–572
    validity and reliability of, 572
Stapedectomy, 523
Stapedius muscle, 37, 511
Stapes, 511
State regulation of the profession, 641–642
Statistical regression, 614
Statistic(s). *See also* Scientific method
    defined, 618
    probability, 618
    techniques for organizing data, 619–620
        measures of central tendency, 620
        measures of variability, 619
Stenosis, 521

Stereotypes, 462
Sternocleidomastoid, 7
Sternohyoid muscle, 12, 13
Sternothyroid muscle, 12, 13
Sternum (breastbone), 5
Stimulability assessment, 216
Stimuli, treatment, 579
Stimulus control in stuttering, 248–249
    adaptation, 249
    adjacency, 249
    audience size, 249
    consistency, 249
Stimulus generalization, 583
Stoma, 301
Stomodeum, 433
Stops, 79, 83, 204
STORCH acronym, 526–527
Strain-strangle voice, 284
Stressed syllable, 88–89
Stretch and flow voice therapy, 325
Stridency deletion, 207, 224
Strident voice, 284
Stridor, 312
Strokes. *See also* Aphasia
    bilingual patient recovery theories, 493
    causes of, 492
    hemorrhagic, 338–339
    ischemic strokes, 338, 339
    recovery in bilinguals, 493
Strong cognition hypothesis, 128
Structure of treatment, degree of, 587
Stuttering. *See also* Fluency
    abnormal motor behaviors, 237
    assessment, 252–254
    associated motor behaviors, 246
    avoidance behaviors, 247
    breathing abnormalities, 246–247
    causes of, 237
    definitions, 238
        based on all types of dysfluencies, 239
        event of stuttering, 238
        limited to certain types of dysfluencies, 239
        moment of stuttering, 238
        person's actions to avoid stuttering, 238
        social role conflict, 238
        in terms of unspecified behaviors, 238
    diagnosis of, 253–254
    family and, 243, 249–250
    incidence of
        defined, 241
        in general population, 241–242
        onset and development of, 242
    loci of, 247–248
    malingered, 265

    motor behaviors (secondary stutterings), 246
    natural recovery and persistence, 244–245
    negative emotions, 247
    onset and development of, 245–246
    personality and, 249, 250
    prevalence of
        concordance rates in twins, 243
        defined, 241
        ethnocultural variables, 244
        familial prevalence, 243
        gender ratio, 242
        in people with brain injuries, 244
        in people with developmental or intellectual disabilities, 244
        socioeconomic variables, 244
    psychogenic, 265
    and social anxiety, 249–250
    stimulus control, 248–249
        adaptation, 248–249
        adjacency, 249
        audience size, 249
        consistency, 249
    and temperament, 250
    theories, 250–251
        avoidance behavior, 251
        brain dysfunction hypotheses, 251
        demands and capacities model, 251
        genetic hypothesis, 250
        leading-edge hypothesis, 251
        mismatch hypotheses, 251
        neurophysiological hypotheses, 250–251
        operant behavior, 251
    treatment, 254–260
        age considerations, 259–260
        direct stuttering reduction methods, 258–259
        fluency reinforcement method, 257
        fluency shaping method (speak-more-fluently), 256–257
        fluent stuttering method (stutter-more-fluently), 255–256
        generalization, maintenance, family training, 260
        goals of, 254–255
        masking and delayed auditory feedback techniques, 257–258
        pause-and-talk (time-out), 258, 259
        pharmacological, 260
        psychological methods, 255
        response cost method, 258–259
Stuttering Severity Instrument–Fourth Edition (SSI-4), 253
Styloglossus muscle, 27
Stylohyoid muscle, 12, 13, 37
Stylopharyngeus muscle, 20
Subcortical aphasia (SA), 348

Subcostal muscle, 7
Subglottal stenosis, 312–313
Subject selection biases, 615
Submucous cleft, 295, 435
Subordinate clause, 106
Substantia nigra, 46, 50
Substitution processes, 203–204
Substitutions, 207
Successive approximation, 583
Suffix, defined, 104
Sulcus, 51
Sulcus cocalis, 315–316
Superficial lamina propria, 15
Superior cerebellar peduncles, 50
Superior cornua, 10, 275
Superior laryngeal artery, 275
Superior laryngeal nerve (SLN), 40
  neuroanatomy, 16
  vocal anatomy and physiology, 275
Superior longitudinal fibers, 61
Superior longitudinal muscle, 27
Superior peduncles, 44
Superior pharyngeal constrictor muscle, 20
Superior (upper) temporal gyrus, 55
Super-supraglottic swallow, 423
Supplementary motor cortex, 16, 54, 342, 343
Supraglottic swallow, 423
Suprahyoid muscles (elevators), 12, 13, 14, 24, 280
Supramarginal gyrus, 55, 347
Suprasegmentals, 88–89
Surgical management of clefts, 440–441
Surveys, 610
Swallowing disorders (dysphagia), 416–424
  assessment, 419–420
  nature and etiology of, 416–417
  normal and disordered swallow, 417–419
    achalasia, 419
      esophageal phase and its disorders, 418–419
      oral phase and its disorders, 418
      oral preparatory phase and its disorders, 417
      pharyngeal phase and its disorders, 418
  treatment, 420–424
    computer applications, 423
    direct treatment, 420–421
    effortful swallow, 423
    exercises to stimulate swallow reflex, 422
    indirect treatment, 422
    Masako maneuver, 422
    medical treatment, 423–424
    Mendelsohn maneuver, 423
    neuromuscular rehabilitation, 423
    oral–motor control exercises, 422
    super-supraglottic swallow, 423
    supraglottic swallow, 423
Swallow maneuvers, 422–423
Syllabics, 78
Syllabification, 78
Syllable awareness, teaching, 181
Syllable interjections, 240
Syllables, 77–78, 224
Syllable structure, patterns, 204
Sylvian fissure (lateral cerebral fissure), 51
Sympathetic branch, 43
Symphysis, 23
Synapses, 31
Syndrome, defined, 444
Synergistic and differential recovery theory, 493
Syntax, 105–106
  African American English, 466–468, 469
  assessment
    adolescents, 172
    elementary-age children, 169, 170
  defined, 105
  developmental milestones
    1–2 years, 112–113
    2–3 years, 114
    3–4 years, 117
    4–5 years, 119
    5–6 years, 120
    6–7 years, 122
    7–8 years, 123
  intellectual disability and, 150
  problems, of SLI, 147
  structures, 105
Syphilis as cause of hearing loss, 526
Systematic Analysis of Language Transcripts (SALT) computer software, 165
s/z ratio, 293

T

Tactile agnosia, 360
Targets of treatment, 583, 585–586, 587
Task shifting, 148
TBI. *See* Traumatic brain injury (TBI)
TDDs. *See* Telecommunication devices for the deaf (TDDs)
Team-oriented approach to evaluation of voice disorders, 286
Teams, working with, 568
Teeth, 24–25
  types of, 25
Teflon injection into vocal folds, 424
Telecommunication devices for the deaf (TDDs), 547
Telegraphic speech, 147

Telepractice, 648
Temperament, and stuttering, 250
Templin Darley Test of Articulation, 439
Temporal auditory processing, 130
Temporal bone, 511
Temporalis muscle, 24
Temporal lobe, 55–56, 514
Temporomandibular joint, 23
Tense/lax qualities, 85
Tense vowels, 84
Tensor tympani, 511
Tensor veli palatini muscle, 21, 22, 436, 511
TEP. *See* Tracheoesophageal puncture (TEP), Blom-Singer
Terminal buttons, 31
Terminal response, 583
Testing, defined, 614. *See also* Assessment; Standardized assessment
Test of Visual Neglect, 377
Test–retest reliability, 600
Thalamus, 49
Theory. *See also* Hypothesis
  articulation skills development
    behavioral theory, 197–198
    generative phonology theory, 198
    linear *vs.* nonlinear phonology theories, 199
    natural phonology theory, 198
    optimality theory, 199
  bilingual patient recovery from strokes, 493
    synergistic and differential recovery theory, 493
  cover-body theory of phonation, 274
  defined, 598
  government binding theory, 127
  language development, 125–132
    behavioral theory, 125–126
    cognitive theory, 127–128, 129–130
    information-processing theory, 128, 130–131
    nativist theory, 126–127
    social interactionism theory, 131–132
  phonology skills development
    behavioral theory, 197–198
    generative phonology theory, 198
    linear *vs.* nonlinear phonology theories, 199
    natural phonology theory, 198
    optimality theory, 199
  stuttering, 250–251
    avoidance behavior, 251
    brain dysfunction hypotheses, 251
    demands and capacities model, 251
    genetic hypothesis, 250
    leading-edge hypothesis, 251

mismatch hypotheses, 251
neurophysiological hypotheses, 250–251
operant behavior, 251
transformational generative theory of grammar, 127
Third ventricle, 49, 61
Thoracic breathing, 293
Thoracic cage (rib cage), 5–6, 7
Thoracic muscles of inspiration, 6–7
Thoracic vertebrae, 5
Threshold of hearing, 532
speech reception, 533
Throat. See Pharynx (throat, pharyngeal cavity)
Throat clearing, 326–327
Thrombus, 338
Thymectomy, 320
Thyroarytenoid, 11, 12, 274
Thyrohyoid muscle, 12, 13
Thyroid angle, 10
Thyroid cartilage, 10, 275, 277
Thyroid notch, 10
Thyromuscularis muscle, 11
Thyroplasty, 328
TIA. See Transient ischemic attacks (TIA)
Tidal volume, 290
Time-out, defined, 583
Time-out (pause-and-talk) stuttering treatment method, 258, 259
Tinnitus, 527
Tip of the tongue, 26
TMA. See Transcortical motor aphasia (TMA)
Toddlers. See also Infants; Preschoolers
assessment of, 164–169
guidelines and procedures, 167
infant–caregiver interaction, 168
language comprehension, 168
language-related skills, 168
late talkers, 167
play activities, 168–169
prelinguistic behavioral deficiencies, 166–167
risk factors for language disorders, 166
verbal communication, 168
cognitive development, 129–130
language developmental milestones, 114–147
morphology, 115–116
pragmatics, 116–117
semantics, 115
syntax, 114
Tokens, 583
Tonar II, 443
Tones, 515
Tongue, 25–27

anatomy, 26
forwardness or retraction, 85
functions, 26
height, 85
muscles, 26–27, 28
Tongue thrust (orofacial myofunctional disorders), 209
Tongue-tie (ankyloglossia), 208
Tonsillectomy, 295
TOSS acronym, 279
Total communication training, 551–552
Total lung capacity, 290
Tourette syndrome, 449–450
Toxoplasmosis, as cause of hearing loss, 526
Trachea, 2, 3
Tracheoesophageal puncture (TEP), Blom-Singer, 302–303
Training of target behaviors, 587
Transcortical motor aphasia (TMA), 342
Transcortical sensory aphasia (TSA), 345–346
Transcranial direct current stimulation, 423
Transcranial magnetic stimulation, 423
Transcription, phonetic, 75–77
Transdisciplinary teams, 568
Transducers, hearing aid, 543
Transfer, and second-language acquisition, 478
Transformational generative theory of grammar, 127
Transgender voice issues, 327–328
Transglottal pressure equalization, 325
Transient ischemic attacks (TIA), 338, 339
Transmitting medium, 91
Transparent messages, 183
Transverse arytenoid muscle, 11, 12
Transverse muscles, 27
Transversus abdominis, 8
Transversus thoracis, 7
Trapezius, 7
Traumatic brain injury (TBI), 379–385
assessment, 154, 382–383
communicative deficits, 383–384
causes of, 154, 380
cognitive and language difficulties, 154
consequences of, 380–382
defined, 153, 379
dementia associated with, 371
diffuse injury, 153
focal injury, 153
immediate effects of, 154
incidence of, 379–380
treatment, 384–385
types of, 380–382
acceleration–deceleration injuries, 381

blast (multisystem) injuries, 381
closed-head (nonpenetrating) injury, 380–381
mild traumatic brain injury, 381
nonacceleration injuries, 381
open-head (penetrating) injury, 380
Traumatic laryngitis, 308
Treacher Collins syndrome, 450
Treatment
aphasia, 337, 354–359
apraxia of speech, 212, 397–398
Asperger's syndrome, 153
autism spectrum disorders, 152
behavioral voice therapy, 322–327
cerebral palsy, 155
childhood apraxia of speech, 212
clefts, 439–443
cluttering, 264
contingencies, 587
defined, 578–579
dementia, 373–374
dysarthria, 210, 414–416
evidence-based practice. See Evidence-based practice
of hearing impairment, 539–552
hormonal therapy, 328
intervention for children in poverty to enrich language skills, 157–158
for language disorders, 174–184
multicultural population communication disorders, 488–494
need for individualized treatment, 590
neurogenic stuttering, 262–263
oral myofunctional therapy, 209
phonation disorders, 298–328
program outline, 588–589
resonance disorders, 297–298
right hemisphere disorder, 378–379
sequence, 586–587
degree of structure, 587
multiple targets, 587
response complexity, 586–587
response modes, 587
shifts in treatment contingencies, 587
training and maintenance, 587
speech sound disorders, 220–228
stuttering, 254–260
swallowing disorders (dysphagia), 420–424
targets, 585–586
traumatic brain injury, 384–385
Trial, defined, 583
Trigeminal nerve (cranial nerve V), 24, 34, 35, 36, 37
damage, and flaccid dysarthria, 406
Trigeminal neuralgia, 37

Trisomy 13, 450
Trochlear nerve (cranial nerve IV), 34, 35
TSA. See Transcortical sensory aphasia (TSA)
TTR. See Type-token ratio (TTR)
Turner syndrome, 451
Turn-taking skills, 110
Twang, 325
Twins, stuttering prevalence and concordance rates, 243
Tympanic membrane (eardrum), 435, 436, 508
Tympanometry, 533
Type-token ratio (TTR), 165–166
Typical score, 620
Typological definitions of aphasia, 340

U

Underextended words, 147
Underextension, 107
Underlying deficits, specific language impairment, 146
Understandability, 201–203
Unilateral paralysis of focal folds, 318
Unilateral upper motor neuron (UUMN) dysarthria, 402, 411–412
Unmarked sounds, 196
Unstressed-syllable deletion, 204
Upper lip, 433
Upper motor neurons, 57
Usher syndrome, 451
Utterances
  acceptable, African American English, 468, 471
  expanded, 356–357
  functions, 108, 113, 114, 115
  mean length of utterance, 165
UUMN. See Unilateral upper motor neuron (UUMN) dysarthria
Uvula, 20

V

Vagus nerve (cranial nerve X)
  damage, and flaccid dysarthria, 407
  functions, 34, 39–40
  neuroanatomy, 16
  structure, 19, 39–40
  vocal anatomy and physiology, 275
Validity
  concurrent, 599
  construct, 599
  content, 600
  of data, 599
  defined, 599
  external, 615–616
  internal, 613–615
  of measurements, 599–600
  predictive (criterion), 599
  of standardized tests, 572
Van Riper's traditional treatment approach, 222–223
Variability
  defined, 619
  measures of, 619
Variables
  classification, 609
  criterion, 609
  dependent, 601, 602
  extraneous (confounding), 601
  independent, 601, 602
Varices, 310
Variegated babbling stage of sound development, 200
Vascular dementia, 371
VCFS. See Velocardiofacial syndrome (VCFS)
Veau-Wardill-Kilner surgery, 440
Velar fronting, 204
Velocardiofacial syndrome (VCFS), 451–452
Velocity, 91, 93
Velopharyngeal closure, 21
Velopharyngeal function assessment of children with clefts, 437–438
Velopharyngeal inadequacy or insufficiency (VPI), 295, 438, 443
Velopharyngeal port, 18
Velum (soft palate)
  function of, 17
  paresis/paralysis, as cause of resonance disorders, 295
  structure, 20–22
Ventricular folds, 13, 274
Verbal behavior, 125, 126
Verbal communication, assessment of, 168
Verbal expression
  expanded utterances, 356–357
  naming, 355–356
Vermis, 50
Vertebrae, 4
Vertebrae foramina, 56
Vertebral arteries, 63
Vertical muscles, 27
Vestibular branch, 513
Vestibular system, 512
Vestibulocochlear nerve. See Acoustic nerve (cranial nerve VIII)
VFE. See Vocal function exercises (VFE)
VHI. See Voice Handicap Index (VHI)
Vibratory motion, 92–93
Videoendoscopy, 286
Videokymography, 289–290
Videostroboscopy, flexible or rigid endoscopy with, 286–287
Visi-Pitch IV, 291
Visual agnosia, 360
Visual aids
  for hypernasality treatment, 297
  for hyponasality treatment, 298
Visually reinforced head turn, 199
Visual reinforcement audiometry, 535
Vital capacity, 290
Vocabulary, semantics of, 106–107
Vocal folds, 11
  anatomy and physiology, 273–275
  function, 9
  hemorrhage, 310
  paralysis of, 317–319
  structure, 13–14
  Teflon injection into, 424
  thickening, 308
Vocal fry, 284
Vocal function exercises (VFE), 325
Vocalic sounds, 84
Vocalis muscle, 11, 13
Vocalization, substitution processes, 203
Vocal nodules, 304–305
Vocal process, 10
Vocal punctuation (juncture), 89
Vocational counselor, 542
Voice
  anatomy and physiology, 273–282
    larynx, 273–280
    voice changes through the life span, 280–282
  behavioral voice therapy, 322–327
    chest resonance, 324
    coughing and throat clearing, 326–327
    hard glottal attack, 326
    integrated implicit–explicit approach, 325–326
    Lessac-Madsen Resonant Voice Therapy, 324
    Lombard effect, 327
    rhythmic breathing, 327
    singhale (inhalation phonation), 326
    stretch and flow, 325
    twang, 325
    vocal function exercises, 325
    yawn–sigh method, 324
  evaluation of disorders, 285–294
    case history, 285
    instrumental evaluation, 286–291
    perceptual evaluation, 291–293
    quality of life evaluation, 293–294
    team-oriented approach, 286
  hearing impairment and voice disorders, 541
  hyperfunctional disorders, 303
  hypofunctional disorders, 303–304
  idiopathic disorders, 317
    paradoxical vocal fold motion disorder, 317

instrumental evaluation, 286–291
  acoustic analysis, 287–289
  acoustic measurements, 291
  aerodynamic measurements, 290
  direct laryngoscopy, 286
  electroglottography, 289
  flexible or rigid endoscopy with videostroboscopy, 286–287
  indirect laryngoscopy (mirror laryngoscopy), 286
  laryngeal electromyography, 289
  videokymography, 289–290
neurological disorders, 317–321
  neurological diseases, 320–321
  paralysis, 317–319
  spasmodic dysphonia, 319–320
perceptual evaluation, 291–293
  basic principles, 291
  loudness assessment, 291
  phonation assessment, 293
  pitch assessment, 291
  rating scales, 291, 292
  resonance assessment, 293
  respiration assessment, 293
phonation disorders, 298–328
  behavioral voice therapy, 322–327
  carcinoma and laryngectomy, 299–303
  gender issues, 327–328
  neurological, 317–321
  physical, 304–317
  psychogenic, 321–322
physical disorders, 304–317
  ankylosis, 317
  contact ulcers, 308
  cysts, 306–307
  gastroesophageal reflux disease, 316
  granuloma, 307
  hemangioma, 307–308
  hyperkeratosis, 311
  laryngeal trauma, 315
  laryngeal web, 314–315
  laryngomalacia, 312
  laryngopharyngeal reflux, 316
  leukoplakia, 311–312
  papilloma, 313–314
  polyps, 305–306
  Reinke's edema, 309
  subglottal stenosis, 312–313
  sulcus vocalis, 315–316
  traumatic laryngitis, 308
  varices, 310
  vocal fold hemorrhage, 310
  vocal fold thickening, 308
  vocal nodules, 304–305
pitch, 282–283
psychogenic disorders, 321–322
  hysterical (conversion) aphonia, 321–322

muscle tension dysphonia, 322
mutational falsetto (puberphonia), 322
quality, 283–284
  breathiness, 284
  defined, 283
  diplophonia, 284
  glottal fry, 284
  harshness, 284
  hoarseness, 283
  strain-strangle, 284
  stridency, 284
quality of life evaluation, 293–294
resonance disorders, 294–298
  assimilative nasality, 296
  cul-de-sac resonance, 296–297
  hypernasality, 295, 297–298
  hyponasality, 296
  treatment, 297–298
training, 550–551
volume, 283
Voice box. *See* Larynx (voice box)
Voiced vowels, 84
Voice Handicap Index (VHI), 293
  Pediatric Voice Handicap Index (pVHI), 294
  VHI-10, 294
Voice onset time, 96
  delay, in stutterers, 250
Voice Related Quality of Life (VRQOL) scale, 294
Voice termination time, 96
Voice therapy, 320, 322, 328. *See also* Behavioral voice therapy
Voicing
  assimilation, 204
  defined, 79
  place-voice-manner analysis, 81
  source, 18
Volume of sound, 89, 283. *See also* Loudness (volume) of sound
von Langenbeck surgery, 441
von Recklinghausen disease, 531
Vowels, 84
  back, 86–87
  central, 86
  chart, 85
  dimensions, 85
  diphthongs, 87
  distinctive feature analysis, 84
  front, 86
  position characteristics, 84–87
  syllable as a unit, 77–78
  voicing of, 196
VPI. *See* Velopharyngeal inadequacy or insufficiency (VPI)
VRQOL. *See* Voice Related Quality of Life (VRQOL) scale
Vygotsky, Lev, 132
V-Y retroposition surgery, 440

W

WA. *See* Wernicke's aphasia (WA)
WAB-R. *See* Western Aphasia Battery–Revised (WAB-R)
Watts, 94, 518
Weak cognition hypothesis, 128
Weak stress of syllables, 88
Weak-syllable deletion, 204
Wernicke-Korsakoff syndrome, 371, 492
Wernicke's aphasia (WA), 56, 344–345
Wernicke's area, 55–56, 344, 345
Western Aphasia Battery–Revised (WAB-R), 350
Wet spirometers, 290
WHO. *See* World Health Organization (WHO)
Whole-word repetition, 239
Williams syndrome (WS), 452
Wilson's disease, 411
Word discrimination test, 533
Word finding problems, 147
Word interjections, 240
Word knowledge, 107
Word recognition test, 533
Word retrieval problems, 147
Working memory
  assessment of, 487
  deficits, 148
World Health Organization (WHO)
  Global Disability Action Plan, 491
  health care for disabled people, 491
  International Classification of Functioning, Disability, and Health–Children and Youth (ICF-CY), 195
World knowledge, 107
World Professional Association for Transgender Health (WPATH), 327
WPATH. *See* World Professional Association for Transgender Health (WPATH)
Writing skills. *See also* Literacy skills
  assessment, 353
    adolescents, 173
  treatment, 357–358
WS. *See* Williams syndrome (WS)

X

Xiphoid process, 5

Y

Yawn–sigh method, 324

Z

Zygomatic major muscle, 28
Zygomatic minor muscle, 28
Zygomatic muscle, 37

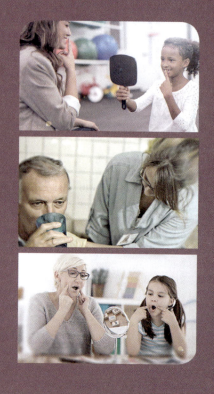

ABOUT THE AUTHORS

Celeste Roseberry-McKibbin received her PhD from Northwestern University. She is a professor of Communication Sciences and Disorders at California State University, Sacramento. Dr. Roseberry-McKibbin is also currently a part-time itinerant speech–language pathologist in the San Juan Unified School District, where she provides direct services to students from preschool through high school. She has worked in educational and medical settings with a wide variety of clients ranging from preschoolers through geriatric patients.

Dr. Roseberry-McKibbin's primary research interests are in the areas of assessment and treatment of culturally and linguistically diverse students with communication disorders, as well as service delivery to students from low-income backgrounds. She has over 70 publications, including 16 books, and has made over 400 presentations at the local, state, national, and international levels. Dr. Roseberry-McKibbin is a fellow of ASHA and winner of ASHA's Certificate of Recognition for Special Contributions in Multicultural Affairs. She received the national presidential Daily Point of Light Award for her service to children in poverty. She lived in the Philippines as the daughter of Baptist missionaries from ages 6 to 17.

M. N. (Giri) Hegde is professor emeritus of communicative sciences and disorders at California State University, Fresno. He holds a master's degree in experimental psychology from the University of Mysore, India, and a post-master's diploma in medical psychology from Bangalore University, India. His doctoral degree in speech–language pathology is from Southern Illinois University in Carbondale.

Dr. Hegde is a specialist in research methods, fluency disorders, language, and treatment procedures in communicative disorders. He has made many professional and scientific presentations to national and international audiences on a wide variety of topics in communicative disorders. He has published many research articles in national and international journals and over 25 critically acclaimed books on a wide range of subjects in speech–language pathology. He has edited nearly 30 books on speech–language pathology. He serves on the editorial board of several national and international journals, including the *Journal of Speech, Language, and Hearing Research*; *Journal of Fluency Disorders*; and *Journal of Speech-Language Pathology and Applied Behavior Analysis*. He has received numerous local, state, and national professional accolades and honors, including the ASHA Fellow Award and the Outstanding Professor Award from California State University, Fresno.

Glen M. Tellis received his PhD from Pennsylvania State University. He is a professor of Communication Sciences and Disorders at Misericordia University in Dallas, Pennsylvania. He is an ASHA Fellow and Board-Certified Fluency Specialist. He has received the Honors of the Pennsylvania Speech-Language Hearing Association as well as Misericordia's Excellence in Scholarship Award. His research interests include fluency disorders, multicultural issues, research designs, treatment efficacy research, advanced digital technology, and clinical outcomes.

Dr. Tellis frequently presents papers at national and international conferences and has published articles that pertain to his areas of specialization. He has also received externally funded grants for his work. He has served as editorial consultant and reviewer for the *Journal of Speech-Language and Hearing Research*, *Journal of Communication Disorders*, *Journal of Fluency Disorders*, and *Journal of Multilingual Communication Disorders*. He has served as a Steering Committee Member for ASHA's Special Interest Group 4 (Fluency Disorders), co-Chair of the Division 4 Leadership Conference, ASHA's Convention Fluency Topic Chair, and Chair of ASHA's Academic Affairs Board.